THE TEACHING FILES FILES Interventional

KEISER UNIVERSITY
2400 Interstate Drive
Lakeland, FL 33805

THE TEACHING FILES: Interventional

Charles T. Burke, MD
Associate Professor
Department of Radiology
University of North Carolina, Chapel Hill
Chapel Hill, North Carolina

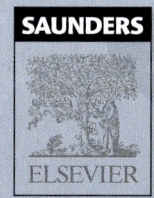

SAUNDERS
ELSEVIER

SAUNDERS
ELSEVIER

1600 John F. Kennedy Blvd.
Ste 1800
Philadelphia, PA 19103-2899

THE TEACHING FILES: INTERVENTIONAL ISBN: 978-1-4160-6260-8

Copyright © 2010 by Saunders, an imprint of Elsevier Inc.

All rights reserved. No part of this publication may be reproduced or transmitted in any form or by any means, electronic or mechanical, including photocopying, recording, or any information storage and retrieval system, without permission in writing from the publisher. Permissions may be sought directly from Elsevier's Rights Department: phone: (+1) 215 239 3804 (US) or (+44) 1865 843830 (UK); fax: (+44) 1865 853333; e-mail: healthpermissions@elsevier.com. You may also complete your request on-line via the Elsevier website at http://www.elsevier.com/permissions.

Notice

Knowledge and best practice in this field are constantly changing. As new research and experience broaden our knowledge, changes in practice, treatment, and drug therapy may become necessary or appropriate. Readers are advised to check the most current information provided (i) on procedures featured or (ii) by the manufacturer of each product to be administered, to verify the recommended dose or formula, the method and duration of administration, and contraindications. It is the responsibility of the practitioner, relying on his or her own experience and knowledge of the patient, to make diagnoses, to determine dosages and the best treatment for each individual patient, and to take all appropriate safety precautions. To the fullest extent of the law, neither the publisher nor the authors assume any liability for any injury and/or damage to persons or property arising out of or related to any use of the material contained in this book.

 The Publisher

Library of Congress Cataloging-in-Publication Data

Burke, Charles T. (Charles Thomas),
 The teaching files: Interventional/Charles T. Burke. — 1st ed.
 p. ; cm.
 ISBN 978-1-4160-6260-8
 1. Interventional radiology—Case studies. I. Title. II. Title: Interventional.
 [DNLM: 1. Radiography, Interventional—Case Reports. WN 200 B9587t 2010]
 RD33.55.B87 2010
 617'.05—dc22 2009034213

Acquisitions Editor: Rebecca Gaertner
Developmental Editor: Colleen McGonigal
Publishing Services Manager: Tina Rebane
Project Manager: Jodi Kaye
Design Direction: Steve Stave

Printed in China

Last digit is the print number: 9 8 7 6 5 4 3 2 1

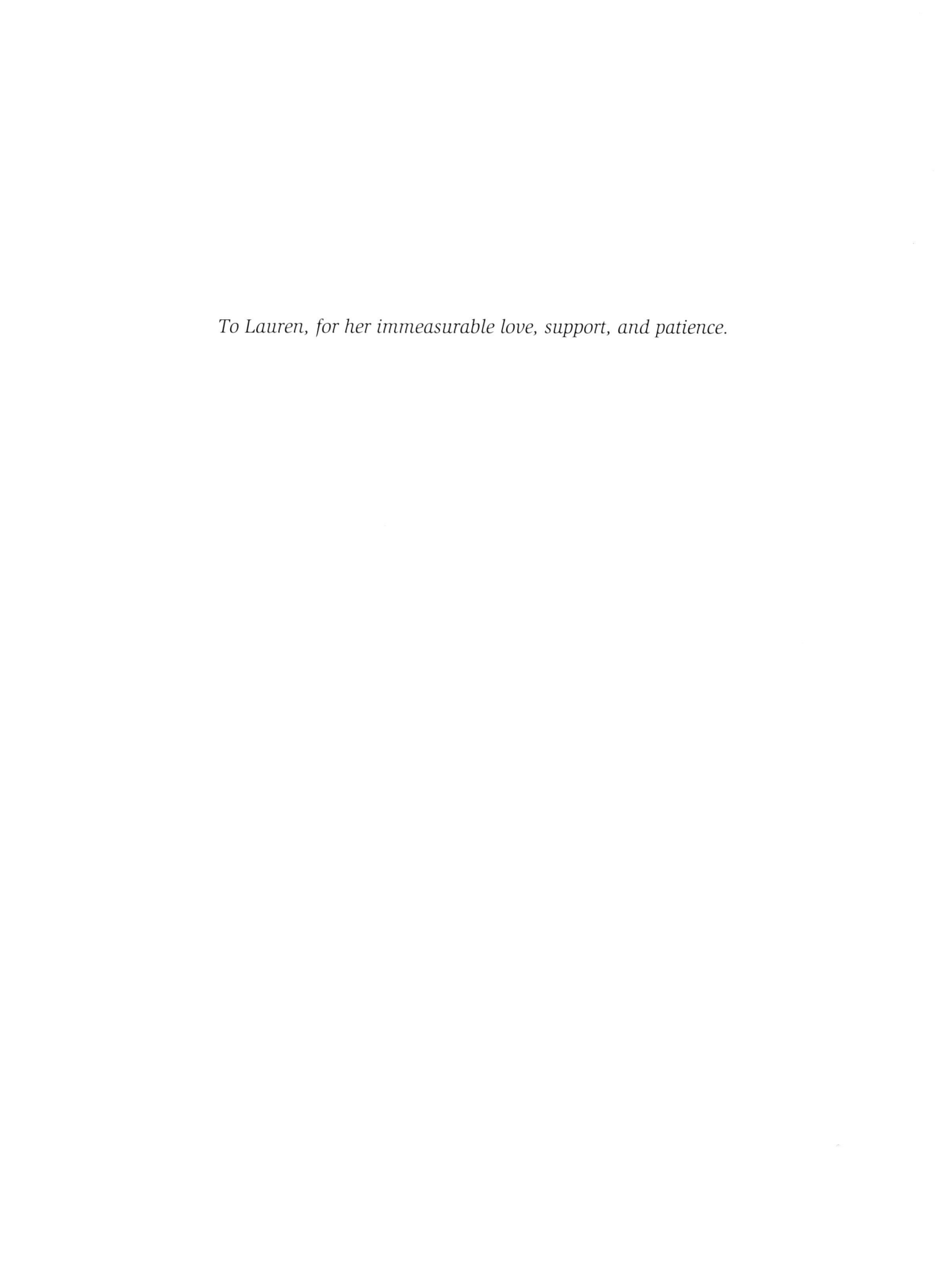

To Lauren, for her immeasurable love, support, and patience.

Contributors

Robert G. Dixon, MD
  Assistant Professor
  Department of Radiology
  University of North Carolina
  Chapel Hill, North Carolina

Susan M. Weeks, MD
  Radiologist
  Wake Radiology
  Raleigh, North Carolina

Preface

"There is no teaching to compare with example"
—Sir Robert Baden-Powell

This book provides an extensive review of a wide range of procedures in interventional radiology illustrated through case examples. Although the cases may be studied in isolation, this book may also be used as a complement to the complete textbook, *Image-Guided Interventions*.

In 2008, Elsevier released, as part of the Expert Radiology series, a comprehensive, two-volume text on the field of interventional radiology, *Image-Guided Interventions*, edited by Matthew A. Mauro, Kieran P.J. Murphy, Kenneth R. Thomson, Anthony C. Venbrux, and Christoph L. Zollikofer. This textbook, written by many of the world's leading experts in interventional radiology, encompasses information about a wide range of procedures commonly performed in the interventional radiology suite in a state-of-the-art and practical format. *The Teaching Files: Interventional* illustrates many of these procedures as "real-world" examples.

I have attempted to bring together cases that illustrate both vascular and nonvascular interventions, combining customary techniques and novel approaches. Each case was identified through an exhaustive search of the University of North Carolina teaching file, looking for examples with instructive imaging and constructive clinical information. I did not shy away from cases with complications and adverse outcomes. Instead, these were included to show how these situations may present and be managed.

As the primary author and editor of this book, I would like to thank my colleagues who helped and supported me through this process and helped contribute to writing of several of the cases. In addition, past and present colleagues performed the majority of the included procedures, and again, I am thankful for their expertise. I would also like to thank the many former residents and fellows who participated in quite a few of these cases and from whom I have learned as much or more about interventional radiology as I have been able to teach.

In conclusion, this is a book about interventional radiology that teaches by examples. The reader may use this book in isolation or as an adjunct to the larger text *Image-Guided Interventions*.

Charles T. Burke, MD

Contents

Cases 1 to 304   2 to 609

Index of Cases   611

Index   617

THE TEACHING FILES

Interventional

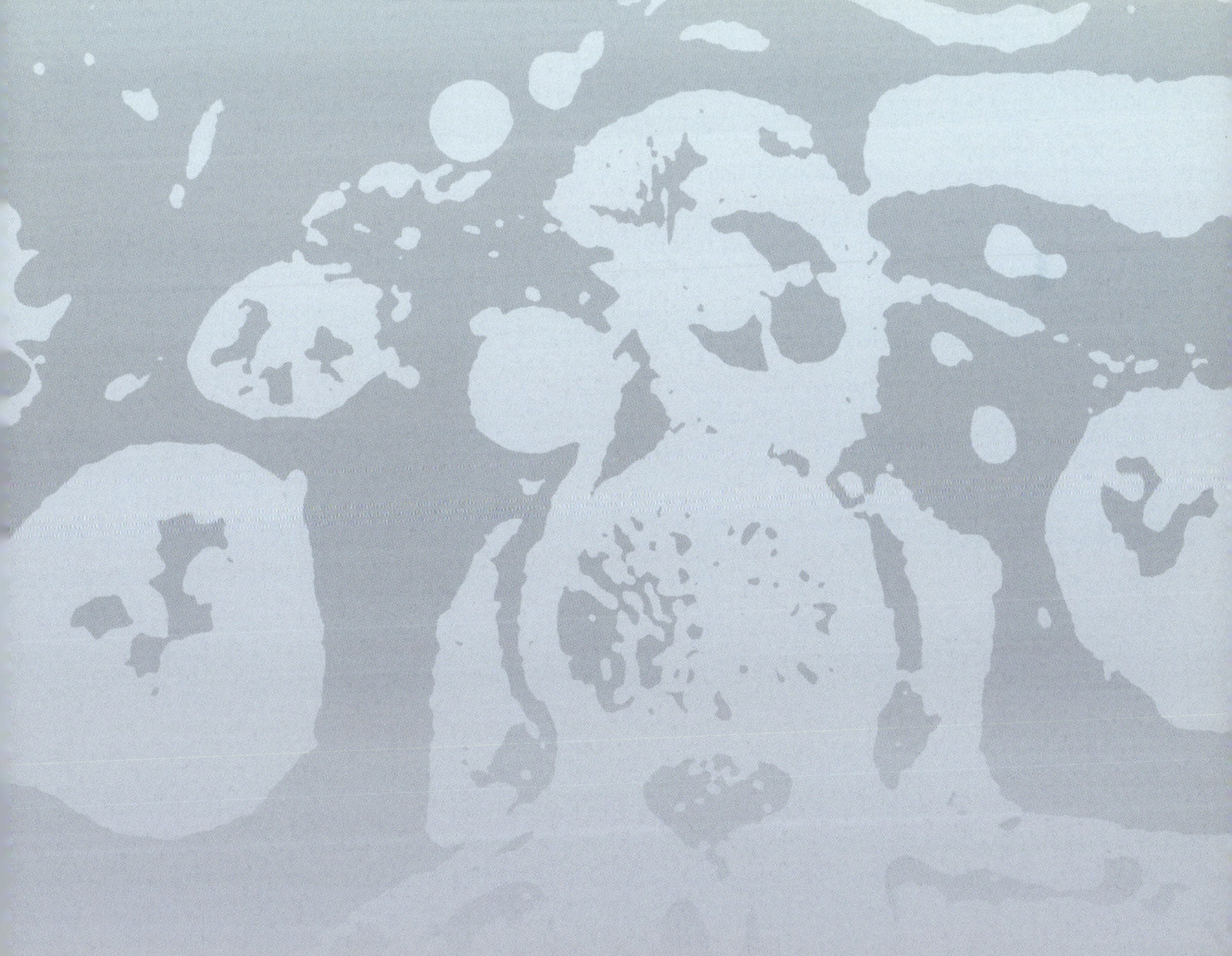

Case 1

DEMOGRAPHICS/CLINICAL HISTORY

A 53-year-old man with bilateral lower extremity claudication, undergoing ultrasound, aortography, and revascularization.

DISCUSSION

History/Indications for Procedure
A 53-year-old man had a history of hypertension and prior myocardial infarction with claudication. He is able to walk approximately 30 feet before the onset of symptoms.

Procedure
Bilateral common iliac artery stenoses

Pre-procedure Imaging
Arterial ultrasound demonstrated elevated systolic acceleration times in the common femoral arteries, which was consistent with inflow obstruction. The ankle/brachial index values were abnormal, measuring 0.90 on the right and 0.80 on the left.

Intraprocedural Findings
Aortogram demonstrates aortoiliac narrowing and diffuse narrowing of the left common iliac artery (Fig. 1). Kissing balloon-expandable iliac stents were placed (Fig. 2), and a self-expanding stent was placed across the distal left common iliac artery (Fig. 3).

Follow-up and Complications
After stent placement, the patient had significant improvement in symptoms and has been able to walk with little leg pain.

Suggested Readings

Bosch JL, Hunink MG: Meta-analysis of the results of percutaneous transluminal angioplasty and stent placement for aortoiliac occlusive disease. Radiology 204:87-96, 1997.

Haulon S, Mounier-Véhier C, Gaxotte V, et al: Percutaneous reconstruction of the aortoiliac bifurcation with the "kissing stents" technique: Long-term follow-up in 106 patients. J Endovasc Ther 9:363-368, 2002.

Klein WM, van der Graaf Y, Seegers J, et al: Dutch iliac stent trial: Long-term results in patients randomized for primary or selective stent placement. Radiology 238:734-744, 2006.

Murphy TP, Ariaratnam NS, Carney WI Jr, et al: Aortoiliac insufficiency: Long-term experience with stent placement for treatment. Radiology 231:243-249, 2004.

Tetteroo E, van der Graaf Y, Bosch JL, et al: Randomised comparison of primary stent placement versus primary angioplasty followed by selective stent placement in patients with iliac-artery occlusive disease. Dutch Iliac Stent Trial Study Group. Lancet 351:1153-1159, 1998.

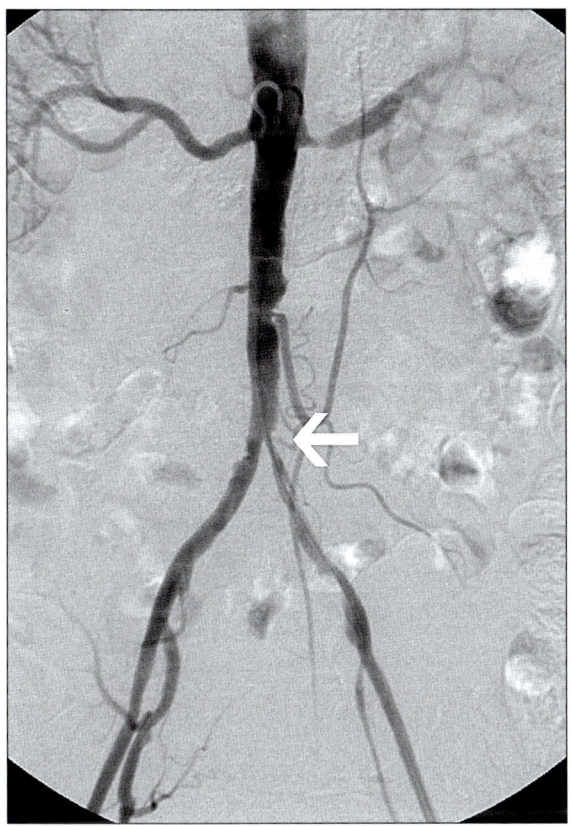

Figure 1. Aortogram demonstrates multifocal atherosclerotic changes. Diffuse aortoiliac disease is present with a high-grade stenosis involving the proximal left common iliac artery *(arrow)*.

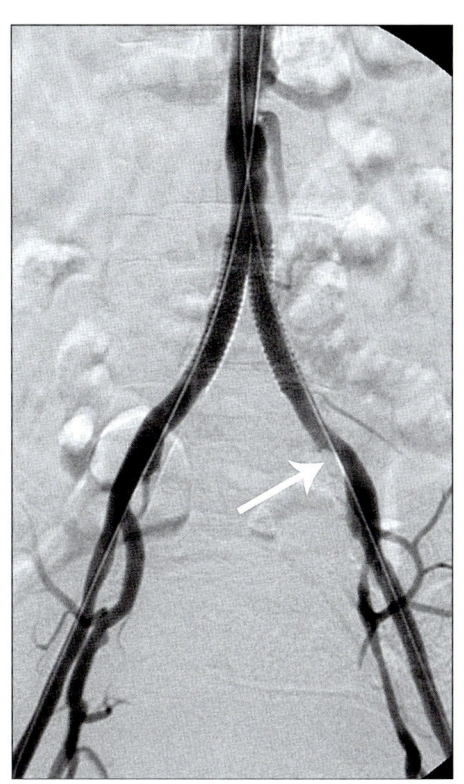

Figure 2. Kissing iliac stents were placed with significant improvement in the common iliac arteries. A focal stenosis of the distal left common iliac artery remains *(arrow)*.

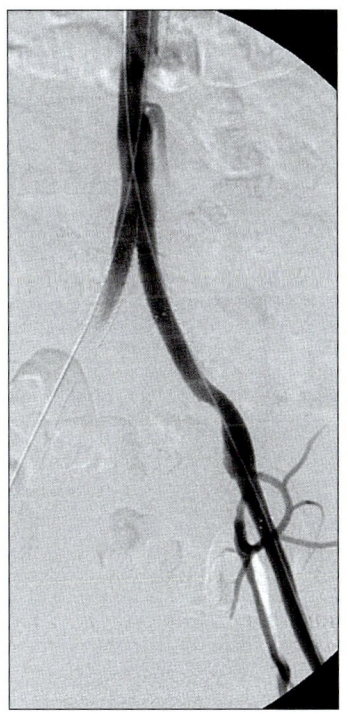

Figure 3. Retrograde injection through the left femoral sheath after distal common iliac artery stenting shows no residual inflow obstruction on the left.

Case 2

DEMOGRAPHICS/CLINICAL HISTORY

A 56-year-old man with blue toe syndrome, undergoing aortography.

DISCUSSION

History/Indications for Procedure
This patient had blue, painful lesions on the right great and second toes; the lesions developed 2 weeks before presentation. The patient also had a 2- to 3-month history of bilateral hip pain while walking.

Procedure
Aortic revascularization

Pre-procedure Imaging
Arterial ultrasound revealed high-velocity arterial signal in the distal aorta consistent with aortic stenosis. The ankle-brachial indexes were 0.81 bilaterally.

Intraprocedural Findings
Abdominal aortogram revealed an irregular, focal stenosis of the infrarenal abdominal aorta (Figs. 1 and 2). The stenosis was treated with the placement of a 10-mm × 29-mm Palmaz balloon expandable stent (Fig. 3).

Suggested Readings
Bosch JL, Hunink MG: Meta-analysis of the results of percutaneous transluminal angioplasty and stent placement for aortoiliac occlusive disease. Radiology 204:87-96, 1997.

Murphy TP, Ariaratnam NS, Carney WI Jr, et al: Aortoiliac insufficiency: Long-term experience with stent placement for treatment. Radiology 231:243-249, 2004.

Case 2   5

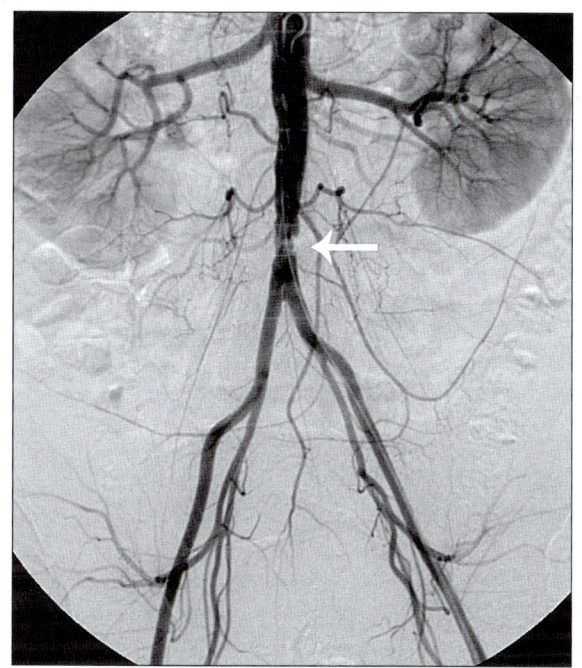

Figure 1. Abdominal aortogram shows a focal, irregular stenosis of the infrarenal abdominal aorta *(arrow)*.

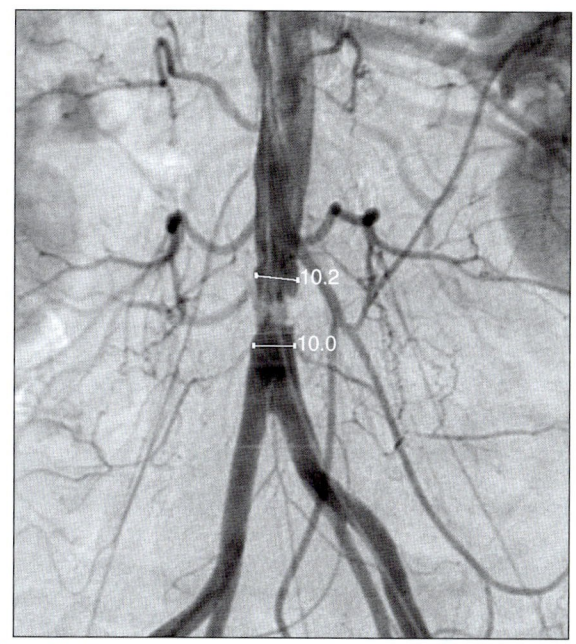

Figure 2. Diameter measurements of the aorta above and below the lesion were performed before stenting.

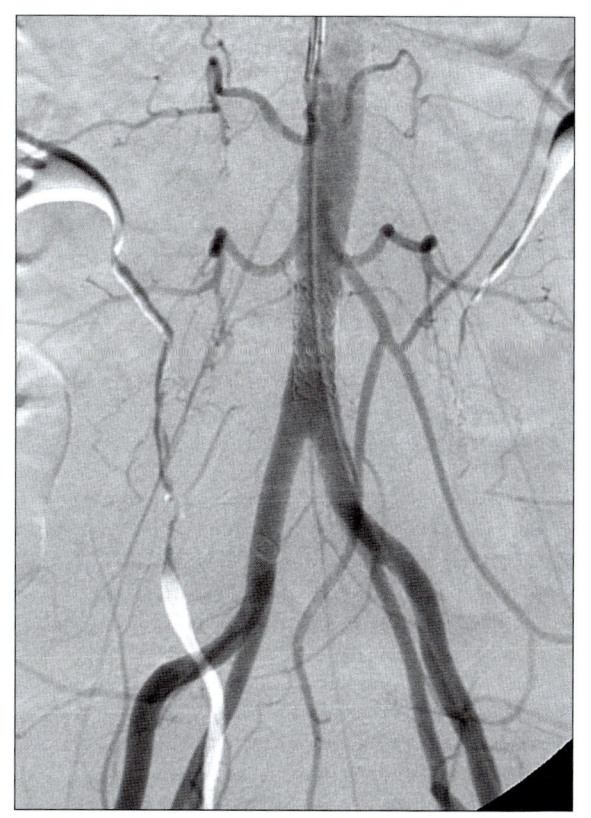

Figure 3. The lesion was treated with the placement of a 10-mm × 29-mm balloon expandable stent.

Case 3

DEMOGRAPHICS/CLINICAL HISTORY

A 63-year-old man with bilateral lower extremity claudication, undergoing ultrasound and aortogram.

DISCUSSION

History/Indications for Procedure
A 63-year-old man presents with bilateral lower extremity claudication at one block. The ankle-brachial indices are decreased bilaterally, measuring 0.47 on the right and 0.54 on the left.

Procedure
Endovascular treatment of aortic stenosis

Pre-procedure Imaging
Arterial ultrasound shows elevated peak systolic velocities in the iliac arteries bilaterally, measuring >500 cm/s on the right and >450 cm/s on the left (Fig. 1).

Intraprocedural Findings
Aortogram shows an irregular stenosis of the infrarenal abdominal aorta (Fig. 2); there is no outflow or runoff disease. The aortic stenosis was treated with the placement of a 10-mm × 39-mm balloon expandable stent (Fig. 3).

Follow-up and Complications
The patient's claudication resolved after stent placement. At follow-up, the ankle-brachial indices had returned to normal, and follow-up ultrasound was normal (Fig. 4).

Suggested Readings
Bosch JL, Hunink MG: Meta-analysis of the results of percutaneous transluminal angioplasty and stent placement for aortoiliac occlusive disease. Radiology 204:87, 1997.

Feugier P, Toursarkissian B, Chevalier JM, et al: Endovascular treatment of isolated atherosclerotic stenosis of the infrarenal abdominal aorta: Long-term outcome. Ann Vasc Surg 17:375, 2003.

Schedel H, Wissgott C, Rademaker J, et al: Primary stent placement for infrarenal aortic stenosis: Immediate and midterm results. J Vasc Interv Radiol 15:353, 2004.

Yilmaz S, Sindel T, Yegin A, et al: Primary stenting of focal atherosclerotic infrarenal aortic stenoses: Long-term results in 13 patients and a literature review. Cardiovasc Intervent Radiol 27:121, 2004.

Case 3   7

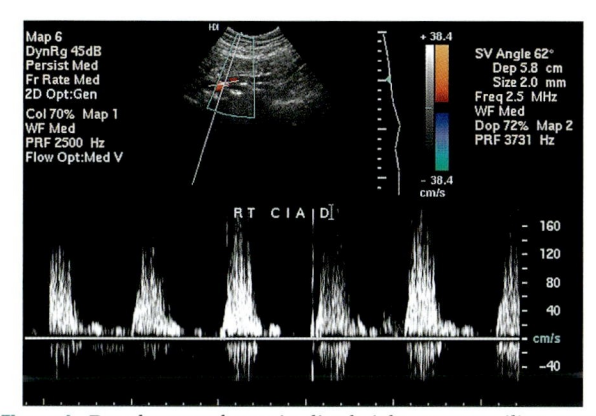

Figure 1. Doppler waveforms in distal right common iliac artery are abnormal with turbulent flow and increased peak systolic velocities.

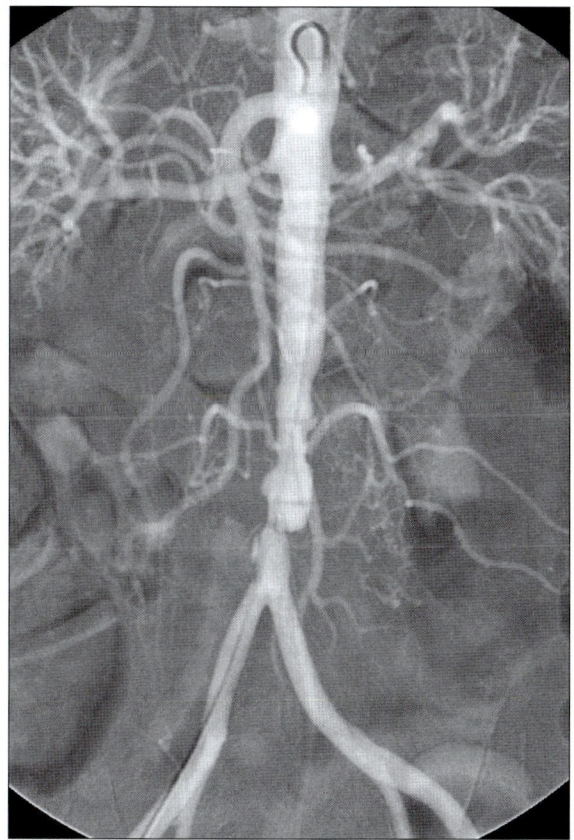

Figure 2. Abdominal aortogram shows focal, high-grade stenosis of distal abdominal aorta. There is also focal stenosis of right renal artery.

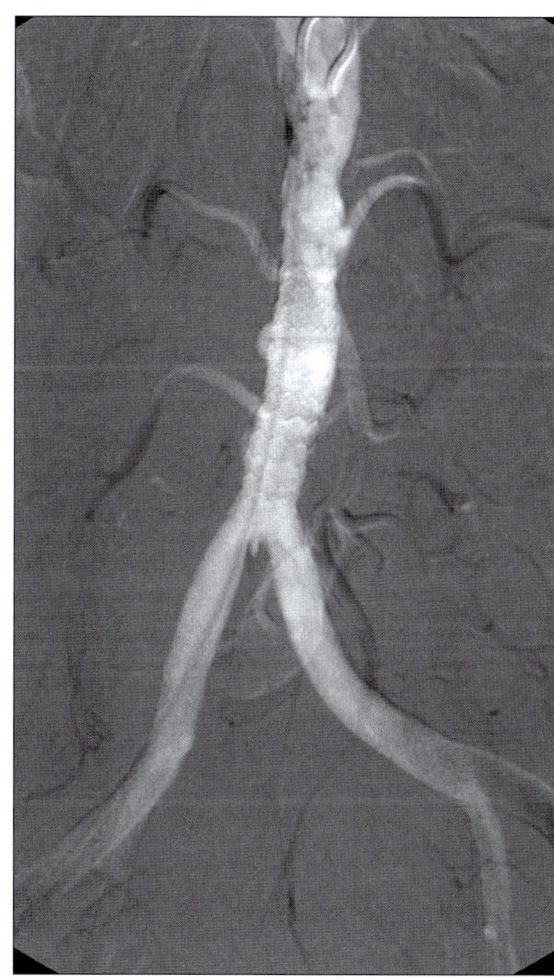

Figure 3. Follow-up aortogram after stent placement, a 10-mm × 39-mm balloon expandable stent (Genesis; Cordis, Warren, NJ).

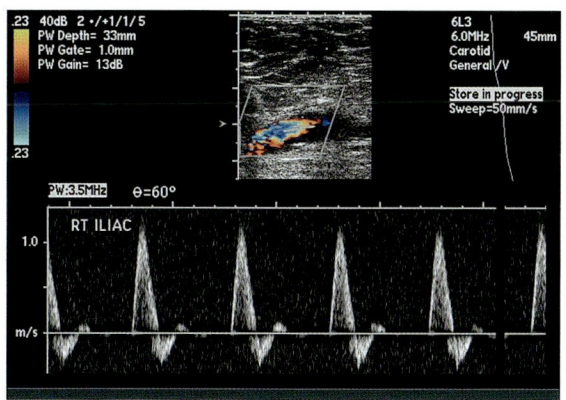

Figure 4. Follow-up ultrasound after stent placement. Doppler waveform of right external iliac artery has normal triphasic appearance.

Case 4

DEMOGRAPHICS/CLINICAL HISTORY

An 80-year-old woman with subclavian steal syndrome, undergoing magnetic resonance angiography (MRA).

DISCUSSION

History/Indications for Procedure
An 80-year-old woman with vertigo and left subclavian artery stenosis.

Procedure
Endovascular treatment of subclavian artery stenosis

Pre-procedure Imaging
MRA demonstrates significant narrowing of the proximal left subclavian artery and a dominant left vertebral artery (Fig. 1).

Intraprocedural Findings
Selective left subclavian artery angiogram demonstrates focal stenosis of the proximal left subclavian artery (Fig. 2). The artery was treated with the primary placement of a 10-mm × 37-mm balloon expandable stent (Fig. 3).

Follow-up and Complications
After stent placement, there was improved flow through the left subclavian artery, with antegrade flow in the left vertebral artery. The patient's vertigo resolved after stent placement.

Suggested Readings
Amor M, Eid-Lidt G, Chati Z, Wilentz JR: Endovascular treatment of the subclavian artery: Stent implantation with or without predilatation. Catheter Cardiovasc Interv 63:364-370, 2004.

Ringelstein EB, Zeumer H: Delayed reversal of vertebral artery blood flow following percutaneous transluminal angioplasty for subclavian steal syndrome. Neuroradiology 26:189-198, 1984.

Woo EY, Fairman RM, Velazquez OC, et al: Endovascular therapy of symptomatic innominate-subclavian arterial occlusive lesions. Vasc Endovascular Surg 40:27-33, 2006.

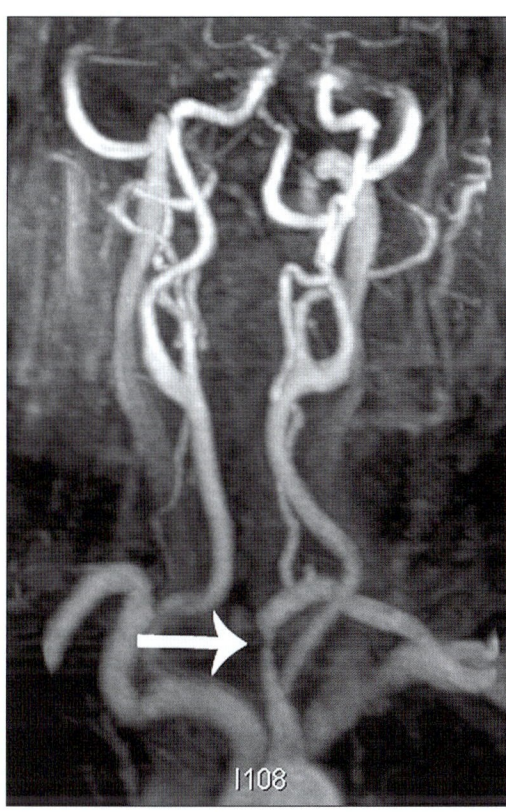

Figure 1. Three-dimensional reconstructed image from the MR angiogram of the neck demonstrates a focal stenosis within the proximal left subclavian artery *(arrow)*. The left vertebral artery is dominant.

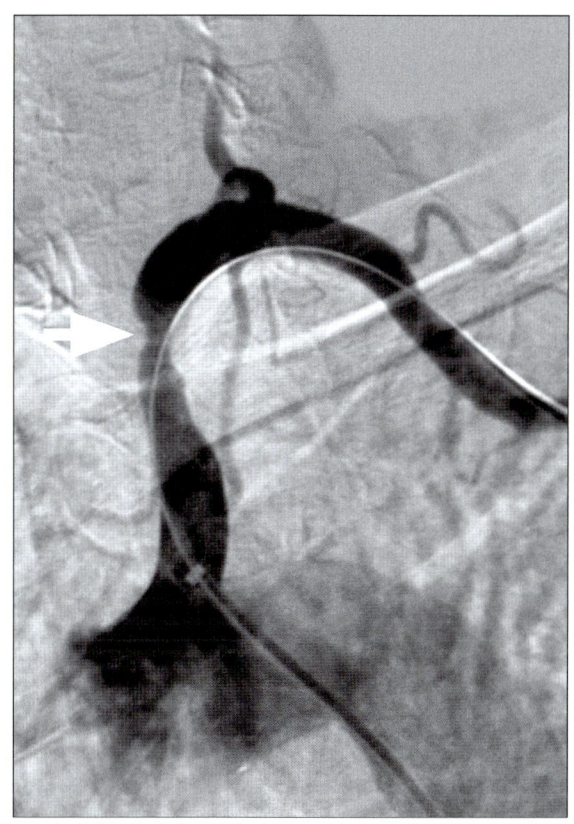

Figure 2. Selective left subclavian arteriogram demonstrates a 70% focal stenosis of the proximal left subclavian artery.

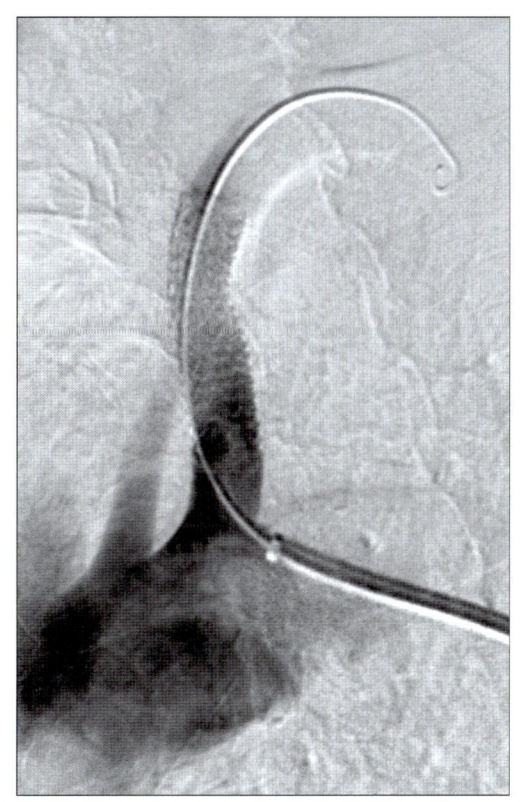

Figure 3. The lesion was treated with the primary placement of a 10-mm × 37-mm balloon expandable stent.

Case 5

DEMOGRAPHICS/CLINICAL HISTORY

A 49-year-old woman with history of progressive vertigo and syncope, undergoing revascularization.

DISCUSSION

History/Indications for Procedure
A 49-year-old woman has a history of progressive vertigo, syncope, uncontrolled hypertension, and smoking.

Procedure
Right subclavian artery occlusion

Intraprocedural Findings
There is complete occlusion of the proximal right subclavian artery with reconstitution just proximal to the origin of the vertebral artery (Figs. 1 and 2). The occlusion was successfully crossed from a right brachial approach and stented with a 6-mm × 17-mm, balloon-expandable stent (Figs. 3 and 4).

Follow-up and Complications
The patient's vertigo improved after stent placement. She is doing well and has required no further subclavian artery intervention.

Suggested Readings

Bates MC, Broce M, Lavigne PS, Stone P: Subclavian artery stenting: Factors influencing long-term outcome. Catheter Cardiovasc Interv 61:5-11, 2004.

De Vries JP, Jager LC, Van den Berg JC, et al: Durability of percutaneous transluminal angioplasty for obstructive lesions of proximal subclavian artery: Long-term results. J Vasc Surg 41:19-23, 2005.

Woo EY, Fairman RM, Velazquez OC, et al: Endovascular therapy of symptomatic innominate-subclavian arterial occlusive lesions. Vasc Endovascular Surg 40:27-33, 2006.

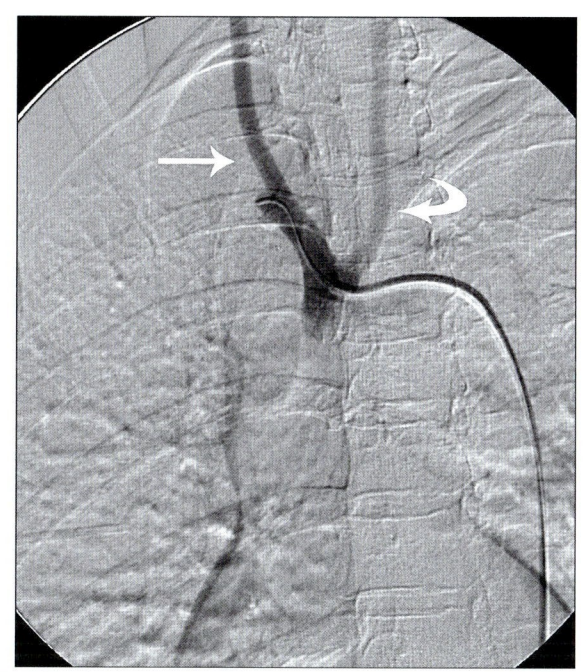

Figure 1. Selective injection of the right subclavian artery demonstrates complete occlusion just beyond the origin of the common carotid *(arrow)*. The left common carotid *(curved arrow)* also can be seen.

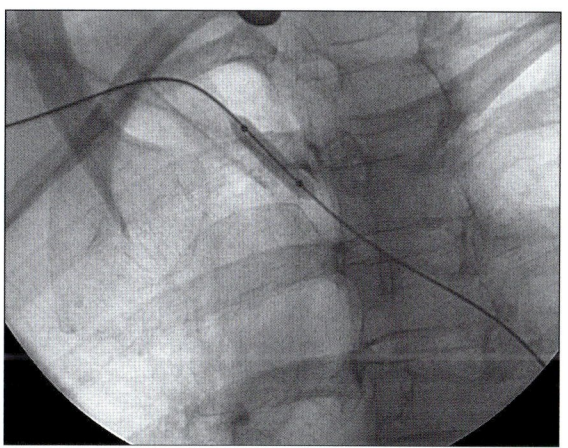

Figure 3. The lesion was crossed, and through-and-through guidewire access was obtained. The lesion was primarily stented with a 6-mm × 17-mm, balloon-expandable stent.

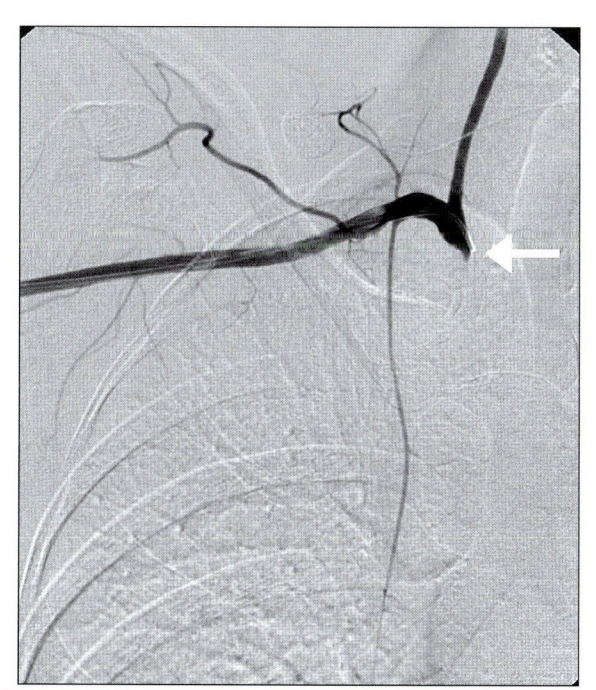

Figure 2. Subclavian angiogram performed from a brachial access demonstrates reconstitution of the subclavian artery just proximal to the origin of the vertebral artery *(arrow)*.

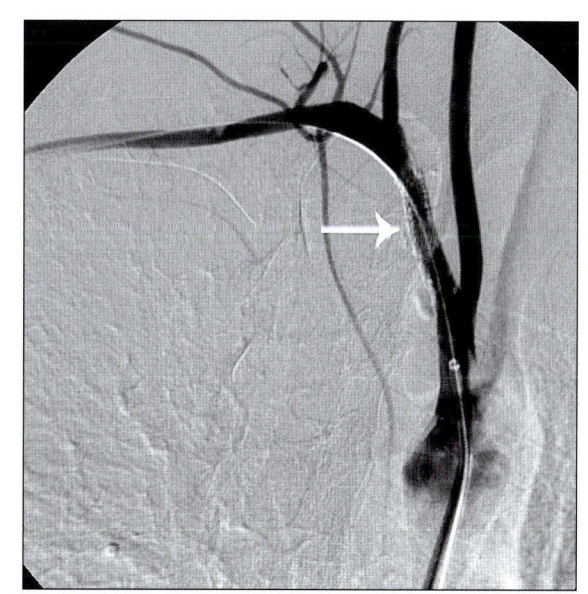

Figure 4. Follow-up angiogram after stent placement demonstrates restoration of flow through the previously occluded segment *(arrow)*.

Case 6

DEMOGRAPHICS/CLINICAL HISTORY

A 47-year-old woman with right upper extremity numbness, undergoing aortography, angiography, and arteriography.

DISCUSSION

History/Indications for Procedure
A 47-year-old woman with a history of coronary artery disease presents with right upper extremity numbness.

Procedure
Percutaneous treatment of right brachiocephalic artery stenosis

Intraprocedural Findings
There is a focal 50% stenosis of the right brachiocephalic artery with an associated 33-mm Hg pressure gradient across the lesion (Fig. 1). The stenosis was primarily stented with a Palmaz 204 stent (Fig. 2).

Follow-up and Complications
Approximately 2.5 years after the stent was placed, the patient developed recurrent right upper extremity numbness. She was referred for repeat arteriogram, which showed intrastent stenosis; the restenosis was successfully treated with balloon angioplasty (Figs. 3 and 4).

Suggested Readings
Bakken AM, Palchik E, Saad WE, et al: Outcomes of endoluminal therapy for ostial disease of the major branches of the aortic arch. Ann Vasc Surg 22:388, 2008.

Bates MC, Broce M, Lavigne PS, et al: Subclavian artery stenting: Factors influencing long-term outcome. Catheter Cardiovasc Intervent 61:5, 2004.

Woo EY, Fairman RM, Velazquez OC, et al: Endovascular therapy of symptomatic innominate-subclavian arterial occlusive lesions. Vasc Endovasc Surg 40:27, 2006.

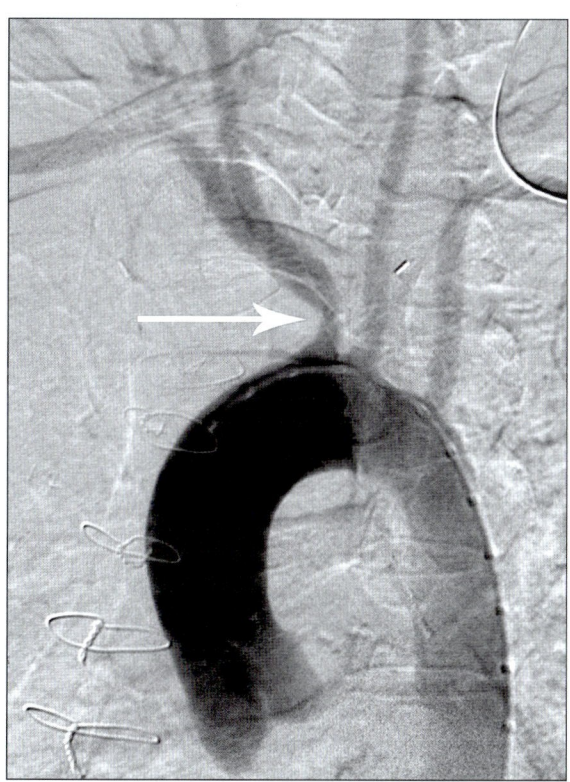

Figure 1. Thoracic aortogram shows focal stenosis of right brachiocephalic artery (arrow). Although stenosis appears mild on angiography, it was associated with significant pressure gradient.

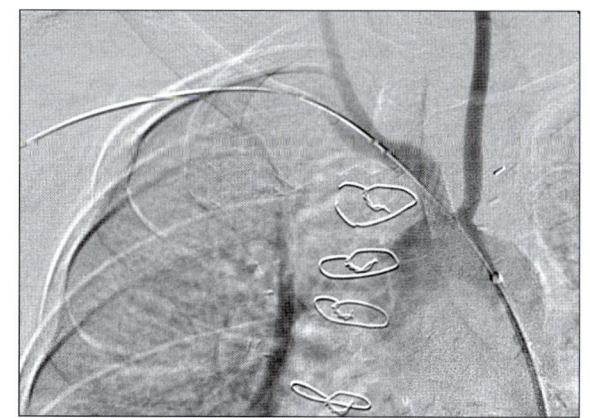

Figure 2. Follow-up angiogram after stent placement shows stent to be appropriately positioned across lesion. There is good flow through the stent.

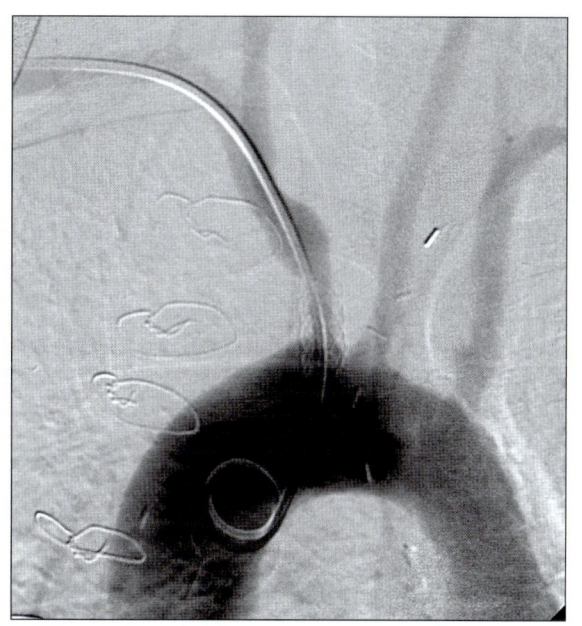

Figure 3. Follow-up arteriogram 2.5 years later, when the patient developed recurrent symptoms. Diffuse narrowing within stent is consistent with intimal hyperplasia.

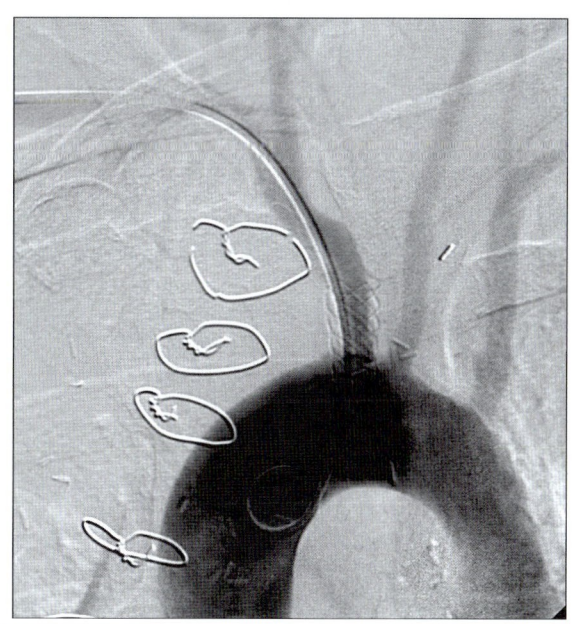

Figure 4. Follow-up angiogram after intrastent balloon angioplasty shows improvement of flow through stent.

Case 7

DEMOGRAPHICS/CLINICAL HISTORY

A 71-year-old woman with left arm pain, undergoing arteriography.

DISCUSSION

History/Indications for Procedure

A 71-year-old woman underwent endovascular stent grafting for contained rupture of the thoracic aorta. The origin of the left subclavian artery was covered by the stent graft, and the patient has had left upper extremity pain since the time of surgery.

Procedure

Left subclavian artery stenting

Pre-procedure Imaging

Arterial ultrasound of the left upper extremity showed post-stenotic waveforms in the subclavian and axillary arteries.

Intraprocedural Findings

Using a left brachial artery approach, the origin of the left subclavian artery was crossed (Figs. 1 and 2). An 8-mm × 30-mm, self-expanding stent was deployed at the origin of the left subclavian artery (Fig. 3), alongside the thoracic stent graft.

Follow-up and Complications

The systolic blood pressure in the left brachial artery increased from 55 mm Hg before stent placement to 99 mm Hg after stent placement (Fig. 4). The patient's symptoms persisted but were significantly improved. Despite the placement of the stent alongside of the thoracic stent graft, no endoleak was seen on follow-up computed tomography.

Suggested Readings

Rehders TC, Petzsch M, Ince H, et al: Intentional occlusion of the left subclavian artery during stent-graft implantation in the thoracic aorta: Risk and relevance. J Endovasc Ther 11:659-666, 2004.

Riesenman PJ, Farber MA, Mendes RR, et al: Coverage of the left subclavian artery during thoracic endovascular aortic repair. J Vasc Surg 45:90-94, 2007.

Scharrer-Pamler R, Kotsis T, Kapfer X, et al: Complications after endovascular treatment of thoracic aortic aneurysms. J Endovasc Ther 10:711-718, 2003.

Case 7   15

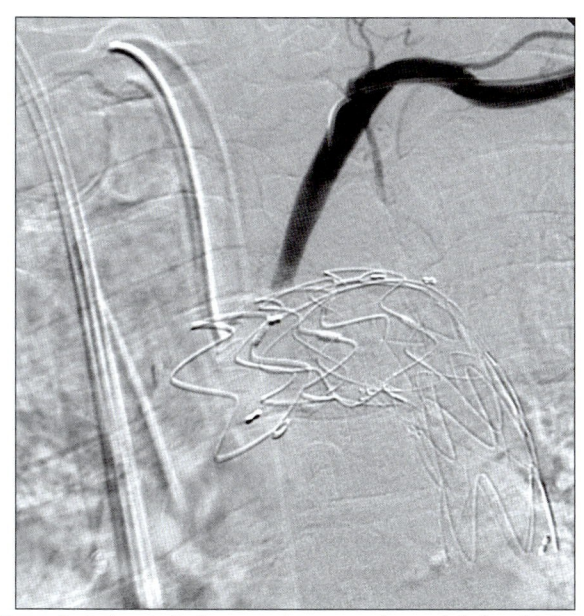

Figure 1. Left subclavian arteriogram using a left brachial approach shows occlusion of the left subclavian artery by the thoracic stent graft.

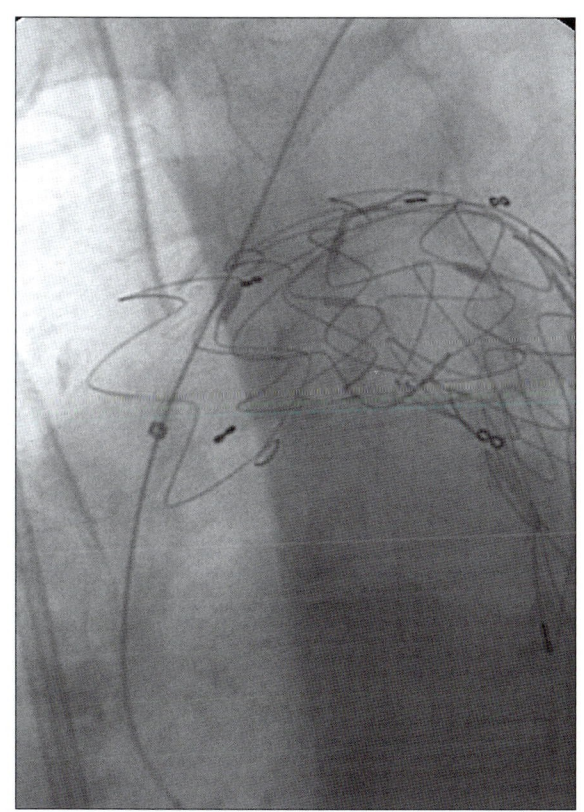

Figure 2. The origin of the subclavian artery was catheterized with a 6-French sheath that was advanced into the ascending thoracic aorta.

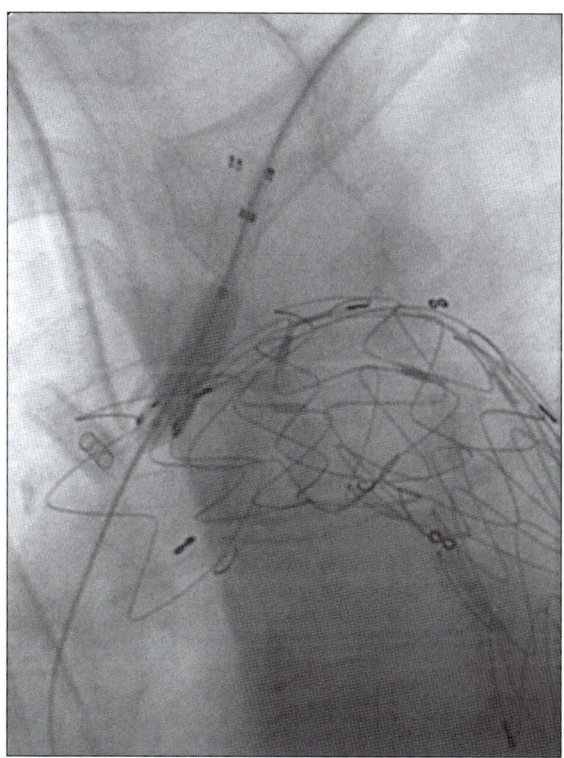

Figure 3. An 8-mm × 30-mm, self-expanding stent was deployed across the origin of the subclavian artery. This arteriogram shows the stent being dilated with a 6-mm balloon.

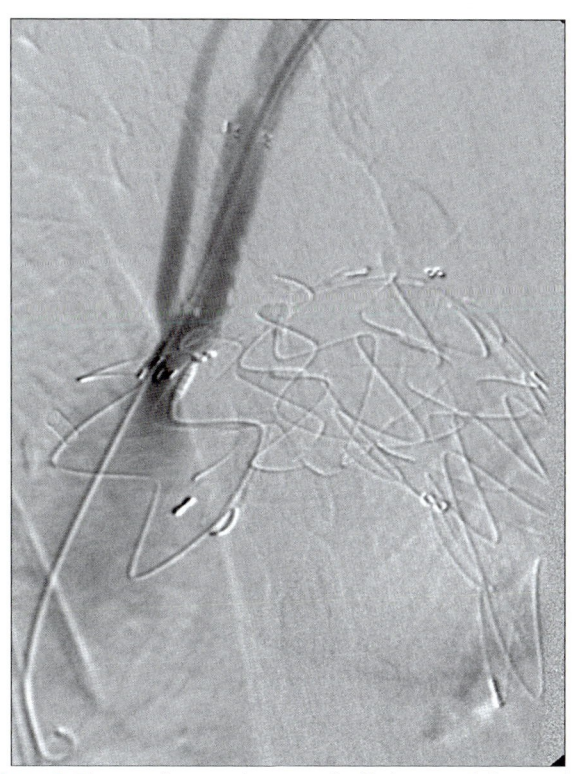

Figure 4. The arteriogram shows markedly improved flow to the left subclavian artery.

Case 8

DEMOGRAPHICS/CLINICAL HISTORY

A 66-year-old woman with intermittent dizziness and loss of balance.

DISCUSSION

History/Indications for Procedure
A 66-year-old woman with intermittent dizziness and loss of balance. There is a 38-mm Hg reduction in systolic blood pressure of the left upper extremity compared with the right.

Procedure
Endovascular management of subclavian steal

Pre-procedure Imaging
Arterial ultrasound shows reversal of flow in the left vertebral artery (Fig. 1). CT angiogram shows a 60% to 70% stenosis of the proximal left subclavian artery (Fig. 2).

Intraprocedural Findings
An 80% stenosis of the proximal left subclavian artery was identified. The stenosis was treated with the primary placement of a 9-mm × 28-mm balloon-expandable stent (Fig. 3).

Follow-up and Complications
The patient's symptoms resolved after the stent placement. Follow-up arterial ultrasound shows restoration of antegrade flow in the left vertebral artery (Fig. 4).

Suggested Readings
Bakken AM, Palchik E, Saad WE, et al: Outcomes of endoluminal therapy for ostial disease of the major branches of the aortic arch. Ann Vasc Surg 22:388-394, 2008.

Brountzos EN, Malagari K, Kelekis DA: Endovascular treatment of occlusive lesions of the subclavian and innominate arteries. Cardiovasc Intervent Radiol 29:503-510, 2006.

Palchik E, Bakken AM, Wolford HY, et al: Subclavian artery revascularization: An outcome analysis based on mode of therapy and presenting symptoms. Ann Vasc Surg 22:70-78, 2008.

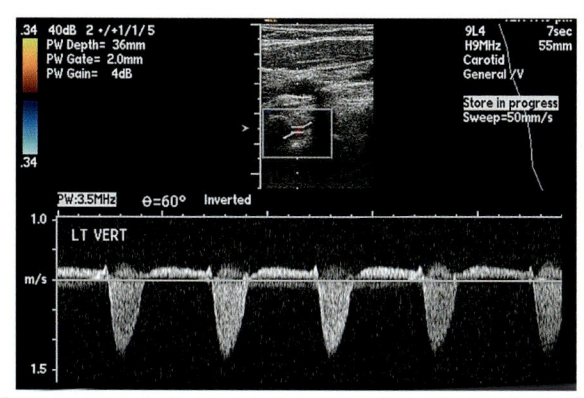

Figure 1. Arterial ultrasound of the left vertebral artery shows reversal of flow during systole.

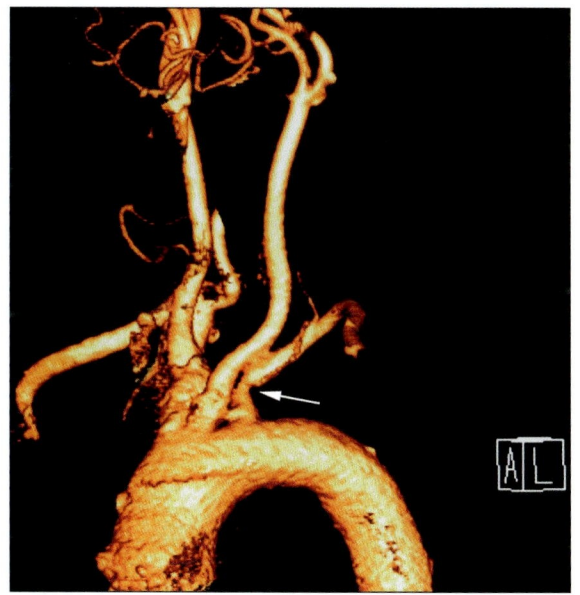

Figure 2. 3-D reconstruction of the aortic arch and great vessels from CT angiogram shows a 60% to 70% stenosis of the proximal left subclavian artery *(arrow)*.

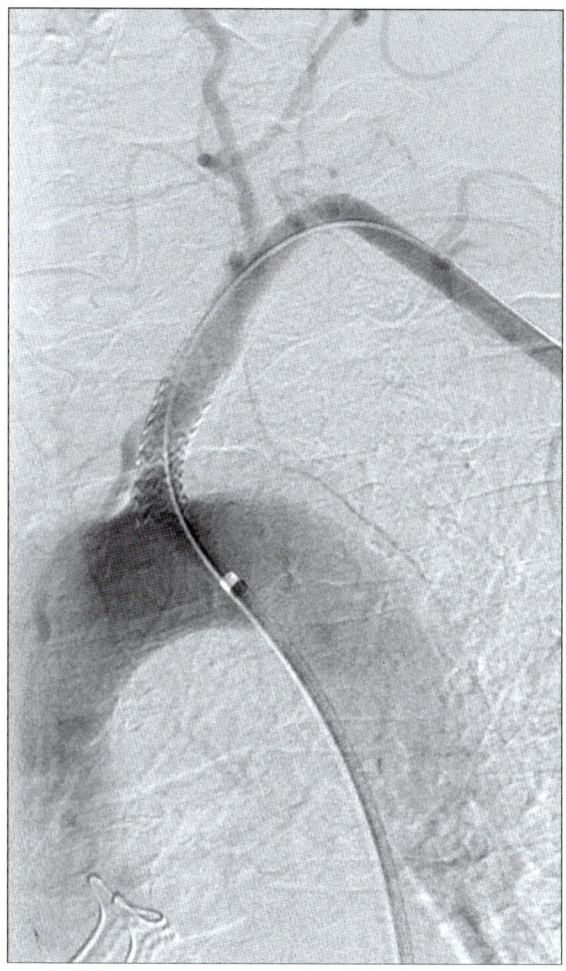

Figure 3. Follow-up arteriogram after stent placement shows no residual narrowing. There is antegrade flow within the left vertebral artery.

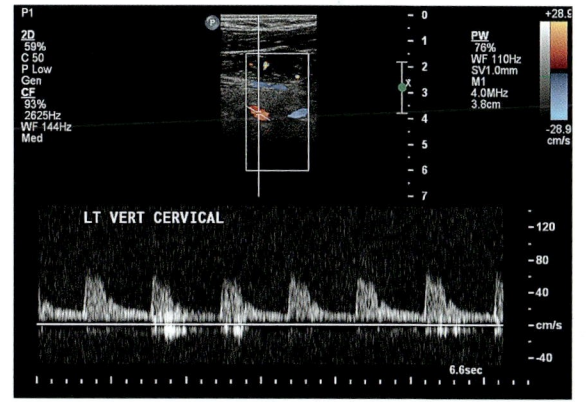

Figure 4. Follow-up arterial ultrasound after stent placement. There is restoration of antegrade flow within the left vertebral artery.

Case 9

DEMOGRAPHICS/CLINICAL HISTORY

A 64-year-old woman with right upper extremity claudication and weakness.

DISCUSSION

History/Indications for Procedure
A 64-year-old woman with right upper extremity claudication and weakness. The right upper extremity pulses are diminished relative to the left.

Procedure
Brachial artery angioplasty

Intraprocedural Findings
There is a focal, high-grade stenosis of the proximal right brachial artery (Fig. 1). The lesion was crossed with a 0.014-inch guidewire and angioplastied with a 4-mm balloon (Fig. 2).

Follow-up and Complications
Follow-up arteriogram following balloon angioplasty shows no residual stenosis or flow-limiting dissection (Fig. 3). Follow-up brachial artery pressures were symmetric bilaterally; follow-up Doppler ultrasound shows no velocity change within the brachial artery at the level of angioplasty.

Suggested Readings

Edwards JM, Porter JM: Upper extremity arterial disease: Etiologic considerations and differential diagnosis. Semin Vasc Surg 11:60-66, 1998.

Greenfield LJ, Rajagopalan S, Olin JW: Upper extremity arterial disease. Cardiol Clin 20:623-631, 2002.

Romanowski, Cam Fairlie NC, Procter AE, et al: Percutaneous transluminal angioplasty of the subclavian and axillary arteries: Initial results and long term follow-up. Clin Radiol 46:104-107, 1992.

Case 9   19

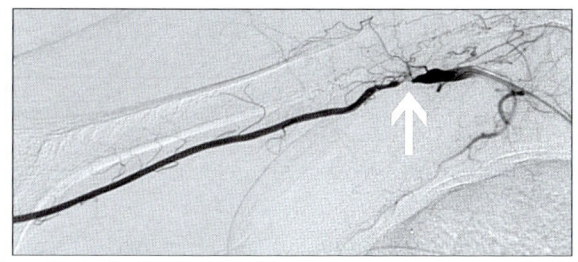

Figure 1. Right upper extremity arteriogram shows a focal, high-grade stenosis *(arrow)* of the proximal brachial artery associated with well-developed arterial collaterals.

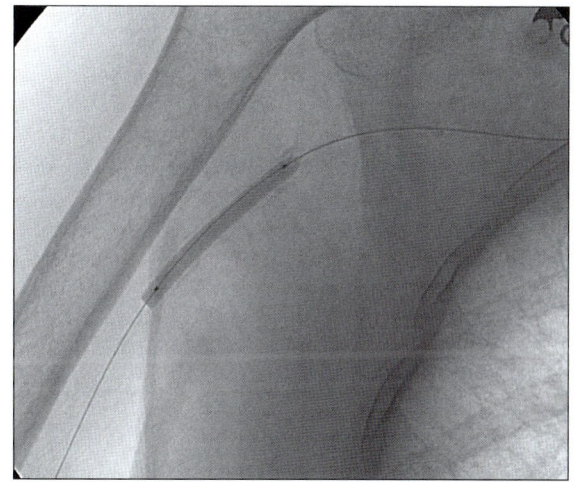

Figure 2. A 4-mm balloon has been inflated across the lesion.

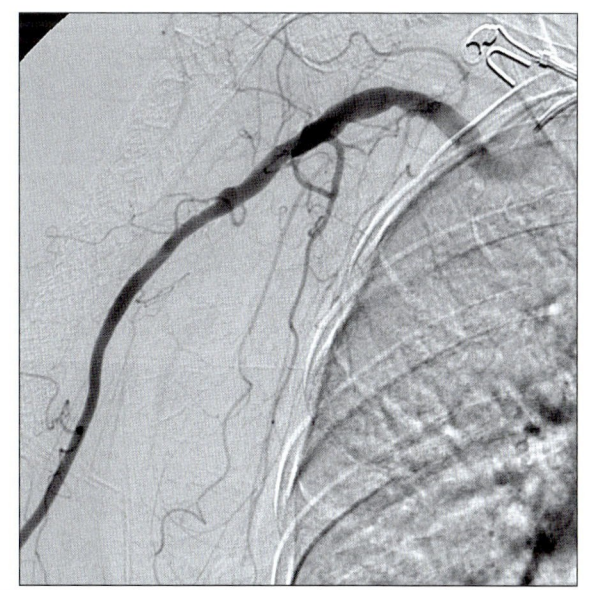

Figure 3. Follow-up arteriogram following balloon angioplasty shows no residual stenosis or dissection at the site of angioplasty.

Case 10

DEMOGRAPHICS/CLINICAL HISTORY

A 56-year-old woman with right upper extremity numbness.

DISCUSSION

History/Indications for Procedure
A 56-year-old woman with numbness in the right hand since a right brachiocephalic fistula was placed 2 weeks earlier. The right hand is cool and weak on physical exam relative to the left.

Procedure
Brachial artery angioplasty

Pre-procedure Imaging
Doppler ultrasound at the right wrist shows diminished waveforms that improve with compression of the fistula.

Intraprocedural Findings
Right upper extremity arteriogram shows a focal, high-grade stenosis of the brachial artery (Fig. 1) and poor flow of the brachial artery distal to the fistula anastamosis (Fig. 2). The lesion was crossed with a 0.014-in wire and dilated using a 4-mm balloon (Fig. 3).

Follow-up and Complications
Follow-up arteriogram after balloon angioplasty shows minimal residual stenosis (Fig. 4). The patient's symptoms improved after the procedure, and after the fistula matured, the patient was able to use it for long-term dialysis access.

Suggested Readings

Malik J, Tuka V, Kasalova Z, et al: Understanding the dialysis access steal syndrome: A review of the etiologies, diagnosis, prevention and treatment strategies. J Vasc Access 9:155-166, 2008.

Suding PN, Wilson SE: Strategies for management of ischemic steal syndrome. Semin Vasc Surg 20:184-188, 2007.

Tordoir JH, Dammers R, van der Sande FM: Upper extremity ischemia and hemodialysis vascular access. Eur J Vasc Endovasc Surg 27:1-5, 2004.

Valji K, Hye RJ, Roberts AC, et al: Hand ischemia in patients with hemodialysis access grafts: Angiographic diagnosis and treatment. Radiology 196:697-701, 1995.

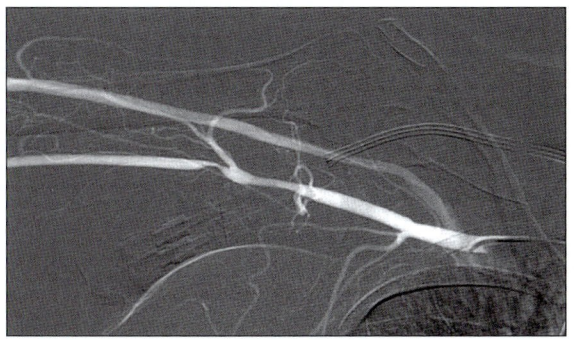

Figure 1. Selective right upper extremity arteriogram shows a focal stenosis of the right brachial artery. There is early opacification of the cephalic vein through the fistula.

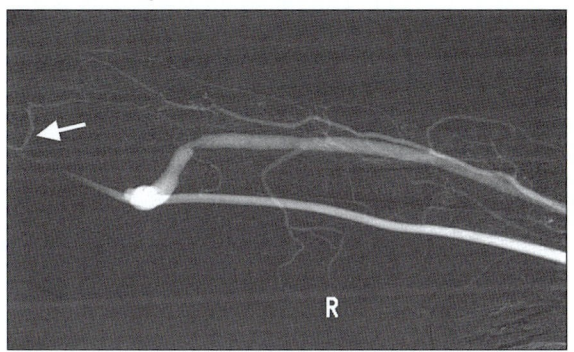

Figure 2. Right upper extremity arteriogram at the level of the arteriovenous anastamosis shows poor perfusion of the brachial artery distal to the anastamosis. There is filling of the distal brachial artery by small collaterals *(arrow)*.

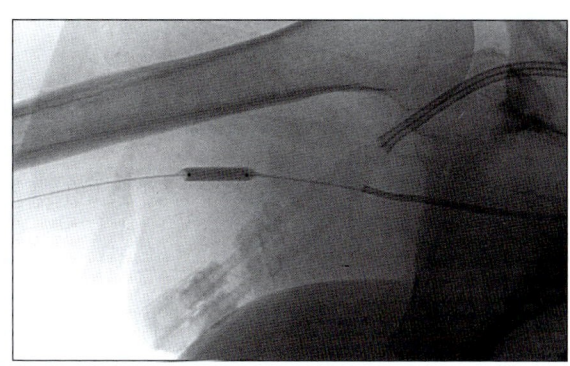

Figure 3. The brachial artery stenosis was dilated using a 4-mm balloon.

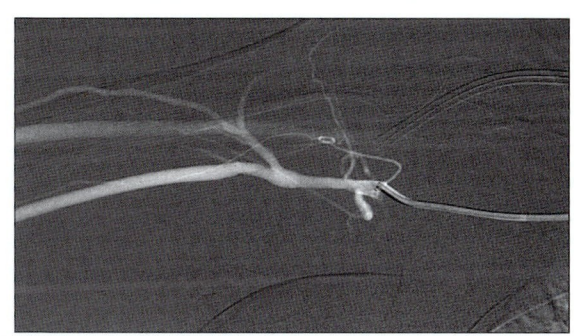

Figure 4. Follow-up arteriogram after balloon angioplasty. There is improved flow to the right arm, with only minimal residual stenosis.

Case 11

DEMOGRAPHICS/CLINICAL HISTORY

A 49-year-old man with right hand numbness, undergoing angiography.

DISCUSSION

History/Indications for Procedure
A 49-year-old carpenter presented with right hand ischemia. The patient had acute onset of pain in the fourth and fifth digits, with white discoloration of these digits.

Procedure
Thrombolysis for hypothenar hammer syndrome

Intraprocedural Findings
The right upper extremity arteriogram shows abrupt tapering and occlusion of the superficial palmar arch, and there are segmental occlusions of the digital arteries of the fourth and fifth digits (Fig. 1). Thrombolysis with tissue plasminogen activator (tPA) was initiated at a rate of 0.5 mg/hr.

Follow-up and Complications
The patient underwent 48 hours of thrombolysis, which uncovered a small aneurysm of the proximal superficial palmar arch (Fig. 2). The patient's symptoms resolved, and he subsequently underwent surgical resection of the aneurysm.

Suggested Readings
Drape JL, Feydy A, Guerini H, et al: Vascular lesions of the hand. Eur J Radiol 56:331-343, 2005.
Ferris BL, Taylor LM Jr, Oyama K, et al: Hypothenar hammer syndrome: Proposed etiology. J Vasc Surg 31:104-113, 2000.
Wong GB, Whetzel TP: Hypothenar hammer syndrome—review and case report. Vasc Surg 35:163-166, 2001.

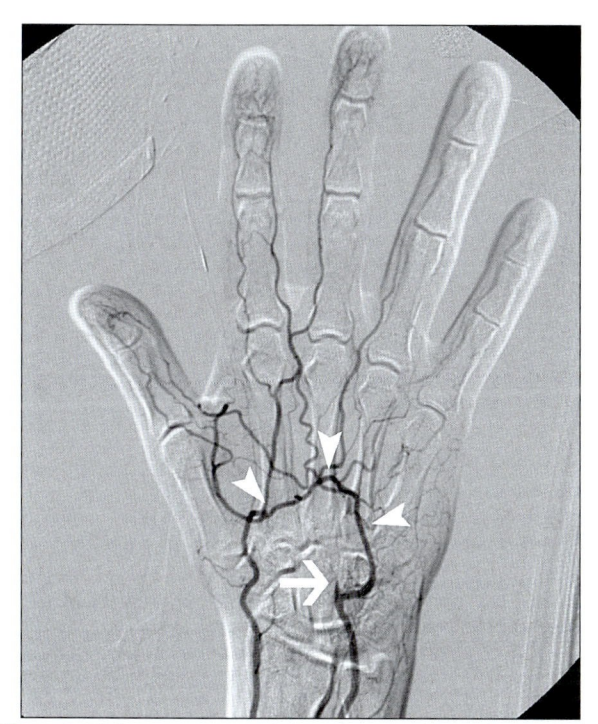

Figure 1. Right upper extremity angiogram shows abrupt occlusion of the superficial palmar arch *(arrow)*. The deep palmar arch remains patent *(arrowheads)*. There is no visible filling of the proper palmar digital arteries of the fourth and fifth digits.

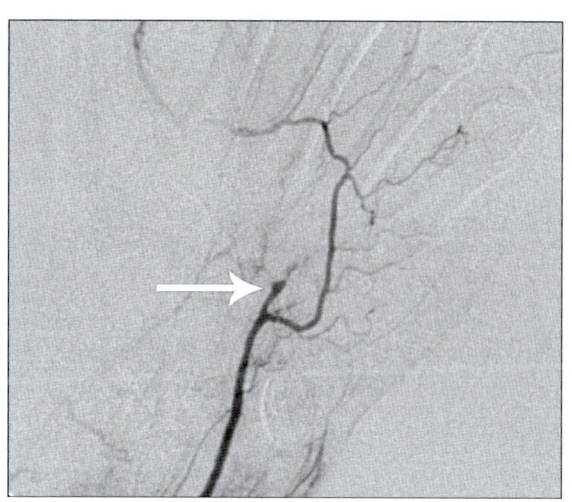

Figure 2. Follow-up right hand arteriogram after 48 hours of thrombolysis shows a small aneurysm within the proximal superficial palmar arch *(arrow)*. The distal superficial palmar arch remains occluded.

Case 12

DEMOGRAPHICS/CLINICAL HISTORY

A 51-year-old woman with a history of sarcoma excision from the right thigh with radiation therapy to this region, undergoing arteriography.

DISCUSSION

History/Indications for Procedure
This patient presented with a 48-hour history of right foot pain. The foot was cool to palpation with reduced distal pulses.

Procedure
Acute superficial femoral artery thrombosis

Pre-procedure Imaging
Arterial ultrasound identified a right superficial femoral artery obstruction (not shown).

Intraprocedural Findings
Right lower extremity arteriography showed segmental occlusion of the distal right superficial femoral artery (Fig. 1). Thrombolytic therapy was initiated.

Follow-up and Complications
The patient underwent 48 hours of thrombolytic therapy. At the conclusion of thrombolysis, an underlying stenosis was uncovered and treated with self-expanding stent placement (Figs. 2 and 3). The patient's symptoms resolved completely.

Suggested Readings

Ouriel K, Veith FJ, Sasahara AA: A comparison of recombinant urokinase with vascular surgery as initial treatment for acute arterial occlusion of the legs. Thrombolysis or Peripheral Arterial Surgery (TOPAS) Investigators. N Engl J Med 338:1105-1111, 1998.

Weaver FA, Comerota AJ, Youngblood M, et al: Surgical revascularization versus thrombolysis for non embolic lower extremity native artery occlusions: Results of a prospective randomized trial. The STILE Investigators. Surgery versus Thrombolysis for Ischemia of the Lower Extremity. J Vasc Surg 24:513-521, 1996.

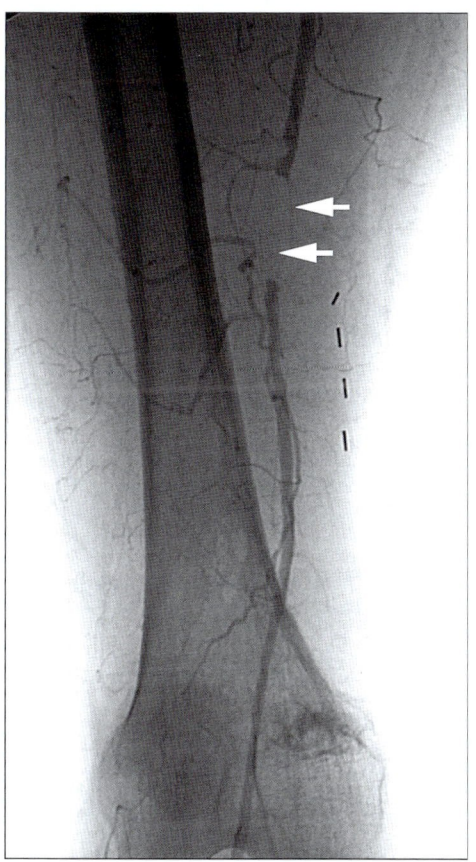

Figure 1. Right lower extremity arteriogram shows segmental occlusion of the distal right superficial femoral artery *(arrows)*. Note the surgical clips from prior soft tissue sarcoma resection.

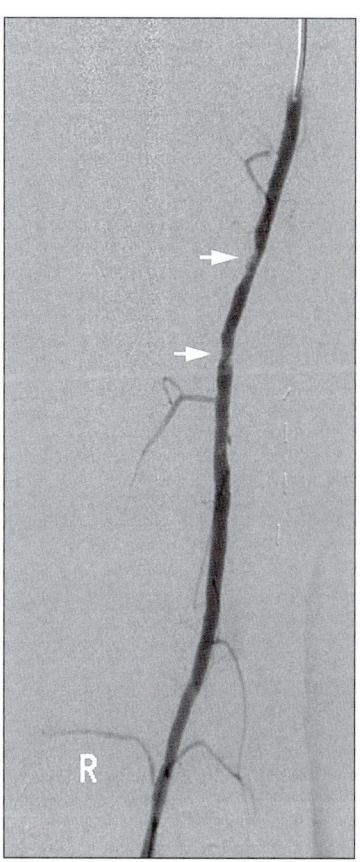

Figure 2. After 48 hours of thrombolytic therapy, flow is restored, uncovering two underlying stenoses *(arrows)*.

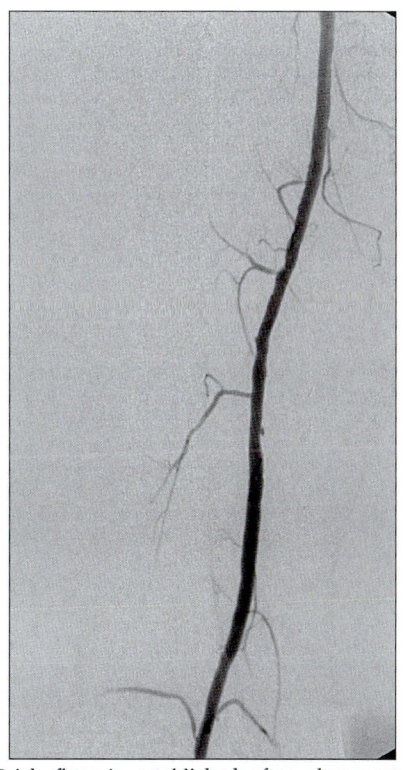

Figure 3. Brisk flow is established after placement of a self-expanding nitinol stent across the underlying stenosis.

Case 13

DEMOGRAPHICS/CLINICAL HISTORY

A 50-year-old woman with left thigh and calf claudication, undergoing arteriography.

DISCUSSION

Procedure
Laser atherectomy of chronically occluded superficial femoral artery

Pre-procedure Imaging
Pre-procedure left lower extremity ankle-brachial index measured 0.52. Arteriogram showed chronic occlusion of the left superficial femoral artery measuring 7 cm in length; there was two-vessel runoff to the foot.

Intraprocedural Findings
A 2.5-mm laser was used for laser atherectomy. Patency of the occluded segment was restored with two passes of the laser catheter.

Suggested Readings
Bates MC, Aburahma AF: An update on endovascular therapy of the lower extremities. J Endovasc Ther 11(Suppl 2):II-107-II-127, 2004.

Lyden SP, Shimshak TM: Contemporary endovascular treatment for disease of the superficial femoral and popliteal arteries: An integrated device-based strategy. J Endovasc Ther 13(Suppl 2):II-41-II-51, 2006.

Wiesinger B, Heller S, Schmehl J, et al: Percutaneous vascular interventions in the superficial femoral artery: A review. Minerva Cardioangiol 54:83-93, 2006.

Case 13   27

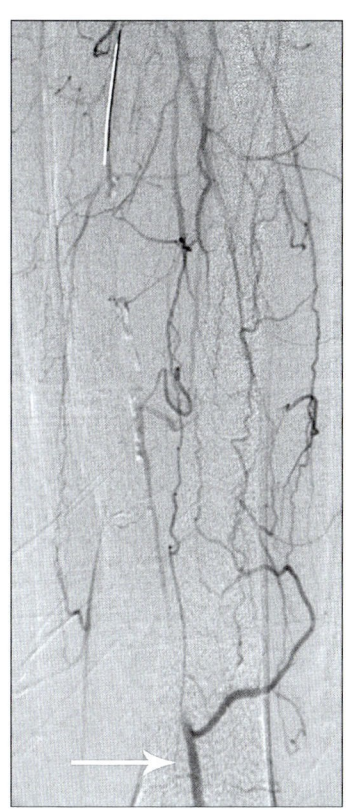

Figure 1. Selective left lower extremity arteriogram shows a 7-cm long occlusion of the superficial femoral artery. There is reconstitution of the above-knee popliteal artery through a collateral *(arrow)*.

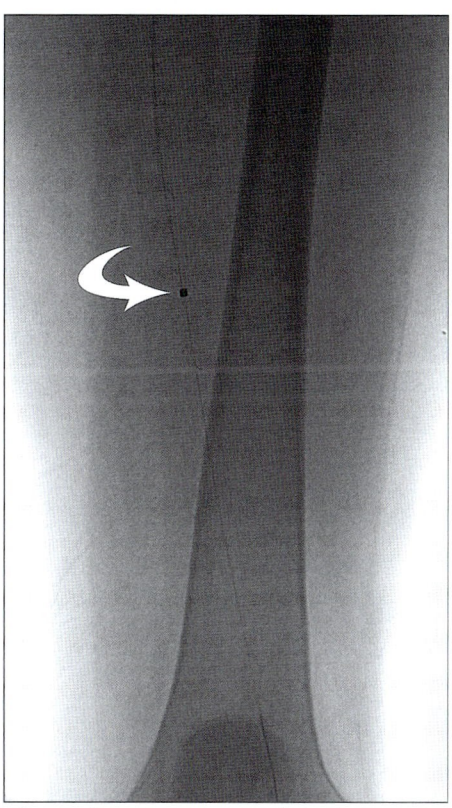

Figure 2. Laser atherectomy was performed. Two passes were made with a 2.5-mm excimer laser *(arrow)*.

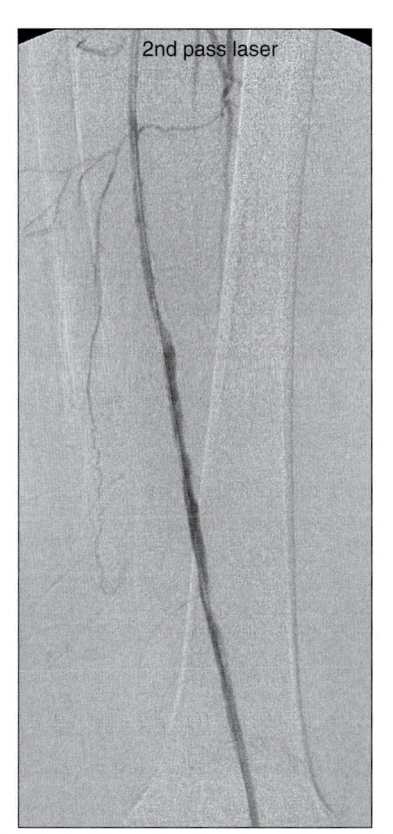

Figure 3. After atherectomy, flow is restored through the previously occluded segment. No angioplasty or stenting was required.

Case 14

DEMOGRAPHICS/CLINICAL HISTORY

A 36-year-old man with a history of Buerger disease, undergoing arteriography.

DISCUSSION

History/Indications for Procedure
This patient underwent a right below-knee amputation for a nonhealing wound at age 31 and now presents with pain and a nonhealing wound in the left great toe.

Procedure
Left lower extremity arterial recanalization

Pre-procedure Imaging
Arterial ultrasound revealed nonpulsatile flow in the posterior tibial artery at the ankle. The left ankle-brachial index measured 0.47.

Intraprocedural Findings
A diagnostic arteriogram shows chronic occlusion of the left superior femoral and popliteal arteries with reconstitution of the posterior tibial artery (Fig. 1). Subintimal recanalization was performed from the proximal superior femoral artery to the posterior tibial artery at the midcalf level (Figs. 2-4).

Follow-up and Complications
Ankle-brachial index the day after the recanalization was 1.2. The left toe wound healed; however, the patient continued to smoke and presented 6 months later with occlusion of the subintimal channel and new left lower extremity ischemia.

Suggested Readings
Bolia A: Percutaneous intentional extraluminal (subintimal) recanalisation of crural arteries. Eur J Radiol 28:199-204, 1998.
Bolia A, Bell PR: Femoropopliteal and crural artery recanalisation using subintimal angioplasty. Semin Vasc Surg 8:253-264, 1995.
Reekers JA, Bolia A: Percutaneous intentional extraluminal (subintimal) recanalisation: How to do it yourself. Eur J Radiol 28:192-198, 1998.
Yilmaz S, Sindel T, Yegin A, et al: Subintimal angioplasty of long SFA occlusions. J Vasc Interv Radiol 14:997-1010, 2003.

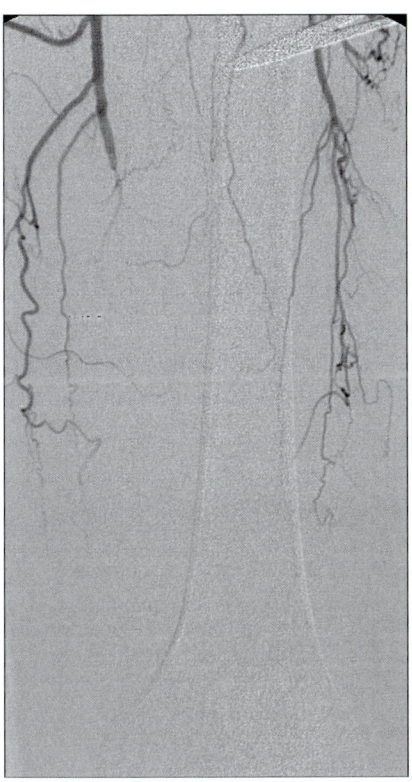

Figure 1. Left lower extremity arteriogram shows chronic occlusion of the proximal left superior femoral artery.

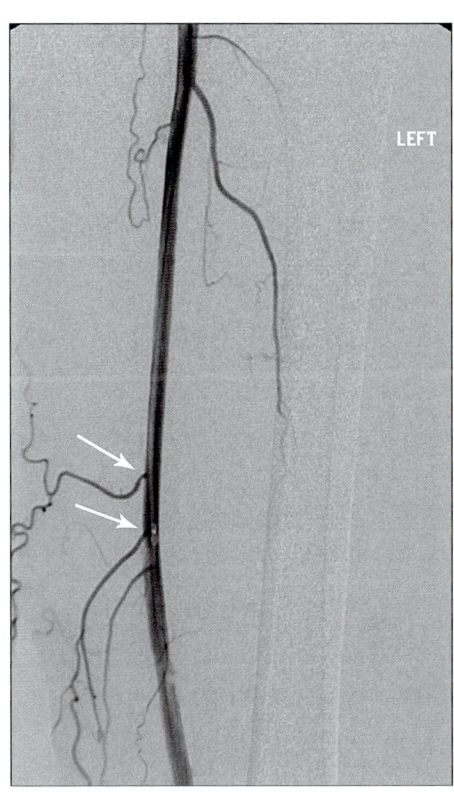

Figure 2. After recanalization, there is brisk flow through the recanalized superior femoral artery. Note the continued filling of superior femoral artery branches *(arrows)*.

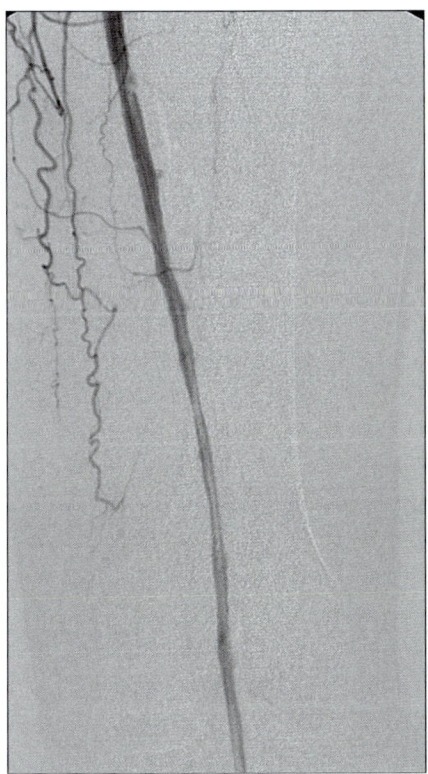

Figure 3. Slightly lower image shows a patent popliteal artery.

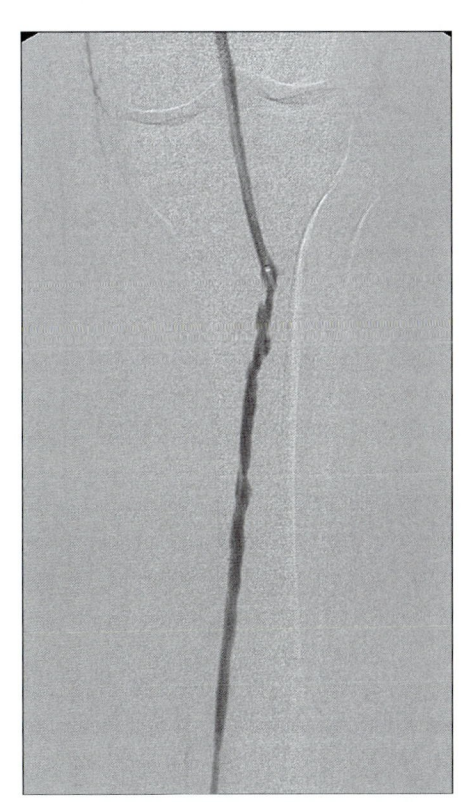

Figure 4. The recanalized segment extends into the posterior tibial artery. There is brisk flow with no opacified collaterals.

Case 15

DEMOGRAPHICS/CLINICAL HISTORY

A 54-year-old man with left lower extremity claudication, undergoing ultrasound, stent placement, arteriography, and angiography.

DISCUSSION

History/Indications for Procedure
A 54-year-old man has a two-block claudication in his left calf.

Procedure
Atherosclerotic disease of the superficial femoral artery

Pre-procedure Imaging
Arterial ultrasound demonstrated a 6-cm long stenosis in the left superficial femoral artery. The ankle-brachial index on the left was diminished at 0.61.

Intraprocedural Findings
A long-segment stenosis involves the distal left superficial femoral artery (Fig. 1). The lesion was treated with a 6-mm × 15-cm Viabahn (Gore & Associates, Flagstaff, AZ) covered stent (Figs. 2 and 3).

Follow-up and Complications
The patient's symptoms improved after stent placement. His symptoms recurred 8 months later, when a focal intrastent stenosis was discovered on repeat angiography (Fig. 4).

Suggested Readings
Jahnke T, Andresen R, Müller-Hülsbeck S, et al: Hemobahn stent-grafts for treatment of femoropopliteal arterial obstructions: Midterm results of a prospective trial. J Vasc Interv Radiol 14:41-51, 2003.

Muradin G, Bosch JL, Stijnen T, Hunink MG: Balloon dilation and stent implantation for treatment of femoropopliteal arterial disease: Meta-analysis. Radiology 221:137-145, 2001.

Schillinger M, Sabeti S, Loewe C, et al: Balloon angioplasty versus implantation of nitinol stents in the superficial femoral artery. N Engl J Med 354:1879-1888, 1006.

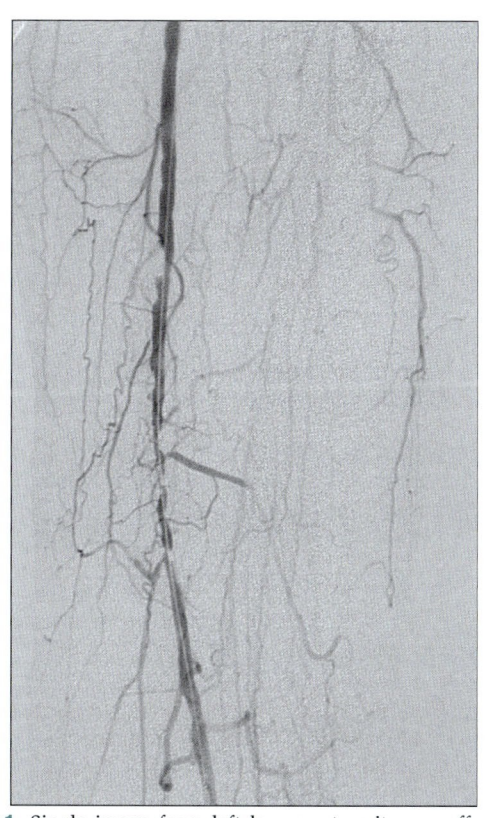

Figure 1. Single image from left lower extremity run-off arteriogram demonstrates a long-segment, irregular stenosis of the distal superficial femoral artery. The entire lesion measured approximately 12 cm long.

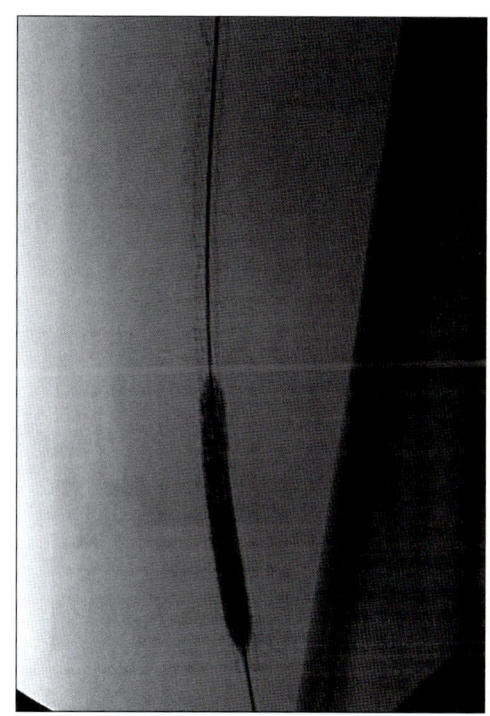

Figure 2. The entire lesion was covered with a 6-mm × 15-cm Viabahn stent. The stent was dilated with a 6-mm balloon.

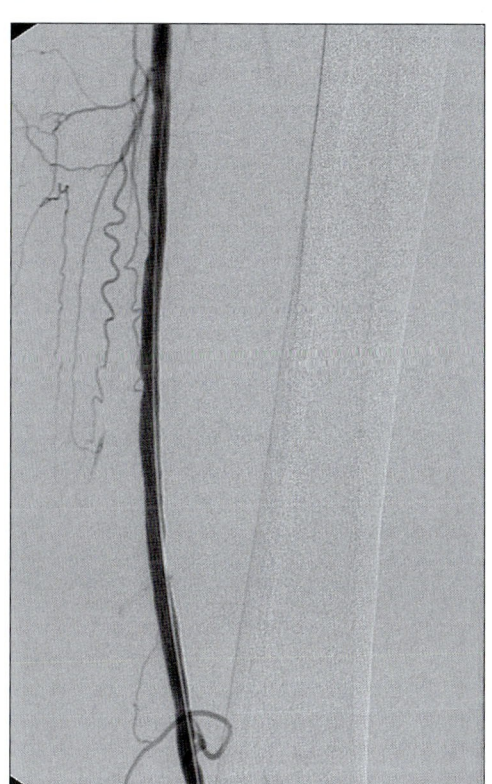

Figure 3. Follow-up angiogram after stent placement shows significantly improved flow through the distal superficial femoral artery.

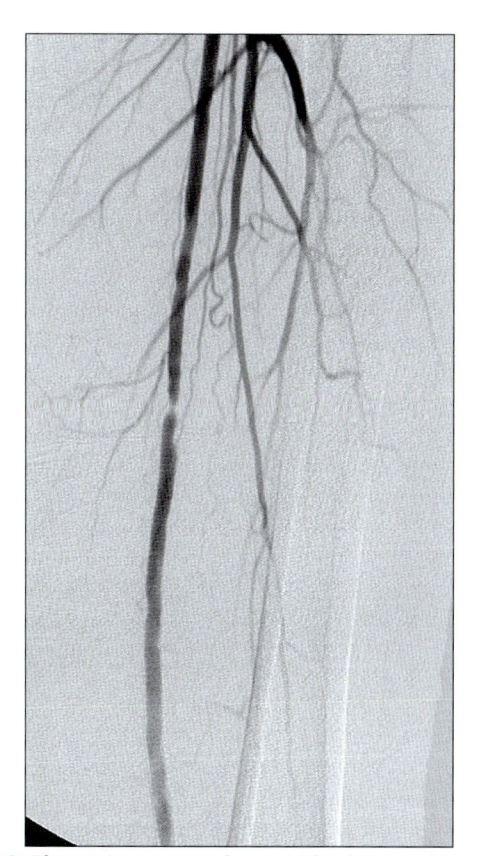

Figure 4. The patient returned 8 months later with recurrent symptoms. A focal intrastent stenosis was discovered. This was successfully treated with balloon angioplasty.

Case 16

DEMOGRAPHICS/CLINICAL HISTORY

A 67-year-old woman with nonhealing ulcer of the right foot, undergoing arteriography.

DISCUSSION

History/Indications for Procedure
A 67-year-old woman presented with a nonhealing ulcer of the right foot.

Procedure
Subintimal recanalization of lower extremity

Pre-procedure Imaging
A diagnostic lower extremity arteriogram (Fig. 1) shows chronic occlusion of the distal right superficial femoral artery and reconstitution of the popliteal artery.

Intraprocedural Findings
The occluded distal superficial femoral artery and popliteal artery were successfully crossed through the subintimal space and dilated with a 6-mm balloon (Figs. 2 and 3). A 6-mm, self-expanding stent was deployed at the reentry point for persistent stenosis after balloon angioplasty (Fig. 4).

Follow-up and Complications
One week after the revascularization procedure, the patient underwent popliteal-to-anterior tibial bypass surgery. The patient went on to transmetatarsal amputation for osteomyelitis with appropriate healing of the transmetatarsal flap.

Suggested Readings
Bolia A, Brennan J, Bell PR: Recanalization of femoropopliteal occlusions: Improving success rate by subintimal recanalization. Clin Radiol 40:325, 1989.

London NJM, Varty K, Sayers RD, et al: Percutaneous transluminal angioplasty for lower limb critical ischaemia. Br J Surg 82:1232, 1995.

Reekers JA, Bolia A: Percutaneous intentional extraluminal (subintimal) recanalisation: How to do it yourself. Eur J Radiol 28:192, 1998.

Yilmaz S, Sindel T, Yegin A, et al: Subintimal angioplasty of long SFA occlusions. J Vasc Interv Radiol 14:997, 2003.

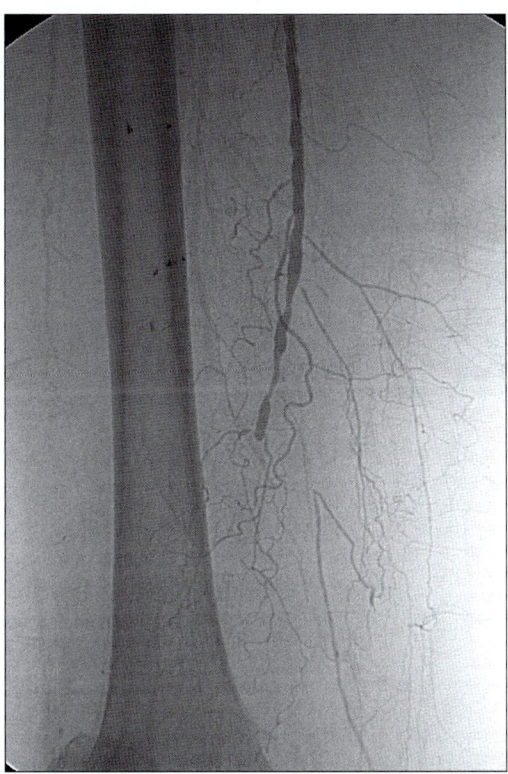

Figure 1. Unsubtracted image from right lower extremity arteriogram shows diffuse atherosclerotic narrowing of mid superior femoral artery with occlusion of distal superior femoral artery and above-knee popliteal artery.

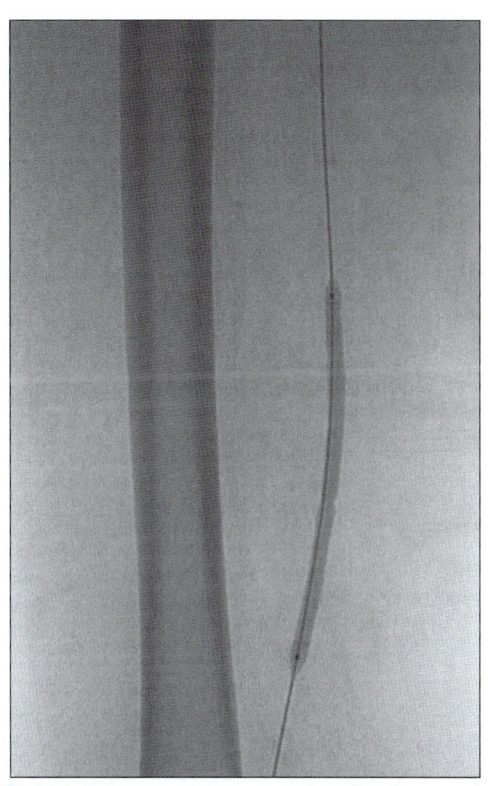

Figure 2. Occluded segment was crossed, and balloon angioplasty was performed.

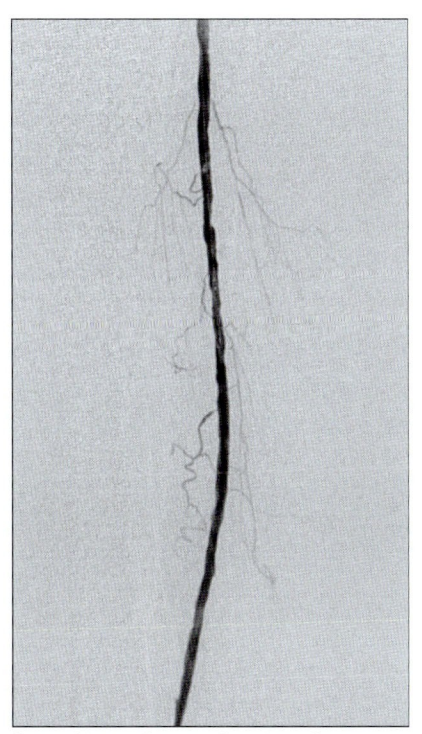

Figure 3. After subintimal recanalization, there is restoration of flow through distal superior femoral artery and popliteal artery.

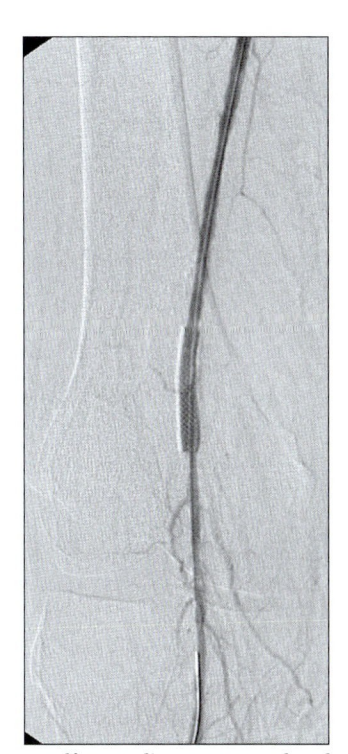

Figure 4. A 6-mm, self-expanding stent was placed at reentry point for persistent stenosis despite repeat angioplasty at this location.

Case 17

DEMOGRAPHICS/CLINICAL HISTORY
An 80-year-old man with long-standing peripheral arterial occlusive disease, undergoing arteriography.

DISCUSSION

History/Indications for Procedure
This patient underwent previous right above-knee amputation for a nonhealing wound and now has a nonhealing ulcer of the left great toe.

Procedure
Recanalization of chronic superficial femoral and popliteal artery occlusion

Pre-procedure Imaging
Doppler ultrasound showed outflow and runoff obstruction of the left lower extremity with monophasic waveform in the posterior tibial artery; the toe pressure was < 10 mm Hg.

Intraprocedural Findings
Diagnostic arteriogram confirmed chronic occlusion of the superior femoral artery (SFA) (Fig. 1) and popliteal arteries with reconstitution of the posterior tibial artery. Subintimal recanalization was performed from the origin of the SFA to the posterior tibial artery.

Follow-up and Complications
After the angioplasty, the left great toe ulcer healed. The patient had no further problems for 2.5 years, at which point he developed new left lower extremity ischemia.

Suggested Readings
Bolia A, Bell PR: Femoropopliteal and crural artery recanalisation using subintimal angioplasty. Semin Vasc Surg 8:253-264, 1995.
London NJ, Srinivasan R, Naylor AR, et al: Subintimal angioplasty of femoropopliteal occlusions: The long term results. Eur J Vasc Surg 8:148-155, 1994.
Reekers JA, Bolia A: Percutaneous intentional extraluminal (subintimal) recanalisation: How to do it yourself. Eur J Radiol 28:192-198, 1998.
Yilmaz S, Sindel T, Yegin A, et al: Subintimal angioplasty of long SFA occlusions. J Vasc Interv Radiol 14:997-1010, 2003.

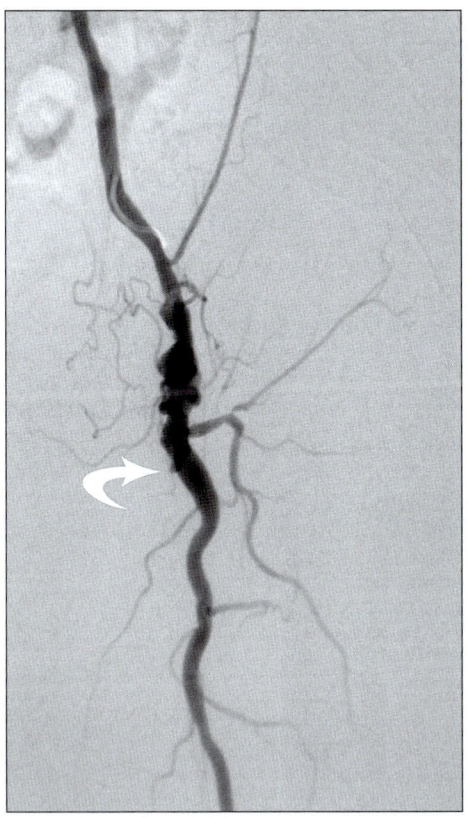

Figure 1. Single image from left lower extremity angiogram shows occlusion of the left SFA. Only a small nubbin of the SFA is present (*arrow*).

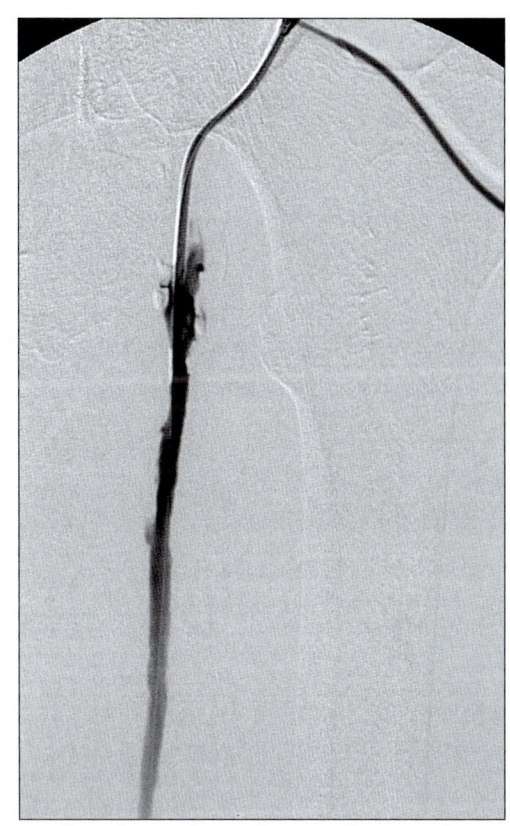

Figure 2. After subintimal recanalization, there is preferential flow within the recanalized SFA.

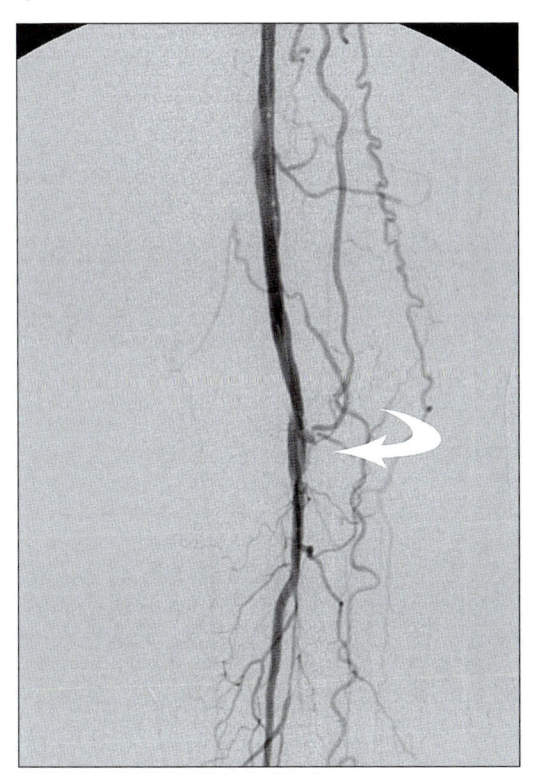

Figure 3. After subintimal recanalization, there is mild irregularity at the reentry point (*arrow*). This did not appear to be flow-limiting.

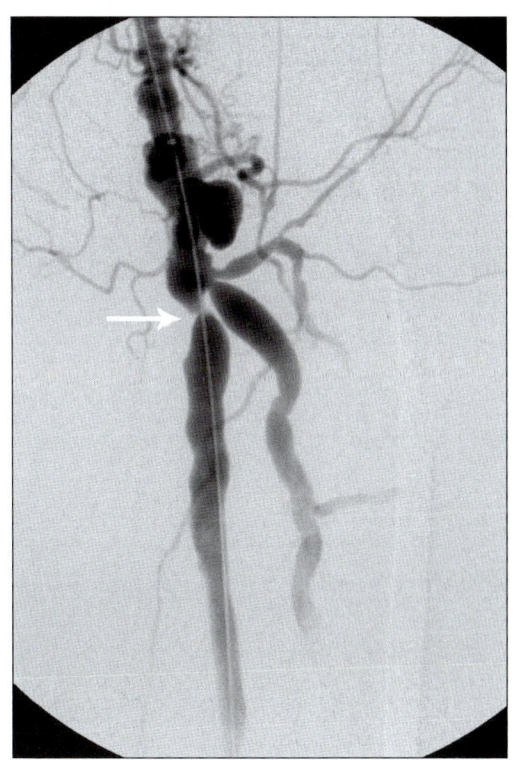

Figure 4. The patient returned 2.5 years after the subintimal recanalization with new left lower extremity ischemia. The subintimal channel remains patent with focal stenosis at the entry site (*arrow*). A second angioplasty was successfully done (not shown).

Case 18

DEMOGRAPHICS/CLINICAL HISTORY

A 65-year-old man with nonhealing ulcer of the left foot.

DISCUSSION

History/Indications for Procedure

A 65-year-old man with a history of chronic, nonhealing ulcer of the left foot. On exam, there is a 1.5-cm × 2-cm ulcer beneath the first metatarsal head.

Procedure

Cryoplasty of superficial femoral artery stenosis

Pre-procedure Imaging

Left lower extremity ABI measured 0.63, and arterial ultrasound shows evidence for high-grade stenosis or occlusion within the superficial femoral artery.

Intraprocedural Findings

Left lower extremity arteriogram shows a focal, high-grade stenosis of the mid-SFA (Fig. 1). The lesion was treated with 5-mm × 6-cm cryoplasty balloon (Polar-cath, Boston Scientific, Nanick, MA) (Figs. 2 and 3).

Follow-up and Complications

Follow-up arteriogram after cryoplasty shows improved flow through the SFA with a non–flow limiting dissection (Fig. 4). The ulcer began granulating after the procedure and eventually healed with conservative management.

Suggested Readings

Fava M, Loyola S, Polydorou A, et al: Cryoplasty for femoropopliteal arterial disease: Late angiographic results of initial human experience. J Vasc Interv Radiol 15:1239-1243, 2004.

Laird J, Jaff MR, Biamino G, et al: Cryoplasty for the treatment of femoropopliteal arterial disease: Results of a prospective, multicenter registry. J Vasc Interv Radiol 16:1067-1073, 2005.

Samson RH, Showalter DP, Lepore M Jr, et al: CryoPlasty of the superficial femoral and popliteal arteries: A reappraisal after 44 months experience. J Vasc Surg 48:634-637, 2008.

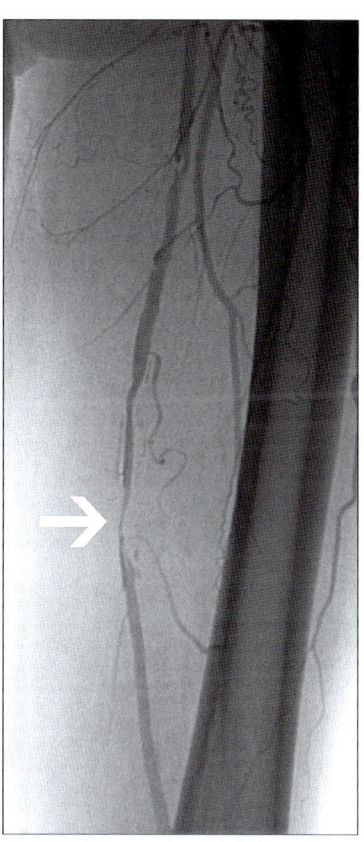

Figure 1. Unsubtracted image from left lower extremity arteriogram shows multilevel disease with a high-grade stenosis in the mid-SFA *(arrow)*.

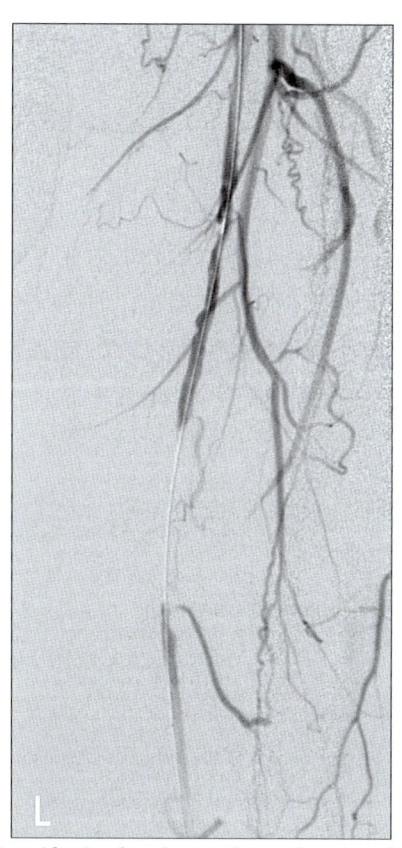

Figure 2. A guidewire has been advanced across the stenosis, causing temporary vessel occlusion.

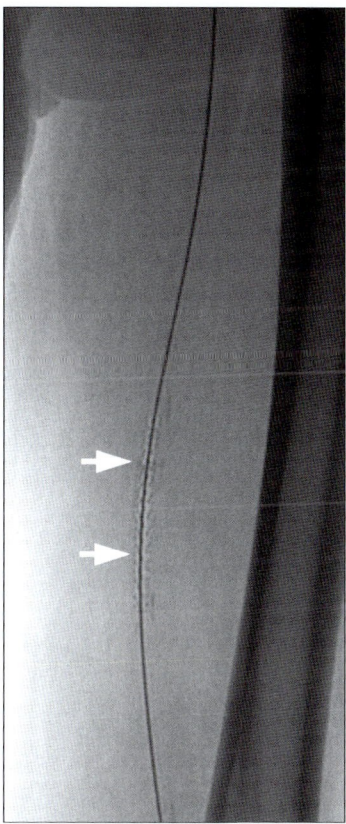

Figure 3. The cryoplasty balloon is inflated *(arrows)*.

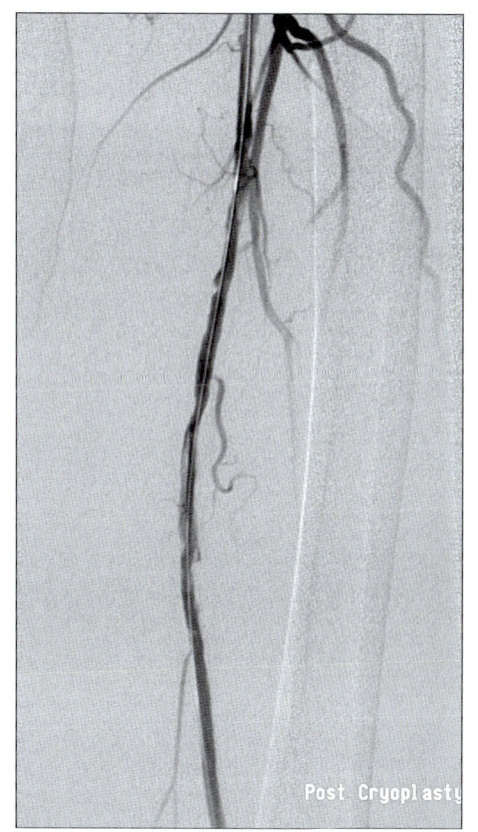

Figure 4. Following cryoplasty, there is improved flow through the mid-SFA. The cryoplasty did result in a non–flow limiting dissection.

Case 19

DEMOGRAPHICS/CLINICAL HISTORY

A 61-year-old man with a nonhealing ulcer on the left lateral foot, undergoing ultrasound, arterial recanalization, and amputation.

DISCUSSION

History/Indications for Procedure
A 61-year-old man with long-standing diabetes has a nonhealing ulcer on the left lateral foot.

Procedure
Subintimal recanalization of the posterior tibial artery

Pre-procedure Imaging
Left lower extremity arterial ultrasound demonstrates severe run-off obstruction. The ankle-brachial index (ABI) on the left was 0.35.

Intraprocedural Findings
There is occlusion of the distal popliteal artery with reconstitution of the posterior tibial artery at the ankle (Fig. 1). Subintimal recanalization of the posterior tibial artery was performed, with restoration of in-line flow to the foot (Fig. 2).

Follow-up and Complications
The left lower extremity ABI improved to 0.73 after the angioplasty (Figs. 3 and 4). The patient subsequently underwent transmetatarsal amputation for gangrene of the left 3 to 5 toes.

Suggested Readings
Bolia A, Sayers RD, Thompson MM, Bell PR: Subintimal and intraluminal recanalisation of occluded crural arteries by percutaneous balloon angioplasty. Eur J Vasc Surg 8:214-219, 1994.

Lazaris AM, Tsiamis AC, Fishwick G, et al: Clinical outcomes of primary infrainguinal subintimal angioplasty in diabetic patients with critical lower limb ischaemia. J Endovasc Ther 11:447-453, 2005.

London NJ, Varty K, Sayers RD, et al: Percutaneous transluminal angioplasty for lower limb critical ischaemia. Br J Surg 82:1232-1235, 1995.

Molloy KJ, Nasim A, London NJ, et al: Percutaneous transluminal angioplasty in the treatment of critical limb ischaemia. J Endovasc Ther 10:298-303, 2003.

Vraux H, Hammer F, Verhelst R, et al: Subintimal angioplasty of tibial vessel occlusions in the treatment of critical limb ischaemia: Midterm results. Eur J Vasc Endovasc Surg 20:441-446, 2000.

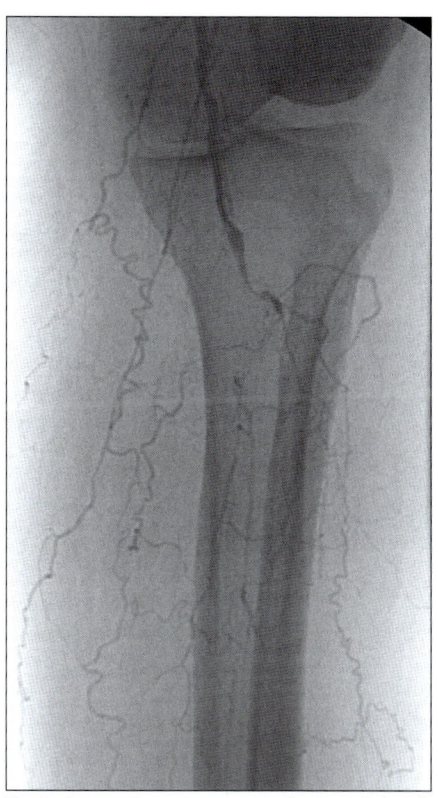

Figure 1. Single image demonstrates occlusion of the distal popliteal artery, just proximal to the origin of the anterior tibial artery.

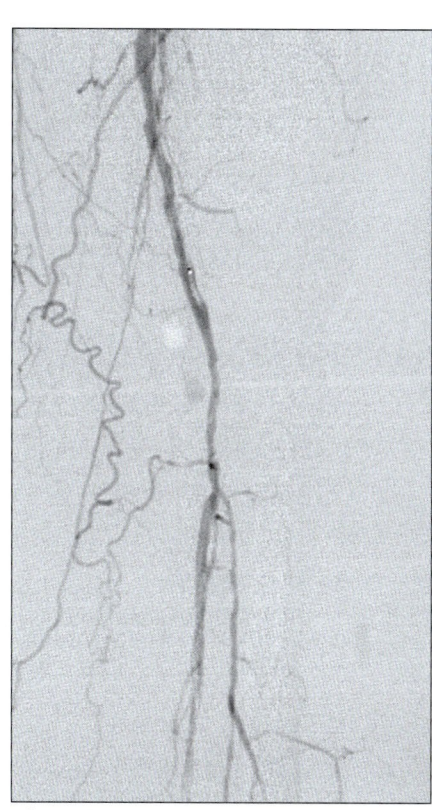

Figure 2. After subintimal recanalization, there is restoration of flow through the tibioperoneal trunk and proximal posterior tibial artery.

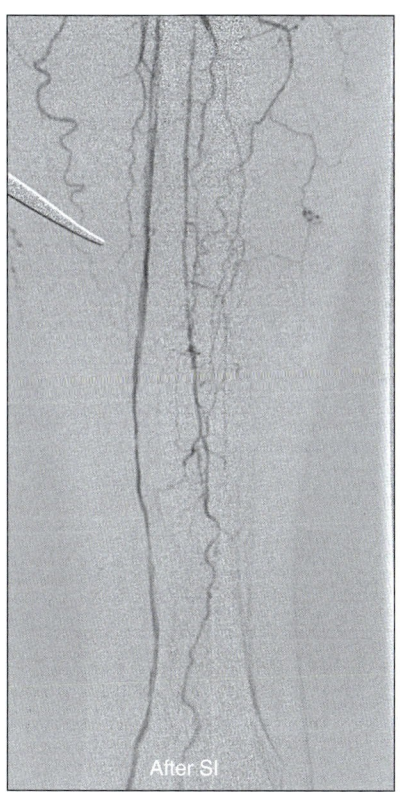

Figure 3. After the initial balloon angioplasty, many stenoses are present in the distal recanalized posterior tibial artery. There is continued filling of many collaterals.

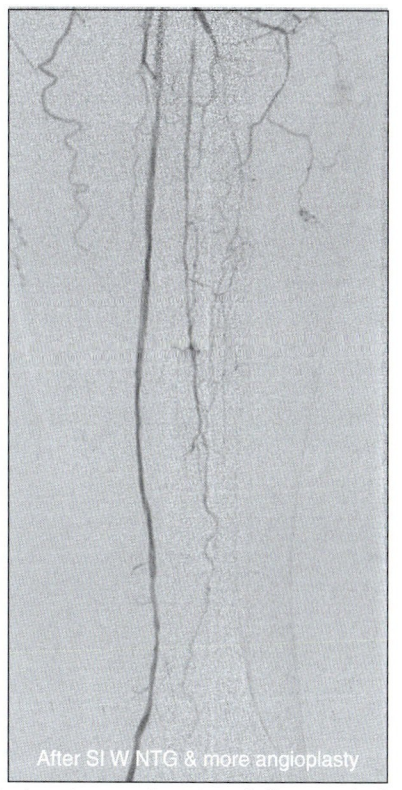

Figure 4. Final angiogram after repeat balloon angioplasty and additional intra-arterial nitroglycerin shows that in-line flow to the right foot has been re-established.

Case 20

DEMOGRAPHICS/CLINICAL HISTORY

A 50-year-old man with calf claudication, undergoing arteriography.

DISCUSSION

History/Indications for Procedure

A 50-year-old man had half-block claudication in the right calf and reported recent onset of occasional pain at rest.

Procedure

Tibioperoneal stenosis angioplasty

Pre-procedure Imaging

The diagnostic arteriogram shows a focal, high-grade stenosis at the origin of the tibial vessels (Fig. 1). The anterior tibial artery is occluded, and the peroneal artery is the dominant run-off vessel.

Intraprocedural Findings

The patient was systemically heparinized, and the stenosis at the origin of the tibial vessels was crossed with a 0.018-inch guidewire. Balloon angioplasty of the stenosis was performed with a 4-mm balloon (Fig. 2).

Follow-up and Complications

The follow-up angiogram after angioplasty shows a good angiographic result (Fig. 3). After the procedure, the patient's symptoms resolved, and he was able to walk without pain.

Suggested Readings

Boyer L, Therre T, Garcier JM, et al: Infra-popliteal percutaneous transluminal angioplasty limb salvage. Acta Radiol 41:73-77, 2000.

Jamsen T, Manninen H, Tulla H, Matsi P: The final outcome of primary infrainguinal percutaneous transluminal angioplasty in 100 consecutive patients with chronic critical limb ischemia. J Vasc Interv Radiol 13:455-463, 2002.

Norgren L, Hiatt WR, Dormandy JA, et al, for the TASC II Working Group: Inter-Society consensus for the management of peripheral arterial disease (TASC II). J Vasc Surg 43(Suppl S):S5-S67, 2007.

Case 20   41

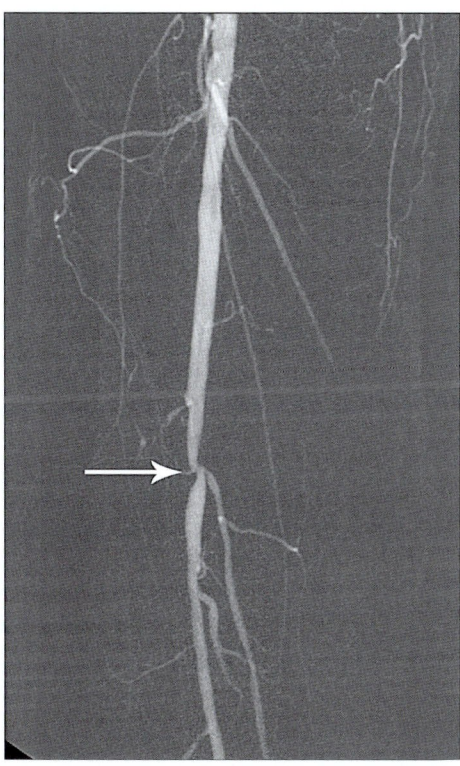

Figure 1. Arteriography of the right lower extremity shows that the anterior tibial artery is occluded. There is a high-grade stenosis at the bifurcation of the tibioperoneal trunk *(arrow)*.

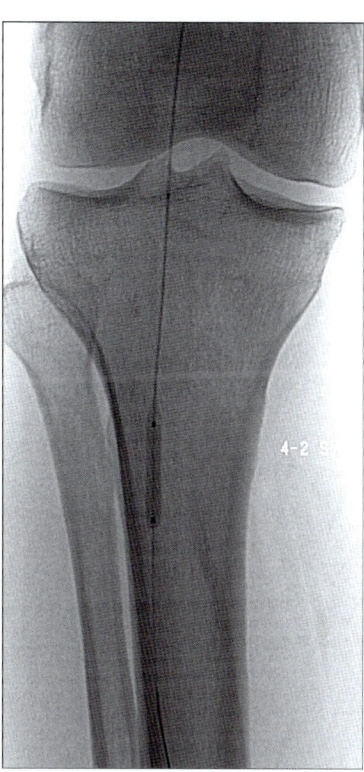

Figure 2. The lesion was crossed with a 0.018-inch guidewire that was advanced into the peroneal artery. Balloon angioplasty was performed with a 4-mm balloon.

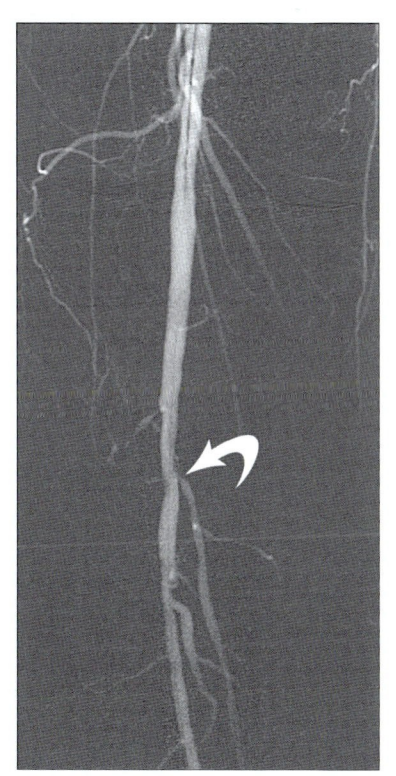

Figure 3. The follow-up angiogram shows minimal residual narrowing at the origin of the peroneal artery. There is persistent stenosis at the origin of the posterior tibial artery *(curved arrow)*. Because the peroneal artery served as the primary run-off vessel, the posterior tibial artery was not treated.

Case 21

DEMOGRAPHICS/CLINICAL HISTORY

An 87-year-old man with bilateral foot ulcers.

DISCUSSION

History/Indications for Procedure
An 87-year-old man with bilateral foot ulcers that have failed to heal with conservative management.

Procedure
Anterior tibial artery recanalization

Pre-procedure Imaging
MR angiogram was performed showing no inflow or outflow obstruction. Conventional arteriogram shows severe run-off disease bilaterally (Fig. 1).

Intraprocedural Findings
The occluded right anterior tibial artery was crossed using the subintimal space. The entire occluded segment was angioplastied with a 3-mm balloon; additional angioplasty of the dorsalis pedis was performed with a 2-mm balloon (Figs. 2–4).

Follow-up and Complications
The patient underwent right great toe amputation. The amputation site healed, and the patient underwent recanalization of the left lower extremity in order to achieve healing of the left foot ulcer.

Suggested Readings

Jamsen T, Manninen H, Tulla H, Matsi P: The final outcome of primary infrainguinal percutaneous transluminal angioplasty in 100 consecutive patients with chronic critical limb ischemia. J Vasc Intervent Radiol 13:455-463, 2002.

Kalra M, Gloviczki P, Bower TC, et al: Limb salvage after successful pedal bypass grafting is associated with improved long term survival. J Vasc Surg 33:6-16, 2000.

London NJ, Varty K, Sayers RD, et al: Percutaneous transluminal angioplasty for lower-limb critical ischemia. Br J Surg 83:135-136, 1996.

Norgen L, Hiatt WR, Dormandy JA: Inter-society consensus for the management of peripheral arterial disease (TASC II). J Vasc Surg 43(Suppl A):1A.116A, S-S5-S67, 2007.

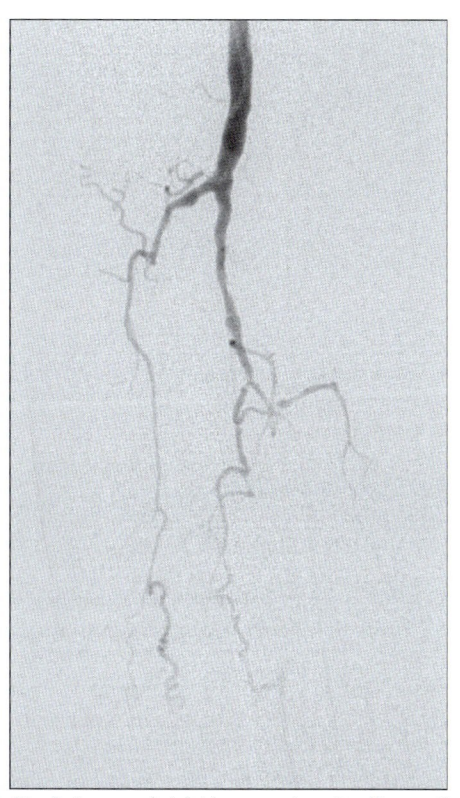

Figure 1. Single image of right lower extremity diagnostic arteriogram shows occlusion of the proximal run-off vessels.

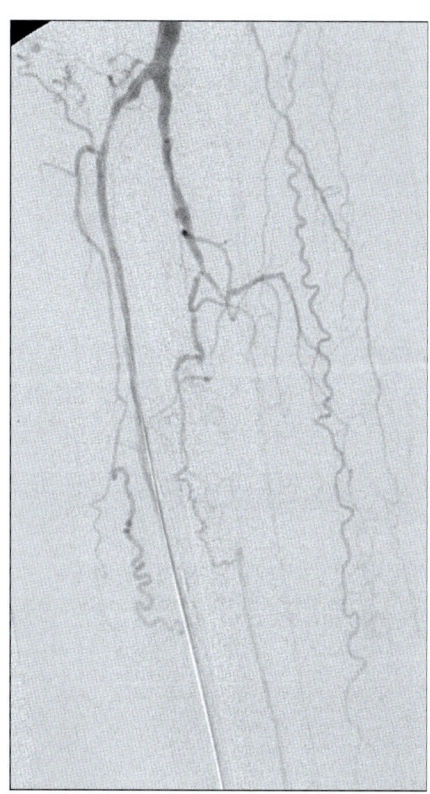

Figure 2. A subintimal racanalization of the anterior tibial artery was performed. Following angioplasty with a 3-mm balloon, flow has been restored.

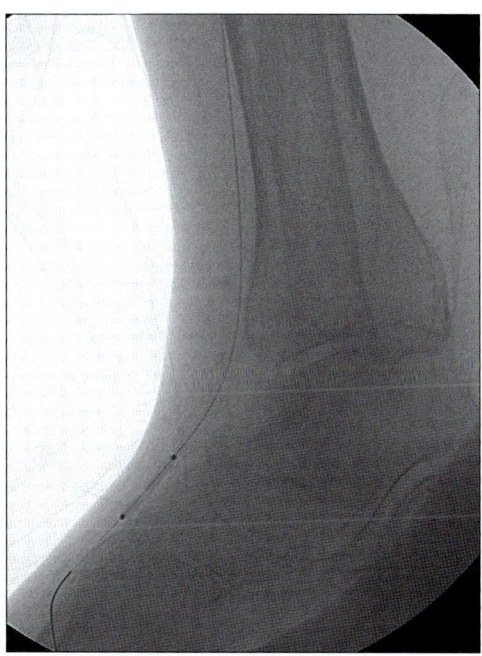

Figure 3. Additional balloon angioplasty at the reentry site in the dorsalis pedis artery was performed with a 2-mm balloon.

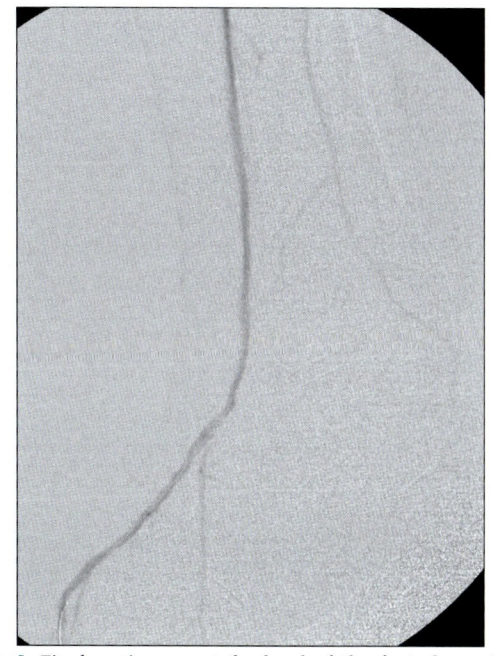

Figure 4. Final angiogram at the level of the foot shows in-line flow to the dorsalis pedis artery.

Case 22

DEMOGRAPHICS/CLINICAL HISTORY

A 61-year-old man with a nonhealing ulcer of the left foot, undergoing arteriography and ultrasonography.

DISCUSSION

History/Indications for Procedure
A 61-year-old man had diabetes and a chronic, nonhealing ulcer of the left foot.

Procedure
Recanalization of occluded posterior tibial artery

Pre-procedure Imaging
Diagnostic arteriography shows complete occlusion of the tibial arteries of the left lower extremity. There is reconstitution of the distal posterior tibial artery just above the ankle (Figs. 1 and 2).

Intraprocedural Findings
The distal posterior tibial artery was accessed with ultrasound, and a 0.018-inch guidewire was advanced retrograde through the subintimal space of the chronically occluded posterior tibial artery. After snaring the guidewire from a femoral access and achieving through-and-through guidewire access, angioplasty of the subintimal tract was performed with a 3-mm balloon.

Follow-up and Complications
After balloon angioplasty, there was restoration of in-line flow to the left foot (Figs. 3 and 4), and the ankle-brachial index (ABI) increased from 0.35 to 0.73. The patient underwent transmetatarsal amputation for gangrenous toes but has not required further amputation.

Suggested Readings

London NJ, Varty K, Sayers RD, et al: Percutaneous transluminal angioplasty for lower-limb critical ischaemia. Br J Surg 82:1232-1235, 1995.

Nydahl S, Hartshorne T, Bell PR, et al: Subintimal angioplasty of infrapopliteal occlusions in critically ischaemic limbs. Eur J Vasc Endovasc Surg 14:212-216, 1997.

Spinosa DJ, Leung DA, Matsumoto AH, et al: Percutaneous intentional extraluminal recanalization in patients with chronic critical limb ischemia. Radiology 232:488-507, 2004.

Vraux H, Hammer F, Verhelst R, et al: Subintimal angioplasty of tibial vessel occlusions in the treatment of critical limb ischaemia: Midterm results. Eur J Vasc Endovasc Surg 20:441-446, 2000.

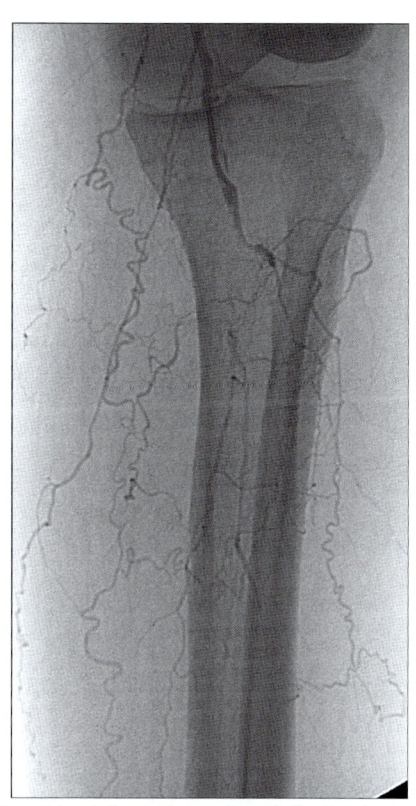

Figure 1. Unsubtracted arteriography of the left lower extremity shows occlusion of the proximal anterior tibial artery and tibioperoneal trunk.

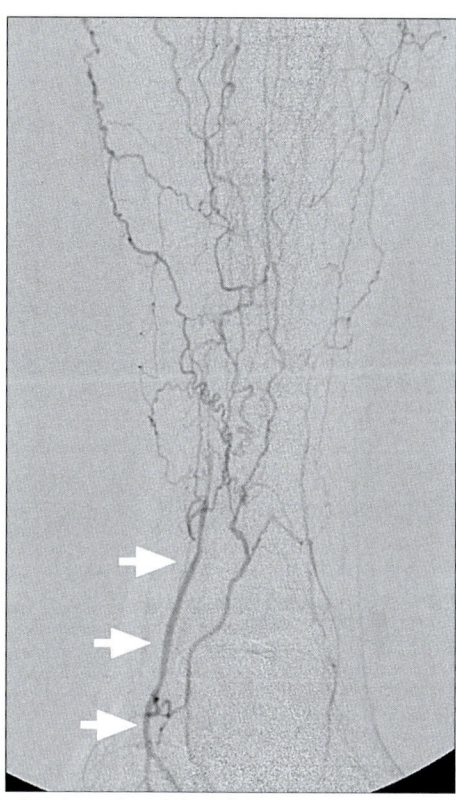

Figure 2. Arteriography of the left lower extremity at the level of the ankle shows numerous arterial collaterals within the distal calf. There is reconstitution of the distal posterior tibial artery *(arrows)*.

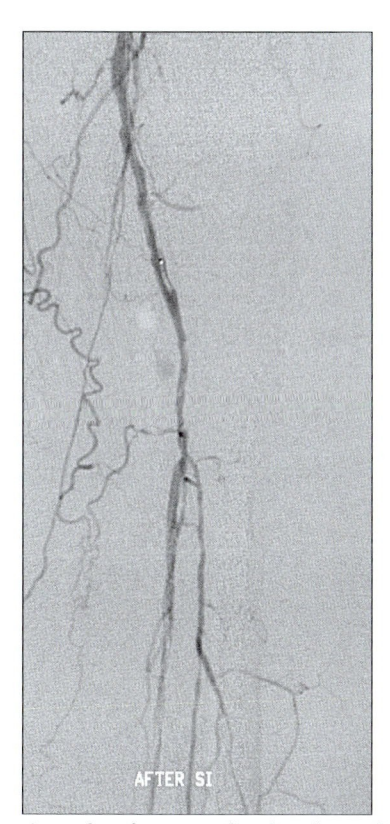

Figure 3. Arteriography after recanalization shows that the tibioperoneal trunk is patent, with restoration of flow in the proximal posterior tibial and peroneal arteries.

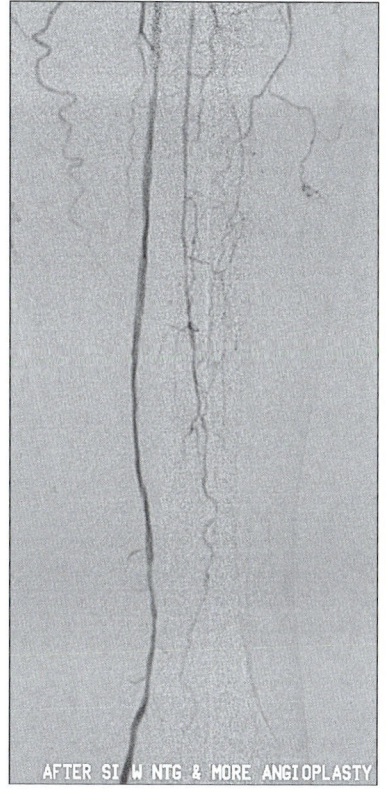

Figure 4. Arteriography after recanalization shows in-line flow through the posterior tibial artery to the foot. There is a marked reduction in arterial collaterals in the left lower leg.

Case 23

DEMOGRAPHICS/CLINICAL HISTORY

A 46-year-old woman with right toe ulceration.

DISCUSSION

History/Indications for Procedure
A 46-year-old woman with a history of type I diabetes and right toe ulcer that has not healed with conservative management.

Procedure
Percutaneous atherectomy for anterior tibial artery stenosis

Pre-procedure Imaging
Right lower extremity ankel-brachial indices were artificially elevated as the result of vessel calcification. No flow could be detected in the right great toe by means of arterial ultrasound.

Intraprocedural Findings
There is an aberrant origin of the right anterior tibial artery (Fig. 1); the anterior tibial artery is the dominant run-off vessel and has a focal, high-grade stenosis (Fig. 2). The stenosis was crossed with a 0.014-in guidewire, and the lesion was treated using the 1.5-mm Diamondback (CSI, Minneapolis, MN) atherectomy catheter.

Follow-up and Complications
After atherectomy, there was minimal residual narrowing at the site of the stenosis and no evidence for dissection or distal embolization (Fig. 3).

Suggested Readings

Sarac TP, Altinel O, Bannazadeh M, et al: Midterm outcome predictors for lower extremity atherectomy procedures. J Vasc Surg 48:885–890, 2008.

Shrikhande GV, McKinsey JF: Use and abuse of atherectomy: Where should it be used?. Semin Vasc Surg 21:204–209, 2008.

Zeller T, Rastan A, Schwarzwalder U, et al: Midterm results after atherectomy-assisted angioplasty of below-knee arteries with use of the Silverhawk device. J Vasc Interv Radiol 15:1391–1397, 2004.

Case 23   47

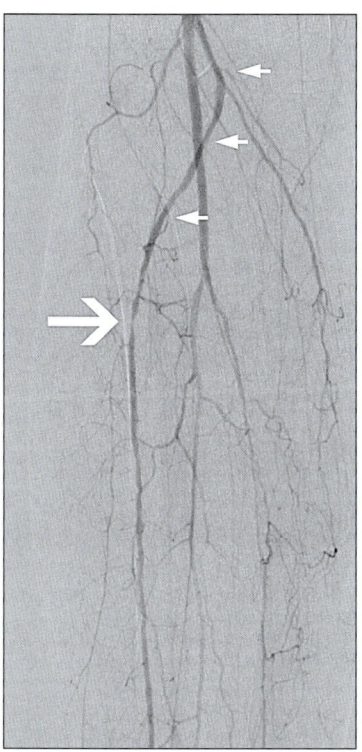

Figure 1. Right lower extremity arteriogram shows an anomalous origin of the anterior tibial artery *(short arrows)*. There is a focal, high-grade stenosis of the proximal anterior tibial artery *(large arrow)*.

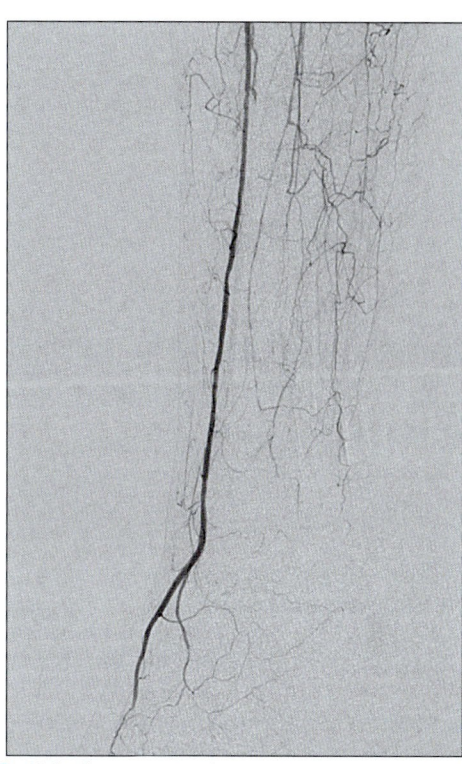

Figure 2. Right lower extremity arteriogram at the level of the ankle shows that the anterior tibial artery is the dominant run-off vessel. There is evidence for diffuse small vessel disease within the foot.

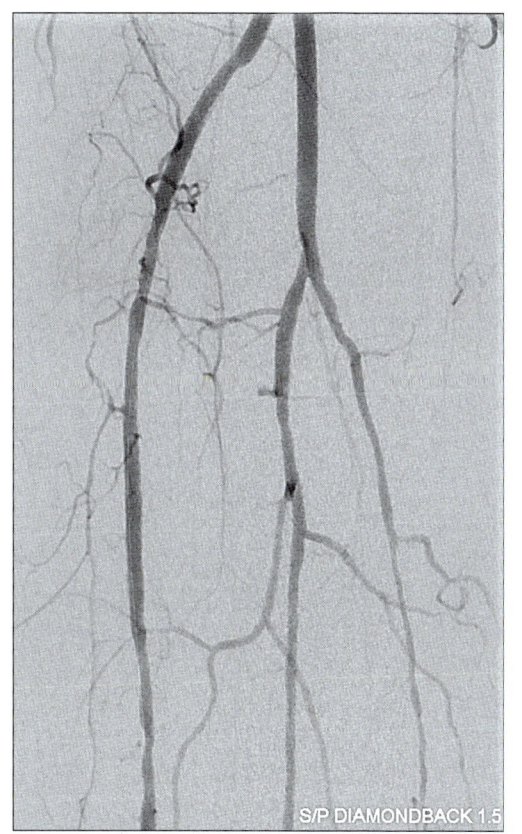

Figure 3. Follow-up arteriogram after atherectomy. There is only minimal residual narrowing at the atherectomy site.

Case 24

DEMOGRAPHICS/CLINICAL HISTORY

A 66-year-old woman with acute, right lower extremity ischemia, undergoing arteriography.

DISCUSSION

History/Indications for Procedure

A 66-year-old woman had an acutely ischemic right lower extremity. She underwent arteriography, performed with right common femoral access 5 days before presentation, and at the conclusion of this procedure, the arteriotomy was closed with an Angio-Seal (St. Jude Medical, St. Paul, MN) closure device.

Procedure

Complication with arterial closure device

Pre-procedure Imaging

Angiography of the right common femoral artery, which was performed through the sheath before placement of an Angio-Seal closure device, shows a stenosis of the distal right common femoral artery (Fig. 1). The right common femoral artery is 6 mm in diameter.

Intraprocedural Findings

Arteriography of the right lower extremity shows a large filling defect in the right common femoral artery (Fig. 2). There is no evidence for distal embolization.

Follow-up and Complications

The common femoral artery was explored surgically, and the collagen plug was found to be intraluminal. The obstruction was removed, and the patient has had no further complications.

Suggested Readings

Carey D, Martin JR, Moore CA, et al: Complications of femoral artery closure devices. Catheter Cardiolvasc Interv 52:3-7, 2001.

Koreny M, Riedmuller E, Nikfarjam M, et al: Arterial puncture closing devices compared with standard manual compression after cardiac catheterization: Systemic review and meta-analysis. JAMA 291:350-357, 2004.

Nikolsky E, Mehran R, Halkin A, et al: Vascular complications associated with arteriotomy closure devices in patients undergoing percutaneous coronary procedures: A meta-analysis. J Am Coll Cardiol 44:1200-1209, 2004.

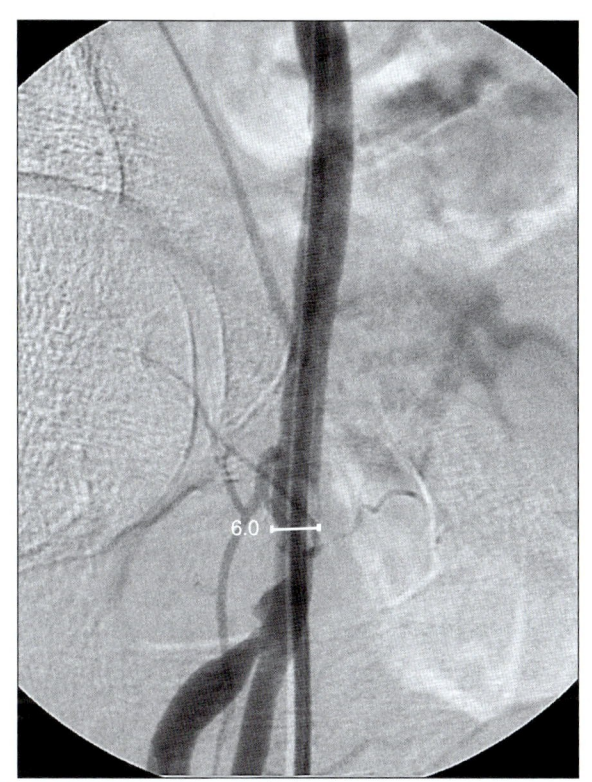

Figure 1. Arteriography of the right common femoral artery was performed through the sheath before placement of the closure device. There is a plaque in the region of the puncture site, and the artery diameter is 6 mm.

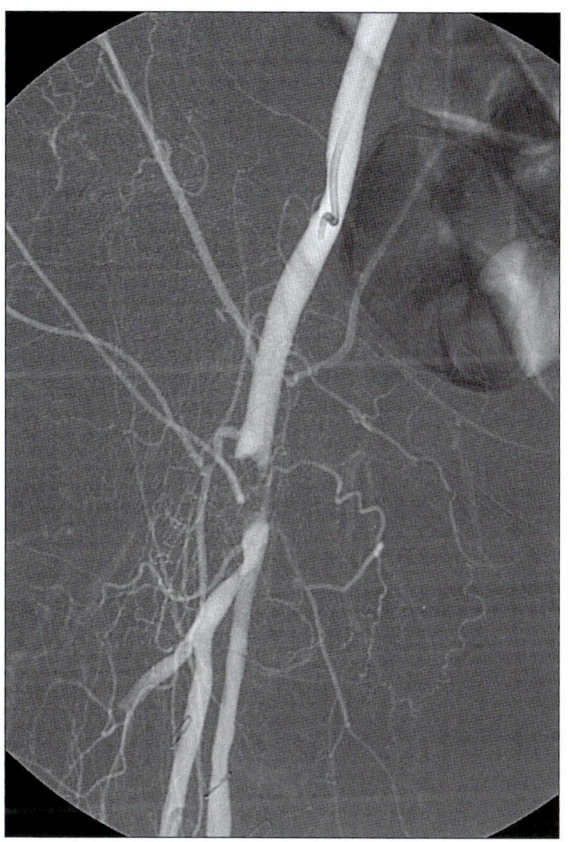

Figure 2. Arteriography of the right lower extremity, performed from a left femoral access site, shows a large filling defect in the right common femoral artery. During surgery, this filling defect was found to be the closure device, which was intraluminal.

Case 25

DEMOGRAPHICS/CLINICAL HISTORY

A 57-year-old man with claudication after diagnostic arteriogram.

DISCUSSION

History/Indications for Procedure
A 57-year-old man presents with right lower extremity claudication 3 days after undergoing a diagnostic hepatic arteriogram. The pain occurs after walking 200 to 300 feet and is relieved by 2 to 3 minutes of rest.

Procedure
Complication with arterial closure device

Pre-procedure Imaging
Arterial ultrasound shows elevated velocity in the right common femoral artery with post-stenotic turbulence. CT angiogram of the right lower extremity shows a focal, short-segment, linear filling defect in the right common femoral artery (Figs. 1 and 2).

Intraprocedural Findings
The patient was taken to the operating room for operative repair. A focal dissection of the common femoral artery was identified (Figs. 3 and 4) and repaired by endarterectomy and patch angioplasty.

Follow-up and Complications
The patient was discharged the following day and was able to ambulate without claudication.

Suggested Readings
Koreny M, Riedmuller E, Nikfardjam M, et al: Arterial puncture closing devices compared with standard manual compression after cardiac catheterization: Systematic review and meta-analysis. JAMA 29:350–357, 2004.

Sanborn TA, Gibbs HH, Brinker JA, et al: A multicenter randomized trail comparing a percutaneous collagen hemostasis device with conventional manual compression after diagnostic angiography and angioplasty. J Invasive Cardiol 11 Suppl B:6B–13B, 1999.

Upponi SS, Ganeshan AG, Warakaulle DR, et al: Angioseal versus manual compression for haemostasis following peripheral vascular diagnostic and interventional procedures: A randomized controlled trial. Eur J Radiol 61:332–334, 2007.

Case 25   51

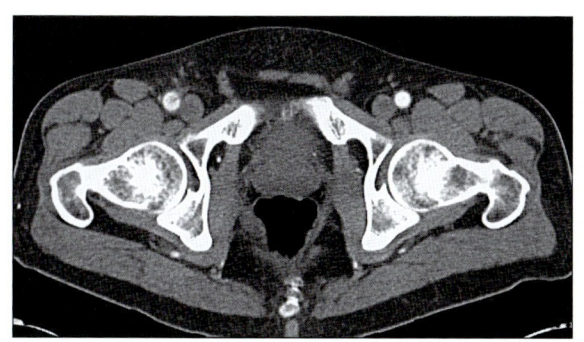

Figure 1. Axial image from CT angiogram shows a linear filling defect in the right common femoral artery.

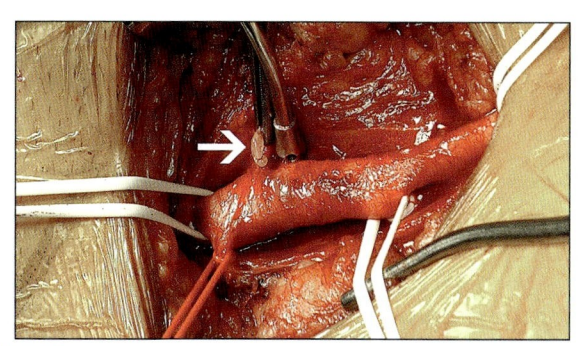

Figure 3. At surgery, the angioseal anchor is found to be located just external to the artery *(arrow)*.

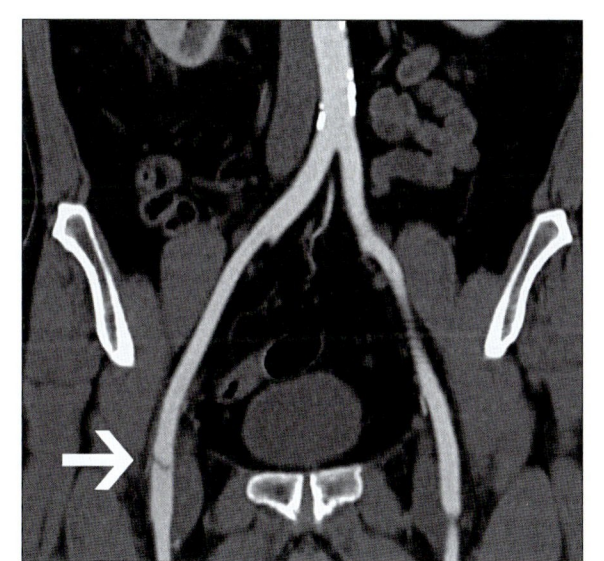

Figure 2. Coronal reconstruction from CT angiogram shows a linear filling defect in the right common femoral artery. The appearance suggests a common femoral artery dissection *(arrow*—collagen footplate of angioseal found just outside the lumen of the artery).

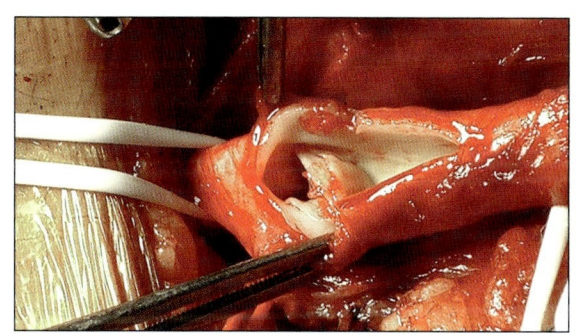

Figure 4. After opening the common femoral artery, a dissection flap is identified, confirming the findings on CT.

Case 26

DEMOGRAPHICS/CLINICAL HISTORY

A 65-year-old man, with right flank pain and decreased urine output, undergoing CT angiography.

DISCUSSION

History/Indications for Procedure
Symptomatic renal artery occlusion in this patient was diagnosed on CT angiography.

Procedure
Renal artery thrombosis

Pre-procedure Imaging
CT angiography shows thrombus within the right renal artery with decreased perfusion of the right kidney (Fig. 1).

Intraprocedural Findings
Angiography shows acute thrombus occluding the right renal artery. After thrombolysis, a high-grade stenosis at the renal artery was uncovered as the causative lesion (Figs. 2-4).

Follow-up and Complications
The patient was discharged home on aspirin and clopidogrel.

Suggested Readings
Bokhari SW, Faxon DP: Current advances in the diagnosis and treatment of renal artery stenosis. Rev Cardiovasc Med 5:204-215, 2004.

Gluck G, Croitoru M, Deleanu D, et al: Local thrombolytic treatment for renal arterial embolism. Eur Urol 38:339-343, 2000.

Leertouwer TC, Gussenhoven EJ, Bosch JL, et al: Stent placement for renal artery stenosis: Where do we stand? A meta-analysis. Radiology 216:78-85, 2000.

Nakayama T, Okaneva T, Kinebuchi Y, et al: Thrombolytic therapy for traumatic unilateral renal artery thrombosis. Int J Urol 13:168-170, 2006.

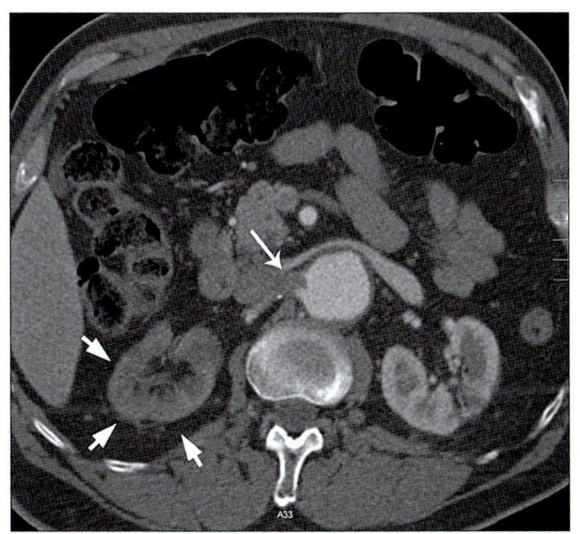

Figure 1. CT shows thrombus in the right main renal artery *(long arrow)*. Note the diminished perfusion of the right kidney *(short arrows)*.

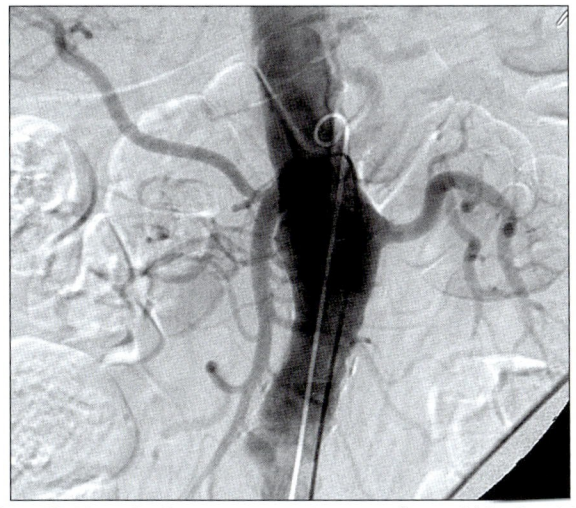

Figure 2. Nonselective aortogram shows no flow within the right renal artery.

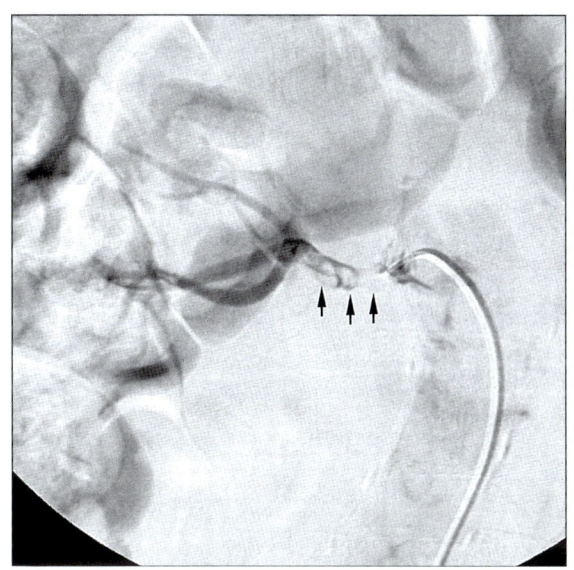

Figure 3. Selective injection of the right renal artery shows acute thrombus in the main renal artery *(arrowheads)*.

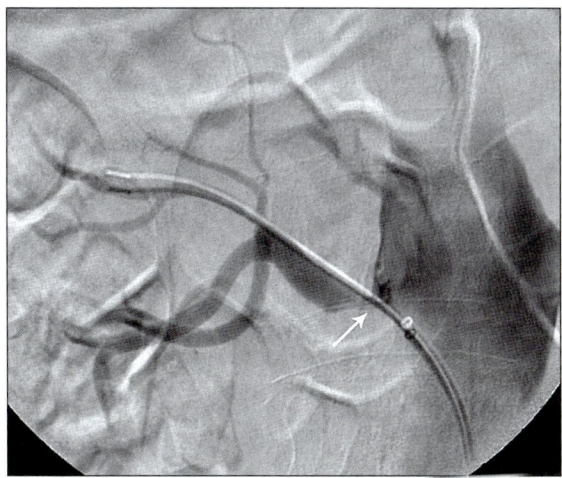

Figure 4. After a pulse-spray of 2 mg of tissue plasminogen activator, the thrombus has resolved, and a high-grade ostial stenosis is identified *(arrow)*. This lesion was treated by placement of a balloon expandable stent (not shown).

Case 27

DEMOGRAPHICS/CLINICAL HISTORY

A 43-year-old man with left renal injury after an assault with a blunt weapon, undergoing CT and arteriography.

DISCUSSION

History/Indications for Procedure
A 43-year-old man presents with a left renal artery injury sustained during an assault with a blunt weapon.

Procedure
Management of acute post-traumatic renal ischemia

Pre-procedure Imaging
A contrast-enhanced CT scan of the abdomen shows poor enhancement of the left kidney, most likely because of a vascular pedicle injury (Fig. 1). There is no active contrast extravasation or evidence of renal parenchymal injury.

Intraprocedural Findings
Abdominal aortogram shows the presence of two left renal arteries, each occluded near its origin. Each renal artery was selectively catheterized (Fig. 2), the guidewire carefully advanced beyond the level of injury, and noncovered balloon expandable stents were deployed (Fig. 3).

Follow-up and Complications
The procedure was complicated by the development of acute thrombus in the lower left renal artery; the thrombus was successfully treated with intra-arterial administration of 4 mg of tissue plasminogen activator. A CT scan of the abdomen performed 2 days after stent placement shows improved perfusion to the left kidney (Fig. 4).

Suggested Readings

Lee JT, White RA: Endovascular management of blunt traumatic renal artery dissection. J Endovasc Ther 9:354, 2002.

Lupattelli T, Basile A, Iozzelli A, et al: Thrombolytic therapy followed by stenting for renal artery dissection secondary to blunt trauma. Emerg Radiol 11:164, 2005.

Memon S, Cheung BY: Long-term results of blunt traumatic renal artery dissection treated by endovascular stenting. Cardiovasc Intervent Radiol 28:668, 2005.

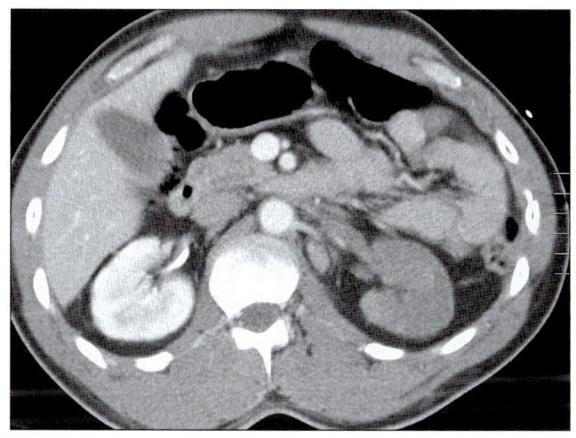

Figure 1. Contrast-enhanced CT scan through kidneys shows markedly diminished enhancement of left kidney consistent with renal pedicle injury. There is no free fluid or evidence of renal parenchymal injury.

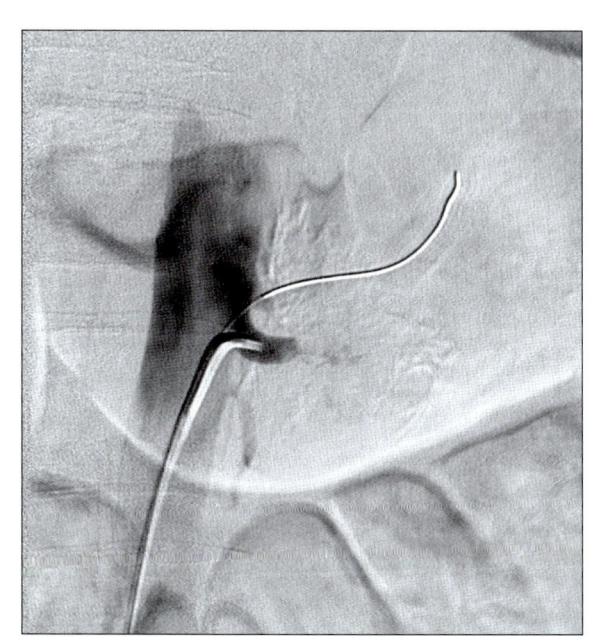

Figure 2. Selective injection of origin of inferior left renal artery. Inferior left renal artery is occluded at its origin. A guidewire already has been inserted across site of injury in the superior left renal artery.

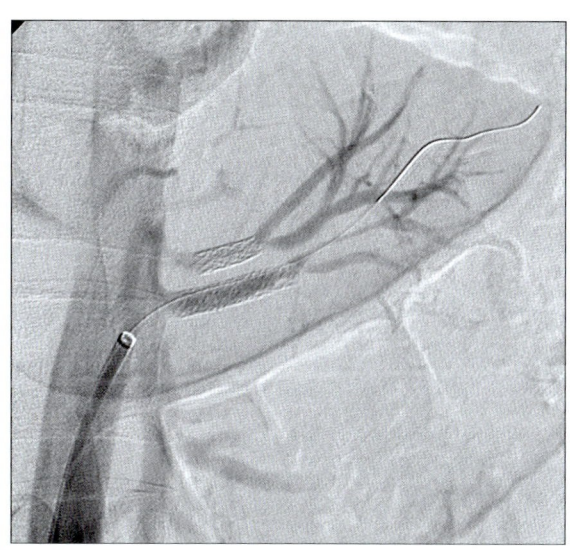

Figure 3. Follow-up arteriogram after stent placement shows reperfusion of left kidney. No extravasation or pseudoaneurysm is seen.

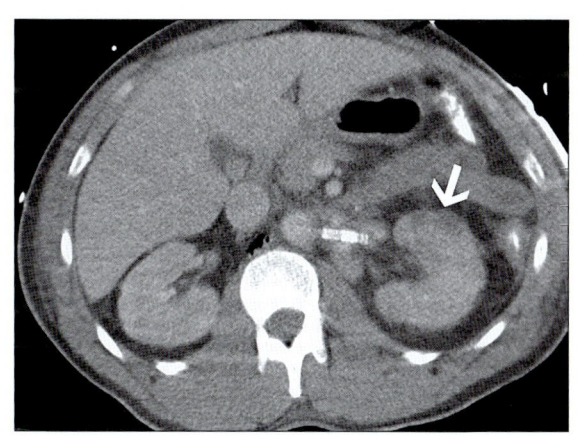

Figure 4. Contrast-enhanced CT scan performed 2 days after renal artery stenting shows two overlapping stents in inferior left renal artery. There is only slightly diminished perfusion of left kidney. An area of hypoperfusion is consistent with small infarct (*arrow*).

Case 28

DEMOGRAPHICS/CLINICAL HISTORY

A 41-year-old man, with long-standing hypertension, undergoing renal arteriography.

DISCUSSION

History/Indications for Procedure

A 41-year-old man with malignant hypertension has experienced daily headaches for the previous 5 years. His blood pressure measurements are usually around 200/130 mm Hg, and he takes three antihypertensive medications.

Procedure

Renal artery stenting

Pre-procedure Imaging

Outside MRI reported bilateral renal artery stenoses (not shown).

Intraprocedural Findings

A renal arteriogram shows a high-grade stenosis at the origin of the left renal artery (Figs. 1 and 2). This was treated with a balloon expandable stent (Fig. 3).

Follow-up and Complications

The patient's blood pressure decreased into normal range immediately after stent placement. The blood pressure remained normal overnight, despite withholding all antihypertensive medications.

Suggested Readings

De Bruyne B, Manoharan G, Pijls NH, et al: Assessment of renal artery stenosis severity by pressure gradient measurements. J Am Coll Cardiol 48:1851-1855, 2006.

Leertouwer TC, Gussenhoven EJ, Bosch JL, et al: Stent placement for renal arterial stenosis: Where do we stand? A meta-analysis. Radiology 216:78-85, 2000.

Plouin PF, Chatellier G, Darne B, et al: Blood pressure outcome of angioplasty in atherosclerotic renal artery stenosis: A randomized trial. Essai Multicentrique Medicaments vs Angioplastie (EMMA) Study Group. Hypertension 31:823-829, 1998.

Van de Ven PJG, Kaatee R, Beutler JJ, et al: Arterial stenting and balloon angioplasty in ostial atherosclerotic renovascular disease: A randomised trial. Lancet 353:282-286, 1999.

van Jaarsveld BC, Krijnen P, Pieterman H, et al: The effect of balloon angioplasty on hypertension in atherosclerotic renal-artery stenosis. Dutch Renal Artery Stenosis Intervention Cooperative Study Group. N Engl J Med 342:1007-1014, 2000.

Case 28   57

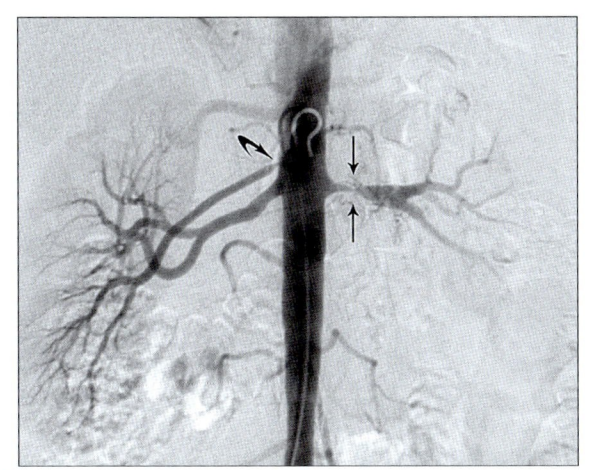

Figure 1. Aortogram shows a high-grade stenosis at the origin of the left renal artery *(straight arrows)*. There also is a stenosis involving an accessory right renal artery *(curved arrow)*.

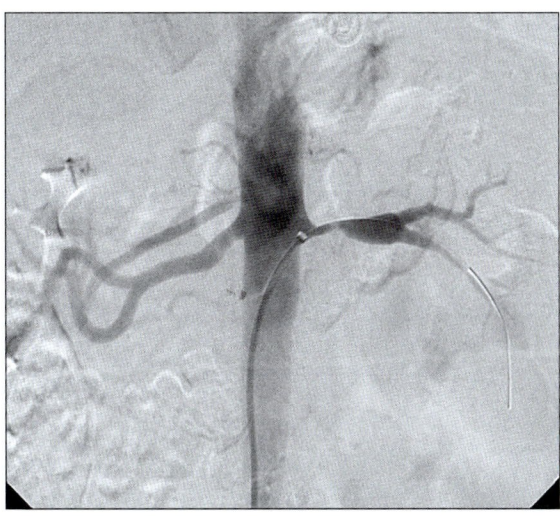

Figure 2. The lesion was crossed with a 0.014-inch wire and predilated with a 3-mm balloon.

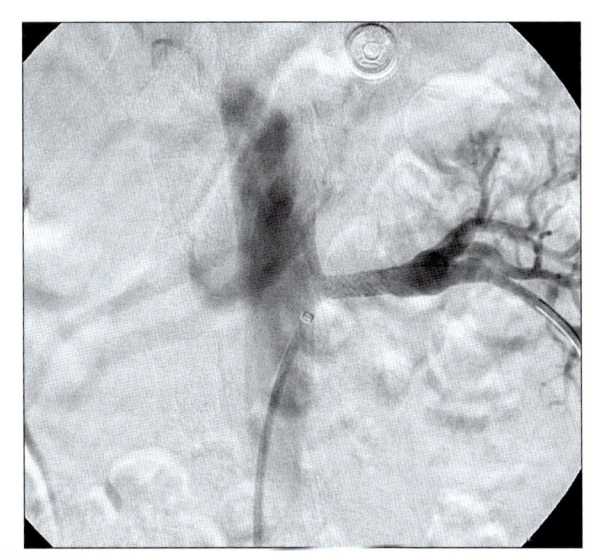

Figure 3. A 6-mm × 18-mm balloon expandable stent was deployed across the lesion

Case 29

DEMOGRAPHICS/CLINICAL HISTORY

A 49-year-old man with aortic dissection and severe hypertension, undergoing computed tomography (CT) angiography, arteriography, catheterization, and stent placement.

DISCUSSION

History/Indications for Procedure
A 49-year-old man had a 10-day history of chest pain caused by an acute type B aortic dissection. The patient has severe hypertension and was placed on intravenous esmolol and Nipride for control.

Procedure
Renal artery stenting in the presence of aortic dissection

Pre-procedure Imaging
CT angiogram demonstrates a type B aortic dissection extending from just distal to the origin of the left subclavian artery to the left common iliac artery. The dissection flap extends into the left renal artery, with decreased enhancement of the left kidney (Fig. 1).

Intraprocedural Findings
The true lumen of the aorta was catheterized, and the left renal arteriogram demonstrates severe narrowing of the proximal left renal artery (Fig. 2). The true lumen of the left renal artery was catheterized (Fig. 3), and a 6-mm × 15-mm, balloon-expandable stent was deployed across the origin of the left renal artery (Fig. 4).

Follow-up and Complications
After the stent placement, the patient was transitioned to oral antihypertensive medications. He eventually underwent endograft placement for aneurysmal aortic enlargement resulting from the aortic dissection.

Suggested Readings
Gaxotte V, Cocheteux B, Haulon S, et al: Relationship of intimal flap to endovascular treatment of malperfusion syndromes in aortic dissection. J Endovasc Ther 10:719-727, 2003.

Vedantham S, Picus D, Sanchez LA, et al: Percutaneous management of ischemic complications in patients with type-B aortic dissection. J Vasc Interv Radiol 14:181-194, 2003.

Slonim SM, Nyman U, Semba CP, et al: Aortic dissection: Percutaneous management of ischemic complications with endovascular stents and balloon fenestration. J Vasc Surg 23:241-253, 1996.

Case 29   59

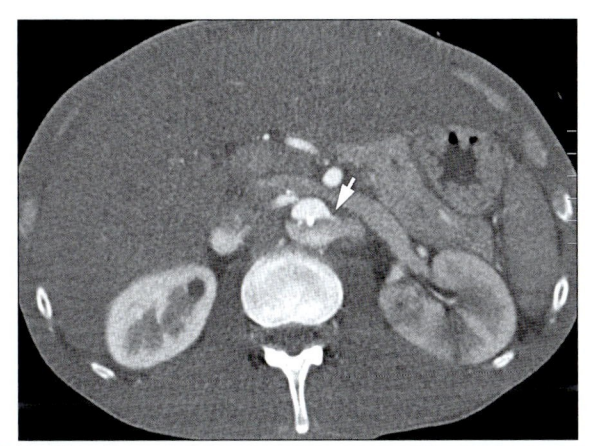

Figure 1. Axial image from the CT angiogram at the level of the left renal artery demonstrates the dissection flap extending into the left renal artery *(arrow)*. There is decreased perfusion of the left kidney.

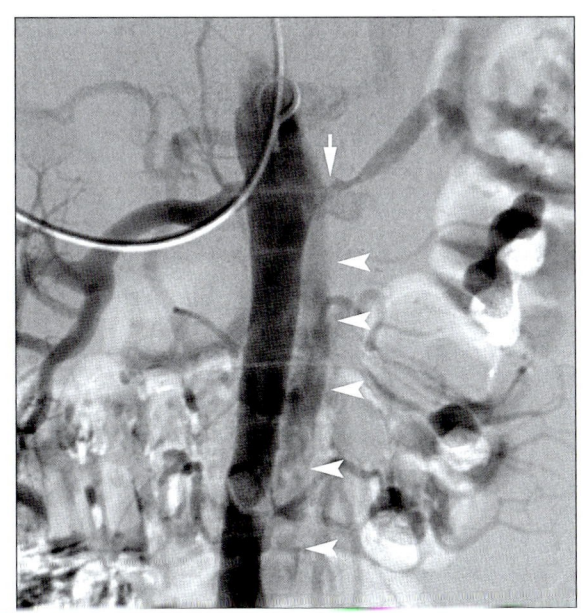

Figure 2. Abdominal aortogram with the catheter in the true lumen demonstrates narrowing of the proximal left renal artery *(arrow)*. There is faint filling of the false lumen of the aorta *(arrowheads)*.

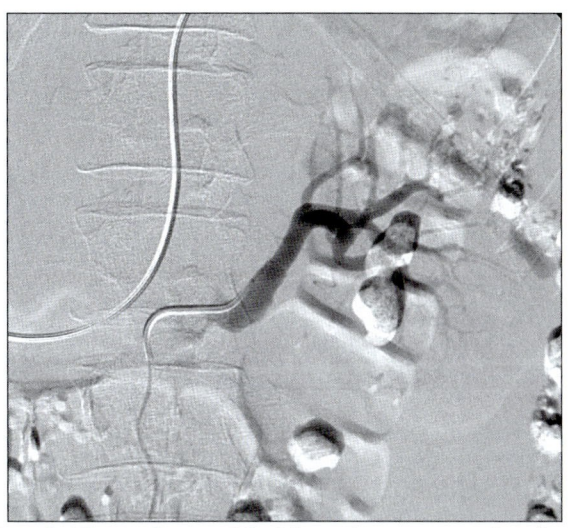

Figure 3. The true lumen of the left renal artery was catheterized.

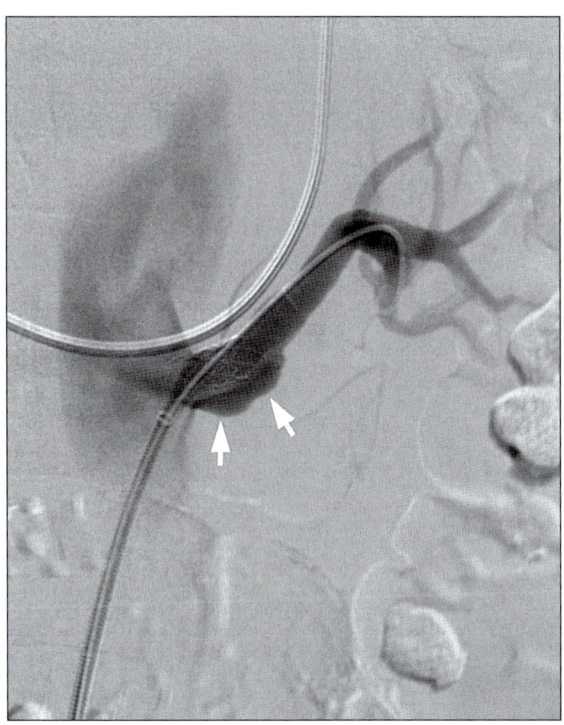

Figure 4. A balloon-expandable stent has been placed, and there is significantly improved perfusion to the left kidney. Notice the continued filling of the false lumen of the left renal artery *(arrows)*.

Case 30

DEMOGRAPHICS/CLINICAL HISTORY

A 29-year-old woman with a 5-year history of hypertension, undergoing angiography.

DISCUSSION

History/Indications for Procedure
This patient presented with uncontrolled hypertension, despite taking three antihypertensive medications.

Procedure
Renal artery angioplasty

Pre-procedure Imaging
Renal ultrasound was performed and showed the kidneys to be symmetric in size (not shown).

Intraprocedural Findings
Irregular beading of the right main renal artery and right upper pole segmental branch indicates fibromuscular dysplasia at these locations (Fig. 1). Both vessels were treated with balloon angioplasty (Figs. 2 and 3).

Follow-up and Complications
One month after percutaneous transluminal angioplasty, the patient's blood pressure was controlled, although she still was taking three antihypertensive medications.

Suggested Readings

Alhadad A, Mattiasson I, Ivancev K, et al: Revascularisation of renal artery stenosis caused by fibromuscular dysplasia: Effects of blood pressure during 7-year follow-up are influenced by duration of hypertension and branch artery stenosis. J Hum Hypertens 19:761-767, 2005.

Mahmud E, Brocato M, Palakodeti V, et al: Fibromuscular dysplasia of renal arteries: Percutaneous revascularization based on hemodynamic assessment with a pressure measurement guidewire. Catheter Cardiovasc Interv 67:434-437, 2006.

Surowiec SM, Sivamurthy N, Rhodes JM, et al: Percutaneous therapy for renal artery fibromuscular dysplasia. Ann Vasc Surg 17:650-655, 2003.

Case 30   61

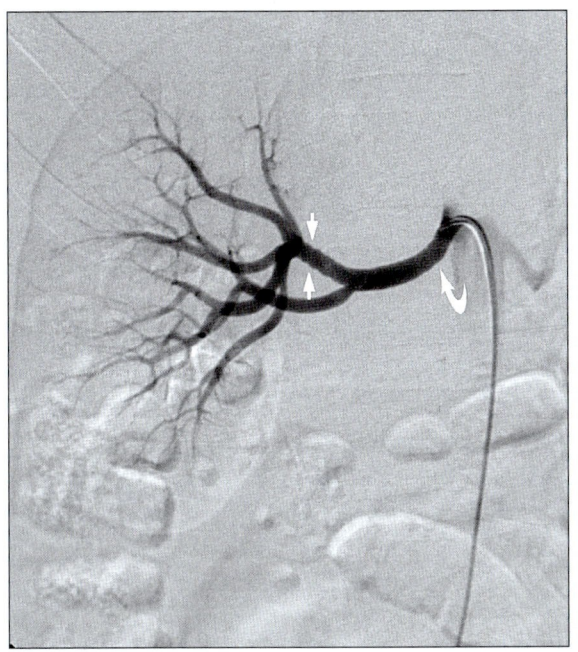

Figure 1. Selective renal arteriogram shows irregular beading of the main renal artery *(curved arrow)* and upper pole segmental branch *(arrows)*. These findings are consistent with fibromuscular dysplasia.

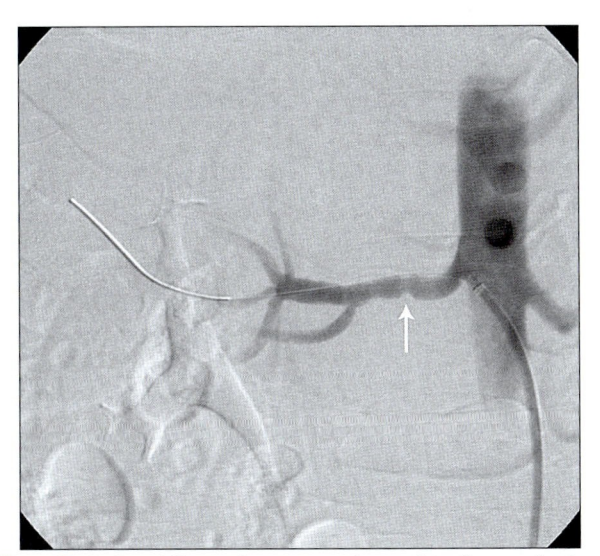

Figure 2. A 6F guiding catheter was advanced to the renal artery origin. A 0.014 inch guidewire was placed across the involved segments. After guidewire placement, the stenosis in the main renal artery is accentuated *(arrow)*.

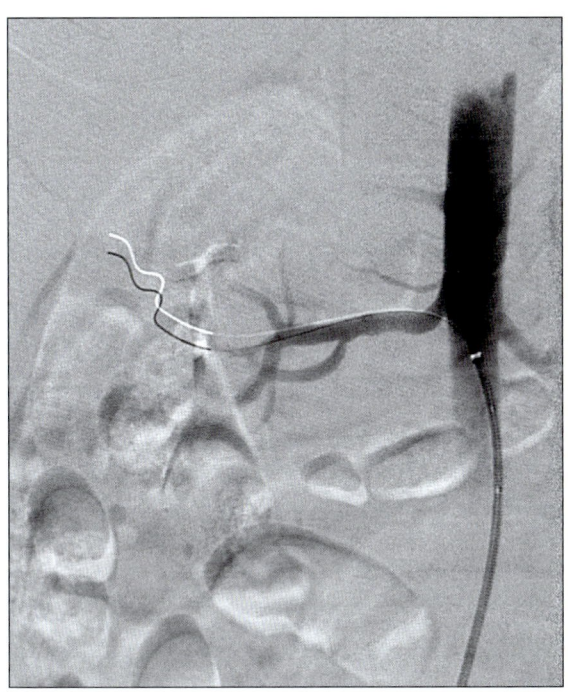

Figure 3. There is an excellent angiographic result after angioplasty.

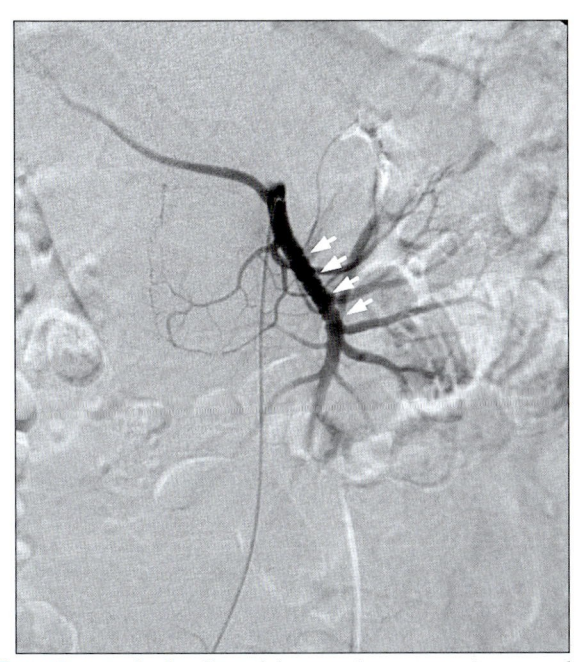

Figure 4. Irregular beading of the superior mesenteric artery also is present *(arrowheads)* indicating fibromuscular dysplasia of the superior mesenteric artery as well.

Case 31

DEMOGRAPHICS/CLINICAL HISTORY

A 60-year-old woman who has decreased urine output after renal transplantation, undergoing ultrasonography and arteriography.

DISCUSSION

History/Indications for Procedure
A 60-year-old who underwent renal transplantation 2 months earlier has decreased urine output.

Procedure
Angioplasty for renal artery stenosis

Pre-procedure Imaging
Doppler ultrasound showed a tardus parvus waveform in the main renal artery.

Intraprocedural Findings
There is a high-grade stenosis at the anastomosis between the transplanted renal artery and the external iliac artery, and there is irregularity of the main renal artery, consistent with fibromuscular dysplasia (FMD) (Figs. 1 and 2). Angioplasty with a 6-mm balloon was performed at the stenosis at the anastomosis and the segment affected by FMD (Fig. 3).

Follow-up and Complications
Angiography after balloon angioplasty shows no residual stenosis at the surgical anastomosis (Fig. 4). The patient's urine output and renal function improved on follow-up, and she has required no further intervention in the 2 years since the angioplasty.

Suggested Readings

Beecroft JR, Rajan DK, Clark TW, et al: Transplant renal artery stenosis: Outcome after percutaneous intervention. J Vasc Interv Radiol 15:1407-1413, 2004.

Pappas P, Zavos G, Kaza S, et al: Angioplasty and stenting of arterial stenosis affecting renal transplant function. Transplant Proc 40:1391-1396, 2008.

Ruggenenti P, Mosconi L, Bruno S, et al: Post-transplant renal artery stenosis: The hemodynamic response to revascularization. Kidney Int 60:309-318, 2001.

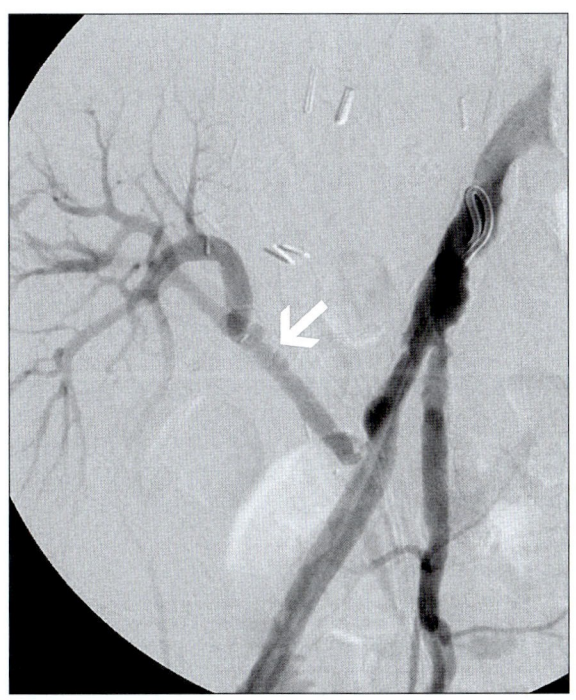

Figure 1. A right iliac arteriogram performed from an ipsilateral approach with the catheter in the right common iliac artery shows a high-grade stenosis at the surgical anastomosis between the right external iliac artery and main renal artery of the transplanted kidney. The beaded appearance of the distal main renal artery is consistent with FMD *(arrow)*.

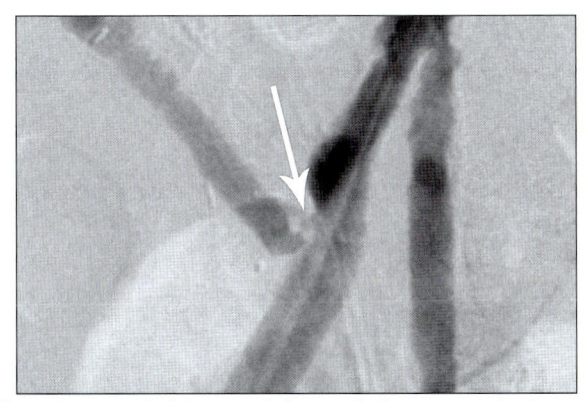

Figure 2. Magnified image of the surgical anastomosis shows a high-grade stenosis between the main renal artery and the external iliac artery *(arrow)*.

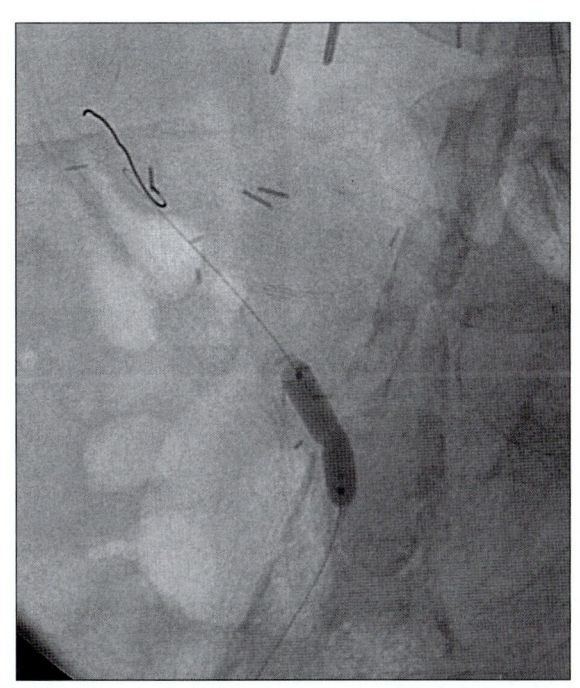

Figure 3. The surgical anastomosis is treated with balloon angioplasty.

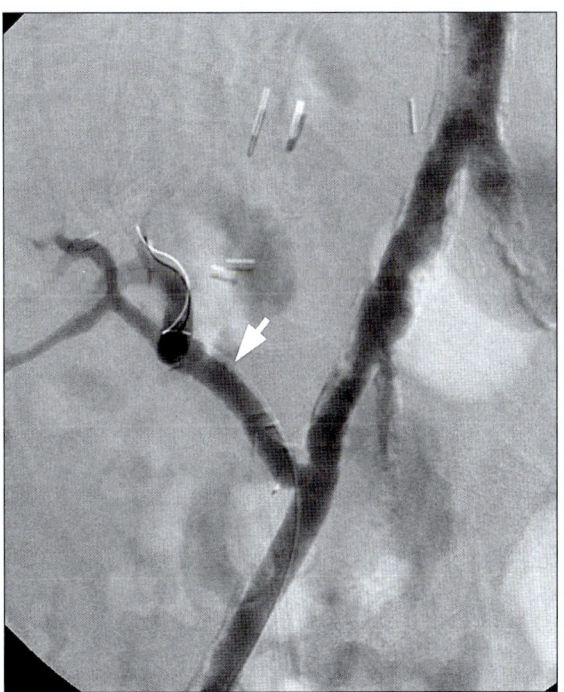

Figure 4. Arteriography after balloon angioplasty shows no residual stenosis at the surgical anastomosis and less irregularity at the site of FMD *(arrow)*.

Case 32

DEMOGRAPHICS/CLINICAL HISTORY

A 13-year-old girl with hypertension.

DISCUSSION

History/Indications for Procedure
A 13-year-old girl with hypertension diagnosed during a routine physical exam. Before starting medication, her blood pressure measured 150/120 mm Hg.

Procedure
Renal angioplasty in a pediatric patient with hypertension

Pre-procedure Imaging
MR angiogram shows a stenosis of the proximal left renal artery (Fig. 1).

Intraprocedural Findings
Renal arteriogram shows a high-grade stenosis of the proximal left renal artery and intersegmental and arcuate artery occlusions in the interpolar region of the left kidney, consistent with fibromuscular dysplasia (Fig. 2). The stenosis was crossed with a 0.014-inch guidewire; the stenosis was dilated using a 4-mm balloon.

Follow-up and Complications
Follow-up arteriogram after balloon angioplasty shows minimal residual stenosis (Fig. 3). The patient's blood pressure returned to normal after the procedure and has remained under control during follow-up.

Suggested Readings
Hughes RJ, Scoble JE, Reidy JF: Renal angioplasty in non-atheromatous renal artery stenosis: Technical results and clinical outcome in 43 patients. Cardiovasc Intervent Radiol 27:435-440, 2004.

McLaren CA, Roebuck DJ: Interventional radiology for renovascular hypertension in children. Tech Vasc Interv Radiol 6:150-157, 2003.

Tullus K, Brennan E, Hamilton G, et al: Renovascular hypertension in children. Lancet 371(9622):1453-1463, 2008.

Tyagi S, Kaul UA, Satsangi DK, et al: Percutaneous transluminal angioplasty for renovascular hypertension in children: Initial and long-term results. Pediatrics 99:44-49, 1997.

Case 32   65

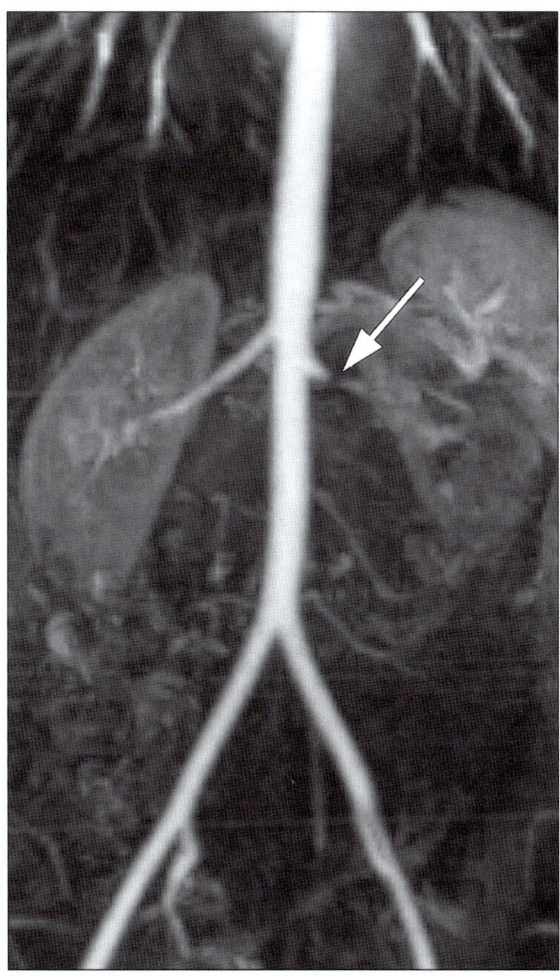

Figure 1. Coronal 3-D reconstruction from MR angiogram shows a focal stenosis of the proximal left renal artery *(arrow)*.

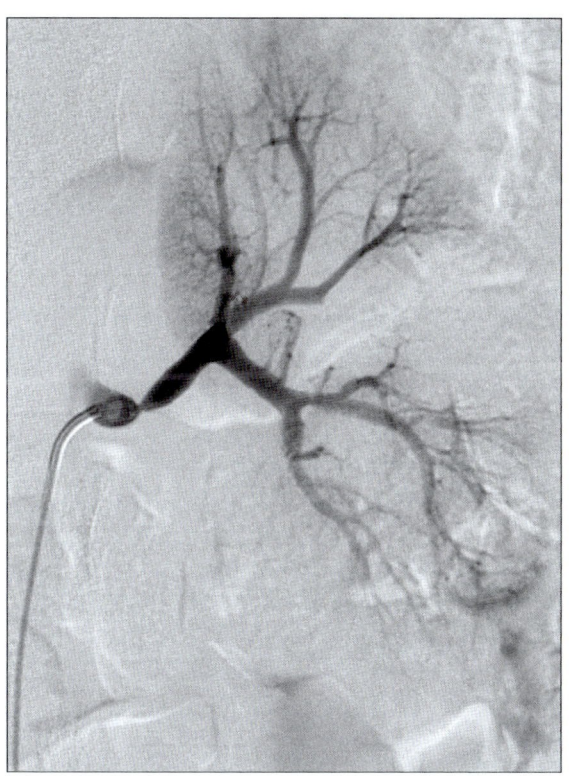

Figure 2. Left renal arteriogram. There is a focal, high-grade stenosis of the proximal left renal artery. In addition, there is occlusion of multiple intersegmental and arcuate arteries within the interpolar region of the left kidney.

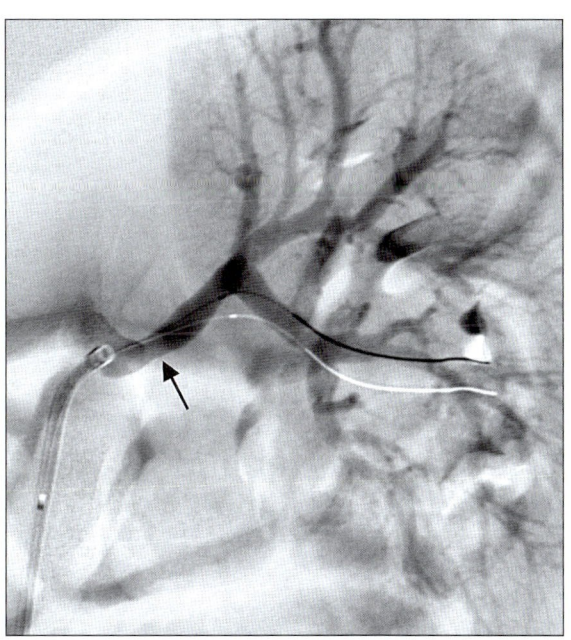

Figure 3. Follow-up arteriogram after balloon angioplasty. There is only mild residual stenosis of the main left renal artery *(arrow)*.

Case 33

DEMOGRAPHICS/CLINICAL HISTORY

A 15-year-old girl with Williams syndrome and hypertension.

DISCUSSION

History/Indications for Procedure
A 15-year-old girl with Williams syndrome presents with hypercalcemia and hypertension despite three-drug therapy.

Procedure
Management of renovascular hypertension in a patient with Williams syndrome

Intraprocedural Findings
Abdominal aortogram shows diffuse narrowing of the abdominal aorta and a focal stenosis of the proximal left renal artery (Figs. 1 and 2). The left renal artery was selectively catheterized and treated via the placement of a 6-mm balloon expandable stent (Fig. 3).

Follow-up and Complications
Follow-up renal arteriogram after stent placement shows minimal residual stenosis at the origin of the left renal artery and mild vasospasm of the main renal artery just distal to the stent (Fig. 4). The patient's hypertension was significantly improved following the procedure.

Suggested Readings
McLaren CA, Roebuck DJ: Interventional radiology for renovascular hypertension in children. Tech Vasc Interv 6:150–157, 2003.

Shroff R, Roebuck DJ, Gordon I, et al: Angioplasty for renovascular hypertension in children: 20-year experience. Pediatrics 118:268–275, 2006.

Tullus K, Brennan E, Hamilton G, et al: Renovascular hypertension in children. Lancet 371:1453–1463, 2008.

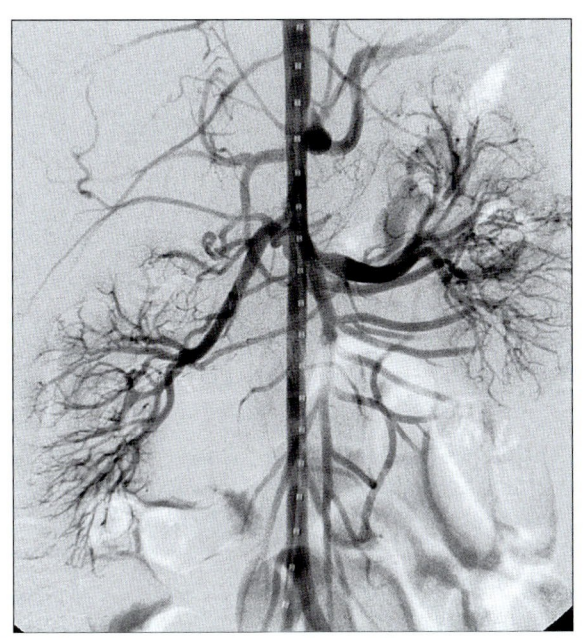

Figure 1. Abdominal aortogram shows diffuse narrowing of the abdominal aorta.

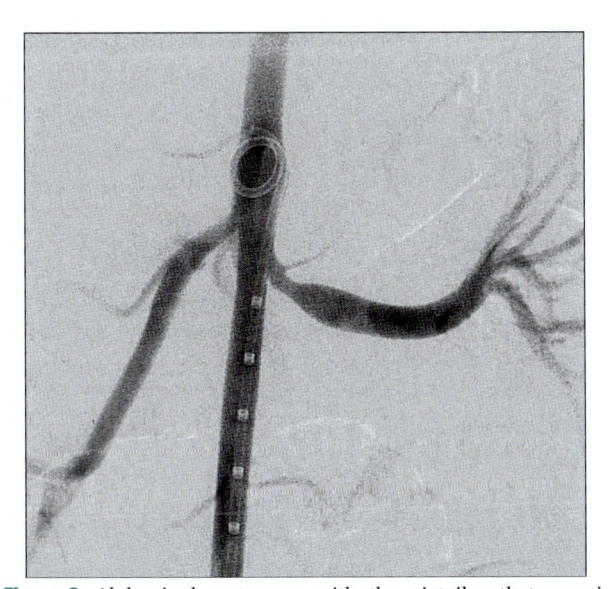

Figure 2. Abdominal aortogram with the pigtail catheter positioned below the origin of the superior mesenteric artery shows a focal stenosis of the left renal artery with post-stenotic dilatation. There is mild narrowing at the origin of the right renal artery.

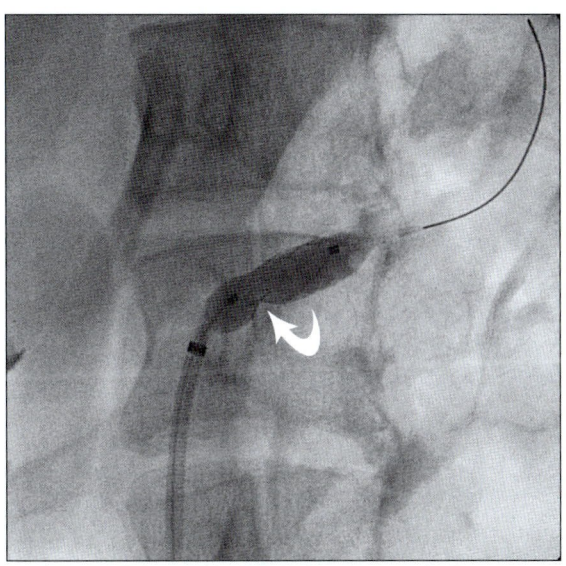

Figure 3. Spot fluoroscopic image during stent deployment. Note the waist in the balloon catheter *(arrow)*, which persisted despite high balloon inflation pressures.

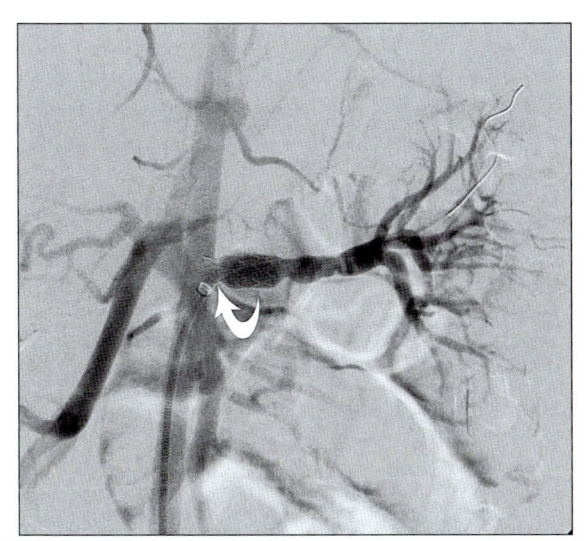

Figure 4. Final arteriogram after stent placement. There is improved blood flow to the left kidney. There is mild constriction of the proximal stent where the balloon could not be fully inflated *(curved arrow)*.

Case 34

DEMOGRAPHICS/CLINICAL HISTORY

An 81-year-old man with acute abdominal pain, undergoing computed tomography (CT) and angiography.

DISCUSSION

History/Indications for Procedure
An 81-year-old man with a history of atrial fibrillation presents with acute left lower quadrant pain.

Procedure
Percutaneous thrombectomy or thrombolysis of superior mesenteric artery embolus

Pre-procedure Imaging
Contrast-enhanced CT shows diffuse mucosal thickening of the ileum and ascending colon. There is an abrupt transition in caliber of the superior mesenteric artery (SMA) at the level of the ileal branches and an intraluminal filling defect (Fig. 1).

Intraprocedural Findings
Superior mesenteric angiogram shows abrupt occlusion of the proximal superior mesenteric artery with reconstitution of distal visceral branches (Figs. 2 and 3). The embolus was treated with the Angiojet (Psosis, Minneapolis, MN) thrombectomy catheter and a 4-hour infusion of thrombolytics.

Follow-up and Complications
The thrombus was successfully cleared from the SMA circulation (Fig. 4). The patient was discharged from the hospital 4 days after therapy with no further abdominal pain and was able to tolerate food.

Suggested Readings
Boyer L, Delorme JM, Alexandre M, et al: Local fibrinolysis for superior mesenteric artery thromboembolism. Cardiovasc Intervent Radiol 17:214-216, 1994.

Clark RA, Gallant TE: Acute mesenteric ischemia: Angiographic spectrum. AJR Am J Roentgenol 142:555-562, 1984.

Oldenburg WA, Lau LL, Rodenberg TJ, et al: Acute mesenteric ischemia: A clinical review. Arch Intern Med 164:1054-1062, 2004.

Simo G, Echenagusia AJ, Camúñez F, et al: Superior mesenteric arterial embolism: Local fibrinolytic treatment with urokinase. Radiology 204:775-779, 1997.

Yamaguchi T, Saeki M, Iwasaki Y, et al: Local thrombolytic therapy for superior mesenteric artery embolism: Complications and long-term clinical follow-up. Radiat Med 17:27-33, 1999.

Case 34   69

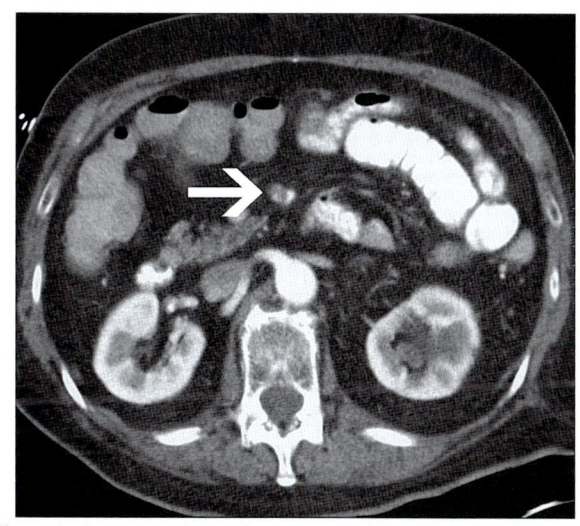

Figure 1. Contrast-enhanced CT shows a filling defect in the proximal SMA consistent with a thrombus or embolus *(arrow)*.

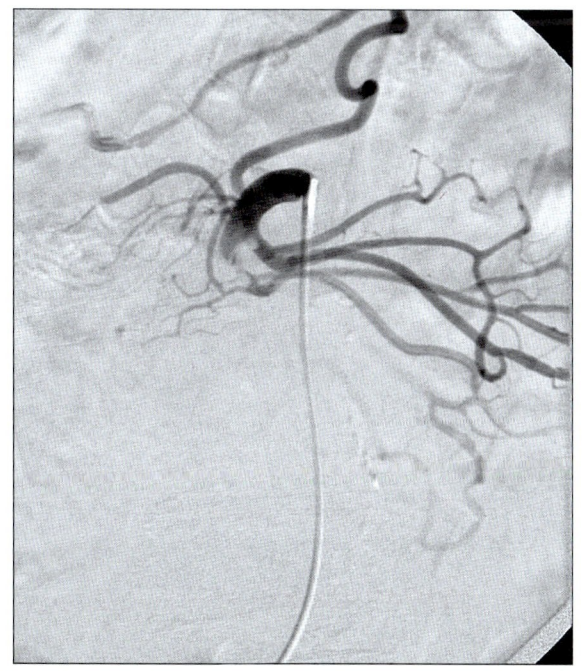

Figure 2. SMA arteriogram shows occlusion of the SMA just beyond the origin of several jejunal branches.

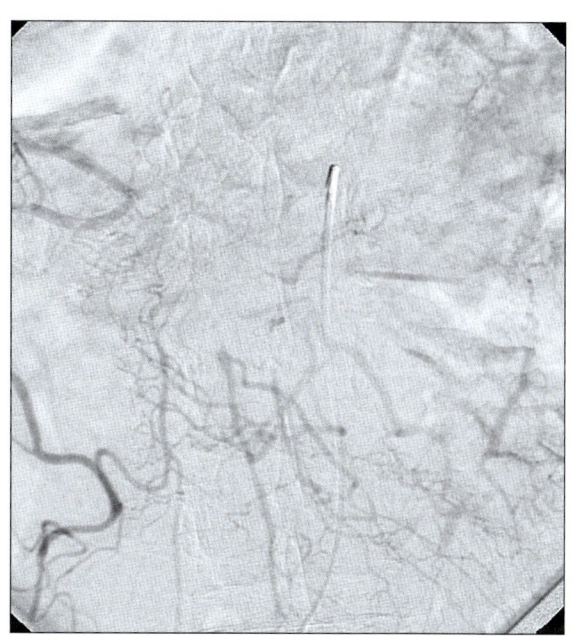

Figure 3. SMA artery injection shows delayed filling of the distal ileal and colic branches of the occluded SMA.

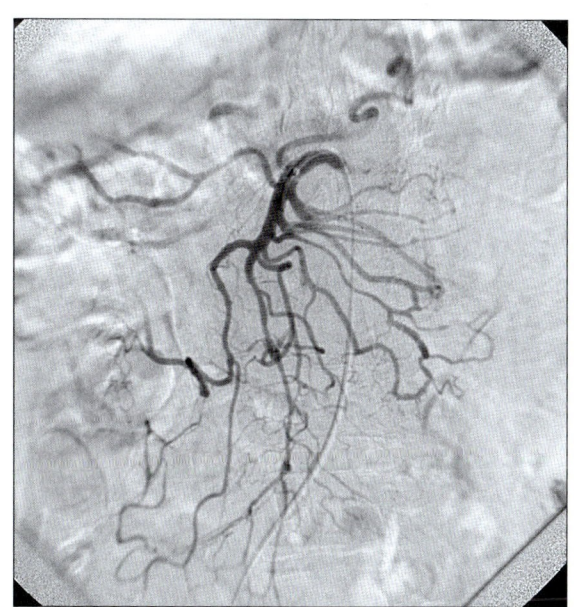

Figure 4. Follow-up SMA arteriogram after mechanical thrombectomy and thrombolytic administration shows restored perfusion through the SMA with improved flow to the ileum and right colon.

Case 35

DEMOGRAPHICS/CLINICAL HISTORY

An 80-year-old man with acute onset of abdominal pain and hemorrhagic diarrhea, undergoing computed tomography (CT) and angiography.

DISCUSSION

History/Indications for Procedure
An 80-year-old man had acute onset of abdominal pain and hemorrhagic diarrhea.

Procedure
Management of acute superior mesenteric artery embolus

Pre-procedure Imaging
Contrast-enhanced CT shows a focal, partially occlusive filling defect in the superior mesenteric artery (Fig. 1). The large and small bowels appeared normal.

Intraprocedural Findings
Visceral angiogram shows a partially occlusive thrombus in the middle of the superior mesenteric artery (SMA) (Figs. 2 and 3). Catheter-directed thrombolytic therapy with tissue plasminogen activator (tPA) was initiated.

Follow-up and Complications
Follow-up arteriogram after 24 hours of thrombolytic therapy shows partial resolution of the thrombus and improved perfusion to the distal branches of the SMA (Fig. 4), and the tPA was discontinued. The patient was asymptomatic and discharged from the hospital 2 days later on oral anticoagulation.

Suggested Readings
Brountzos EN, Critselis A, Magoulas D, et al: Emergency endovascular treatment of a superior mesenteric artery occlusion. Cardiovasc Intervent Radiol 24:57-60, 2001.
Clark RA, Gallant TE: Acute mesenteric ischemia: Angiographic spectrum. AJR Am J Roentgenol 142:555-562, 1984.
Oldenburg WA, Lau LL, Rodenberg TJ, et al: Acute mesenteric ischemia: A clinical review. Arch Intern Med 164:1054-1062, 2004.
Simó G, Echenagusia AJ, Camúñez F, et al: Superior mesenteric arterial embolism: Local fibrinolytic treatment with urokinase. Radiology 204:775-779, 1997.

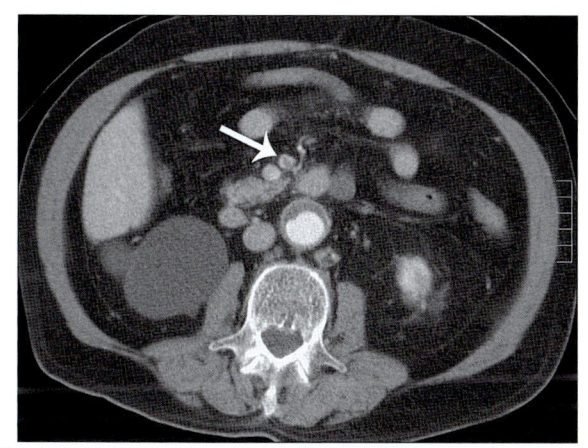

Figure 1. Contrast-enhanced CT shows a focal filling defect in the SMA (arrow).

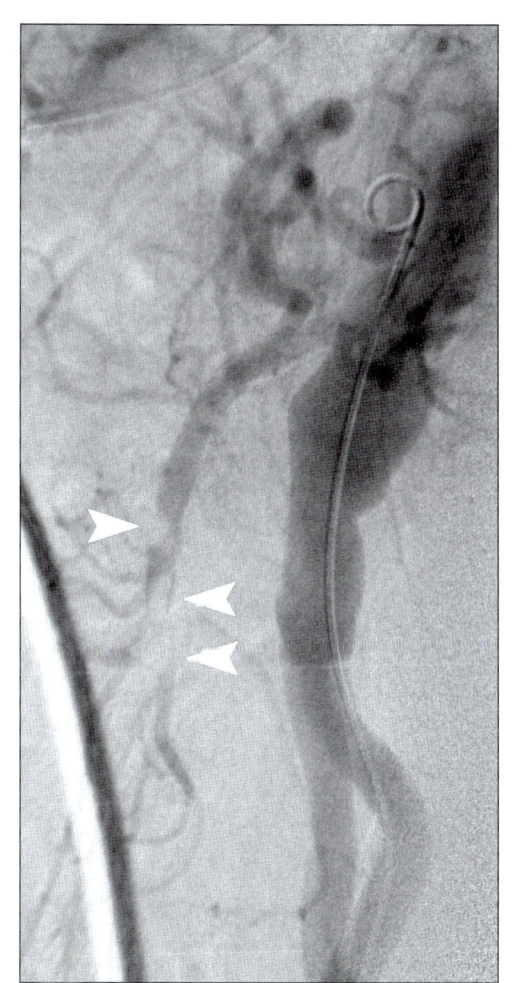

Figure 2. Lateral abdominal aortogram shows a large filling defect in the SMA at the level of the jejunal and ileal branches (arrowheads).

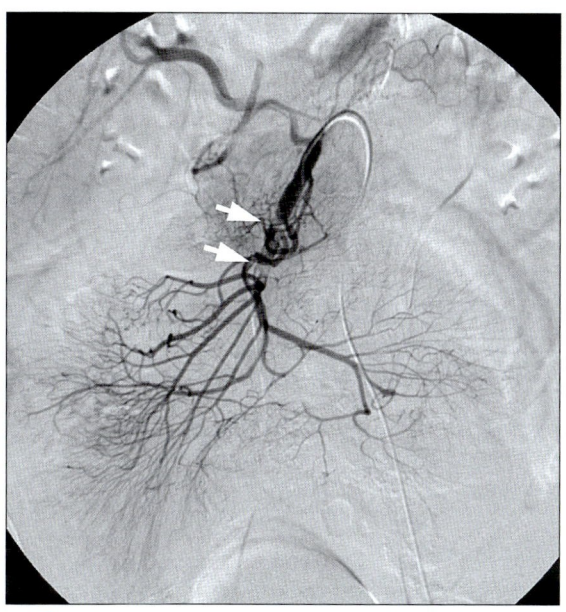

Figure 3. Selective superior mesenteric arteriogram in the anteroposterior projection shows a partially occlusive thrombus in the SMA (arrows). There is poor distal perfusion, especially to the middle jejunal region.

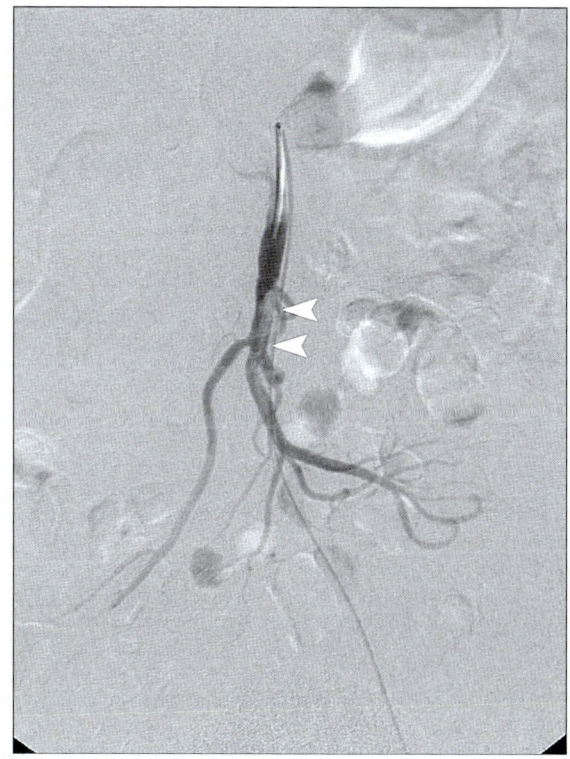

Figure 4. Follow-up SMA after 24 hours of thrombolysis shows partial resolution of the SMA thrombus (arrowheads). There was improved distal perfusion, and the tPA infusion was stopped.

Case 36

DEMOGRAPHICS/CLINICAL HISTORY

A 77-year-old woman with a history of peripheral vascular disease and intermittent, severe abdominal pain exacerbated by eating, undergoing ultrasound, magnetic resonance angiography (MRA), and stent placement.

DISCUSSION

History/Indications for Procedure
A 77-year-old woman has a history of peripheral vascular disease with intermittent, severe abdominal pain and nausea. Her symptoms are exacerbated by eating, and she has developed an aversion to food.

Procedure
Chronic mesenteric ischemia

Pre-procedure Imaging
Arterial ultrasound examination revealed elevated velocities at the origin of the celiac and superior mesenteric arteries, corresponding to more than 70% stenosis. MRA demonstrates high-grade stenoses of the proximal celiac and superior mesenteric arteries (Fig. 1) and stenosis at the origin of the inferior mesenteric artery.

Intraprocedural Findings
High-grade stenoses were identified at the origin of the celiac and superior mesenteric arteries. The celiac artery was treated with a 6-mm × 15-mm, balloon-expandable stent, and the superior mesenteric artery was treated with a 6-mm × 24-mm, self-expanding nitinol stent (Figs. 2 and 3).

Follow-up and Complications
The patient's abdominal pain, nausea, and vomiting resolved after stent placement. The patient did develop a left brachial artery pseudoaneurysm at the arterial access site that required surgical repair.

Suggested Readings

Leung, et al: Endovascular interventions for acute and chronic mesenteric ischemia. In Baum S, Pentecost MJ (eds): Abrams' Angiography: Interventional Radiology. Philadelphia, Lippincott Williams & Wilkins, 2005, pp 398-414.

Cognet F, Ben Salem D, Dranssart M, et al: Chronic mesenteric ischemia: Imaging and percutaneous treatment. Radiographics 22:863-879, 2002.

Matsumoto AH, Angle JF, Spinosa DJ, et al: Percutaneous transluminal angioplasty and stenting in the treatment of chronic mesenteric ischemia: Results and longterm followup. J Am Coll Surg 194(Suppl):S22-S31, 2002.

Razavi M, Chung HH: Endovascular management of chronic mesenteric ischemia. Tech Vasc Interv Radiol 7:155-159, 2004.

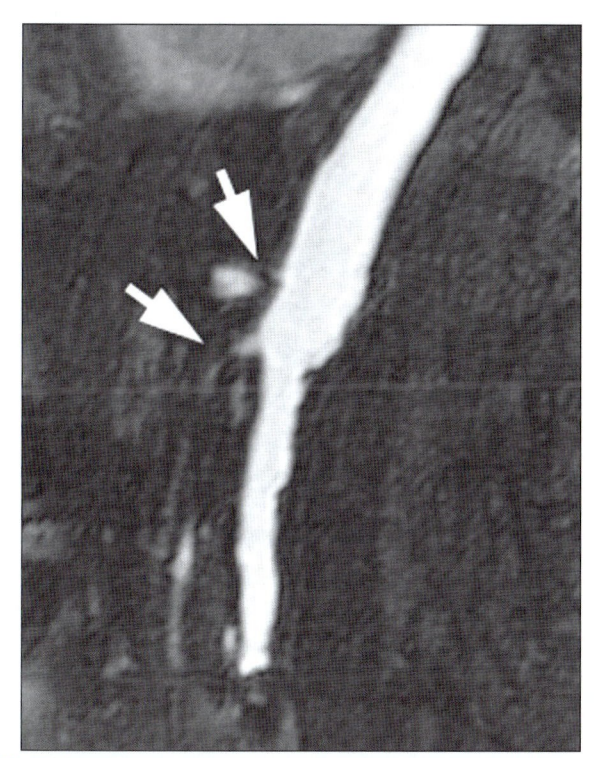

Figure 1. Selected sagittal image from contrast-enhanced MRA of the abdomen demonstrates high-grade stenoses at the origins of the celiac and superior mesenteric arteries *(arrows)*.

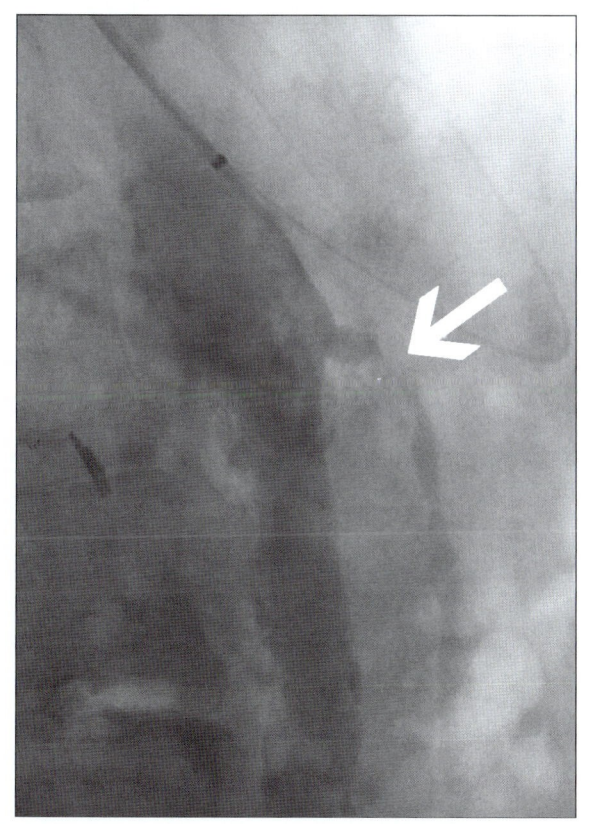

Figure 2. Sagittal aortogram after catheterization of the celiac artery shows a guidewire across the celiac artery stenosis. The high-grade superior mesenteric artery stenosis *(arrow)* can be seen.

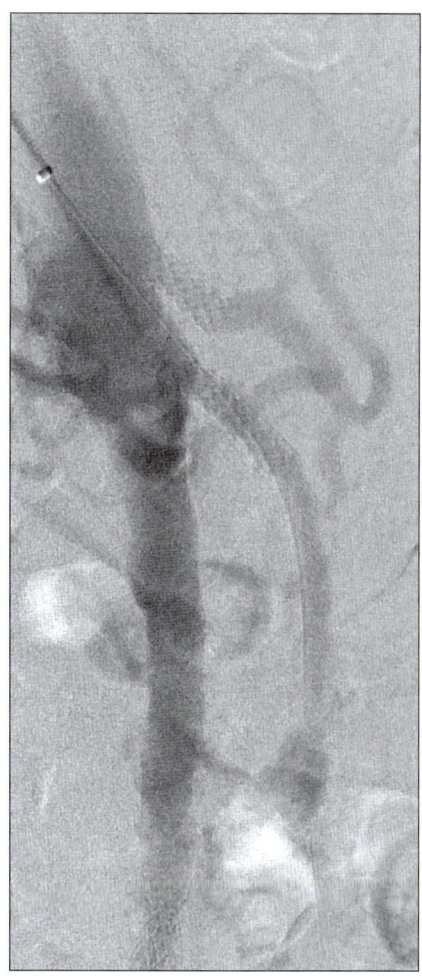

Figure 3. Completion aortogram after stent placement demonstrates improved flow in the celiac and superior mesenteric arteries.

Case 37

DEMOGRAPHICS/CLINICAL HISTORY

A 79-year-old woman with postprandial abdominal pain and weight loss.

DISCUSSION

History/Indications for Procedure
A 79-year-old woman with a 10-month history of postprandial pain and weight loss.

Procedure
Superior mesenteric artery stent placement

Pre-procedure Imaging
Arterial ultrasound (not shown) shows that the origin of the superior mesenteric artery (SMA) is occluded with reconstitution 1.5 cm distally. There is also evidence for stenosis at the origin of the celiac trunk.

Intraprocedural Findings
The occluded SMA was confirmed, and collateral arterial supply through the arc of Riolen was identified (Figs. 1 and 2). The occluded segment of the SMA was crossed (Fig. 3) and primarily stented with a 6-mm × 17-mm balloon expandable stent (Fig. 4).

Follow-up and Complications
Following the stent placement, the patient's symptoms resolved, and she is able to tolerate food with no pain.

Suggested Readings
Cognet F, Ben Salem D, Dranssart M, et al: Chronic mesenteric ischemia: Imaging and percutaneous treatment. Radiographics 22:863–879, 2002.

Matsumoto AH, Angle JF, Spinosa DJ, et al: Percutaneous transluminal angioplasty and stenting in the treatment of chronic mesenteric ischemia: Results and long-term follow-up. J Am Coll Surg 194:S22–S31, 2002.

Razavi M, Chung HH: Endovascular management of chronic mesenteric ischemia. Tech Vasc Interv Radiol 7:155–159, 2004.

Case 37   75

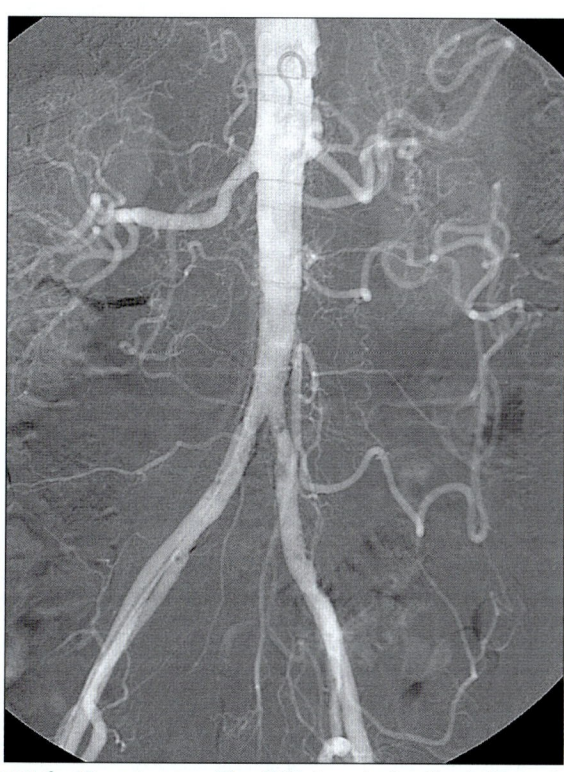

Figure 1. AP aortogram. The SMA is not visualized. There is a prominent arc of Riolen identified.

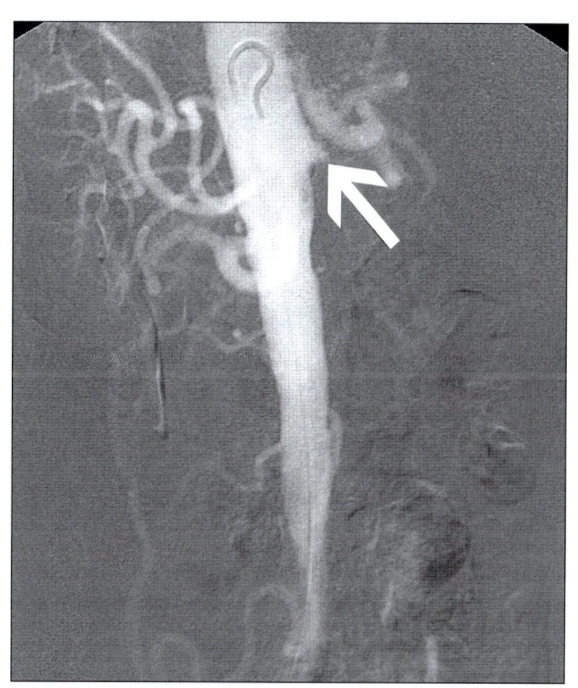

Figure 2. Lateral aortogram. The SMA is occluded at its origin (arrow).

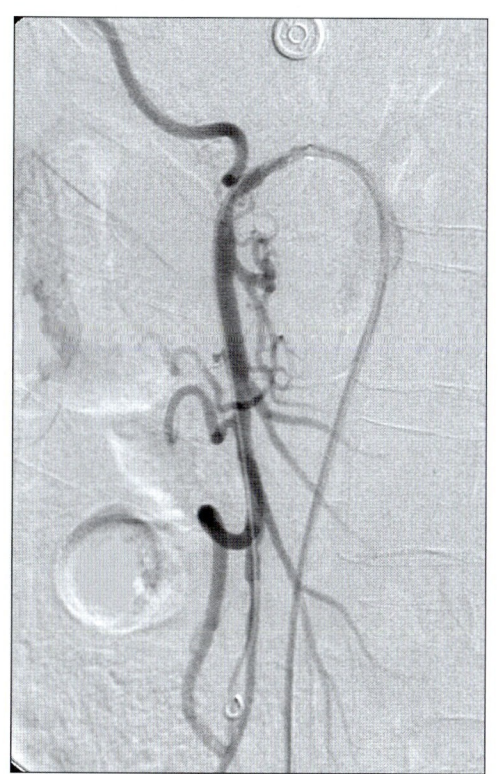

Figure 3. The occluded segment of the SMA was crossed and a guidewire has been advanced into the distal SMA. This is a follow-up angiogram following pre-dilatation with a 3-mm balloon.

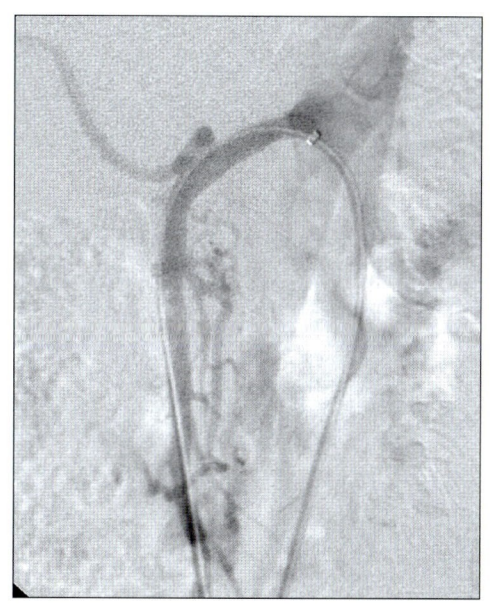

Figure 4. Final angiogram. A balloon expandable stent has been deployed and there is significantly improved flow through the SMA.

Case 38

DEMOGRAPHICS/CLINICAL HISTORY

A 56-year-old woman with left upper extremity claudication and rest pain, undergoing aortography.

DISCUSSION

History/Indications for Procedure
This patient had long-standing Takayasu's arteritis with worsening left upper extremity claudication and rest pain.

Procedure
Left subclavian artery stenosis secondary to Takayasu's arteritis

Pre-procedure Imaging
The patient had a CT scan at an outside hospital (not shown). This study did not reveal any wall enhancement or other evidence for active disease in the aorta or great vessels.

Intraprocedural Findings
Arch aortogram shows a focal, high-grade stenosis of the proximal left subclavian artery and mild irregularity of the right subclavian artery (Fig. 1). The lesion was successfully angioplastied with a 6-mm balloon (Figs. 2 and 3).

Follow-up and Complications
The patient's symptoms resolved after the angioplasty. She has remained asymptomatic for 3 years since percutaneous transluminal angioplasty.

Suggested Readings
Johnston SL, Lock RJ, Gompels MM: Takayasu arteritis: A review. J Clin Pathol 55:481-486, 2002.

Kumar S, Mandalam KR, Rao VRK, et al: Percutaneous transluminal angioplasty in nonspecific aortoarteritis (Takayasu's disease): Experience of 16 cases. Cardiovasc Intervent Radiol 12:321-325, 1990.

Sharma S, Rajani M, Talwar KK: Angiographic morphology in nonspecific aortoarteritis (Takayasu's arteritis): A study of 126 patients from North India. Cardiovasc Intervent Radiol 15:160-165, 1992.

Yamato M, Lecky JW, Hiramatsu K, et al: Takayasu's arteritis: Radiographic and angiographic findings in 59 patients. Radiology 161:329-334, 1986.

Case 38   77

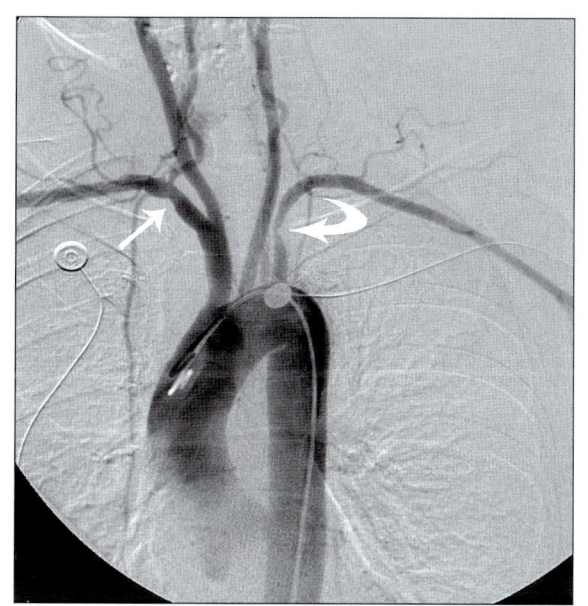

Figure 1. Arch aortogram shows a focal, high-grade stenosis of the proximal left subclavian artery *(curved arrow)*. There also is mild irregularity of the right subclavian artery *(arrow)*.

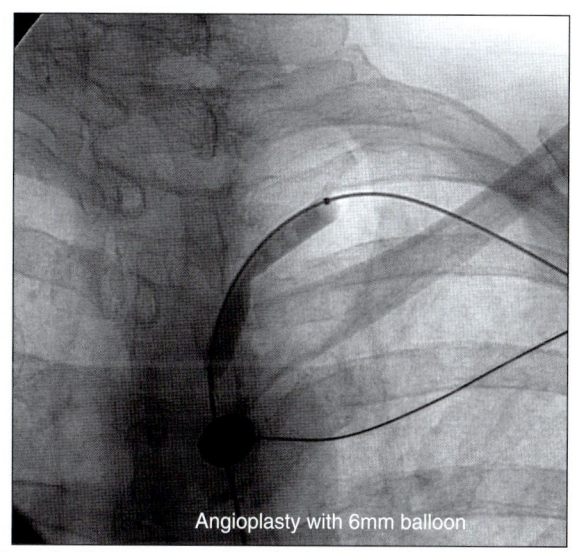

Figure 2. The lesion was dilated with a 6-mm balloon.

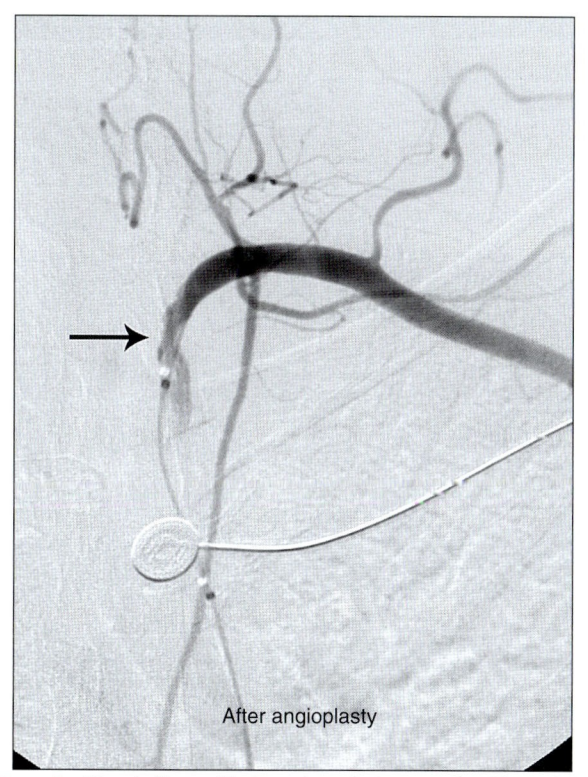

Figure 3. After balloon dilation, there is improved caliber of the vessel with a small, non–flow-limiting dissection at the angioplasty site *(arrow)*.

Case 39

DEMOGRAPHICS/CLINICAL HISTORY

A 55-year-old woman with abdominal pain and weight loss, undergoing magnetic resonance angiography (MRA), aortography, and stent placement.

DISCUSSION

History/Indications for Procedure
A 55-year-old woman had abdominal pain and weight loss. She has a history of Takayasu's vasculitis.

Procedure
Chronic mesenteric ischemia

Pre-procedure Imaging
MRA demonstrated severe stenosis at the origins of several aortic branch vessels, including the celiac, superior mesenteric, and right renal arteries.

Intraprocedural Findings
A lateral aortogram demonstrated a high-grade stenosis at the origin of the celiac and superior mesenteric arteries (Fig. 1), and contrast injection was used to determine the position of the stent before deployment (Fig. 2). The proximal superior mesenteric artery was primarily stented with a 7-mm × 15-mm, balloon-expandable stent.

Follow-up and Complications
The patient's abdominal pain improved after the stent placement (Fig. 3). She did well for 1 year, when she developed recurrent symptoms and intrastent stenosis, for which she was treated by ileomesenteric bypass.

Suggested Readings

Leung et al: Endovascular interventions for acute and chronic mesenteric ischemia. In Baum S, Pentecost MJ (eds): Abrams' Angiography: Interventional Radiology. Philadelphia, Lippincott Williams & Wilkins, 2005, pp 398-414.

Behar JV, et al: Endovascular interventions for chronic mesenteric ischemia. In Pearce WH, Yao JST, Matsumura JS (eds): Trends in Vascular Surgery. Chicago, Precept Press, 2002, pp 237-247.

Cognet F, Ben Salem D, Dranssart M, et al: Chronic mesenteric ischemia: Imaging and percutaneous treatment. Radiographics 22:863-879, 2002.

Razavi M, Chung HH: Endovascular management of chronic mesenteric ischemia. Tech Vasc Interv Radiol 7:155-159, 2004.

Matsumoto AH, Angle JF, Spinosa DJ, et al: Percutaneous transluminal angioplasty and stenting in the treatment of chronic mesenteric ischemia: Results and longterm followup. J Am Coll Surg 194(Suppl):S22-S31, 2002.

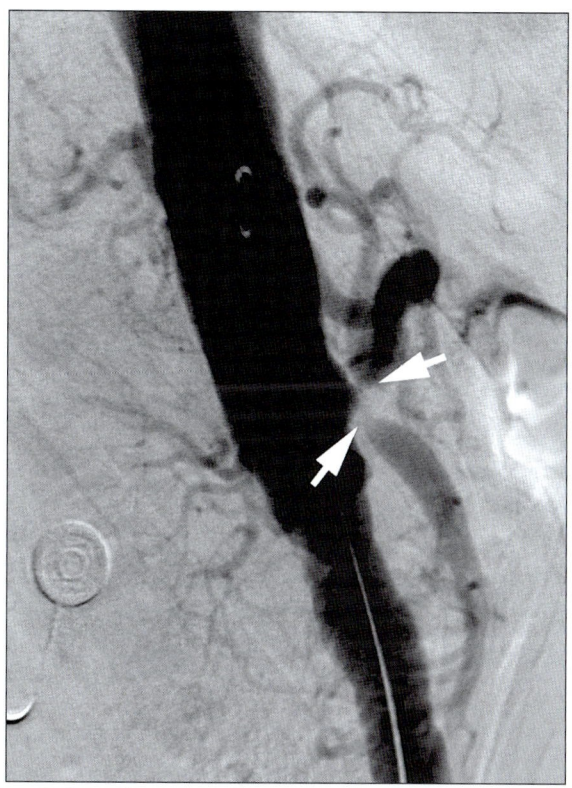

Figure 1. Lateral aortogram demonstrates high-grade stenoses at the origin of the superior mesenteric and celiac arteries *(arrows)*. Notice that the celiac arises from the proximal superior mesenteric artery.

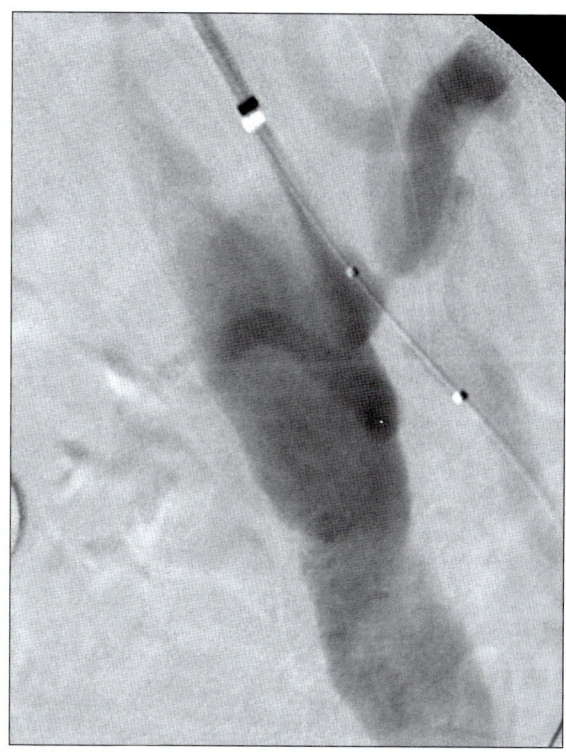

Figure 2. Contrast injection was used to evaluate the position of the stent before deployment.

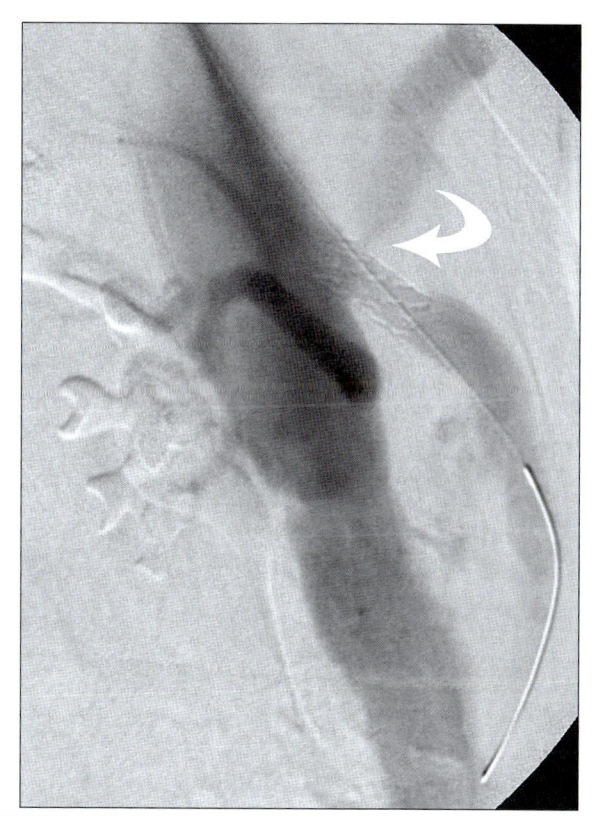

Figure 3. Follow-up contrast injection after stent placement shows significant improvement in flow through the superior mesenteric artery. The celiac artery continues to fill through the interstices of the stent *(arrow)*.

Case 40

DEMOGRAPHICS/CLINICAL HISTORY

A 26-year-old man shot near the right knee with a high-caliber pistol, undergoing angiography.

DISCUSSION

History/Indications for Procedure
This patient developed increasing swelling and pain of the medial right thigh while being evaluated in the emergency department.

Procedure
Management of post-traumatic popliteal arterial injury

Pre-procedure Imaging
A CT angiogram of the lower extremities revealed a bilobed pseudoaneurysm arising from the above-knee popliteal artery (Fig. 1).

Intraprocedural Findings
A right lower extremity angiogram confirms the presence of a bilobed popliteal pseudoaneurysm (Fig. 2). The injury was treated by placing a 7-mm × 5-cm Viabahn (Gore, Flagstaff, AZ) covered stent across the site of injury (Fig. 3).

Follow-up and Complications
The swelling resolved, and the patient had an uneventful recovery from the gunshot wound.

Suggested Readings
Criado E, Marston WA, Ligush J, et al: Endovascular repair of peripheral aneurysms, pseudoaneurysms, and arteriovenous fistulas. Ann Vasc Surg 11:256-263, 1997.

Mavili E, Donmez H, Ozcan N, et al: Endovascular treatment of lower limb penetrating arterial traumas. Cardiovasc Intervent Radiol 30:1124-1129, 2007.

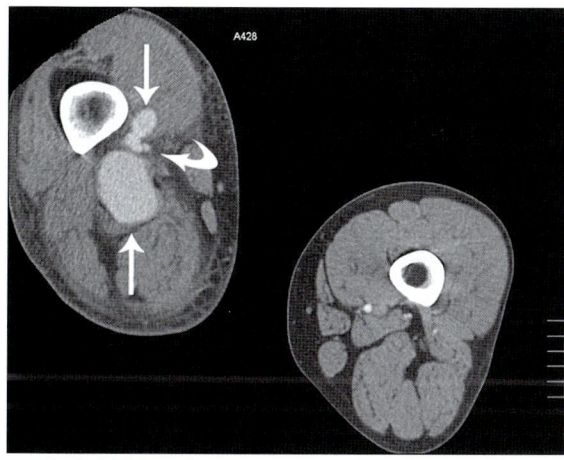

Figure 1. Axial image from CT angiography shows a bilobed pseudoaneurysm *(straight arrows)* involving the proximal right popliteal artery *(curved arrow)*.

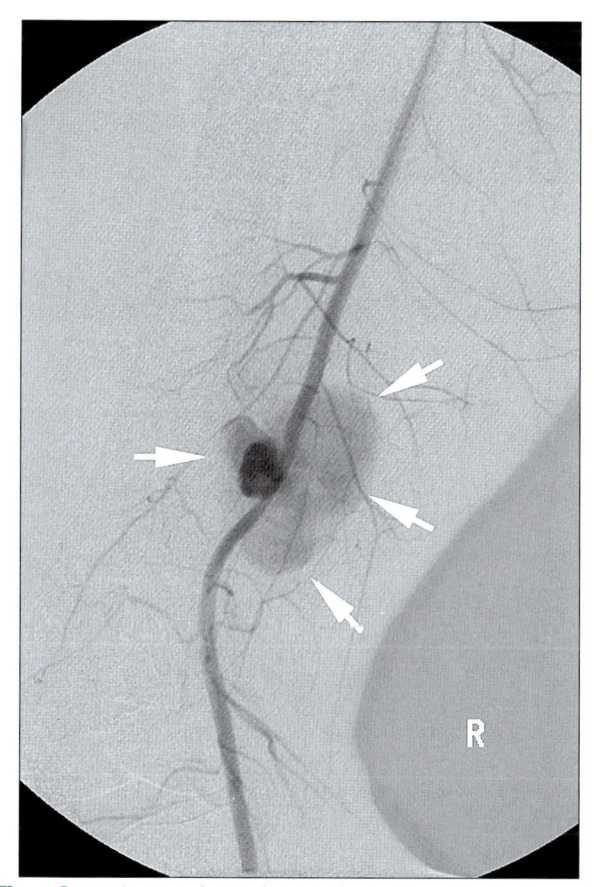

Figure 2. Angiogram shows the pseudoaneurysm *(arrows)*.

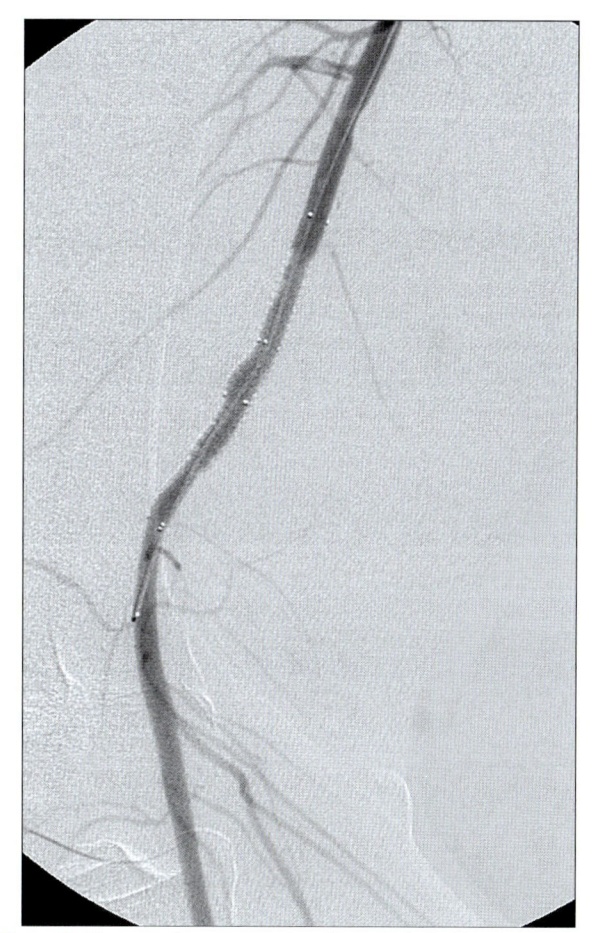

Figure 3. The pseudoaneurysm has been occluded by the covered stent.

Case 41

DEMOGRAPHICS/CLINICAL HISTORY
A 23-year-old man with a traumatic arteriovenous fistula caused by a gunshot wound, undergoing angiography.

DISCUSSION
History/Indications for Procedure
A 23-year-old man was shot through the left thigh with a 32-caliber handgun approximately 10 months earlier. He has pain and occasional numbness along the medial aspect of the left thigh.

Procedure
Endovascular management of arteriovenous fistula

Intraprocedural Findings
There is a pseudoaneurysm of the proximal superficial femoral artery with a fistula to the femoral vein (Fig. 1). A 10-mm × 60-mm Fluency covered stent (Bard Peripheral Vascular, Tempe, AZ) was placed across the pseudoaneurysm, closing the fistula (Figs. 2 and 3).

Follow-up and Complications
The patient's symptoms improved after arteriovenous fistula closure. The stent has remained patent for 1 year after implantation.

Suggested Readings
Hanks SE, Pantecost MJ: Angiography and transcatheter treatment of extremity trauma. Semin Intervent Radiol 9:20-25, 1992.

Semba CP, Dake MD: Stent-graft therapy for subclavian artery aneurysms and fistulas: Single-center mid-term results. J Vasc Interv Radiol 11:578-584, 2000.

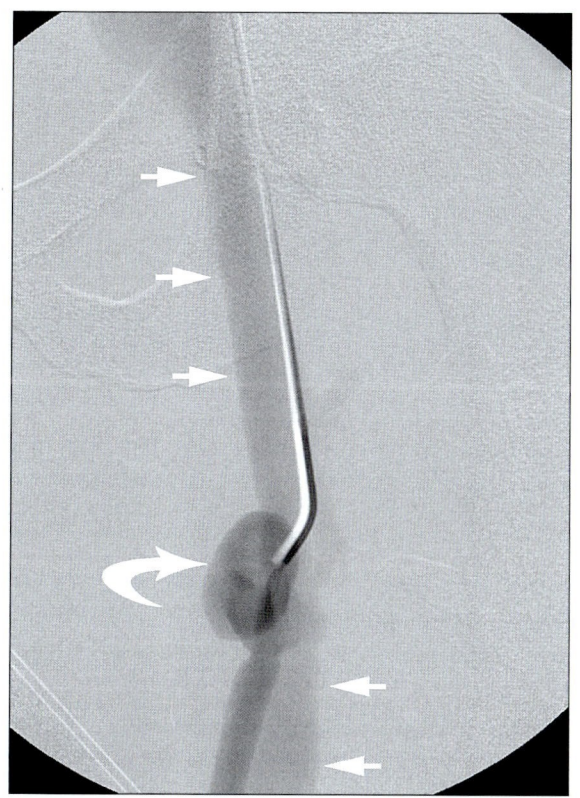

Figure 1. Selective injection of the left superficial femoral artery shows the pseudoaneurysm *(curved arrow)* and simultaneous filling of the femoral vein *(short arrows)*.

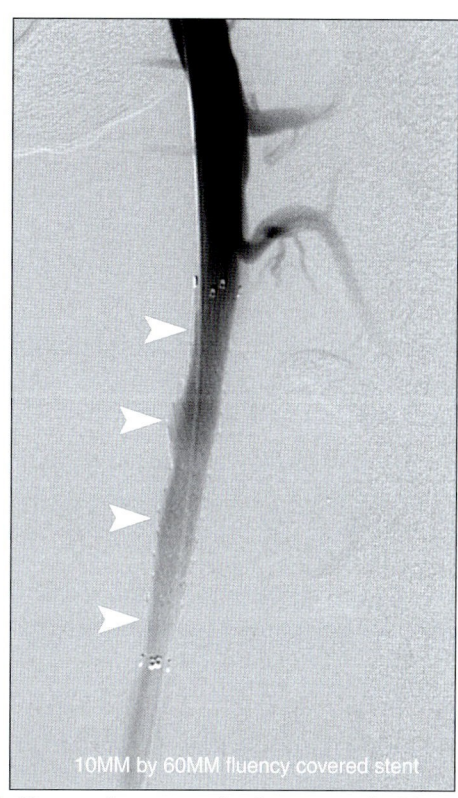

Figure 2. The pseudoaneurysm has been covered with a 10- × 60-mm Fluency covered stent *(arrowheads)*. The arteriovenous fistula is no longer seen.

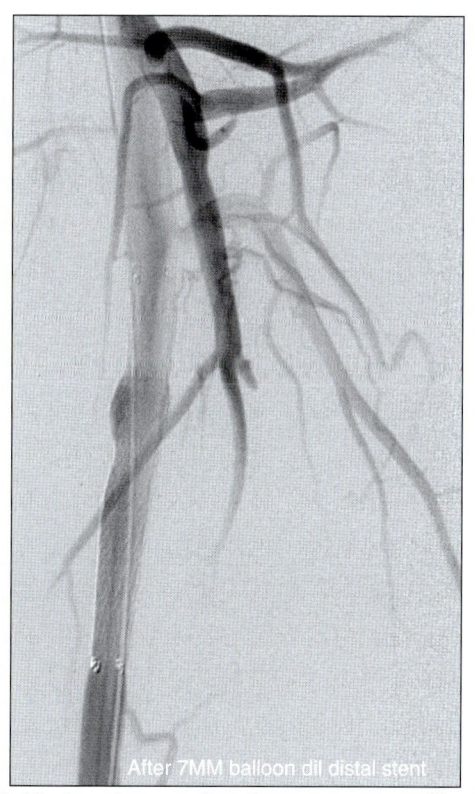

Figure 3. Final angiogram after the stent was postdilated. The pseudoaneurysm is excluded, with no further filling of the arteriovenous fistula.

Case 42

DEMOGRAPHICS/CLINICAL HISTORY

A 42-year-old man with a gunshot wound to the back of the left leg.

DISCUSSION

History/Indications for Procedure
A 42-year-old man shot in the back of the left leg with a 35-mm pistol at close range. On physical exam, a bruit is present over the left popliteal fossa

Procedure
Coil embolization for traumatic lower extremity arteriovenous fistula

Pre-procedure Imaging
Arterial ultrasound shows elevated end-diastolic velocities within the left popliteal artery, suggesting an arteriovenous fistula (Fig. 1).

Intraprocedural Findings
Left lower extremity arteriogram shows a pseudoaneurysm arising from a sural branch of the popliteal artery with an associated arteriovenous fistula (Figs. 2 and 3). The sural artery was selectively catheterized and embolized with coils (Fig. 4).

Follow-up and Complications
The patient was observed overnight and the following day was able to ambulate without assistance. At 1 month's follow-up, the patient had continued mild left lower extremity edema; there was no evidence for recurrence of the fistula.

Suggested Readings
Hanks SE, Pantecost MJ: Angiography and transcatheter treatment of extremity trauma. Semin Intervent Radiol 9:20-25, 1992.

Lopera JE, Suri R, Cura M, et al: Crural artery traumatic injuries: Treatment with embolization. Cardiovasc Intervent Radiol 31:550-557, 2008.

Mavili E, Donmez H, Ozcan N, et al: Endovascular treatment of lower limb penetrating arterial traumas. Cardiovasc Intervent Radiol 30:1124-1129, 2007.

Teitelbaum GP, Reed RA, Larsen D, et al: Microcatheter embolization of non-neurologic traumatic vascular lesions. J Vasc Interv Radiol 4:149-154, 1993.

Case 42   85

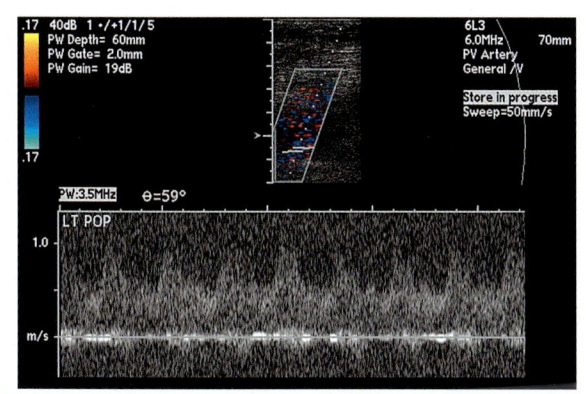

Figure 1. Arterial ultrasound over the left popliteal artery shows elevated end-diastolic velocities in the left popliteal artery, suggesting possible arteriovenous fistula.

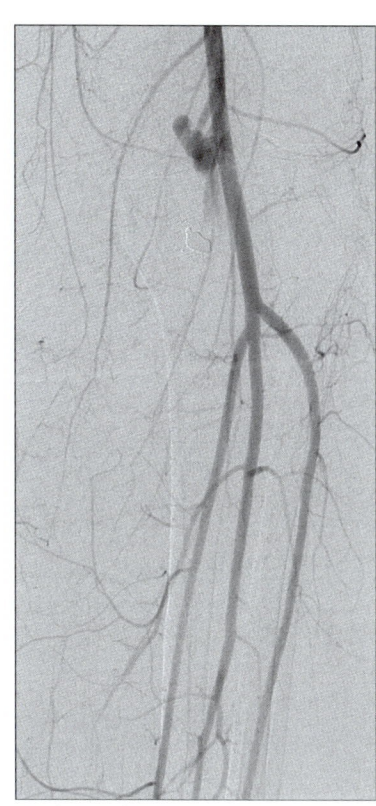

Figure 2. Image from left lower extremity arteriogram shows a pseudoaneurysm arising from a sural branch of the left popliteal artery. The vessels are otherwise normal.

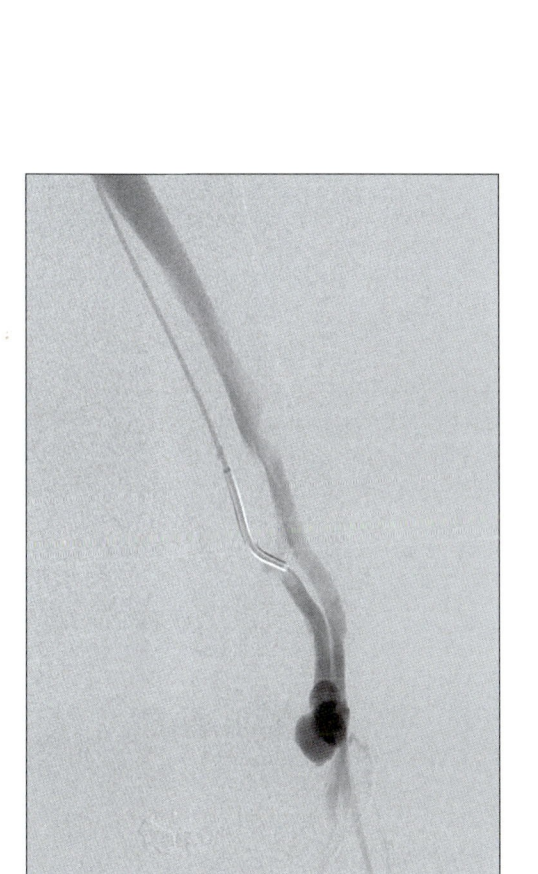

Figure 3. Selective injection of the injured sural branch again shows the presence of the pseudoaneurysm. There is also brisk filling of the popliteal vein, indicating the presence of an arteriovenous fistula.

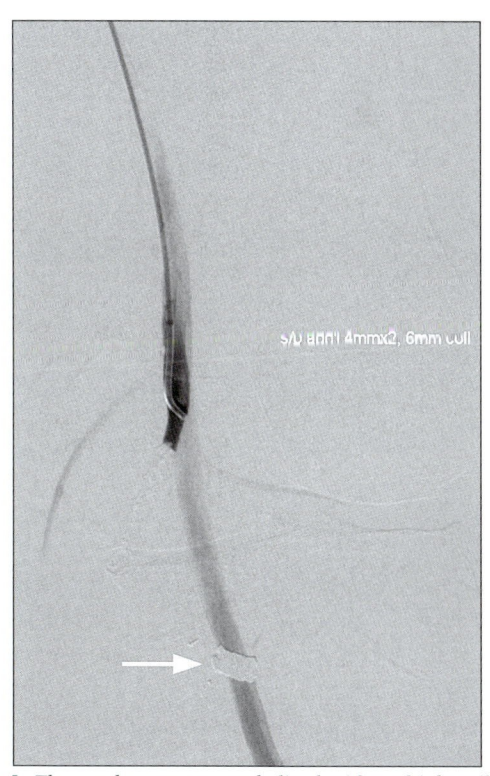

Figure 4. The sural artery was embolized with multiple coils. The filling defect over the lower popliteal artery (*arrow*) is a subtraction artifact from the bullet fragment.

Case 43

DEMOGRAPHICS/CLINICAL HISTORY

A 26-year-old man with a gunshot wound to the neck, undergoing arteriography.

DISCUSSION

History/Indications for Procedure
This patient sustained a gunshot wound to the base of the right neck.

Procedure
Endovascular repair of traumatic upper extremity arterial injury

Pre-procedure Imaging
An arteriogram performed at an outside hospital (not shown) revealed an injury to the right subclavian artery with an associated arteriovenous fistula (AVF) to the right internal jugular vein.

Intraprocedural Findings
There is focal irregularity of the proximal right subclavian artery (Fig. 1) with a subclavian artery to internal jugular vein AVF (Fig. 2; see Fig. 1). The injured subclavian artery was treated with a 10-mm × 5-cm Viabahn-covered stent (Fig. 3).

Follow-up and Complications
There were no immediate complications. The patient has since been lost to follow-up.

Suggested Readings
Hilfiker PR, Razavi MK, Kee ST, et al: Stent-graft therapy for subclavian artery aneurysms and fistulas: Single-center mid-term results. J Vasc Interv Radiol 11:578-584, 2000.

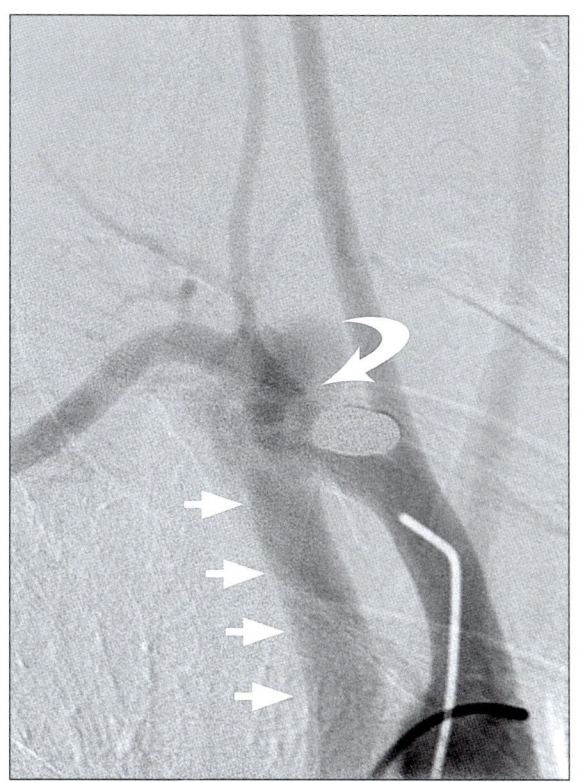

Figure 1. Right upper extremity arteriogram shows focal injury of the proximal right subclavian artery *(curved arrow)* with fistulous communication to the right internal jugular vein *(arrows)*.

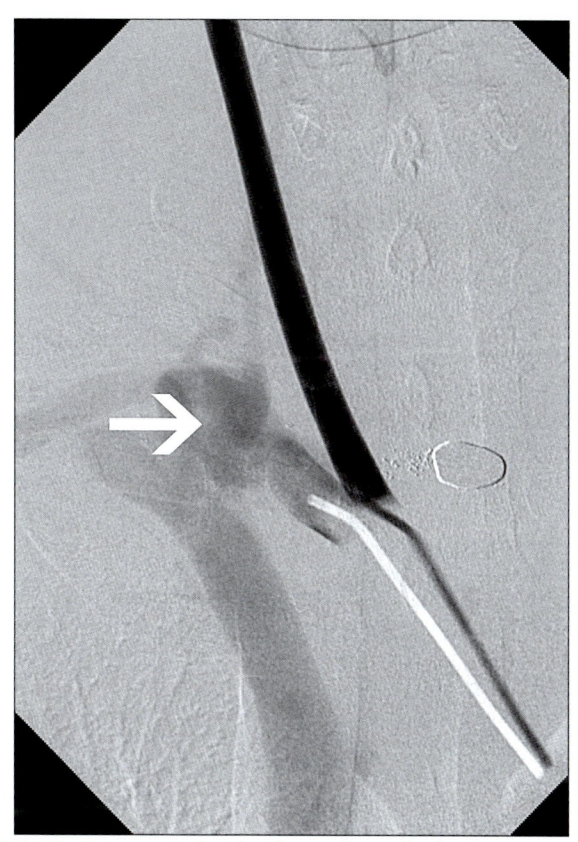

Figure 2. Anteroposterior view better shows the fistulous communication with the internal jugular vein *(arrow)*.

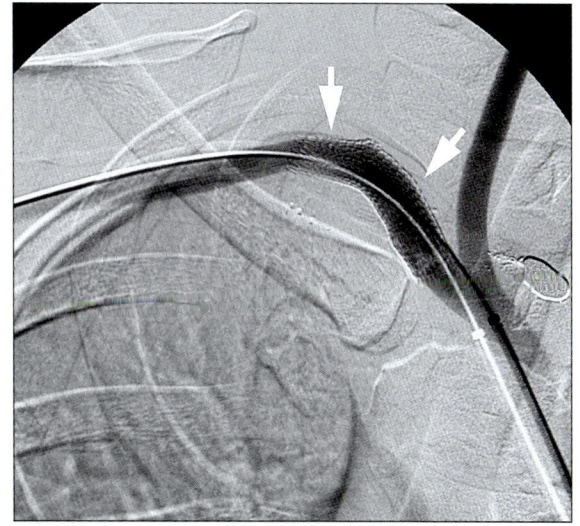

Figure 3. After stent-graft placement *(arrows)*, the pseudoaneurysm and AVF have been successfully excluded.

Case 44

DEMOGRAPHICS/CLINICAL HISTORY

A 38-year-old man who sustained a gunshot wound to the left lower extremity with subsequent surgical plating for fracture nonunion, undergoing angiography.

DISCUSSION

History/Indications for Procedure
This patient developed a pulsatile mass in the left lower extremity 2 weeks after surgical repair of a fracture nonunion.

Procedure
Embolization of post-traumatic anterior tibial artery pseudoaneurysm

Pre-procedure Imaging
Doppler ultrasound of the left lower extremity showed a pseudoaneurysm of the anterior tibial artery (not shown).

Intraprocedural Findings
There is a pseudoaneurysm arising from the anterior tibial artery (Figs. 1 and 2). The pseudoaneurysm was occluded with fibered coils deployed across the site of injury (Fig. 3).

Follow-up and Complications
Doppler ultrasound performed the day after the embolization showed thrombosis of the pseudoaneurysm (not shown).

Suggested Readings

Hanks SE, Pantecost MJ: Angiography and transcatheter treatment of extremity trauma. Semin Intervent Radiol 9:20-25, 1992.

Panetta T, Sclafani SJ, Goldstein AS, et al: Percutaneous transcatheter embolization for arterial trauma. J Vasc Surg 2:54-65, 1985.

Rosa P, O'Donnell SD, Goff JM, et al: Endovascular management of a peroneal artery injury due to a military fragment wound. Ann Vasc Surg 17:678-681, 2003.

Case 44   89

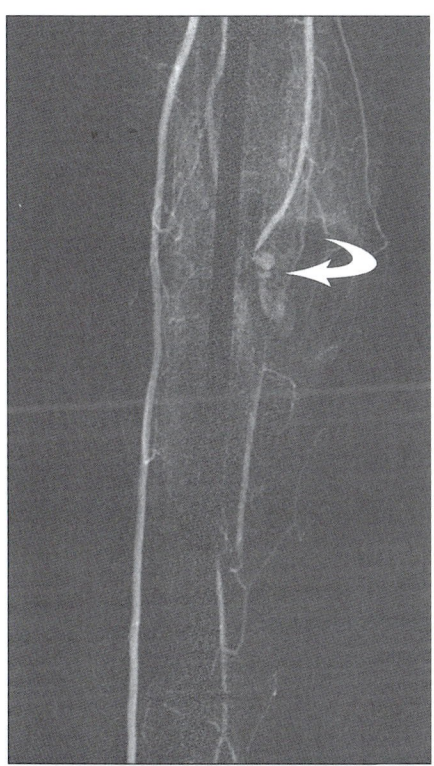

Figure 1. Nonselective angiogram shows discontinuity of the anterior tibial artery with early filling of a pseudoaneurysm *(curved arrow)*. Note the mass effect of the pseudoaneurysm.

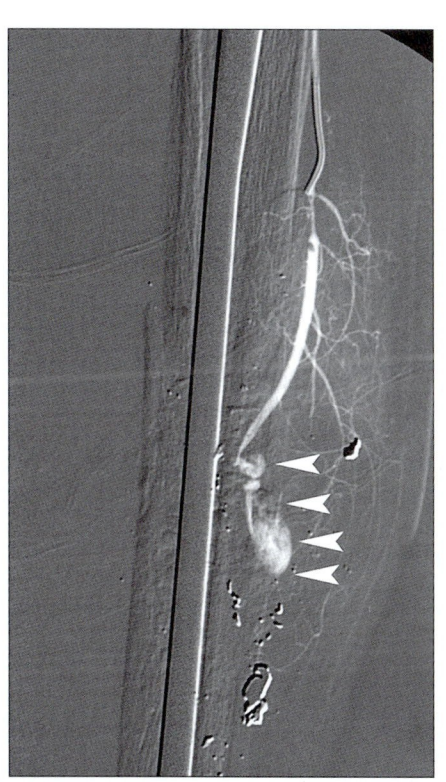

Figure 2. Selective catheterization of the anterior tibial artery shows better opacification of the pseudoaneurysm *(arrowheads)*.

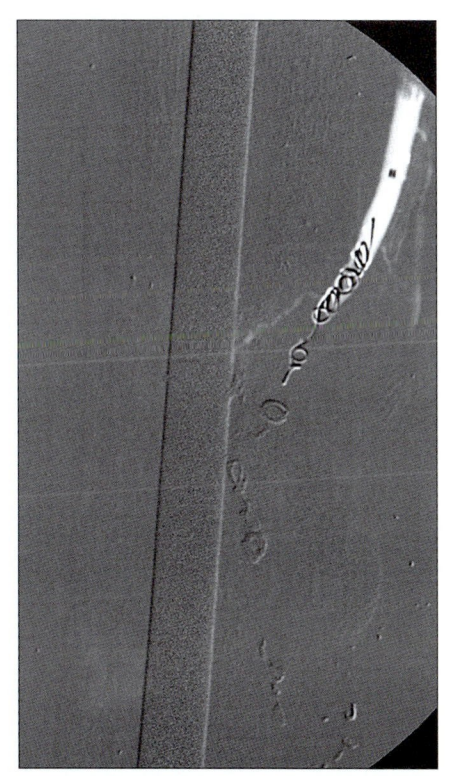

Figure 3. The anterior tibial artery was catheterized beyond the site of injury, and coils were deployed back across the site of injury.

Case 45

DEMOGRAPHICS/CLINICAL HISTORY

A 22-year-old man with a post-traumatic pseudoaneurysm of the dorsalis pedis artery, undergoing ultrasonography and arteriography.

DISCUSSION

History/Indications for Procedure

A 22-year-old man with mild hemophilia B developed a pseudoaneurysm of the dorsalis pedis artery after trauma to the foot while running. The pseudoaneurysm has been slowly enlarging and now is more than 3 cm in diameter.

Procedure

Embolization of post-traumatic dorsalis pedis artery pseudoaneurysm

Pre-procedure Imaging

Doppler ultrasound shows a bilobed pseudoaneurysm; one lobe is 2.2 × 2.2 cm, and the other is 2.7 × 1.7 cm. There is active blood flow within the pseudoaneurysm (Fig. 1).

Intraprocedural Findings

The dorsalis pedis artery supplies the pseudoaneurysm and is occluded distal to the pseudoaneurysm (Figs. 2 and 3). The dorsalis pedis artery was embolized with several coils (Fig. 4).

Follow-up and Complications

A follow-up ultrasound scan confirmed the successful thrombosis of the pseudoaneurysm.

Suggested Readings

Hanks SE, Pantecost MJ: Angiography and transcatheter treatment of extremity trauma. Semin Intervent Radiol 9:20-25, 1992.

Panetta T, Sclafani S, Goldstein AS, Phillips TF: Percutaneous transcatheter embolization for arterial trauma. J Vasc Surg 2:54-64, 1985.

Case 45   91

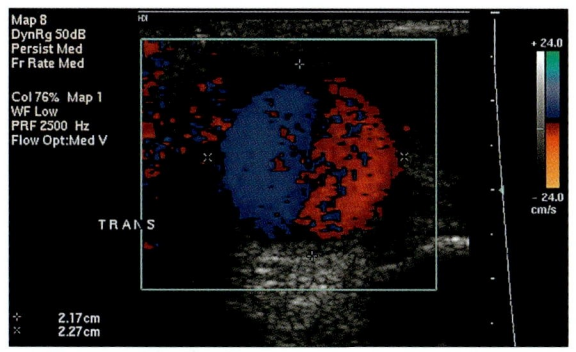

Figure 1. Color Doppler ultrasound shows the typical yin-yang pattern of flow within the pseudoaneurysm.

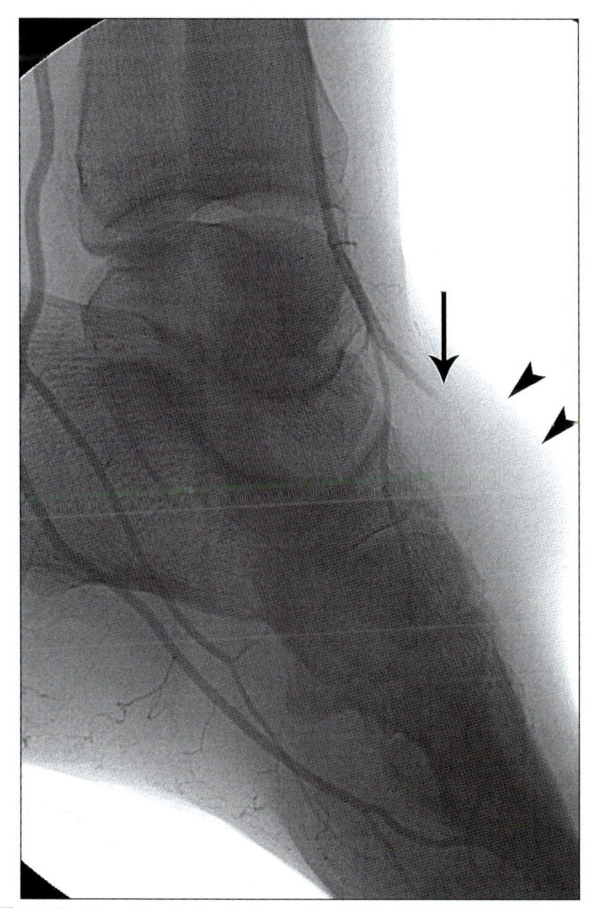

Figure 2. Unsubtracted arteriography of the lower extremity shows no flow in the distal dorsalis pedis artery *(arrow)*. There is soft tissue swelling over the pseudoaneurysm *(arrowheads)*.

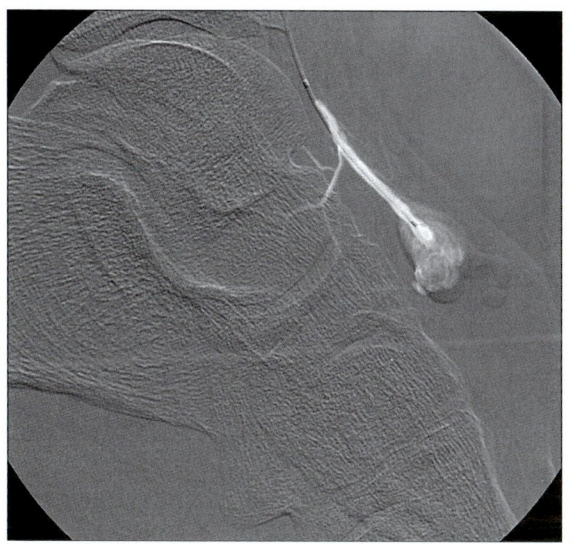

Figure 3. A microcatheter has been advanced into the pseudoaneurysm. Selective contrast injection shows filling of the pseudoaneurysm with no visible outflow.

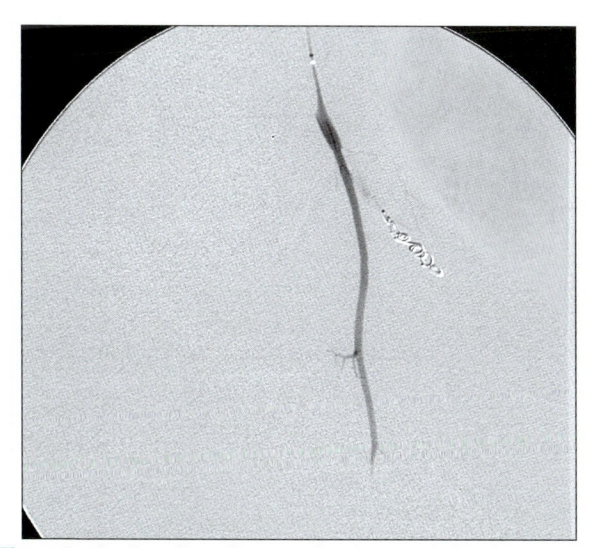

Figure 4. The dorsalis pedis artery has been embolized with coils. No further filling of the pseudoaneurysm is seen on the follow-up angiogram.

Case 46

DEMOGRAPHICS/CLINICAL HISTORY

A 26-year-old man involved in motor vehicle accident.

DISCUSSION

History/Indications for Procedure
A 26-year-old man involved in a motor vehicle accident with decreased left lower extremity pulses.

Procedure
Percutaneous stent placement in the setting of lower extremity traumatic dissection

Pre-procedure Imaging
Radiograph of the left femur shows a comminuted fracture of the distal femur (Fig. 1).

Intraprocedural Findings
There is an intimal flap within the distal superficial femoral artery, resulting in a high-grade stenosis (Fig. 2). The dissection was treated with the placement of a 5-mm × 15-mm balloon expandable stent (Genesis, Cordis, Miami, FL) (Figs. 3 and 4).

Follow-up and Complications
The patient underwent multiple debridements of the left lower extremity, eventually necessitating through-the-knee amputation. The patient went on to heal at the amputation site.

Suggested Readings
Hanks SE, Pantecost MJ: Angiography and transcatheter treatment of extremity trauma. Semin Intervent Radiol 9:20-25, 1992.

McCorkell SJ, Harley JD, Morishima MS, et al: Indications for angiography in extremity trauma. AJR Am J Roentgenol 145:1245-1247, 1985.

Case 46   93

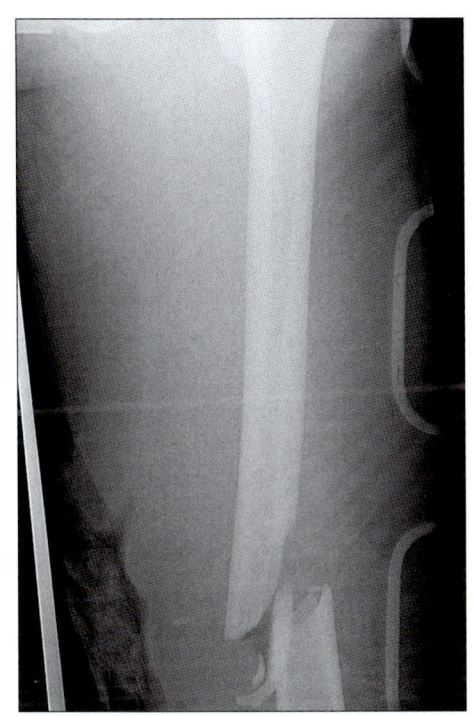

Figure 1. AP radiograph of the left femur shows a comminuted fracture through the distal left femur.

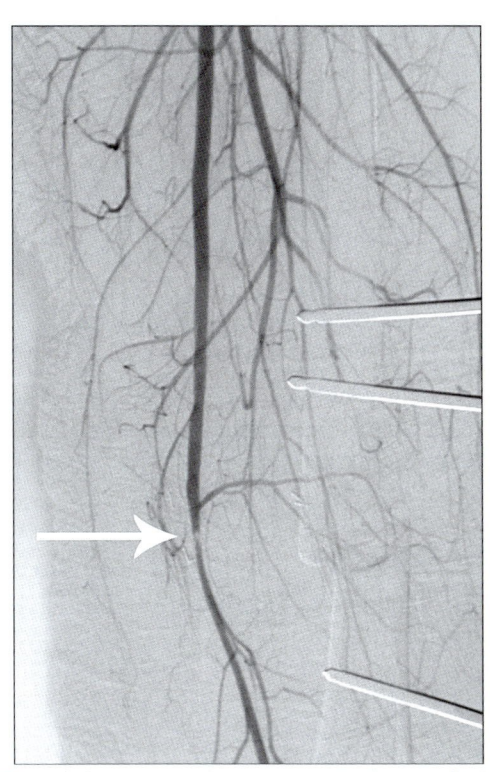

Figure 2. Left lower extremity arteriogram shows a high-grade stenosis of the distal left superficial femoral artery due to a post-traumatic dissection *(arrow)* at the level of the femur injury.

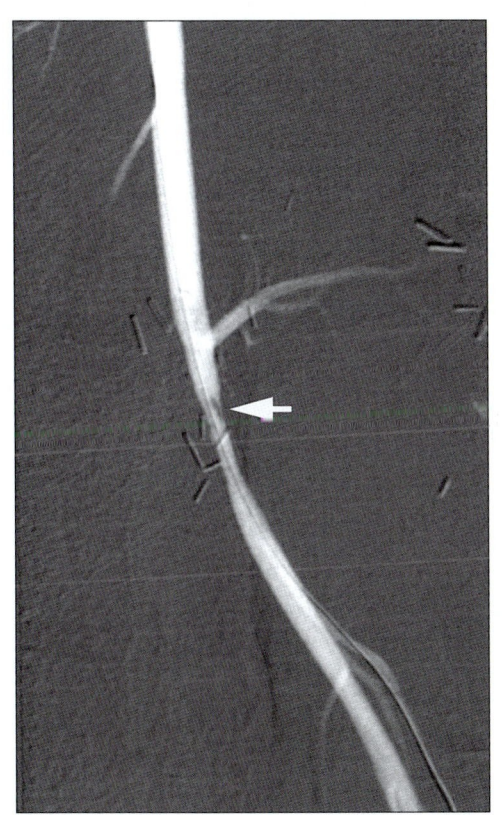

Figure 3. The lesion was gently predilated with a partially inflated 5-mm balloon. Follow-up angiogram shows the continued presence of the intimal flap resulting in persistent luminal narrowing *(arrow)*.

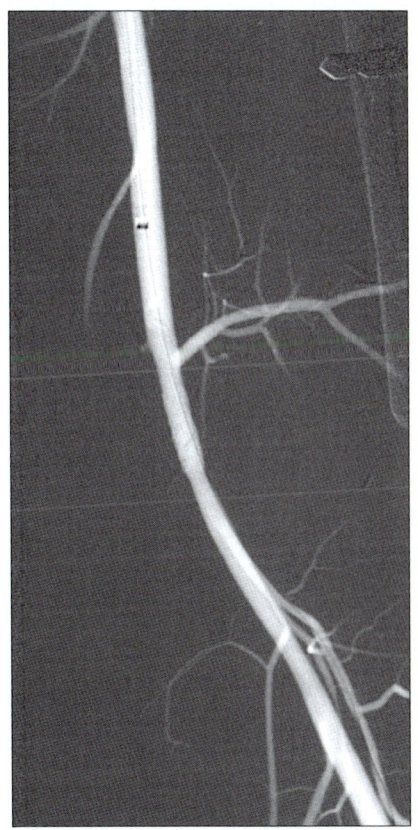

Figure 4. The traumatic dissection was treated with the placement of a 5- × 15-mm balloon expandable stent.

Case 47

DEMOGRAPHICS/CLINICAL HISTORY

A 21-year-old man who was involved in a roll-over motor vehicle accident, undergoing radiography, computed tomography (CT), arteriography, and embolization.

DISCUSSION

History/Indications for Procedure
A 21-year-old man was involved in a roll-over motor vehicle accident. The patient was hemodynamically unstable on presentation to the emergency department.

Procedure
Pelvic hemorrhage caused by trauma

Pre-procedure Imaging
A plain radiograph of the pelvis demonstrated fractures of the left acetabulum and left inferior pubic ramus. Contrast-enhanced CT demonstrated intramuscular hematoma along the left pelvic sidewall and a small amount of active contrast extravasation adjacent to the pubic symphysis (Fig. 1).

Intraprocedural Findings
Pelvic arteriogram demonstrated a focus of contrast extravasation arising from a branch of the anterior division of the right internal iliac artery (Figs. 2 and 3). The anterior division of the right internal iliac artery was embolized with Gelfoam (Fig. 4).

Follow-up and Complications
The patient's hemoglobin level remained stable after the embolization. He was treated for his other injuries and discharged from the hospital 2 weeks after admission.

Suggested Readings
Lang EK: Transcatheter embolization of pelvic vessels for control of intractable hemorrhage. Radiology 140:331-339, 1981.

Yoon W, Kim JK, Jeong YY, et al: Pelvic arterial hemorrhage in patients with pelvic fractures: Detection with contrast-enhanced CT. Radiographics 24:1591-1605, 2004.

Case 47   95

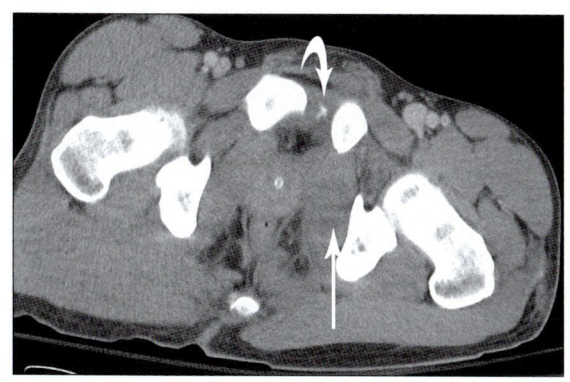

Figure 1. Single image from a pelvic CT scan demonstrates asymmetric enlargement of the left obturator internus muscle *(straight arrow)*. A small focus of contrast extravasation is seen adjacent to the pubic symphysis *(curved arrow)*.

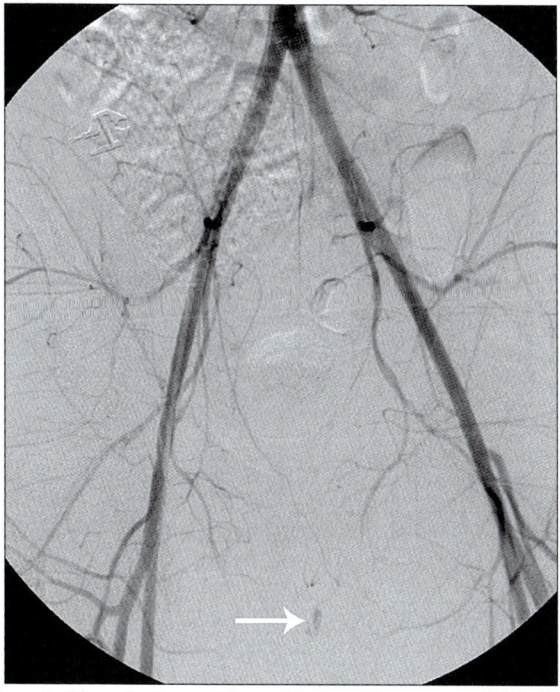

Figure 2. Nonselective pelvic arteriogram shows a small blush of contrast near the midline of the pelvis, which is consistent with active hemorrhage *(arrow)*.

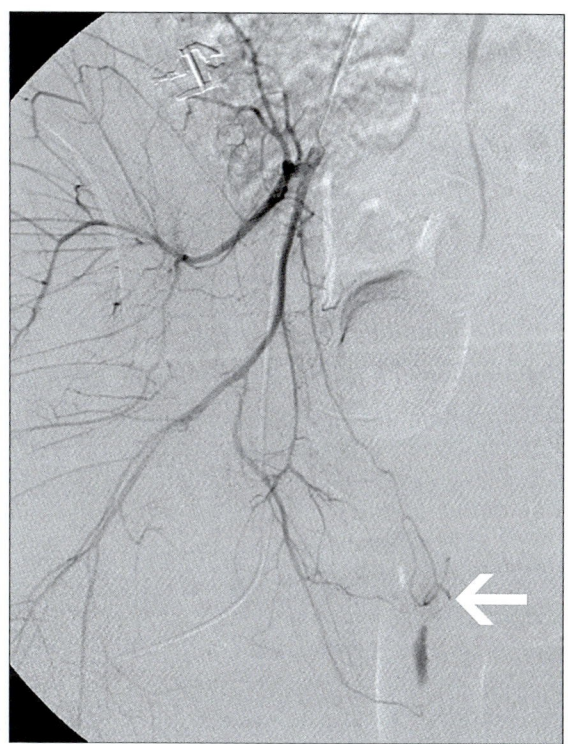

Figure 3. Selective injection of the right internal iliac artery localizes the source of hemorrhage to a branch of the anterior division of the internal iliac artery *(arrow)*.

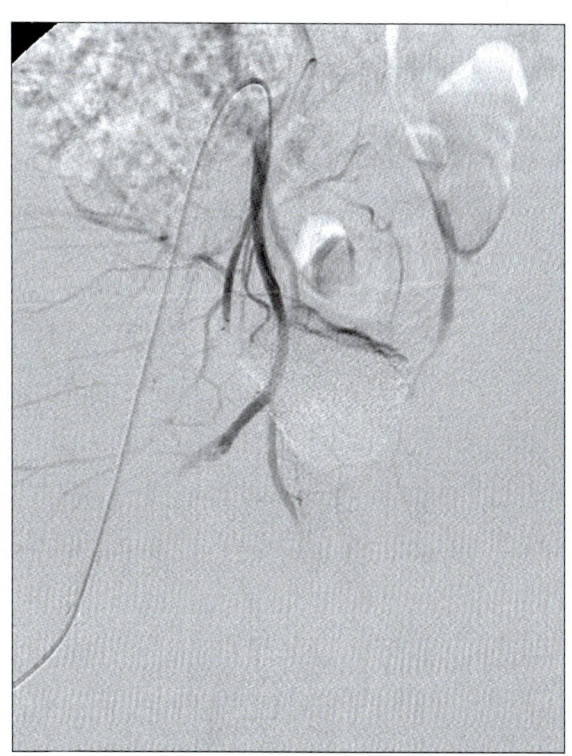

Figure 4. Injection after embolization demonstrates stasis of flow within the anterior division of the right internal iliac artery.

Case 48

DEMOGRAPHICS/CLINICAL HISTORY

A 34-year-old woman with a history of neurofibromatosis who presented with shortness of breath and hypotension, undergoing arteriography under fluoroscopic guidance.

DISCUSSION

History/Indications for Procedure
A 34-year-old woman with a history of neurofibromatosis, who underwent cesarean section 6 days earlier, presents with shortness of breath and hypotension. Placement of a right-sided chest tube returned a large volume of blood.

Procedure
Endovascular management of thyrocervical aneurysm

Pre-procedure Imaging
Computed tomography of the chest before chest tube placement showed a large, right hemothorax, and no contrast extravasation was seen.

Intraprocedural Findings
Right upper extremity arteriogram shows an aneurysm arising from the thyrocervical trunk with active extravasation (Figs. 1 and 2). The aneurysm was selectively catheterized and packed with coils (Fig. 3).

Follow-up and Complications
The patient continued to have a large volume of bloody output from the chest tube, and a repeat arteriogram showed continued aneurysm filling and extravasation due to continued perfusion by numerous arterial collaterals. The aneurysm and area of extravasation were punctured directly under fluoroscopy and embolized with a direct injection of thrombin (Fig. 4); the bleeding was controlled, and the follow-up arteriogram 1 month later showed persistent occlusion of the aneurysm.

Suggested Readings
Arai K, Sanada J, Kurozumi A, et al: Spontaneous hemothorax in neurofibromatosis treated with percutaneous embolization. Cardiovasc Intervent Radiol 30:477-479, 2007.

Oderich GS, Sullivan TM, Bower TC, et al: Vascular abnormalities in patients with neurofibromatosis syndrome type I: Clinical spectrum, management, and results. J Vasc Surg 46:475-484, 2007.

Sueyoshi E, Sakamoto I, Nakashima K, et al: Visceral and peripheral arterial pseudoaneurysms. AJR Am J Roentgenol 185:741-749, 2005.

Case 48   97

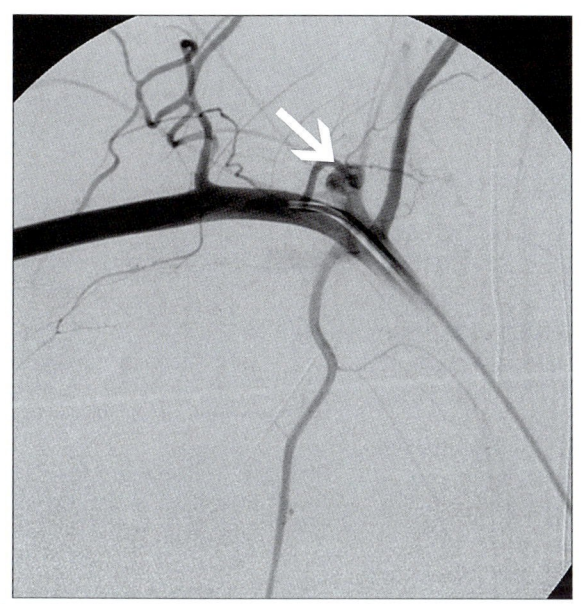

Figure 1. Right subclavian arteriogram shows an aneurysm arising from the thyrocervical trunk *(arrow)*. No active extravasation was seen on this injection.

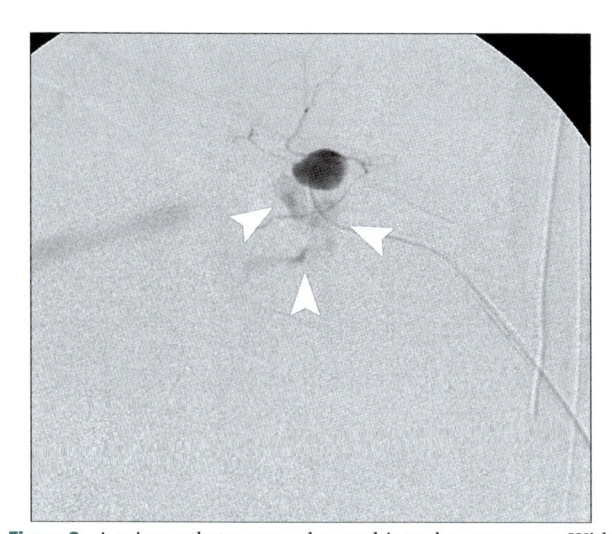

Figure 2. A microcatheter was advanced into the aneurysm. With a gentle injection into the aneurysm, active extravasation is visualized extending into the upper thorax *(arrowheads)*.

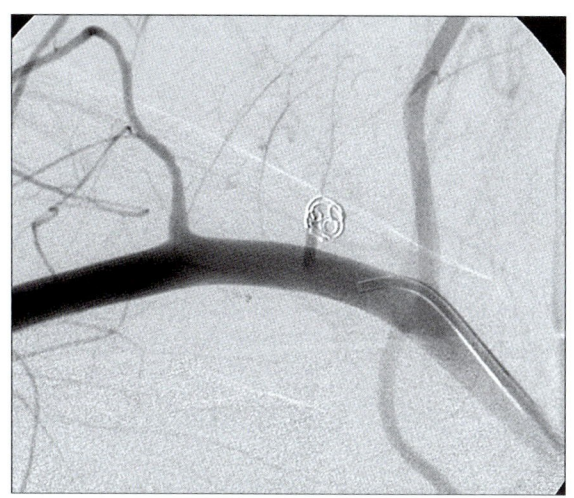

Figure 3. The aneurysm was packed with coils, and no further extravasation was seen.

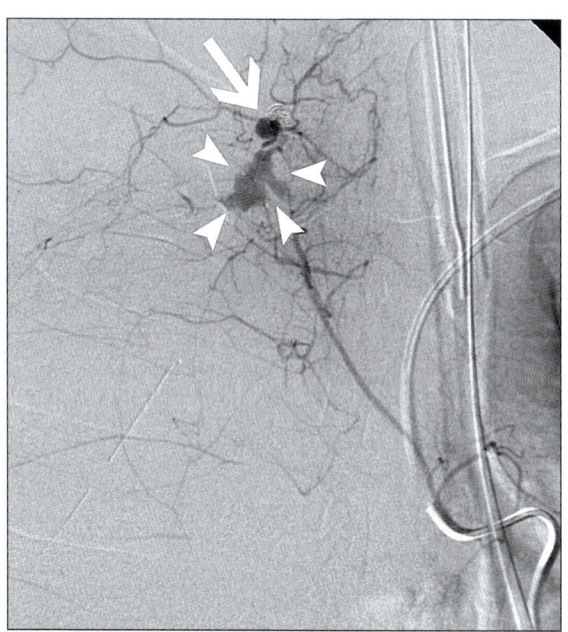

Figure 4. A follow-up arteriogram was performed the next day because of continued bloody output from the chest tube. Selective injection of the right superior intercostal artery shows filling of the aneurysm *(arrow)* through collaterals with active extravasation *(arrowheads)*.

Case 49

DEMOGRAPHICS/CLINICAL HISTORY

A 59-year-old woman with a left subclavian artery aneurysm, undergoing computed tomography (CT) angiography.

DISCUSSION

History/Indications for Procedure
A 59-year-old woman had a left subclavian artery aneurysm incidentally diagnosed at another hospital while undergoing a thoracic aortogram that required a left brachial approach. The aneurysm has been followed with CT, and the patient has been asymptomatic relative to the aneurysm.

Procedure
Endovascular repair of subclavian artery aneurysm

Pre-procedure Imaging
CT angiogram shows a 2.9-cm saccular aneurysm (Fig. 1) arising from the proximal left subclavian artery that has enlarged since the previous CT study. The aneurysm contains some mural thrombus and arises just distal to the origin of the left vertebral artery (Fig. 2).

Intraprocedural Findings
The aneurysm was identified, and to protect against retrograde flow after stent placement, the internal mammary, thyrocervical trunk, and ascending cervical arteries were embolized with coils (Fig. 3). A 6-mm × 22-mm, covered, balloon-expandable stent (Atrium Medical, Hudson, NH) was placed across the aneurysm (Fig. 4).

Follow-up and Complications
Follow-up arteriogram after covered-stent placement showed no further filling of the aneurysm. The patient was started on enoxaparin (Lovenox) and later converted to Coumadin for long-term anticoagulation.

Suggested Readings
Davidovic LB, Markovic DM, Pejkic SD, et al: Subclavian artery aneurysms. Asian J Surg 26:7-11, 2003.
Onal B, Ilgit ET, Kosar S, et al: Endovascular treatment of peripheral vascular lesions with stent-grafts. Diagn Interv Radiol 11:170-174, 2005.
Peynircioglu B, Ergun O, Hazirolan T, et al: Stent-graft applications in peripheral non-atherosclerotic arterial lesions. Diagn Interv Radiol 14:40-50, 2008.

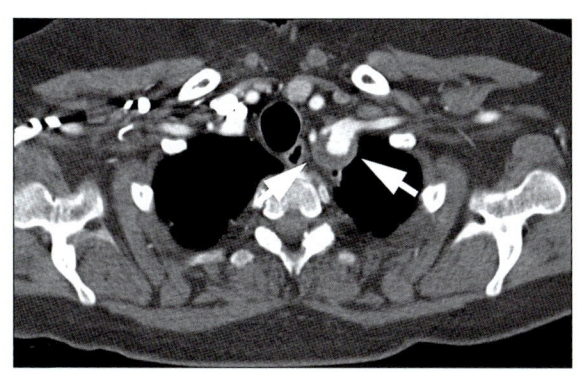

Figure 1. Axial CT angiogram shows a saccular aneurysm of the proximal left subclavian artery *(arrow)*.

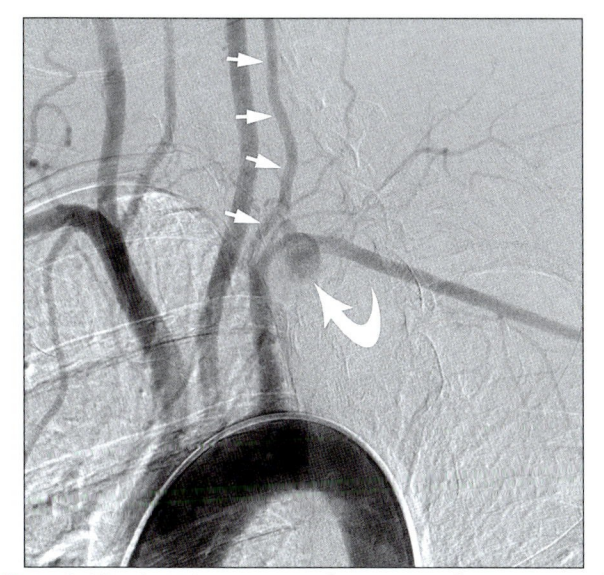

Figure 2. The thoracic aortogram shows a saccular aneurysm of the proximal left subclavian artery *(curved arrow)*. The aneurysm arises just distal to the origin of the left vertebral artery *(short arrows)*.

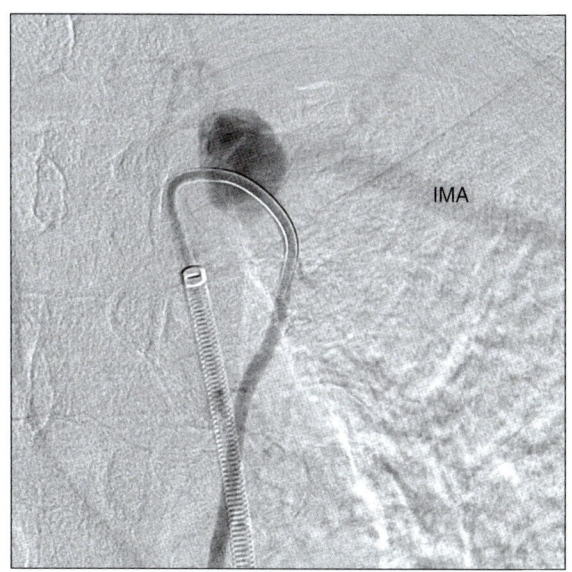

Figure 3. The left internal mammary artery has been selectively catheterized. All adjacent branch vessels were embolized with coils to prevent an endoleak after coverage of the aneurysm.

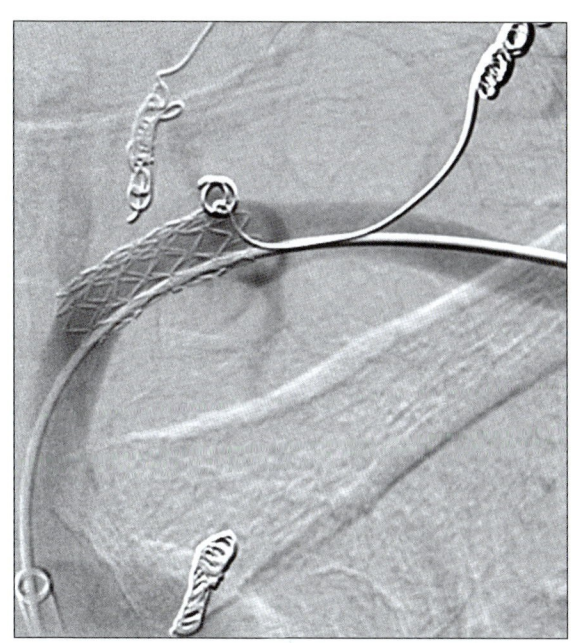

Figure 4. The adjacent branch vessels have been embolized with coils. A balloon-expandable stent-graft has been deployed across the neck of the aneurysm. No further filling of the aneurysm is seen.

Case 50

DEMOGRAPHICS/CLINICAL HISTORY

A 50-year-old woman with a history of pelvic angiosarcoma and hematuria.

DISCUSSION

History/Indications for Procedure
A 50-year-old woman with prior resection of angiosarcoma and pelvic radiation presents with gross hematuria after cystoscopic ureteral stent exchange.

Procedure
Stent-graft placement for arterial pseudoaneurysm secondary to pelvic radiation

Pre-procedure Imaging
Contrast-enhanced MRI performed 1 month earlier shows abnormal enhancing soft tissue along the left pelvic sidewall (Fig. 1). Antegrade nephrostogram performed at the time of the initial nephrostomy placement shows large filling defects in the renal pelvis and ureter, consistent with blood clots, and complete obstruction of the distal left ureter.

Intraprocedural Findings
Pelvic arteriogram shows mild narrowing of the left external iliac artery; within the area of stenosis, there is filling of a small pseudoaneurysm (Fig. 2). An 8-mm × 4-cm covered stent (Fluency, Bard, Tempe, AZ) was deployed across the pseudoaneurysm (Fig. 3).

Follow-up and Complications
The patient had no further episodes of hematuria. The patient returned and, while the nephrostomy was being internalized, a long-segment stricture of the distal ureter was identified (Fig. 4); the patient has since been managed using cystoscopic ureter stent exchanges.

Suggested Readings
Araki T, Nagata M, Araki T, et al: Endovascular treatment of ureteroarterial fistulas with stent-grafts. Radiat Med 26:372–375, 2008.

Feuer DS, Ciocca RG, Nackman GB, et al: Endovascular management of ureteroarterial fistula. J Vasc Surg 30:1146–1149, 1999.

Krambeck AE, DiMarco DS, Gettman MT, et al: Ureteroiliac artery fistula: Diagnosis and treatment algorithm. Urology 66:990–994, 2005.

Case 50   101

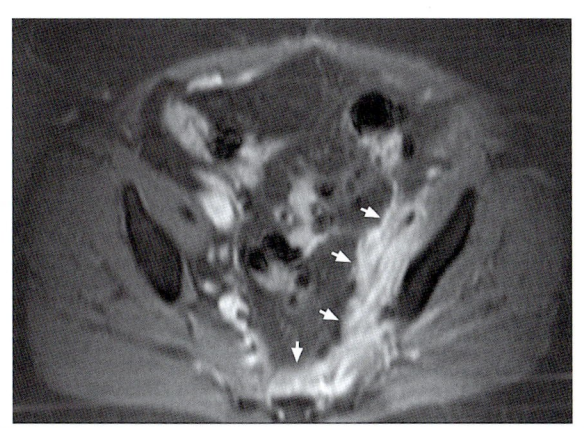

Figure 1. Axial T1, post-contrast, fat-saturated MR image through the pelvis shows diffuse abnormal enhancing soft tissue along the left pelvic sidewall and presacral space *(arrows)*.

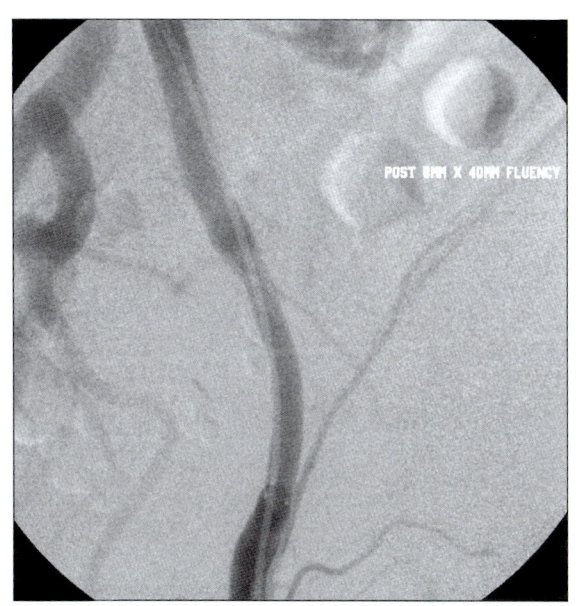

Figure 3. The pseudoaneurysm was successfully excluded with the placement of an 8-mm × 4-cm covered stent.

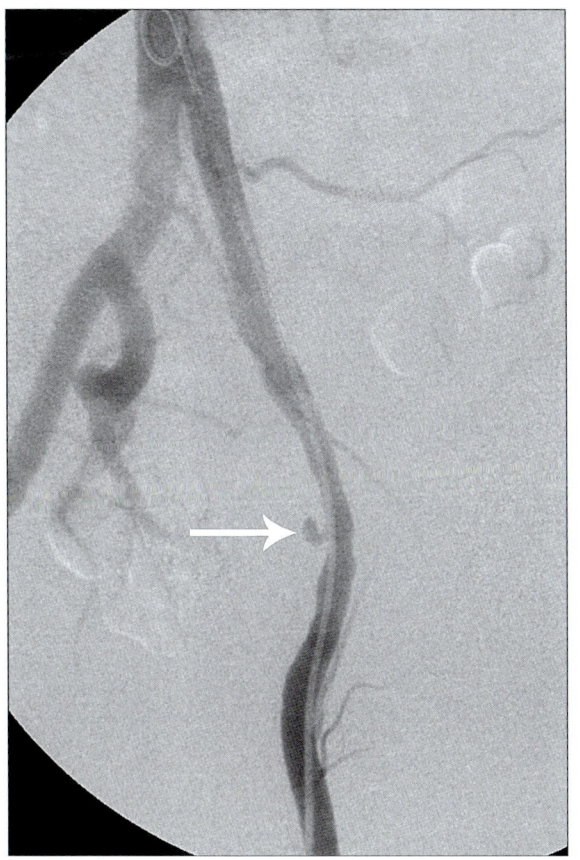

Figure 2. Pelvic arteriogram. There is a mild, smooth stenosis of the left external iliac artery consistent with a radiation-induced stricture. There is a small pseudoaneurysm *(arrow)* arising from the medial wall of the distal left external iliac artery, a likely site of the arterial–ureteral fistula.

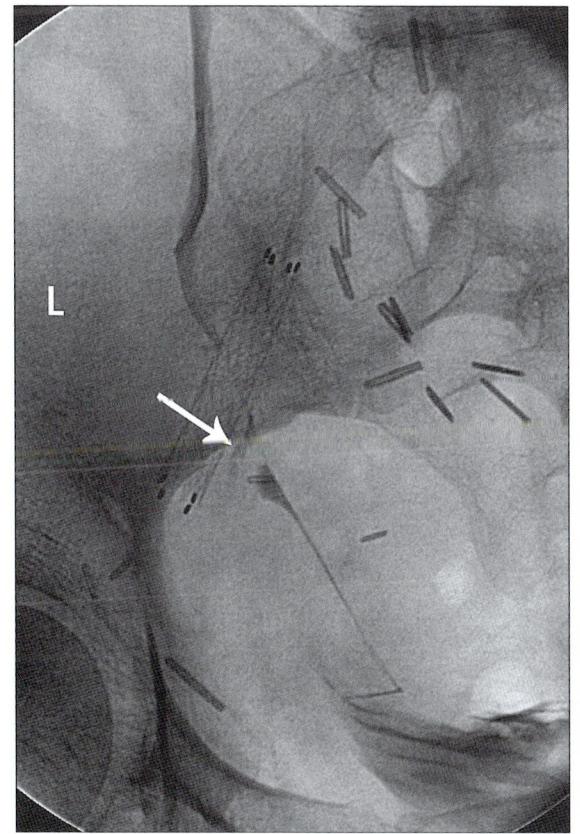

Figure 4. Antegrade urogram performed from a catheter positioned in the distal left ureter shows a long-segment, high-grade stricture of the distal left ureter. There is a small amount of extravasation from the distal left ureter *(arrow)*.

Case 51

DEMOGRAPHICS/CLINICAL HISTORY

A 35-year-old man with postoperative pseudoaneurysm of the celiac trunk, undergoing CT angiogram and arteriography.

DISCUSSION

History/Indications for Procedure

A 35-year-old man underwent a complex total gastrectomy and esophagojejunostomy for gastric carcinoma. At the time of surgery, the patient required thromboembolectomy of the celiac, hepatic, and splenic arteries, and a small pseudoaneurysm was identified on postoperative CT.

Procedure

Endovascular management of celiac trunk pseudoaneurysm

Pre-procedure Imaging

A CT angiogram performed 6 weeks after surgery shows a 2.5-cm × 2.5-cm pseudoaneurysm adjacent to the celiac trunk and proximal splenic artery (Fig. 1). The pseudoaneurysm has enlarged since the prior study.

Intraprocedural Findings

A celiac arteriogram shows the neck of the pseudoaneurysm to arise from the celiac trunk, at the origin of the splenic artery (Fig. 2). The splenic artery was embolized with coils (Fig. 3), and an 8-mm balloon-expandable covered stent was placed across the defect in the celiac trunk (Fig. 4).

Follow-up and Complications

A completion arteriogram showed no further filling of the pseudoaneurysm, and follow-up CT showed successful thrombosis of the pseudoaneurysm. Subsequent abdominal CT scans showed complete resolution of the pseudoaneurysm.

Suggested Readings

Basile A, Lupattelli T, Magnano M, et al: Treatment of a celiac trunk aneurysm close to the hepato-splenic bifurcation by using hepatic stent-graft implantation and splenic artery embolization. Cardiovasc Intervent Radiol 30:126, 2007.

Onal B, Ilgit ET, Kosar S, et al: Endovascular treatment of peripheral vascular lesions with stent-grafts. Diagn Intervent Radiol 11:170, 2005.

Rossi M, Rebonato A, Greco L, et al: Endovascular exclusion of visceral artery aneurysms with stent-grafts: Technique and long-term follow-up. Cardiovasc Intervent Radiol 31:36, 2008.

Case 51   103

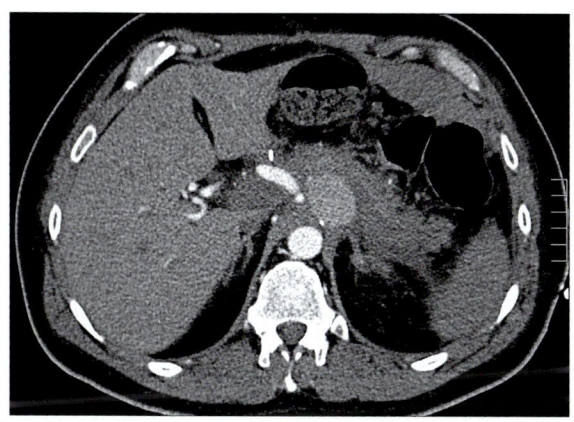

Figure 1. Contrast-enhanced CT scan of abdomen shows 2.5-cm pseudoaneurysm just to the left of the celiac trunk, at the level of the origin of the splenic artery.

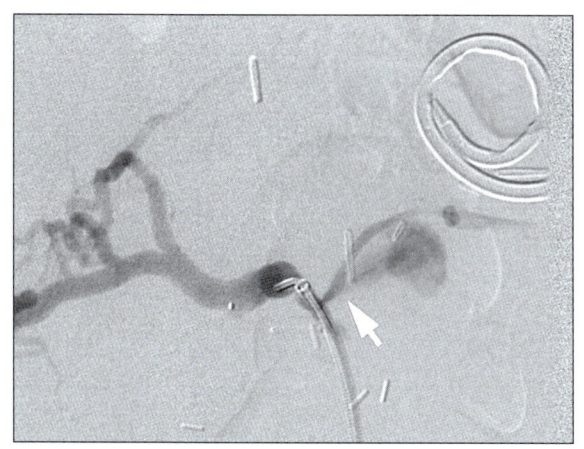

Figure 2. Celiac arteriogram shows filling of pseudoaneurysm from a rent in the celiac trunk *(arrow)*, at the origin of the splenic artery.

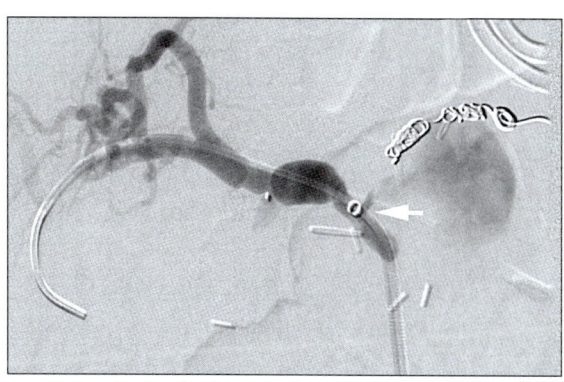

Figure 3. Proximal splenic artery has been completely embolized with coils. There is continued filling of pseudoaneurysm from the rent in the celiac trunk *(arrow)*.

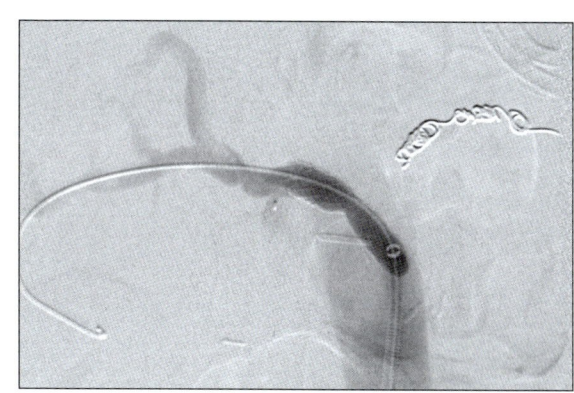

Figure 4. Defect in celiac trunk has been covered with balloon-expandable stent graft. There is no further filling of pseudoaneurysm.

Case 52

DEMOGRAPHICS/CLINICAL HISTORY

A 53-year-old woman with chronic hepatitis C, hepatic cirrhosis, and an incidental finding of splenic artery aneurysm, undergoing computed tomography (CT), arteriography, and embolization.

DISCUSSION

History/Indications for Procedure
A 53-year-old woman has chronic hepatitis C and hepatic cirrhosis. She had a splenic artery aneurysm incidentally discovered on a CT scan performed for other reasons.

Procedure
Splenic artery aneurysm

Pre-procedure Imaging
Contrast-enhanced CT demonstrates a 4-cm × 4-cm splenic artery aneurysm (Fig. 1).

Intraprocedural Findings
A large, saccular aneurysm involves the main splenic artery (Fig. 2). The artery distal to the aneurysm was catheterized with a microcatheter, and the main splenic artery was embolized with coils starting distal to the aneurysm and ending proximal to the aneurysm (Figs. 3 and 4).

Follow-up and Complications
The splenic artery aneurysm was thrombosed on follow-up CT. There was partial infarction of the spleen, likely due to distal migration of one of the coils.

Suggested Readings
Grego FG, Lepidi S, Ragazzi R, et al: Visceral artery aneurysms: A single center experience. Cardiovasc Surg 11:19-25, 2003.

Sueyoshi E, Sakamoto I, Nakashima K, et al: Visceral and peripheral arterial pseudoaneurysms. AJR Am J Roentgenol 185:741-749.

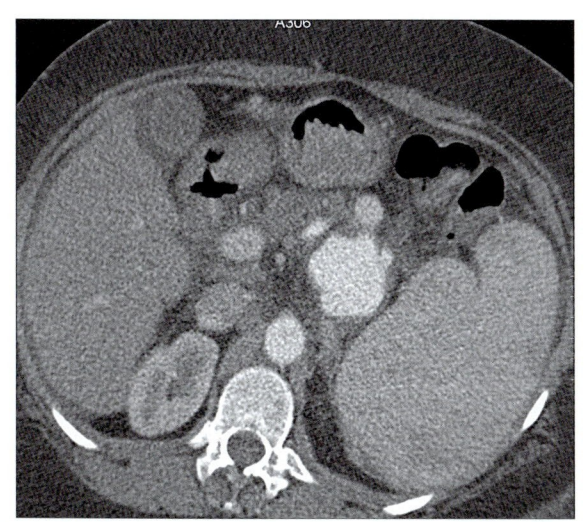

Figure 1. Contrast-enhanced CT demonstrates a saccular aneurysm of the main splenic artery. The aneurysm wall is slightly irregular, although there is no evidence for associated hemorrhage.

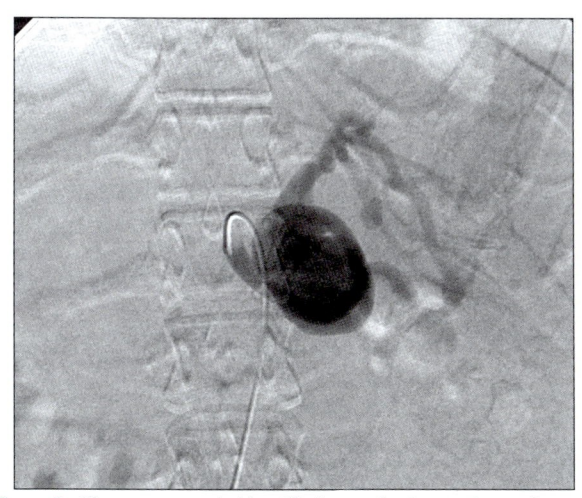

Figure 2. The aneurysm is identified on splenic arteriography.

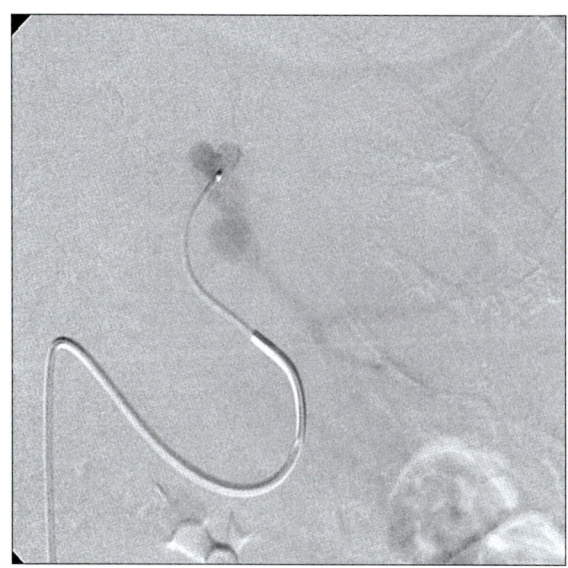

Figure 3. The splenic artery distal to the aneurysm is catheterized with a microcatheter.

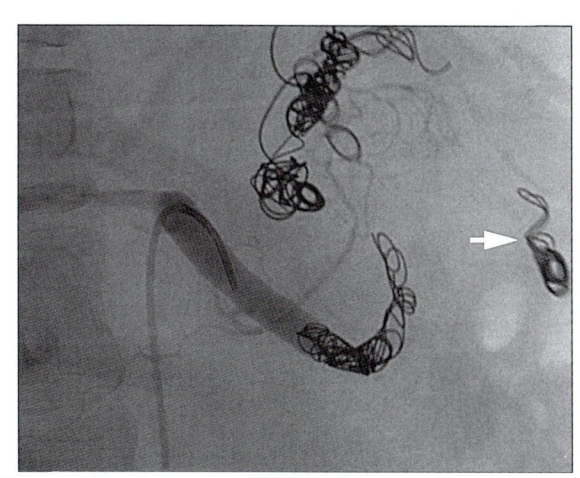

Figure 4. The splenic artery was embolized with coils starting distal to the aneurysm and ending just proximal to the aneurysm. One of the coils migrated distally *(arrow)*, which resulted in partial infarction of the spleen.

Case 53

Robert G. Dixon, MD

DEMOGRAPHICS/CLINICAL HISTORY

A 68-year-old woman with history of Crohn's disease and COPD on chronic steroids, found to have multiple hepatic aneurysms of uncertain etiology.

DISCUSSION

History/Indications for Procedure
A 68-year-old woman with 3 days of abdominal pain found to have multiple aneurysms with associated dissections involving the hepatic arteries, including a pseudoaneurysm arising from the left hepatic artery.

Procedure
Percutaneous thrombin injection of hepatic artery pseudoaneurysm

Pre-procedure Imaging
CT of the abdomen identified hemoperitoneum and a pseudoaneurysm arising from the left hepatic artery (Fig. 1).

Intraprocedural Findings
Ultrasound allowed visualization of the pseudoaneurysm, with a small neck at the inferior aspect (Fig. 2). This was targeted with a 22-gauge needle, allowing injection of thrombin (Fig. 3).

Follow-up and Complications
CT performed 1 day later showed thrombosis of the aneurysm (Fig. 4).

Suggested Readings
Krueger K, Zaehringer M, Lackner K: Percutaneous treatment of a splenic artery pseudoaneurysm by thrombin injection. J Vasc Interv Radiol 16:1023–1025, 2005.

Philleaul F, Beuf O: Diagnosis of splanchnic artery aneurysms and pseudoaneurysms, with special reference to contrast enhanced 3D magnetic resonance angiography: A review. Acta Radiol 45: 702–708, 2004.

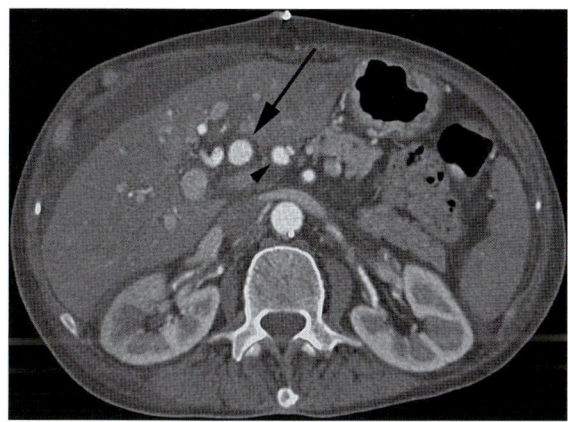

Figure 1. CT of the abdomen demonstrates a pseudoaneurysm arising from the left hepatic artery *(arrow)*. Note the dissection of the ectatic common hepatic artery *(arrowhead)*.

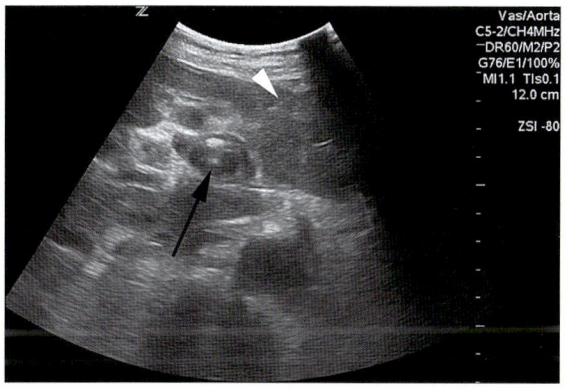

Figure 3. Ultrasound showing a 22-gauge needle *(arrowhead)* entering from an anterior approach, with the tip of the needle *(arrow)* in the pseudoaneurysm. Thrombin injection has been initiated, with early thrombus formation seen adjacent to the needle tip.

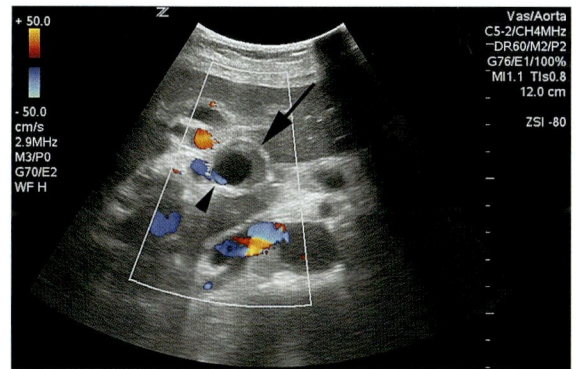

Figure 2. Ultrasound with color flow Doppler shows the pseudoaneurysm *(arrow)* with a small neck along its caudal margin *(arrowhead)*.

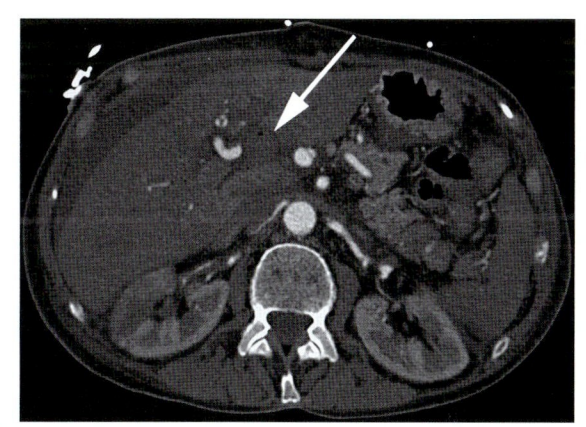

Figure 4. CT performed 1 day later shows thrombosis of the pseudoaneurysm *(arrow)*.

Case 54

DEMOGRAPHICS/CLINICAL HISTORY

A 63-year-old man with a 7.3-cm infrarenal abdominal aortic aneurysm undergoing endovascular aneurysm repair, evaluated with CT.

DISCUSSION

History/Indications for Procedure
The aneurysm has exceeded the 5- to 5.5-cm diameter threshold, when the risk of rupture increases, and intervention becomes indicated (Fig. 1).

Procedure
Endovascular repair of abdominal aortic aneurysm

Pre-procedure Imaging
Contrast-enhanced CT was performed to determine whether the patient is a candidate for endograft placement, including assessment of the diameter, length, and angulation of the aneurysm neck; size of the aneurysm; and size, degree of calcification, and tortuosity of the iliac arteries.

Intraprocedural Findings
A Zenith stent graft (Cook, Bloomington, IN) was placed. After endograft placement, an aortogram was performed to evaluate for endoleak or other stent graft–related complications (Fig. 2).

Follow-up and Complications
After stent graft placement, the aneurysm was followed with cross-sectional imaging to assess aneurysm size and potential complications, such as the presence of an endoleak (Figs. 3 and 4).

Suggested Readings
Brewster DC, Cronenwett JL, Hallett JW, et al: Guidelines for the treatment of abdominal aortic aneurysms. J Vasc Surg 37:1106-1117, 2003.

Drury D, Michaels JA, Jones L, et al: Systematic review of recent evidence for the safety and efficacy of elective endovascular repair in the management of infrarenal abdominal aortic aneurysm. Br J Surg 92:937-946, 2005.

EVAR trial participants: Endovascular aneurysm repair versus open repair in patients with abdominal aortic aneurysm (EVAR trial 1): Randomised controlled trial. Lancet 365:2179-2186, 2005.

Rose J: Stent grafts for unruptured abdominal aortic aneurysms: Current status. Cardiovasc Intervent Radiol 29:332-343, 2006.

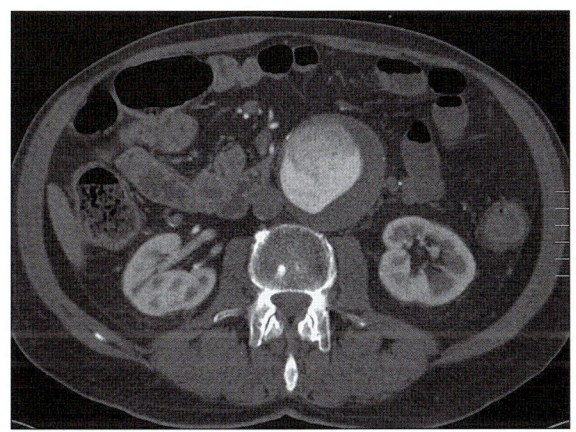

Figure 1. Selected image from CT before aneurysm repair. The aneurysm sac measures 7.3 cm in diameter.

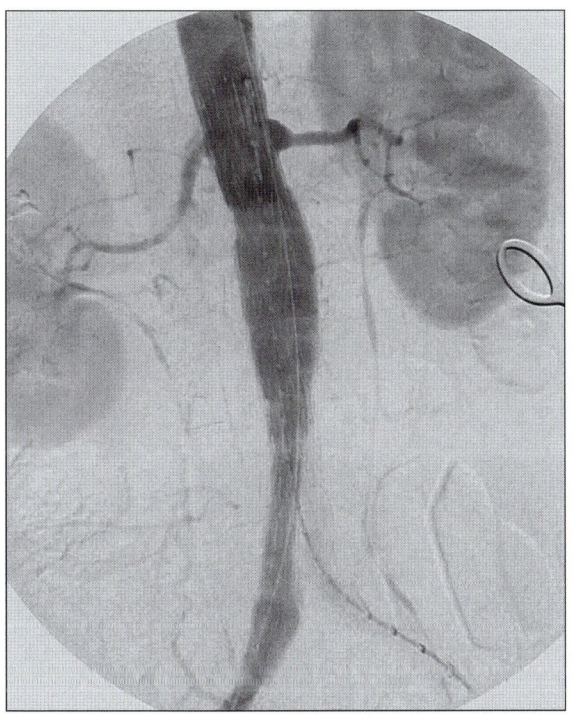

Figure 2. Post–stent graft placement aortogram shows exclusion of the aneurysm sac with no visible endoleak.

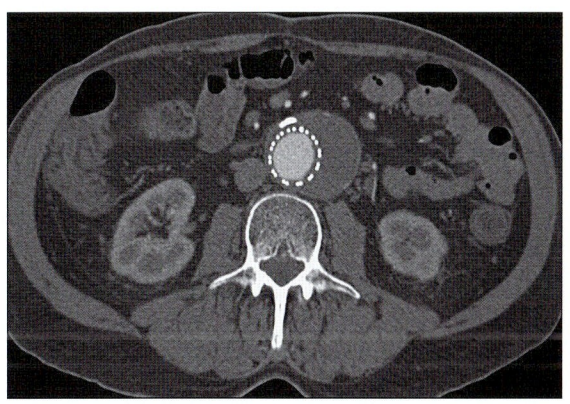

Figure 3. CT scan performed 8 months after stent graft was placed shows thrombosis of the aneurysm sac and no endoleak. The aneurysm sac size decreased from 7.3 to 5.8 cm.

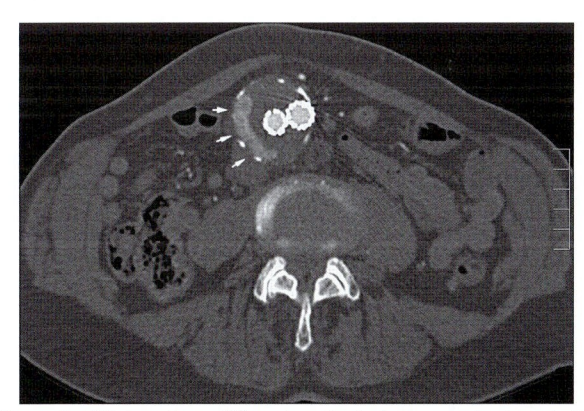

Figure 4. CT scan in a different patient shows contrast material within the aneurysm sac after stent graft placement *(arrowheads)*. This finding is indicative of an endoleak.

Case 55

DEMOGRAPHICS/CLINICAL HISTORY

A 70-year-old woman with a ruptured abdominal aortic aneurysm.

DISCUSSION

History/Indications for Procedure
A 70-year-old woman with known abdominal aortic aneurysm presents to the emergency department with sudden onset of left flank pain and hypotension.

Procedure
Endovascular repair of ruptured abdominal aortic aneurysm

Pre-procedure Imaging
Contrast-enhanced CT of the abdomen shows a 6.4-cm abdominal aortic aneurysm. There is irregularity of the left anterolateral aneurysm wall and a large retroperitoneal hematoma (Fig. 1).

Intraprocedural Findings
The abdominal aortic aneurysm was treated with the placement of an Excluder (Gore, Flagstaff, AZ) stent graft. Midline abdominal laparotomy was performed at the time of repair for abdominal decompression and hematoma evacuation (Figs. 2,3).

Follow-up and Complications
The patient was discharged from the hospital 9 days after aneurysm repair. She has done well since; recent CT (Fig. 4) shows the aneurysm sac has nearly completely resolved.

Suggested Readings
Harkin DW, Dillon M, Blair PH, et al.: Endovascular ruptured abdominal aortic aneurysm repair (EVRAR): A systematic review. Eur J Vasc Endovasc Surg 34:673–681, 2007.

Hoornweg LL, Wisselink W, Vahl A, et al.: The Amsterdam Acute Aneurysm Trial: Suitability and application rate for endovascular repair of ruptured abdominal aortic aneurysms. Eur J Vasc Endovasc Surg 33:679–683, 2007.

Greco G, Egorova N, Anderson PL, et al.: Outcomes of endovascular treatment of ruptured abdominal aortic aneurysms. J Vasc Surg 43:45–59, 2006.

Visser JJ, van Sambeek MR, Hamza TH, et al.: Ruptured abdominal aortic aneurysms: Endovascular repair versus open surgery—systemic review. Radiology 245:122–129, 2007.

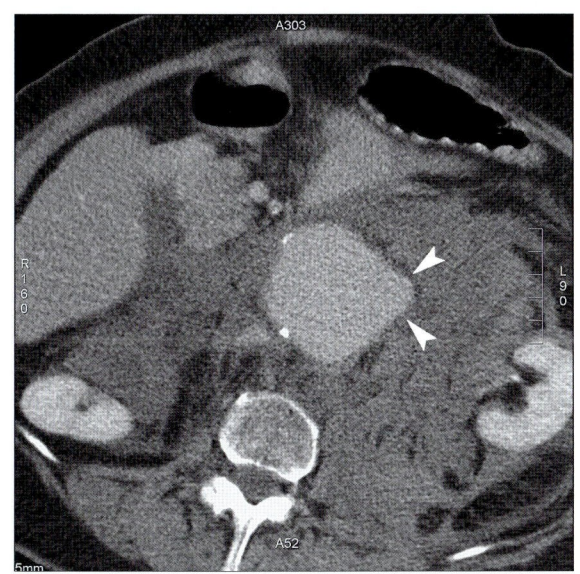

Figure 1. Contrast-enhanced CT shows an infrarenal abdominal aortic aneurysm. In this image, there is protuberance of the left lateral wall *(arrowheads)* and a large retroperitoneal hematoma.

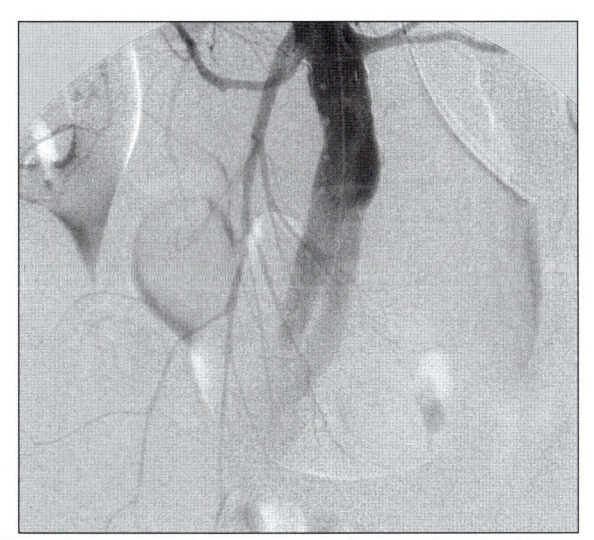

Figure 2. Intraoperative aortogram after stent graft placement shows an adequate seal at the proximal attachment site.

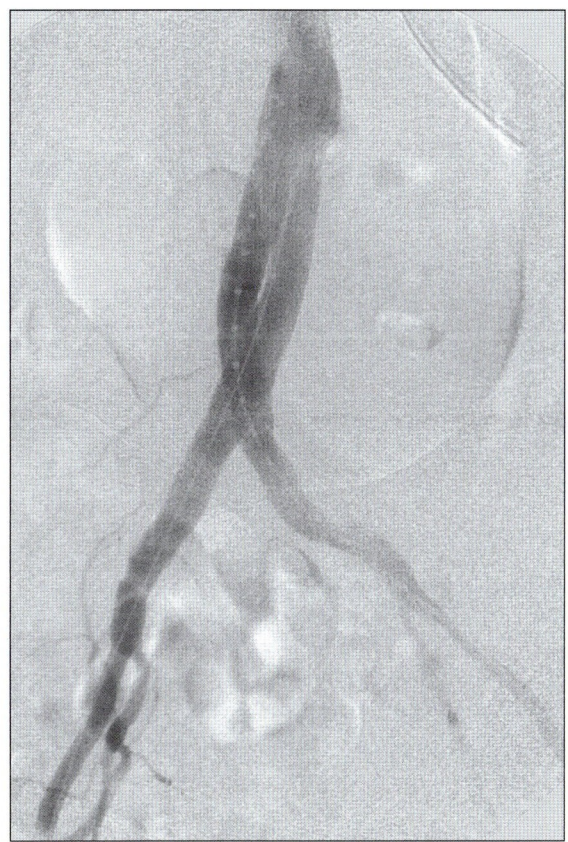

Figure 3. Intraoperative aortogram after stent graft placement shows exclusion of the ruptured aneurysm. No endoleak was seen.

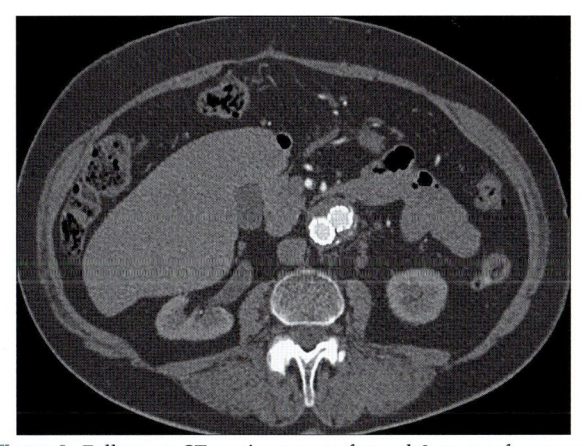

Figure 4. Follow-up CT angiogram performed 2 years after aneurysm repair shows minimal residual aneurysm sac.

Case 56

DEMOGRAPHICS/CLINICAL HISTORY

A 64-year-old man with a mycotic pseudoaneurysm associated with an aortoenteric fistula, undergoing CT and aortogram.

DISCUSSION

History/Indications for Procedure

A 64-year-old man presents with fever and pain 2 weeks after endograft placement for ruptured aortic plaque. After admission to the hospital, the patient became hypotensive, requiring emergent aortic repair.

Procedure

Endograft placement, aortoenteric fistula repair

Pre-procedure Imaging

CT scan shows heterogeneous soft tissue around the abdominal aorta (Fig. 1) with obscuration of the fat plane with the duodenum, which is concerning for an aortoenteric fistula. There is an aortic pseudoaneurysm below the inferior attachment site of the aortic endograft (Fig. 2).

Intraprocedural Findings

An intraoperative aortogram showed an aortic pseudoaneurysm arising just inferior to the previously placed tube graft. A rifampin-soaked, bifurcated aortic stent graft (Aneuryx, Medtronic, Santa Rosa, CA) was placed (Fig. 3).

Follow-up and Complications

The patient was discharged from the hospital 2 weeks later, but returned with abdominal pain. A follow-up CT scan showed gas within the endograft (Fig. 4), indicating graft infection; the patient was taken emergently to the operating room for a right axillobifemoral artery bypass graft, and aortic resection and primary closure of the duodenal defect was performed 3 days later.

Suggested Readings

Armonstrong PA, Back MR, Wilson JS, et al: Improved outcomes in the recent management of secondary aortoenteric fistula. J Vasc Surg 42:660, 2005.

Bergqvist D, Bjorck M, Nyman R: Secondary aortoenteric fistula after endovascular aortic interventions: A systematic literature review. J Vasc Interv Radiol 19:163, 2008.

Burks JA Jr, Faries PL, Gravereaux EC, et al: Endovascular repair of bleeding aortoenteric fistulas: A 5-year experience. J Vasc Surg 34:1055, 2001.

Hagspiel KD, Turba UC, Bozlar U, et al: Diagnosis of aortoenteric fistulas with CT angiography. J Vasc Interv Radiol 18:497, 2007.

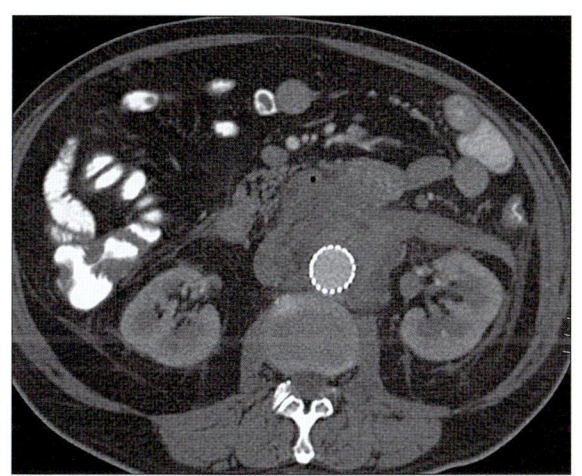

Figure 1. Contrast-enhanced CT scan of abdomen shows heterogeneous soft tissue around aortic stent graft. There is loss of the fat plane between the aorta and duodenum, raising the suspicion of an aortoenteric fistula.

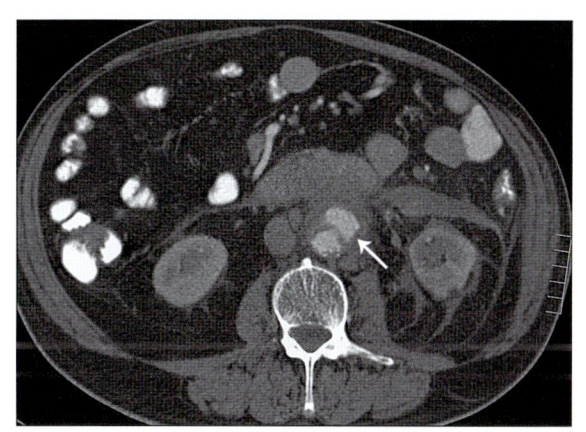

Figure 2. Contrast-enhanced CT scan of abdomen at level just below aortic tube graft shows pseudoaneurysm arising from anterolateral wall of abdominal aorta *(arrow)*.

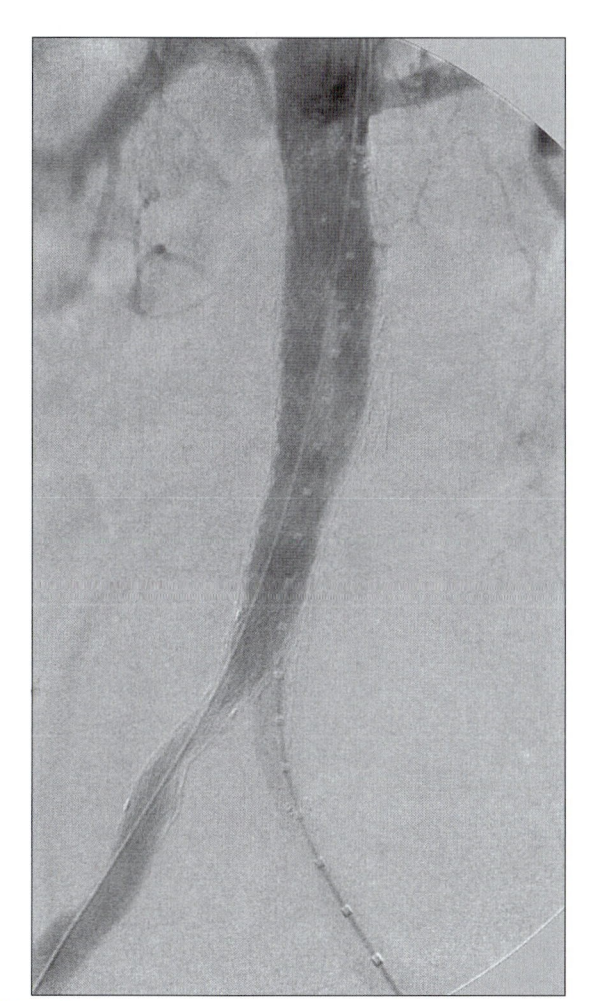

Figure 3. Intraoperative aortogram after stent graft placement. There has been exclusion of aortic pseudoaneurysm, and no endoleak is seen.

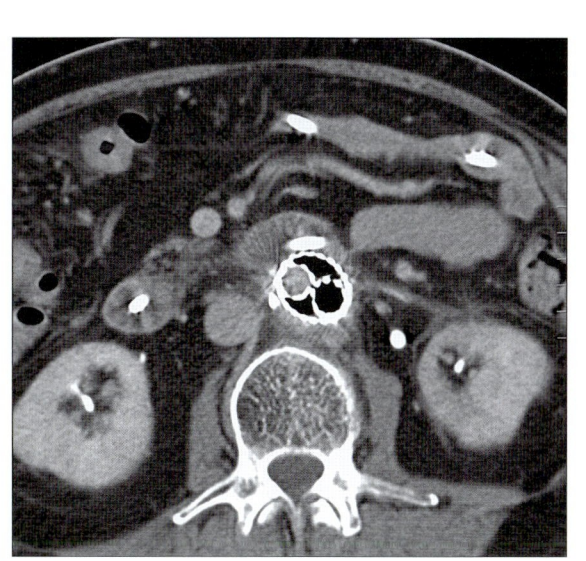

Figure 4. Follow-up CT scan 2 months after endograft placement shows air within lumen of stent graft, a finding concerning for persistent aortoenteric fistula.

Case 57

DEMOGRAPHICS/CLINICAL HISTORY

An 80-year-old man with a 6.4-cm juxtarenal abdominal aortic aneurysm undergoing endovascular aneurysm repair.

DISCUSSION

History/Indications for Procedure
An 80-year-old man had a 6.4-cm juxtarenal abdominal aortic aneurysm.

Procedure
Endovascular repair of juxtarenal aortic aneurysm

Pre-procedure Imaging
Contrast-enhanced computed tomography (CT) demonstrates a juxtarenal abdominal aortic aneurysm (Fig. 1). The aneurysm extends to the right common iliac artery bifurcation, and the patient underwent preoperative embolization of the right internal iliac artery.

Intraprocedural Findings
The abdominal aortic aneurysm was treated using a fenestrated endograft. The graft had small rings sewn into the fabric that identified the sites of the fenestrations (Fig. 2), and through these rings the renal arteries were cannulated and stented with balloon-expandable covered stents.

Follow-up and Complications
Follow-up CT demonstrated exclusion of the aneurysm sac without endoleak (Figs. 3 and 4). The patient's renal function has remained stable, and the renal artery stents have remained patent.

Suggested Readings

Haddad F, Greenberg RK, Walker E, et al: Fenestrated endovascular grafting: The renal side of the story. J Vasc Surg 41:181-190, 2005.

Rockman C: Reducing complications by better case selection: Anatomic considerations. Semin Vasc Surg 17:298-306, 2004.

Zarins CK, Bloch DA, Crabtree T, et al: Stent graft migration after endovascular aneurysm repair: Importance of proximal fixation. J Vasc Surg 38:1264-1272, 2003;discussion 1272.

Case 57   **115**

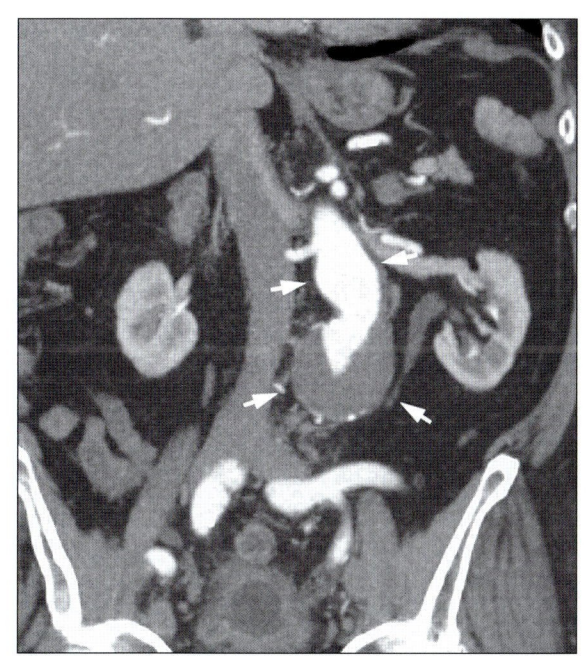

Figure 1. Coronal image from a contrast-enhanced CT scan demonstrates a juxtarenal aortic aneurysm. The aneurysm has a bilobed configuration *(arrows)*.

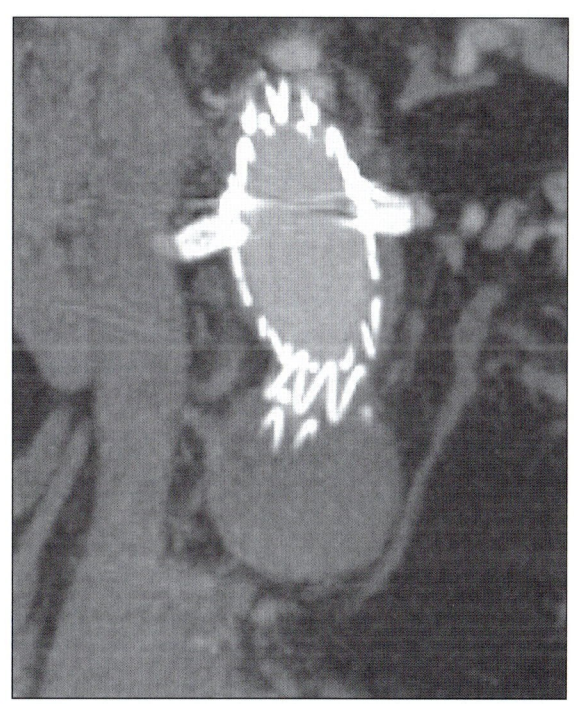

Figure 3. Coronal image from the contrast-enhanced CT scans 1 month after stent-graft placement demonstrates the stent graft extending to the level of the superior mesenteric artery with a bilateral renal stent in place. No endoleak occurred.

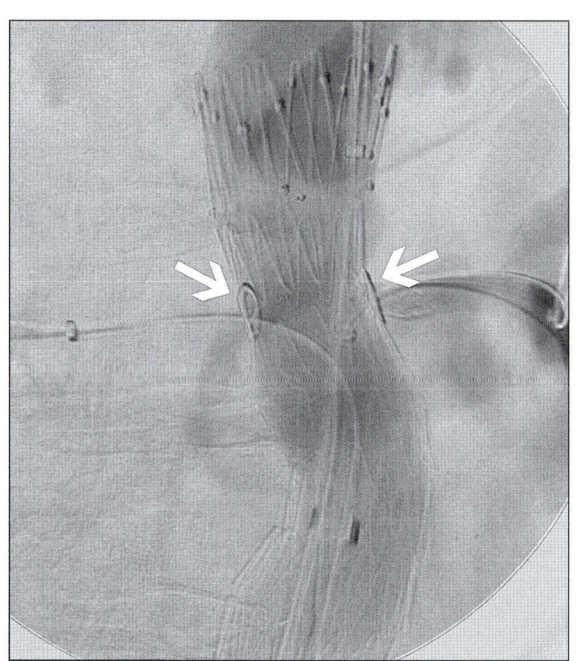

Figure 2. Image from an intraoperative aortogram during graft placement shows the small rings *(arrows)* that were sewn to the fabric of the graft to identify the site of fenestration. The renal arteries have been cannulated through the rings for covered stent placement.

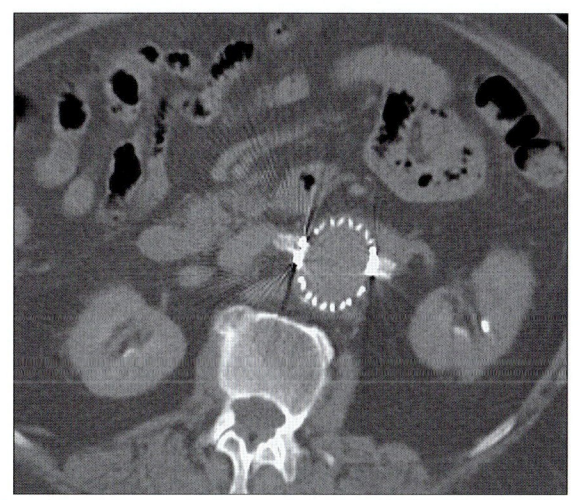

Figure 4. Axial image on follow-up CT confirms the presence of bilateral renal stents that have been placed through the fabric of the endograft.

Case 58

DEMOGRAPHICS/CLINICAL HISTORY

An 85-year-old man with a 6.5-cm juxtarenal abdominal aortic aneurysm.

DISCUSSION

History/Indications for Procedure
An 85-year-old man with a 6.5-cm juxtarenal abdominal aortic aneurysm.

Procedure
Endovascular repair of juxtarenal abdominal aortic aneurysm

Pre-procedure Imaging
Contrast-enhanced CT of the abdomen shows a 6.5-cm juxtarenal abdominal aortic aneurysm (Fig. 1).

Intraprocedural Findings
A Zenith stent-graft (Cook, Bloomington, IN) was modified with the addition of bilateral fenestrations, marked with radiopaque wire sutured to the graft. After partial deployment of the stent-graft, the renal arteries were catheterized through the fenestrations, and bilateral, covered balloon-expandable stents were deployed in the renal arteries (Figs. 2,3).

Follow-up and Complications
The patient was observed in the ICU the night of the procedure for treatment for postoperative hypotension; the patient recovered uneventfully and was discharged from the hospital on postoperative day number 8. Follow-up CT of the abdomen shows exclusion of the aneurysm, with no evidence for endoleak (Fig. 4).

Suggested Readings

Chuter TA: Fenestrated and branched stent-grafts for thoracoabdominal, pararenal and juxtarenal aortic aneurysm repair. Semin Vasc Surg 20:90–96, 2007.

Muhs BE, Verhoeven EL, Zeebregts CJ, et al.: Mid-term results of endovascular aneurysm repair with branched and fenestrated endografts. J Vasc Surg 44:9–15, 2006.

Rockman C: Reducing complications by better case selection: Anatomic considerations. Semin Vasc Surg 17:298–306, 2004.

Case 58   117

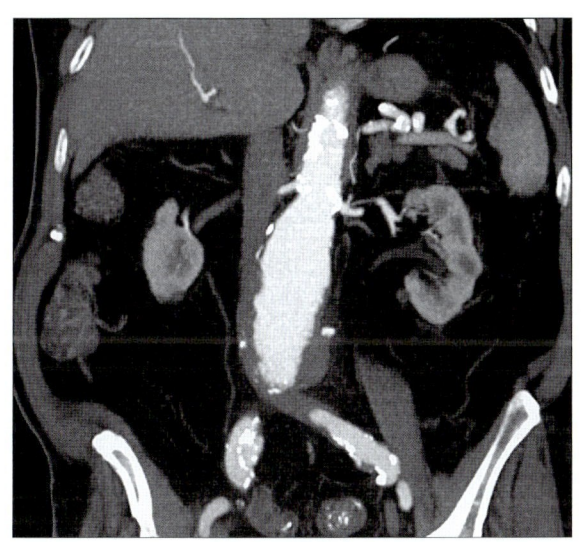

Figure 1. Coronal reconstruction from contrast-enhanced CT shows the presence of a juxtarenal abdominal aortic aneurysm.

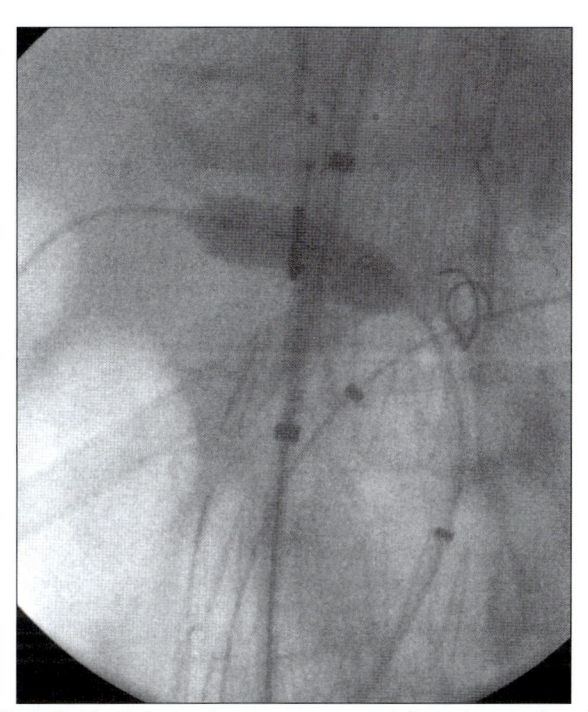

Figure 3. The right renal artery was successfully catheterized, and a balloon-expandable covered stent was deployed.

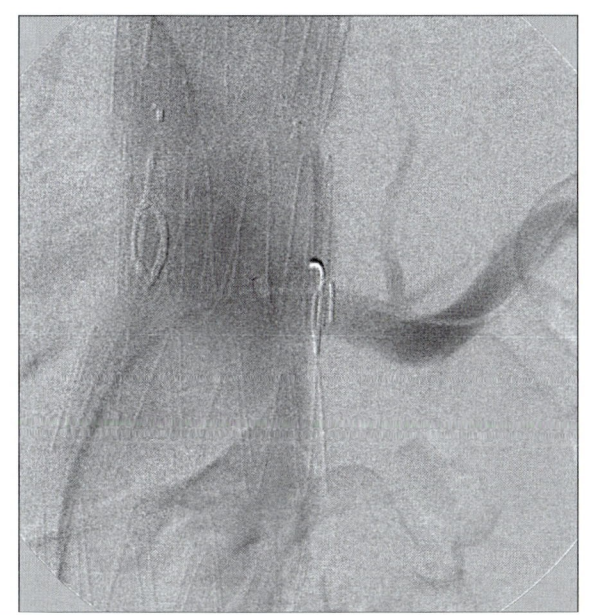

Figure 2. Intraoperative angiogram shows the successful catheterization of the left renal artery through the marked graft fenestration.

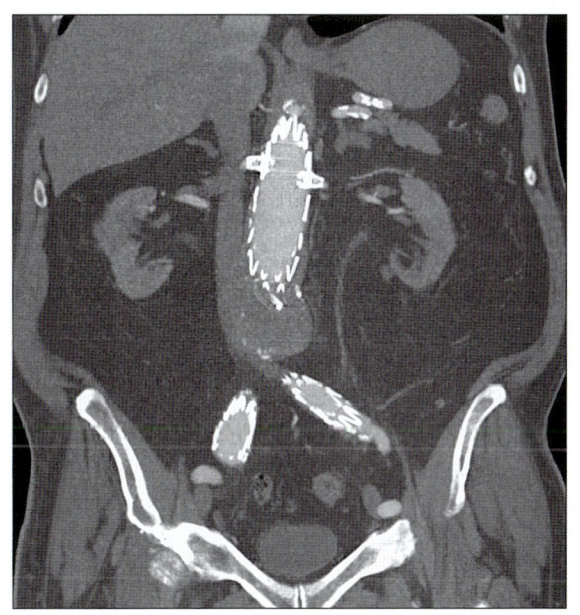

Figure 4. Follow-up contrast-enhanced abdominal CT shows the presence of the renal artery stents through the stent-graft fenestrations.

Case 59

DEMOGRAPHICS/CLINICAL HISTORY

An 84-year-old man with endoleak and enlarging aneurysm sac on surveillance CT imaging.

DISCUSSION

History/Indications for Procedure
In this patient status post–endovascular abdominal aortic aneurysm repair, surveillance CT scan shows contrast material within the aneurysm sac and a slight increase in aneurysm sac size.

Procedure
Management of abdominal endoleak after endovascular abdominal aortic aneurysm repair

Pre-procedure Imaging
Contrast-enhanced CT scan shows contrast material within the aneurysm sac (i.e., endoleak) (Fig.1). The endoleak was classified as type Ia by angiography (not shown).

Intraprocedural Findings
The sac was accessed using a translumbar approach under CT guidance (Fig. 2). Direct sac injection showed filling of the aneurysm sac (Fig. 3). The endoleak was embolized using a combination of platinum coils and n-butyl-cyanoacrylate (nBCA).

Follow-up and Complications
Follow-up CT 3 months after endoleak embolization confirms persistent obliteration of the endoleak (Fig. 4). The aneurysm sac size stabilized.

Suggested Readings
Baum RA, Cope C, Fairman RM, et al: Translumbar embolization of type 2 endoleaks after endovascular repair of abdominal aortic aneurysms. J Vasc Interv Radiol 12:111-116, 2001.

Stavropoulos SW, Marin H, Fairman RM, et al: Recurrent endoleak detection and measurement of aneurysm size with CTA after coil embolization of endoleaks. J Vasc Interv Radiol 16:1313-1317, 2005.

Veith FJ, Baum RA, Ohki T, et al: Nature and significance of endoleaks and endotension: Summary of opinions expressed at an international conference. J Vasc Surg 35:1029-1035, 2002.

Case 59   119

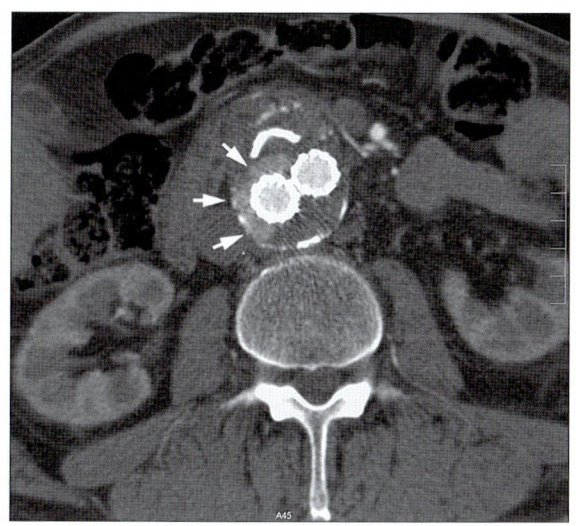

Figure 1. Axial image from contrast-enhanced CT shows enhancement in the aneurysm sac anterior and lateral to the right iliac limb of the endograft *(arrowheads)*.

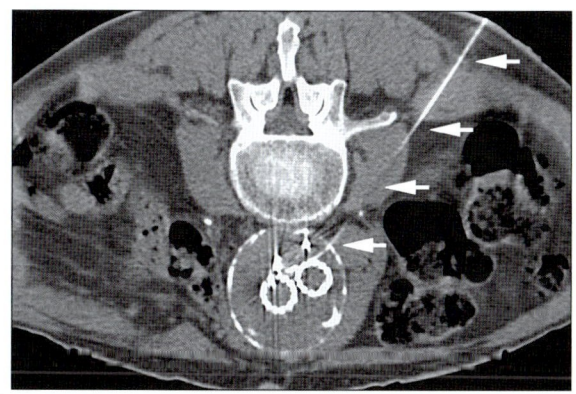

Figure 2. The aneurysm sac was accessed directly with a right translumbar approach using CT guidance.

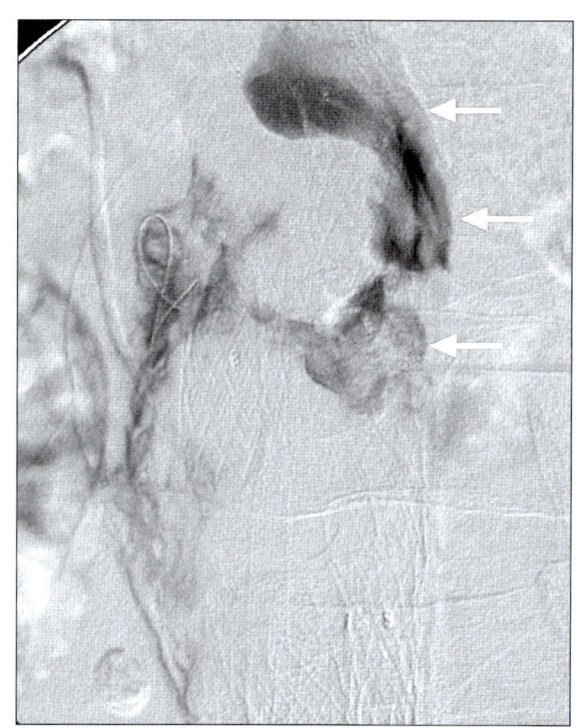

Figure 3. Sac injection shows filling of the aneurysm sac with contrast material tracking along the endograft *(arrows)* to the proximal attachment site.

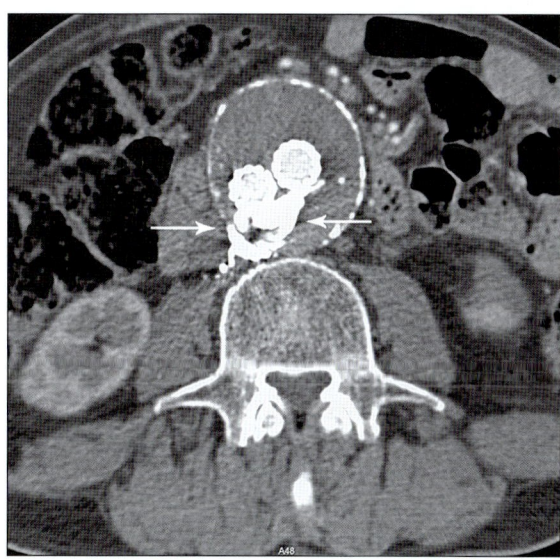

Figure 4. CT performed 3 months after the embolization shows high-density material corresponding to the *n*BCA posterior to the endograft *(arrows)*. No endoleak was present, and the aneurysm sac size had stabilized.

Case 60

DEMOGRAPHICS/CLINICAL HISTORY

A 77-year-old man with an endoleak after endovascular abdominal aortic aneurysm repair, undergoing computed tomography (CT), arteriography, and embolization.

DISCUSSION

History/Indications for Procedure
A 77-year-old man had endovascular aneurysm repair at an outside hospital 1 year earlier. The aneurysm sac has continued to enlarge, despite branch vessel embolization at an outside facility.

Procedure
Type II endoleak repair

Pre-procedure Imaging
Contrast-enhanced CT shows a type II endoleak with opacification within the aneurysm sac adjacent to several lumbar arteries and the inferior mesenteric artery (Fig. 1).

Intraprocedural Findings
Right iliac arteriogram demonstrates filling of the aneurysm sac through the right iliolumbar artery (Fig. 2). The aneurysm sac was catheterized with a microcatheter, and the endoleak was embolized with *n*-butyl cyanoacrylate and coils (Fig. 3).

Follow-up and Complications
CT scan performed 1 year after embolization demonstrates occlusion of the endoleak (Fig. 4). The aneurysm sac size has decreased.

Suggested Readings
Baum RA, Carpenter JP, Golden MA, et al: Treatment of type 2 endoleaks after endovascular repair of abdominal aortic aneurysms: Comparison of transarterial and translumbar techniques. J Vasc Surg 35:23-29, 2002.

Baum RA, Stavropoulos SW, Fairman RM, Carpenter JP: Endoleaks after endovascular repair of abdominal aortic aneurysms. J Vasc Interv Radiol 14(Pt 1):1111-1117.

Chernyak V, Rozenblit AM, Patlas M, et al: Type II endoleak after endoaortic graft implantation: Diagnosis with helical CT arteriography. Radiology 240:885-893, 2006.

Stavropoulos SW, Marin H, Fairman RM, et al: Recurrent endoleak detection and measurement of aneurysm size with CTA after coil embolization of endoleaks. J Vasc Interv Radiol 16:1313-1317, 2005.

Case 60   121

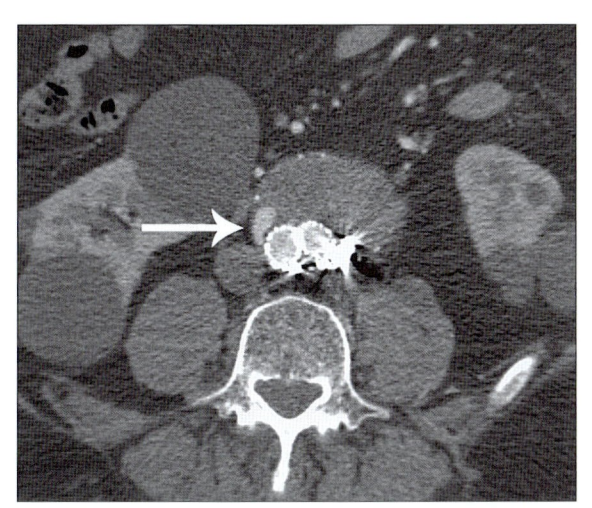

Figure 1. Contrast-enhanced, axial CT image demonstrates a small focus of enhancement within the aneurysm sac that is consistent with a type II endoleak *(arrow)*. Coils are present on the opposite side of the aneurysm sac from a previously attempted endoleak embolization.

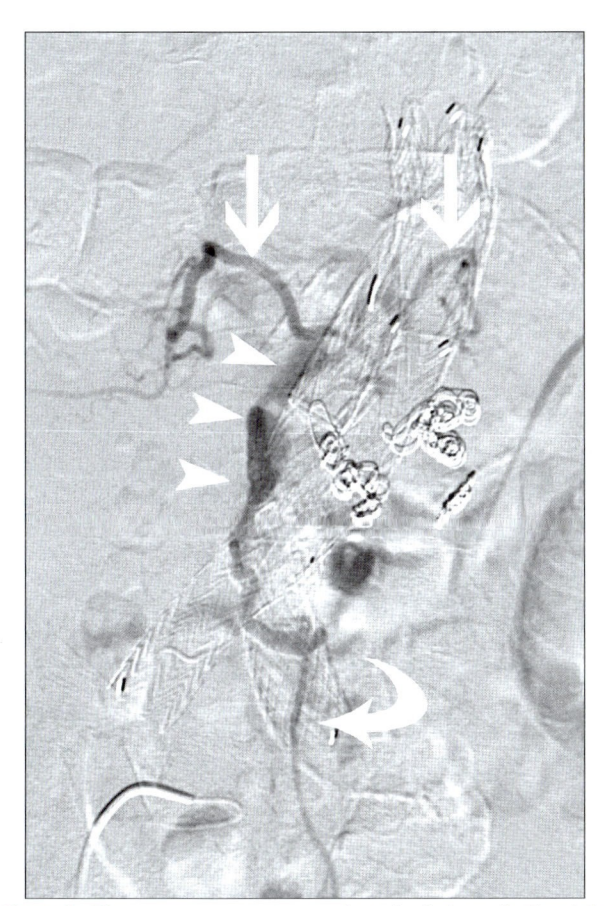

Figure 2. The aneurysm sac was catheterized through the right iliolumbar artery. Contrast injection into the aneurysm sac demonstrates the endoleak *(arrowheads)* with opacification of many efferent lumbar arteries *(arrows)* and the middle sacral artery *(curved arrow)*.

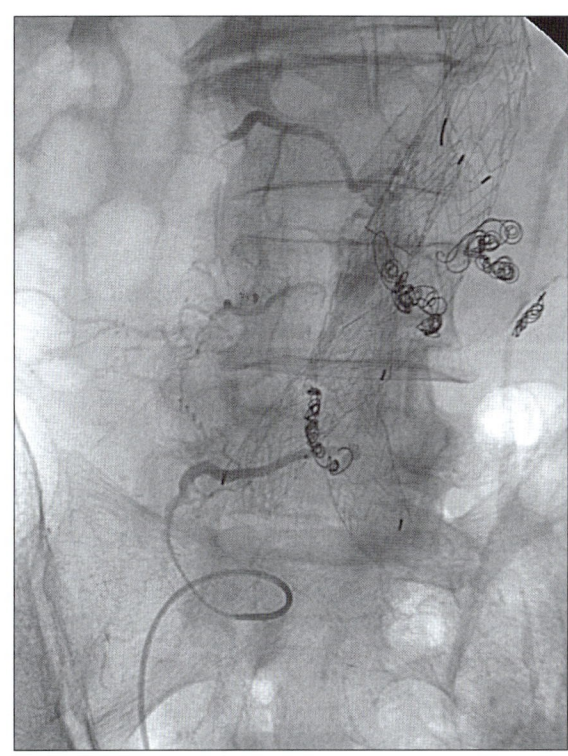

Figure 3. The endoleak was embolized with a combination of *n*-butyl cyanoacrylate and coils.

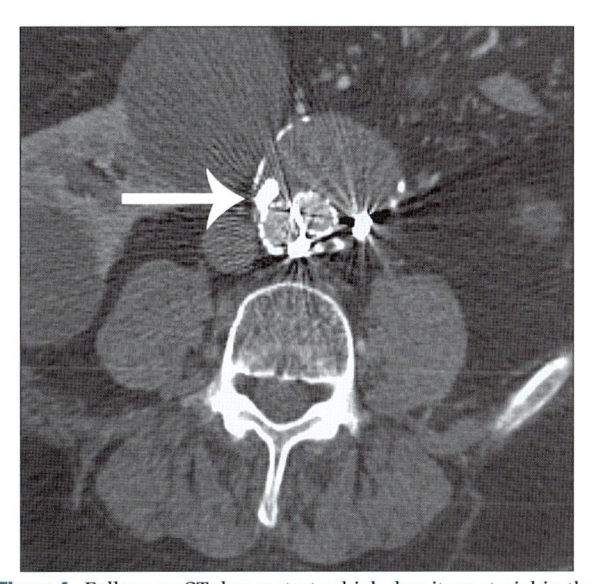

Figure 4. Follow-up CT demonstrates high-density material in the aneurysm sac at the site of the endoleak *(arrow)*. There was no residual endoleak, and the aneurysm sac has decreased in size.

Case 61

DEMOGRAPHICS/CLINICAL HISTORY

An 84-year-old man with a persistent endoleak after endovascular abdominal aortic aneurysm repair, undergoing computed tomography (CT) and arteriography.

DISCUSSION

History/Indications for Procedure
An 84-year-old man underwent endovascular abdominal aortic aneurysm repair 14 months earlier. A persistent endoleak was identified on surveillance imaging.

Procedure
Translumbar embolization of type II endoleak

Pre-procedure Imaging
Contrast-enhanced CT shows contrast enhancement within the right lateral aspect of the aneurysm sac, which is consistent with an endoleak (Fig. 1). The size of the aneurysm sac has remained stable, with a 5.5-cm diameter.

Intraprocedural Findings
Translumbar access to the aneurysm sac was obtained at the level of the endoleak (Fig. 2). The aneurysm sac pressure was elevated, with a systolic pressure of 80 mm Hg. The efferent collaterals were embolized with coils, and the endoleak was embolized with a combination of coils and *n*-butyl-2-cyanoacrylate (NBCA) glue (Trufill, Cordis, Milami Lakes, FL) (Fig. 3).

Follow-up and Complications
No further endoleak was identified on follow-up imaging. Contrast-enhanced CT performed 11 months after embolization shows significant streak artifact within the aneurysm sac from the platinum coils (Fig. 4), but no endoleak is seen, and the aneurysm sac size has begun to shrink.

Suggested Readings
Baum RA, Carpenter JP, Golden MA, et al: Treatment of type 2 endoleaks after endovascular repair of abdominal aortic aneurysms: Comparison of transarterial and translumbar techniques. J Vasc Surg 35:23-29, 2002.

Higashiura W, Greenberg RK, Katz E, et al: Predictive factors, morphologic effects, and proposed treatment paradigm for type II endoleaks after repair of infrarenal abdominal aortic aneurysms. J Vasc Interv Radiol 18:975-981, 2007.

Silverberg D, Baril DT, Ellozy SH, et al: An 8-year experience with type II endoleaks: Natural history suggests selective intervention is a safe approach. J Vasc Surg 44:453-459, 2006.

Stavropoulos SW, Marin H, Fairman RM, et al: Recurrent endoleak detection and measurement of aneurysm size with CTA after coil embolization of endoleaks. J Vasc Interv Radiol 16:1313-1317, 2005.

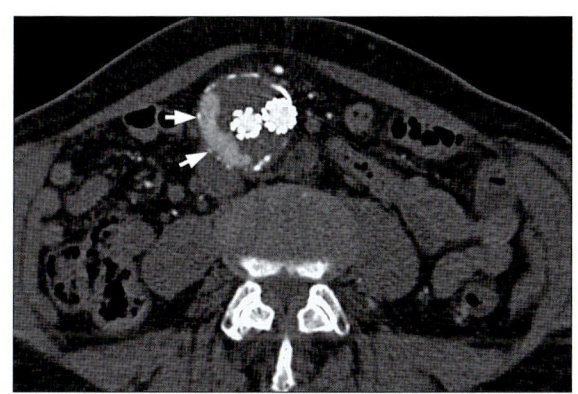

Figure 1. Contrast-enhanced CT shows a large endoleak within the right lateral aspect of the aneurysm sac *(arrows)*.

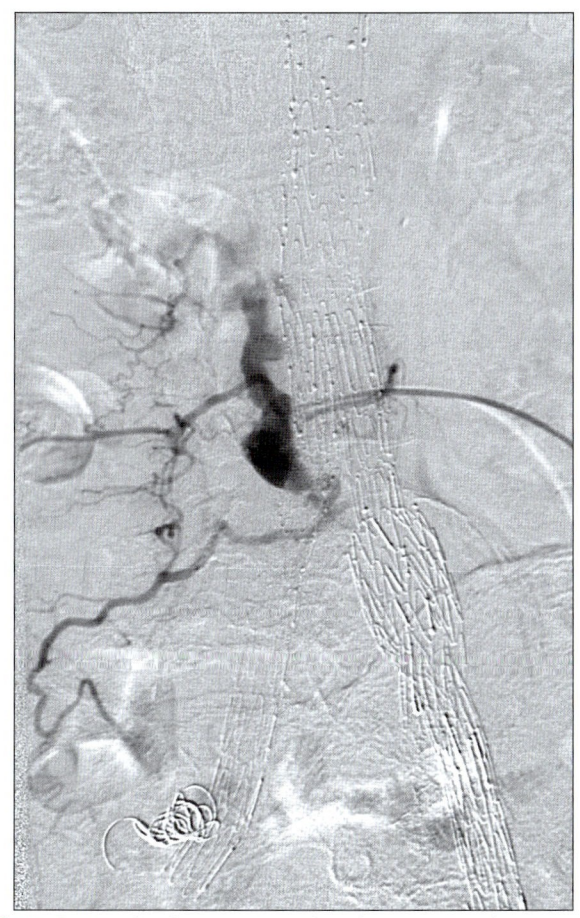

Figure 2. Translumbar arteriography shows a complex type II endoleak with filling of multiple lumbar collaterals.

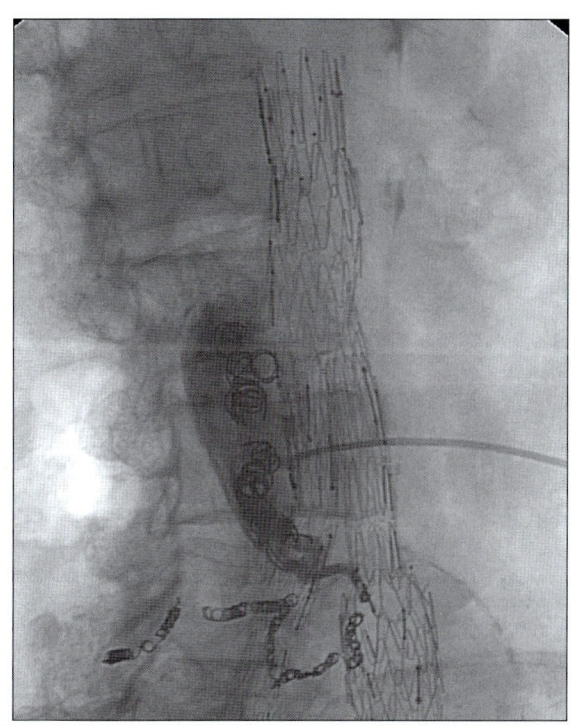

Figure 3. The efferent lumbar arteries were embolized with coils, and the aneurysm sac was embolized with a combination of coils and glue.

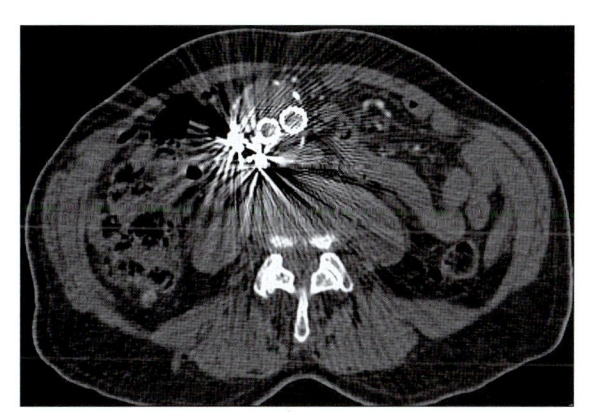

Figure 4. Contrast-enhanced CT 11 months after endoleak embolization shows a significant artifact from the coils in the aneurysm sac, limiting evaluation for a small endoleak. The aneurysm sac size has begun to shrink and is now 4.7 cm in diameter.

Case 62

DEMOGRAPHICS/CLINICAL HISTORY

A 71-year-old man with persistent type II endoleak 2 years after endovascular aneurysm repair, undergoing computed tomography (CT) and arteriography.

DISCUSSION

History/Indications for Procedure
A 71-year-old man has persistent type II endoleak 2 years after endovascular aneurysm repair.

Procedure
Transarterial embolization of type II endoleak

Pre-procedure Imaging
Contrast-enhanced CT of the abdomen shows a small, type II endoleak in the anterior aneurysm sac (Fig. 1). The aneurysm sac diameter had remained stable at 5.4 cm.

Intraprocedural Findings
Superior mesenteric arteriogram showed filling of the aneurysm sac through an enlarged arc of Riolan. The aneurysm sac was catheterized with a microcatheter through the arc of Riolan (Fig. 2), and the endoleak was embolized with *n*-butyl cyanoacrylate (Fig. 3).

Follow-up and Complications
The endoleak was occluded on follow-up CT (Fig. 4). At the last follow-up examination, the aneurysm sac had started to decrease in size, and there was no evidence of recurrent endoleak.

Suggested Readings

Baum RA, Stavropoulos SW, Fairman RM, Carpenter JP: Endoleaks after endovascular repair of abdominal aortic aneurysms. J Vasc Interv Radiol 14:1111-1117, 2003.

Chernyak V, Rozenblit AM, Patlas M, et al: Type II endoleak after endoaortic graft implantation: Diagnosis with helical arteriography. Radiology 240:885-893, 2006.

Veith FJ, Baum RA, Ohki T, et al: Nature and significance of endoleaks and endotension: Summary of opinions expressed at an international conference. J Vasc Surg 35:1029-1035, 2002.

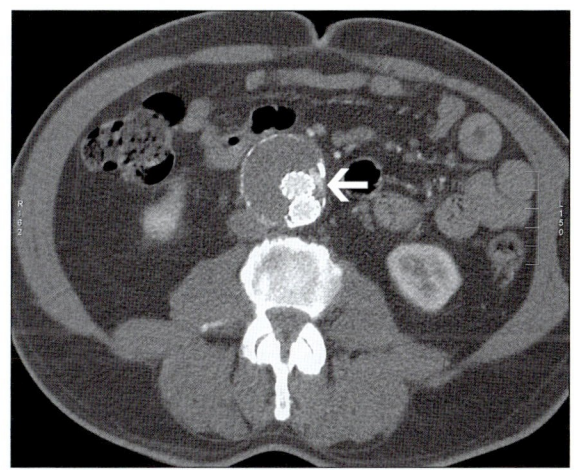

Figure 1. Contrast-enhanced CT 2 years after endograft placement shows a focal area of enhancement in the anterior aneurysm sac *(arrow)*. Based on the location, a type II endoleak through the inferior mesenteric artery was suspected.

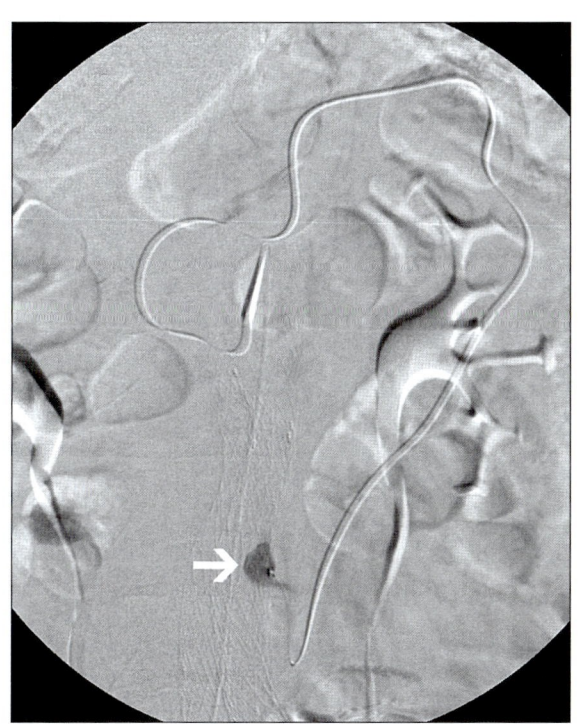

Figure 2. A 3-French microcatheter was used to selectively catheterize the aneurysm sac through the arc of Riolan. Injected contrast has opacified the endoleak *(arrow)*.

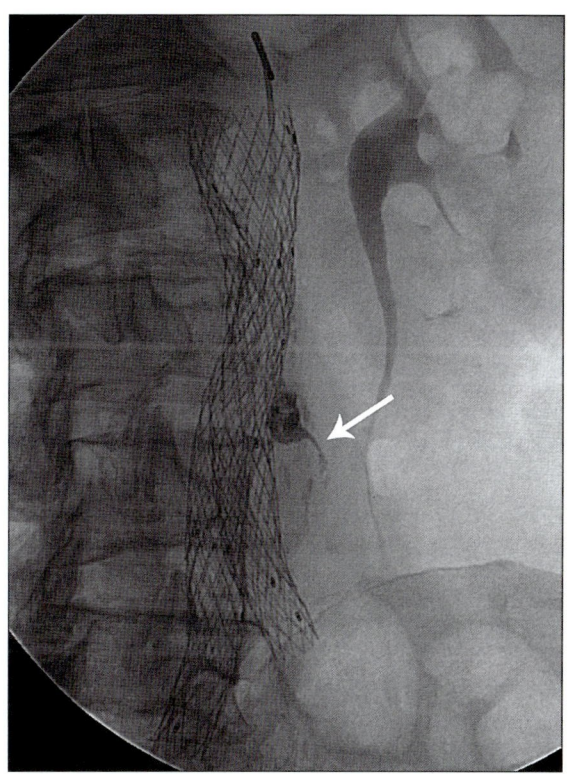

Figure 3. The endoleak was embolized with *n*-butyl cyanoacrylate. There is a small tail of glue extending into the proximal inferior mesenteric artery *(arrow)*, which did not result in any complication.

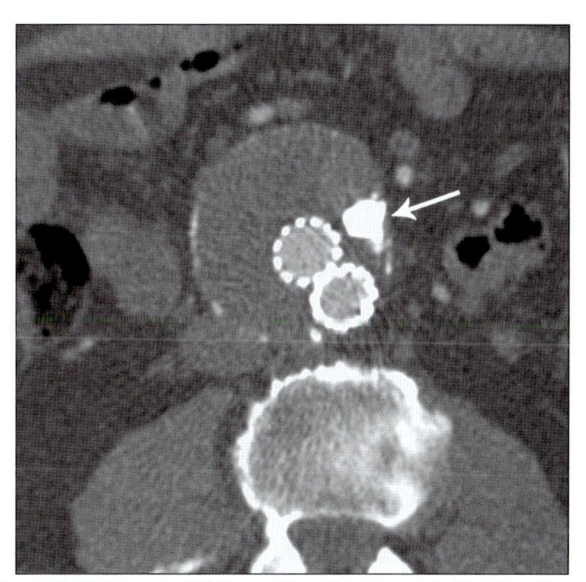

Figure 4. Follow-up CT 3 months after the embolization shows the high-density glue in the region of the previously identified endoleak *(arrow)*. No residual endoleak was seen.

Case 63

DEMOGRAPHICS/CLINICAL HISTORY

A 77-year-old man who underwent endovascular abdominal aortic aneurysm repair with endoleak identified on CT.

DISCUSSION

History/Indications for Procedure

A 77-year-old man underwent endovascular aneurysm repair 4 years earlier for an enlarging 5-cm abdominal aortic aneurysm. The aneurysm sac had reduced in size, although now it is beginning to enlarge.

Procedure

Diagnosis and management of type Ib endoleak

Pre-procedure Imaging

Contrast-enhanced CT of the abdomen shows the presence of an endoleak at the level of the aortic bifurcation (Fig. 1). Because of the proximity to a lumbar artery, the leak was thought most likely to represent a type II endoleak.

Intraprocedural Findings

Translumbar access to the aneurysm sac was obtained with CT guidance; translumbar aortogram shows the lumbar vessel to be an efferent vessel and the leak to be a type Ib from the left iliac attachment site (Fig. 2).

Follow-up and Complications

The leak at the distal attachment site was confirmed by left iliac arteriogram (Fig. 3). The patient had an extension piece added to the left iliac limb (Fig. 4); over the next 4 years, the aneurysm sac has continued to shrink and there has been no recurrent endoleak.

Suggested Readings

Baum RA, Stavropoulos SW, Fairman RM, et al.: Endoleaks after endovascular repair of abdominal aortic aneurysms. J Vasc Interv Radiol 14:1111–17, 2003.

Veith FJ, Baum RA, Ohki T, et al.: Nature and significance of endoleaks and endotension: Summary of opinions expressed at an international conference. J Vasc Surg 35:1029–35, 2002.

White GH, Yu W, May J, et al.: Endoleak as a complication of endoluminal grafting of abdominal aortic aneurysm: Classification, incidence, diagnosis, and management. J Endovasc Surg 4:152–68, 1997.

Case 63   127

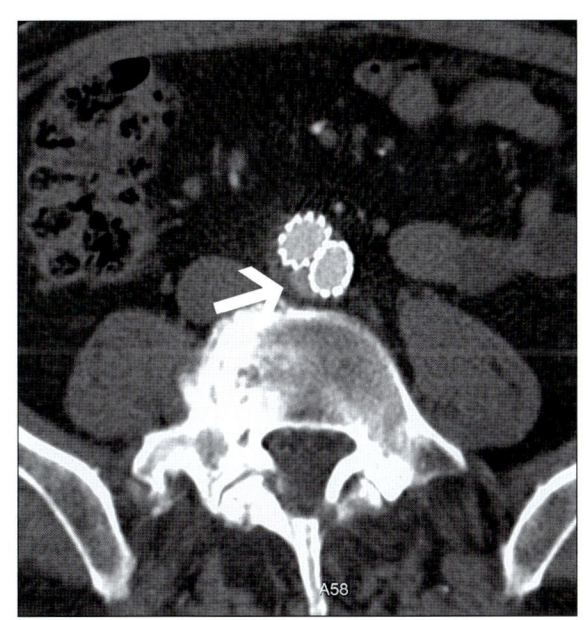

Figure 1. Contrast-enhanced CT shows enhancement within the aneurysm sac posterior to the iliac limbs *(arrow)*. This was initially thought to be a type II endoleak.

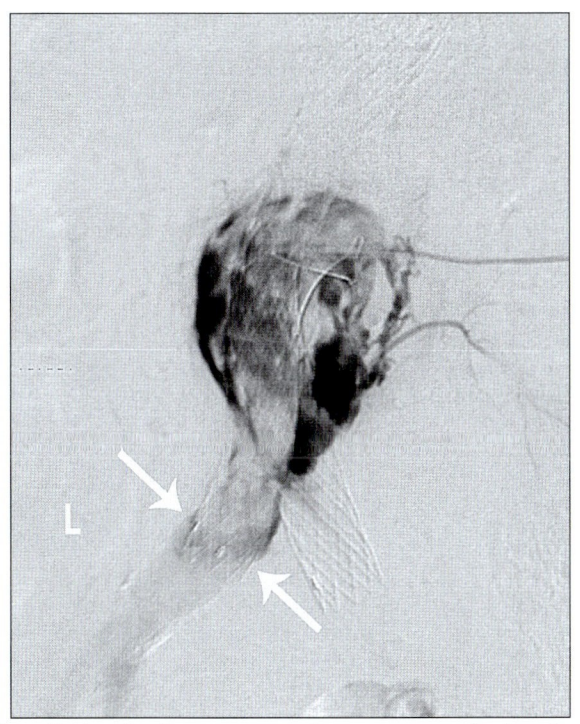

Figure 2. Translumbar aortogram shows contrast refluxing along the left iliac limb *(arrows)*, indicating the presence of a type Ib endoleak. A prominent lumbar artery is seen; this is most likely an efferent vessel.

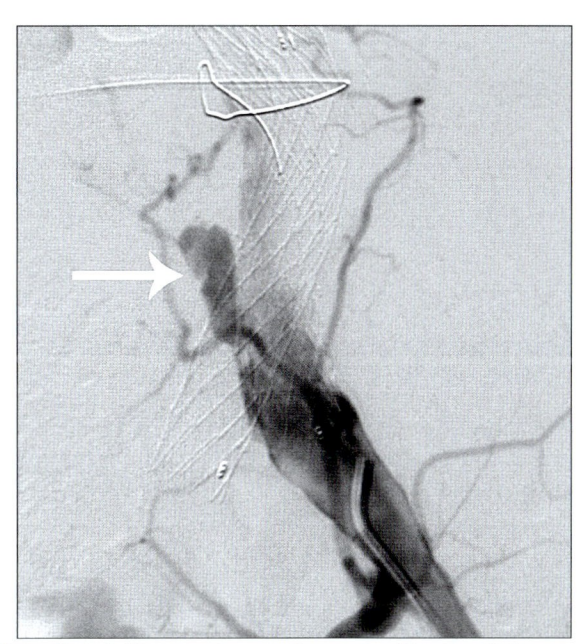

Figure 3. Left iliac arteriogram shows opacification of the aneurysm sac *(arrow)* around the left iliac limb, confirming the type Ib endoleak.

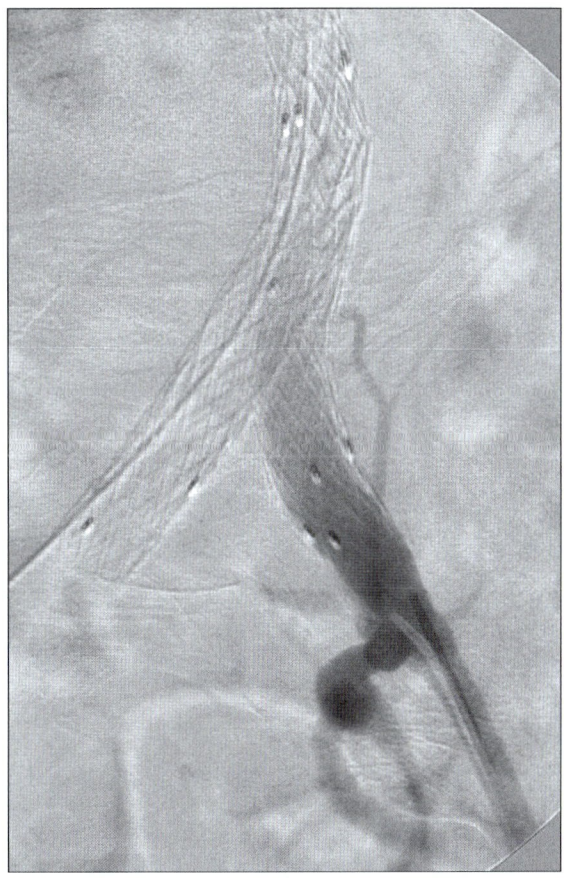

Figure 4. Intraoperative angiogram after placement of a left iliac extension. The distal attachment site has been successfully sealed.

Case 64

DEMOGRAPHICS/CLINICAL HISTORY

A 77-year-old man with dehiscence of the right iliac limb, 3 years after endovascular aneurysm repair.

DISCUSSION

History/Indications for Procedure
A 77-year-old man with dehiscence of the right iliac limb, 3 years after endovascular aneurysm repair with a Vanguard stent graft. The patient also reports new-onset claudication of the right lower extremity.

Procedure
Late endovascular management of endograft failure

Pre-procedure Imaging
Contrast-enhanced CT shows the separation of the right iliac limb from the main body of the stent graft. The right iliac limb is occluded (Fig. 1), and the aneurysm sac size has increased.

Intraprocedural Findings
A catheter was advanced through the right iliac limb into the aneurysm sac, and a pressure measurement was obtained; the aneurysm sac pressure was elevated, measuring 108/77 (95) mm Hg (Fig. 2). The thrombosed right iliac limb was treated using catheter directed thrombolysis, and a Wallgraft (Boston Scientific, Natick, MA) was used to cover the type III endoleak.

Follow-up and Complications
The aneurysm sac remained stable in follow-up, with no evidence of recurrent endoleak (Fig. 3). Ten months later, the right iliac limb re-thrombosed, and the patient underwent placement of a femoral-femoral bypass graft (Fig. 4).

Suggested Readings

Carpenter JP, Neschis DG, Fairman RM, et al: Failure of endovascular abdominal aortic aneurysm graft limbs. J Vasc Surg 33:296–302, 2001.

Carroccio A, Faries PL, Morrissey NJ, et al: Predicting iliac limb occlusions after bifurcated aortic stent grafting: Anatomic and device-related causes. J Vasc Surg 36:679–684, 2002.

Tillich M, Hausegger KA, Tiesenhausen K, et al: Helical CT angiography of stent-grafts in abdominal aortic aneurysms: Morphologic changes and complications. Radiographics 19:1573–1583, 1999.

Case 64   129

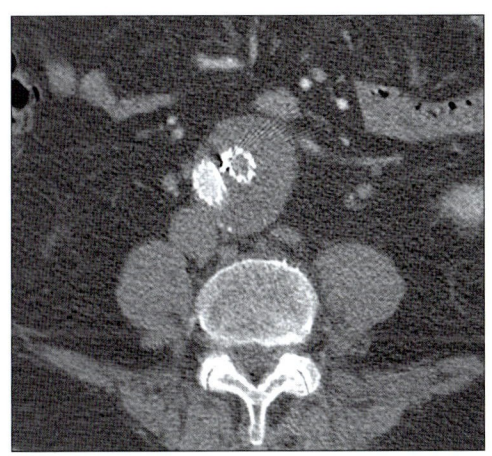

Figure 1. Contrast-enhanced CT through the iliac limbs shows thrombosis of the right iliac limb.

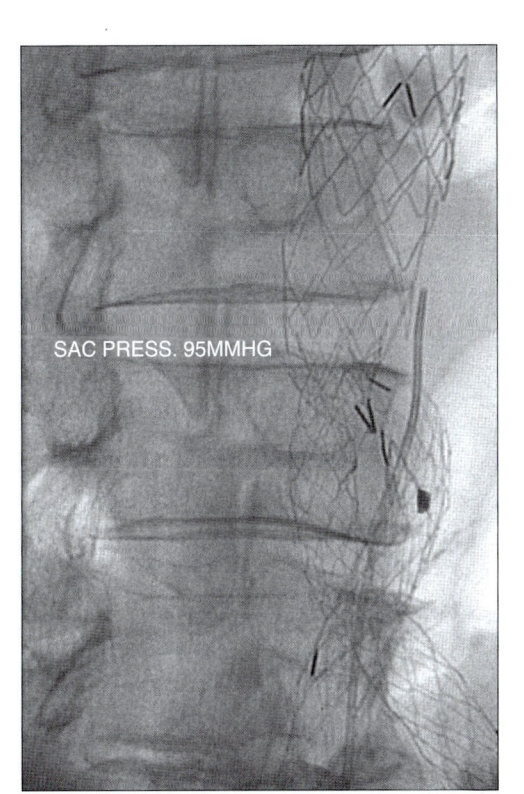

Figure 2. The right iliac limb has been successfully catheterized. An aortic sac pressure is obtained through the diagnostic catheter.

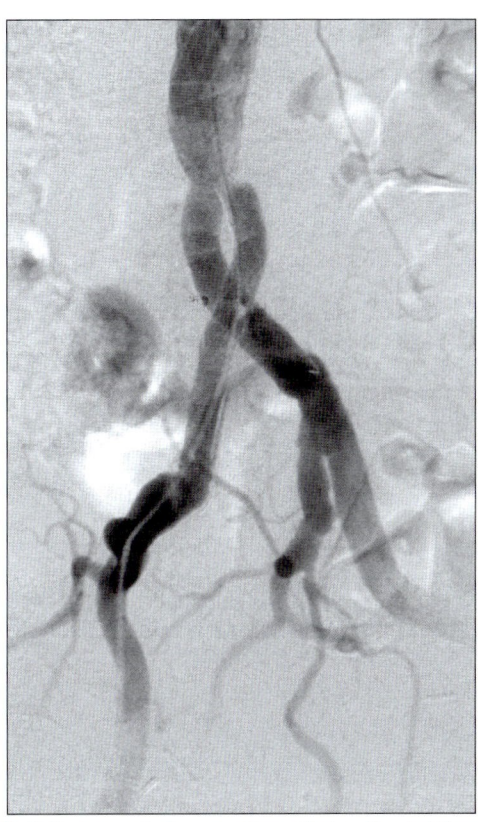

Figure 3. Follow-up arteriogram after catheter-directed thrombolysis. There is restoration of flow to the right iliac limb. No contrast is seen extravasating into the aortic aneurysm.

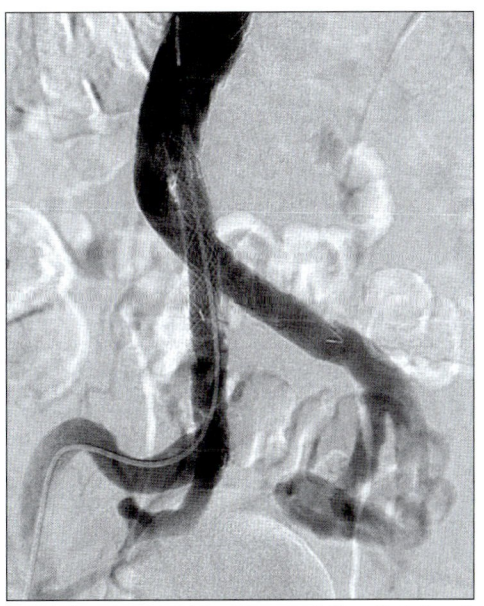

Figure 4. Final aortogram. The distracted iliac limb has been repaired with the placement of a Wallgraft.

Case 65

DEMOGRAPHICS/CLINICAL HISTORY

A 72-year-old man with aortic arch aneurysm identified on chest radiograph.

DISCUSSION

History/Indications for Procedure
A 72-year-old man with aortic arch aneurysm identified on chest radiograph. The patient underwent prior surgical repair of a suprarenal abdominal aortic aneurysm 13 years earlier.

Procedure
Endovascular repair for diverticulum of Kommerell aneurysm

Pre-procedure Imaging
CT angiogram shows an aberrant right subclavian artery with a dilated diverticulum of Kommerell (Figs. 1 and 2). There is a thrombosed aneurysm of the proximal right subclavian, measuring 11 cm × 6 cm × 7 cm.

Intraprocedural Findings
In preparation for endograft placement, the patient underwent left carotid-to-subclavian artery bypass 1 week prior. A TAG (Gore, Flagstaff, AZ) thoracic stent graft was deployed just distal to the origin of the left subclavian artery (Fig. 3), and the proximal left subclavian artery was embolized with coils.

Follow-up and Complications
The patient had a protracted hospital course following the endograft placement as a result of severe deconditioning. Follow-up CT angiogram shows occlusion of the right subclavian artery aneurysm without evidence for endoleak (Fig. 4).

Suggested Readings
Brown KE, Eskandari MK, Matsumura JS, et al: Short and midterm results with minimally invasive endovascular repair of acute and chronic thoracic aortic pathology. J Vasc Surg 47:714–22, 2008.

Corral JS, Zuniga CG, Sanchez JB, et al: Treatment of aberrant right subclavian artery aneurysm with endovascular exclusion and adjunctive surgical bypass. J Vasc Interv Radiol 14:789–92, 2003.

Fisher RG, Whignham CJ, Trinh C: Diverticula of Kommerell and aberrant subclavian arteries complicated by aneurysms. Cardiovasc Intervent Radiol 28:553–60, 2005.

Kopp R, Wizgall I, Kreuzer E, et al: Surgical and endovascular treatment of symptomatic aberrant right subclavian artery (arteria lusoria). Vascular 15:84–91, 2007.

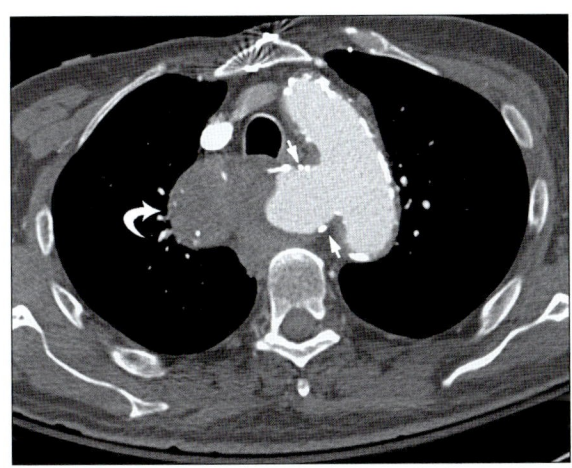

Figure 1. CT angiogram through the aortic arch shows a large diverticulum of Kommerell *(straight arrows)* and thrombosed aberrant right subclavian artery aneurysm *(curved arrow)*.

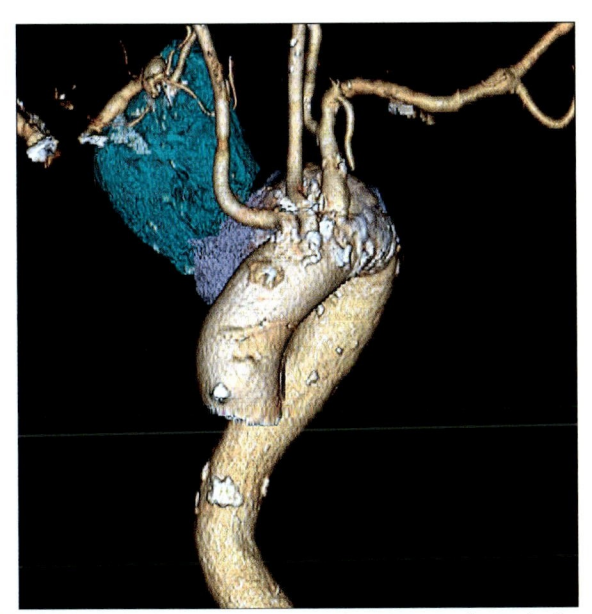

Figure 2. A 3-D reconstruction from CT angiogram shows the large diverticulum and thrombosed right subclavian artery aneurysm *(green)*.

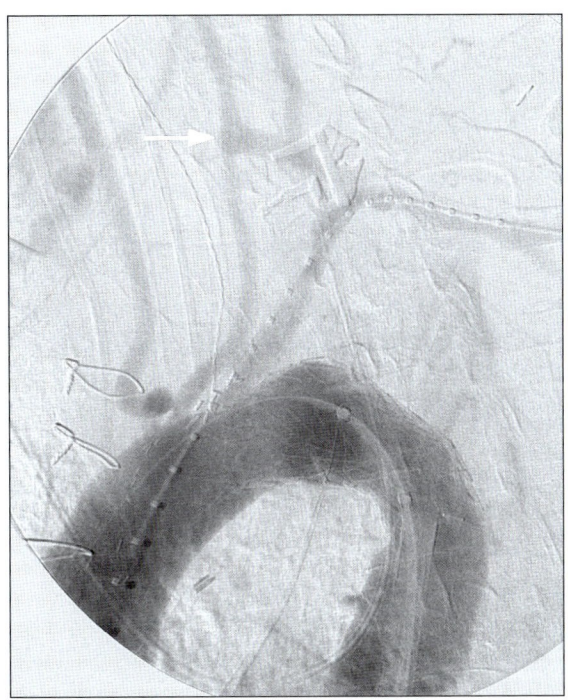

Figure 3. Arch aortogram after endograft placement shows an endograft across the origin of the aberrant right subclavian artery. A left carotid-to-subclavian bypass is present *(arrow)*, and the proximal left subclavian artery was embolized after endograft placement.

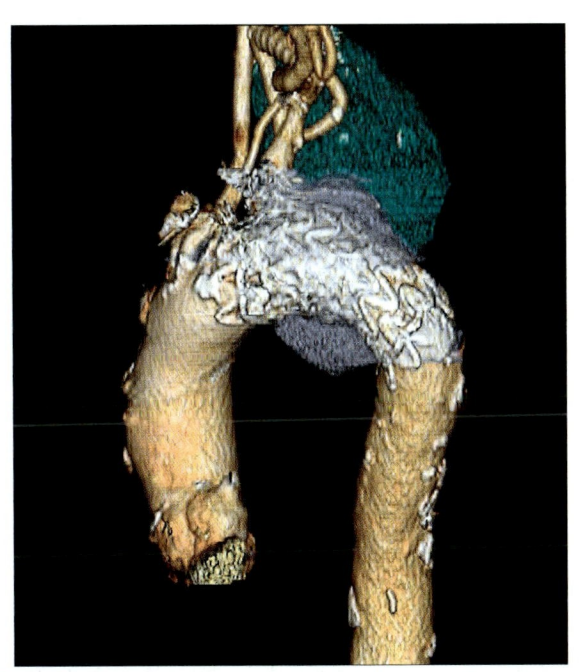

Figure 4. A 3-D reconstruction from follow-up CT angiogram shows the endograft across the origin of the aberrant right subclavian artery. On the source images, no flow was seen in the diverticulum of Kommerell.

Case 66

DEMOGRAPHICS/CLINICAL HISTORY

An 18-year-old girl who sustained an acute traumatic aortic injury in a high-speed motor vehicle collision, undergoing computed tomography (CT) and arteriography.

DISCUSSION

History/Indications for Procedure
An 18-year-old girl was involved in a motor vehicle collision. In addition to the aortic injury, she sustained a severe closed head injury.

Procedure
Endovascular management of acute traumatic aortic injury

Pre-procedure Imaging
Contrast-enhanced CT of the chest shows a pseudoaneurysm arising from the anterior wall of the proximal descending thoracic aorta (Fig. 1).

Intraprocedural Findings
Intraoperative thoracic aortogram confirms the presence of a post-traumatic aortic pseudoaneurysm (Fig. 2). Three overlapping, 23-mm diameter, thoracic stent grafts (Gore TAG, Flagstaff, AZ) were placed across the origin of the left subclavian artery, with the distal attachment site distal to the pseudoaneurysm (Fig. 3).

Follow-up and Complications
The patient was discharged from the hospital 1 month after admission, and she underwent rehabilitation for the traumatic brain injury. Follow-up thoracic CT angiogram 1 month after endograft placement showed resolution of the periaortic hematoma and no endoleak with the stent graft (Fig. 4).

Suggested Readings
Lin PH, Bush RL, Zhou W, et al: Endovascular treatment of traumatic thoracic aortic injury—should this be the new standard of treatment? J Vasc Surg 43:22A-29A, 2006.

Ott MC, Stewart TC, Lawlor DK, et al: Management of blunt thoracic aortic injuries: Endovascular stents versus open repair. J Trauma 56:565-570, 2004.

Peterson BG, Matsumura JS, Morasch MD, et al: Percutaneous endovascular repair of blunt thoracic aortic transection. J Trauma 59:1062-1065, 2005.

Rousseau H, Dambrin C, Marcheix B, et al: Acute traumatic aortic rupture: A comparison of surgical and stent-graft repair. J Thorac Cardiovasc Surg 129:1050-1055, 2005.

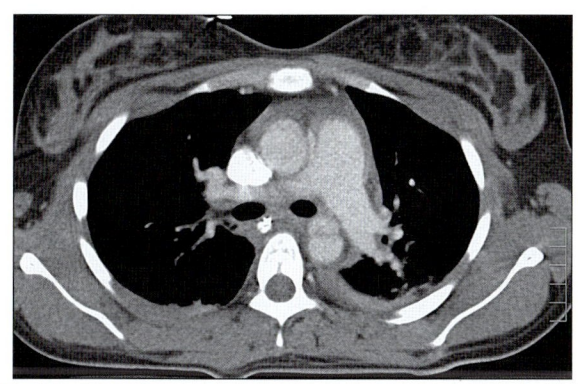

Figure 1. CT angiogram shows a pseudoaneurysm arising from the anterior wall of the proximal descending thoracic aorta *(arrow)*.

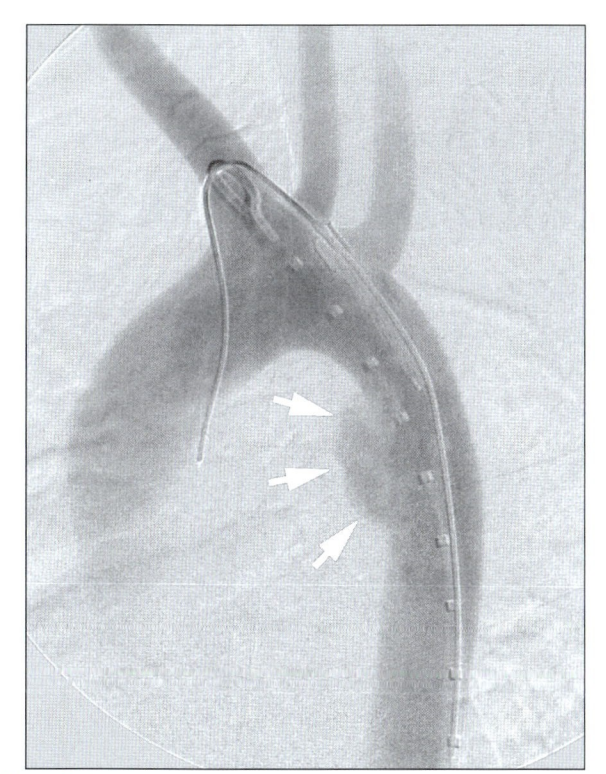

Figure 2. Intraoperative thoracic aortogram confirms the presence of an acute traumatic aortic injury *(arrows)* approximately 1 cm distal to the origin of the left subclavian artery.

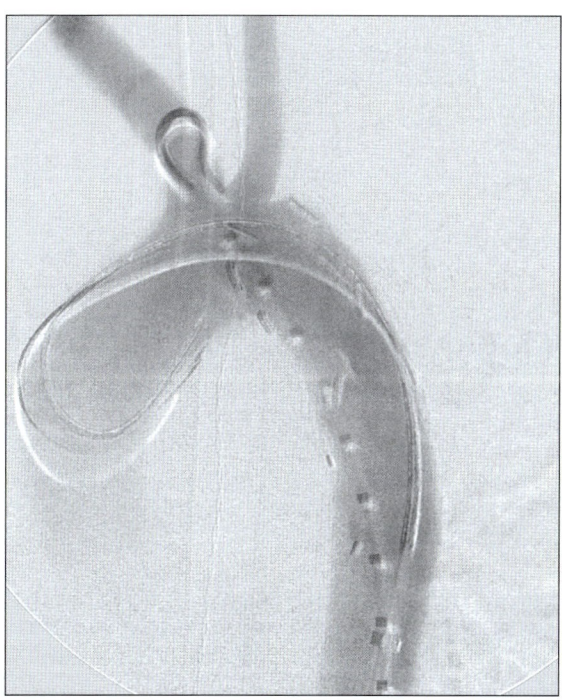

Figure 3. The aortogram after endograft placement shows the pseudoaneurysm is no longer opacified, and there is a lack of filling of the left subclavian artery. The proximity of the injury to the left subclavian artery required covering the artery's origin by the stent graft *(arrow)*.

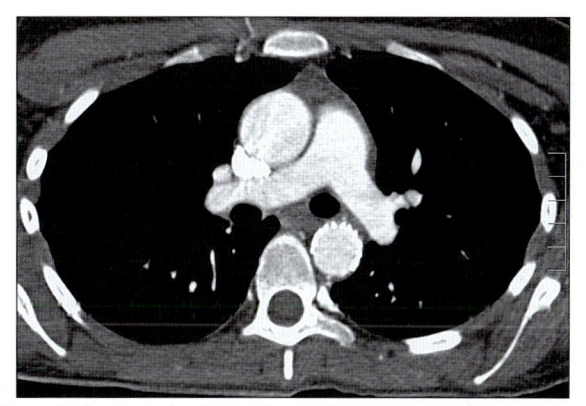

Figure 4. One month after endovascular repair, the CT angiogram shows an endograft in the proximal descending thoracic aorta. The pseudoaneurysm and periaortic hematoma have resolved.

Case 67

DEMOGRAPHICS/CLINICAL HISTORY

A 61-year-old woman with an acute traumatic aortic injury after a motor vehicle accident, undergoing computed tomography (CT).

DISCUSSION

History/Indications for Procedure

A 61-year-old woman, who was in a motor vehicle accident, had many injuries, including a closed head injury, acute traumatic aortic injury, splenic laceration, and multiple rib and pelvic fractures.

Procedure

Thoracic endograft for acute traumatic aortic injury

Pre-procedure Imaging

Contrast-enhanced CT of the chest shows a contained, extraluminal collection of contrast filling from the superiolateral wall of the proximal descending thoracic aorta (Fig. 1), consistent with an acute traumatic aortic injury.

Intraprocedural Findings

A 31-mm × 10-cm TAG (Gore, Flagstaff, AZ) endovascular stent graft was deployed at the level of the left subclavian across the injured segment of the thoracic aorta (Fig. 2). No leak was identified on the aortogram after placement of the endograft.

Follow-up and Complications

Follow-up CT of the chest 3 weeks after endovascular repair shows the stent graft within the proximal descending thoracic aorta (Figs. 3 and 4). There is no further filling of the aortic pseudoaneurysm.

Suggested Readings

Dunham MB, Zygun D, Petrasek P, et al: Endovascular stent grafts for acute blunt aortic injury. J Trauma 56:1173-1178, 2004.

Risenman PJ, Farber MA, Mendes RR, et al: Endovascular repair of lesions involving the descending thoracic aorta. J Vasc Surg 42:1063-1074, 2005.

Wheatley GH, Gurbuz AT, Rodriguez-Lopez JA, et al: Midterm outcome in 158 consecutive Gore TAG thoracic endoprostheses: Single center experience. Ann Thorac Surg 81:1570-1577, 2006.

Case 67   135

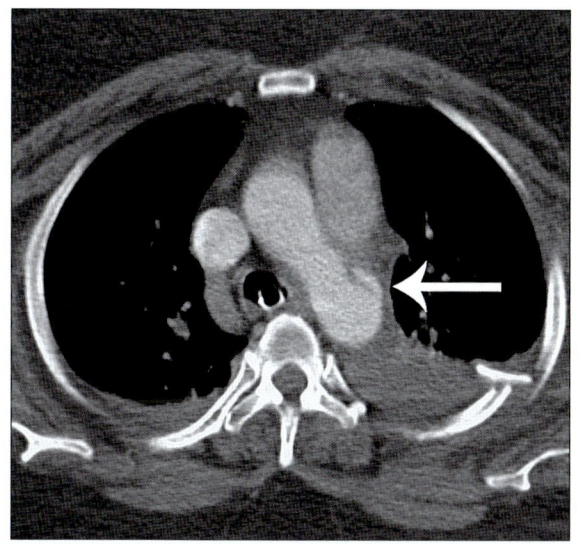

Figure 1. Axial, contrast-enhanced CT through the aortic arch shows a focal pseudoaneurysm along the anterior wall of the aorta (arrow). There is also a left pleural effusion and left-sided rib fractures.

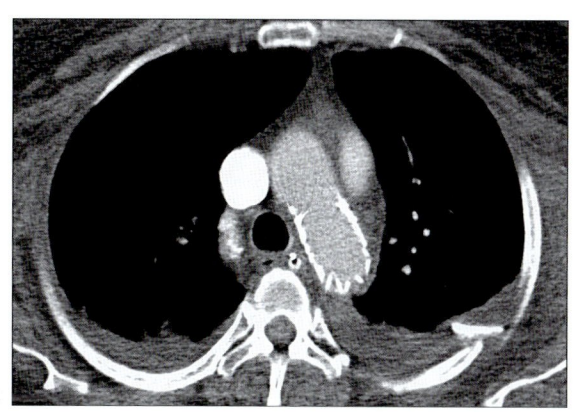

Figure 3. Contrast-enhanced CT performed 3 weeks after the endograft placement shows exclusion of the pseudoaneurysm. There has been nearly complete resolution of the mediastinal hematoma.

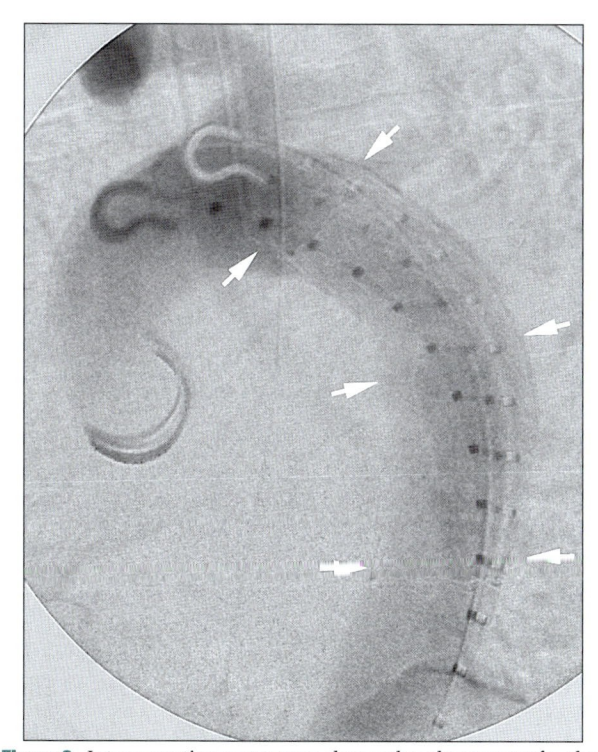

Figure 2. Intraoperative aortogram shows the placement of a thoracic endograft (arrows) across the site of injury.

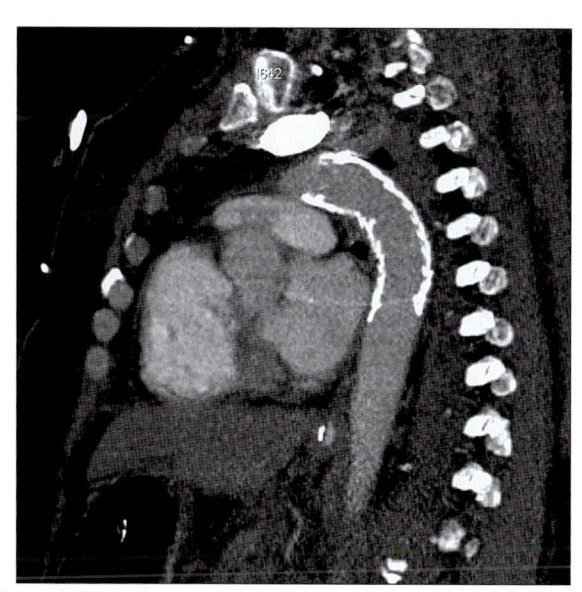

Figure 4. Sagittal reconstruction shows the presence of the endograft. The proximal attachment site crosses the origin of the left subclavian artery. Despite this, the patient had no symptoms of left upper extremity ischemia.

Case 68

DEMOGRAPHICS/CLINICAL HISTORY

A 27-year-old man with aortic transection after a motor vehicle accident, undergoing computed tomography (CT), angiography, and aortography.

DISCUSSION

History/Indications for Procedure
A 27-year-old man had an aortic transection after a motor vehicle accident. Attempted surgical repair was aborted after the patient developed respiratory distress, and the site of injury was wrapped in Teflon and BioGlue.

Procedure
Endovascular repair of acute traumatic aortic injury

Pre-procedure Imaging
A CT angiogram of the thorax shows postoperative changes to the proximal descending thoracic aorta (Fig. 1) and mediastinal hemorrhage.

Intraprocedural Findings
A thoracic stent graft was placed across the site of injury (Fig. 2). After placement, aortography and CT angiography show no evidence of an endoleak (Fig. 3).

Follow-up and Complications
The patient recovered from the motor vehicle accident and was discharged from the hospital. Four years later, he developed hypertension and claudication due to stent narrowing from intimal hyperplasia (Fig. 4).

Suggested Readings
Amabile P, Collart F, Gariboldi V, et al: Surgical versus endovascular treatment of traumatic thoracic aortic rupture. J Vasc Surg 40:873-879, 2004.

Kasirajan K, Heffernan D, Langsfeld M: Acute thoracic aortic trauma: A comparison of endoluminal stent grafts with open repair and nonoperative management. Ann Vasc Surg 17:589-595, 2003.

Peterson BG, Matsumura JS, Morasch MD, et al: Percutaneous endovascular repair of blunt thoracic aortic transection. J Trauma 59:1062-1065, 2005.

Sayed S, Thompson MM: Endovascular repair of the descending thoracic aorta: Evidence for the change in clinical practice. Vascular 13:148-157, 2005.

Case 68   137

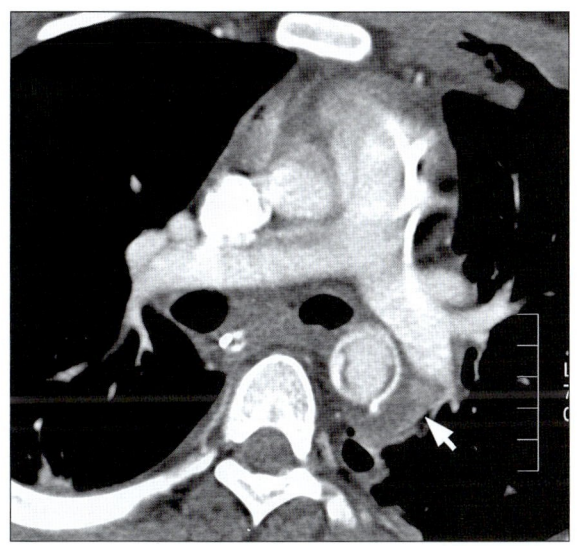

Figure 1. Axial, contrast-enhanced CT shows high-density material surrounding the aortic wall from the Teflon and BioGlue placed at the outside hospital. Periaortic, mediastinal hemorrhage (*arrow*) can be seen.

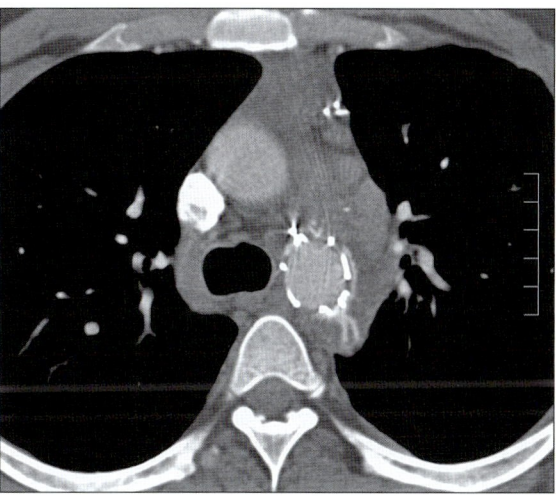

Figure 3. Contrast-enhanced, axial CT through the proximal descending thoracic aorta shows the endograft in place. The high-density Teflon is clearly visible.

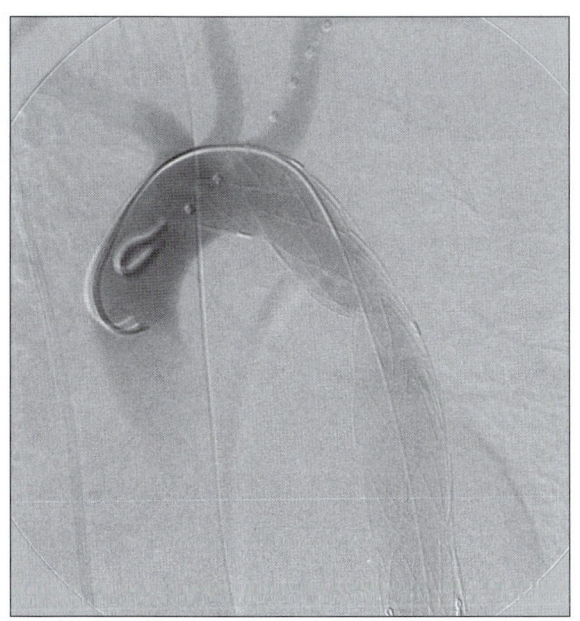

Figure 2. After stent graft placement, intraoperative thoracic aortography was performed through a flush catheter placed by means of a left brachial artery approach. The endograft covers the site of injury, and there is no evidence of an endoleak.

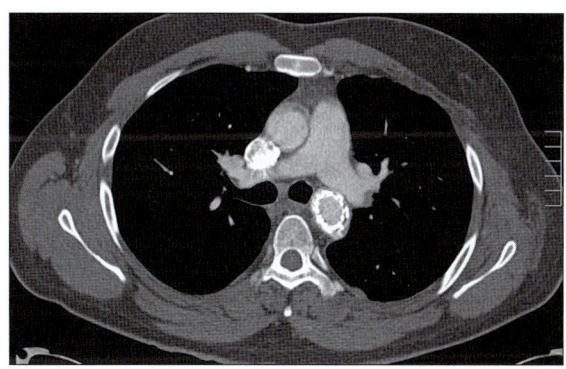

Figure 4. CT angiogram 4 years after endograft placement shows resolution of the mediastinal hematoma. An additional stent has been placed within the graft to treat the intragraft stenosis.

Case 69

DEMOGRAPHICS/CLINICAL HISTORY

A 52-year-old woman with a history of a type A aortic dissection and left lower extremity claudication.

DISCUSSION

History/Indications for Procedure
A 52-year-old woman who has undergone prior ascending aortic repair for type A aortic dissection. She presents with left lower extremity claudication.

Procedure
Stent-graft placement for lower extremity ischemia secondary to dissection

Pre-procedure Imaging
Contrast-enhanced CT shows an aortic dissection that extends from the aortic arch into the left common iliac artery (Figs. 1 and 2).

Intraprocedural Findings
Abdominal aortogram from the true lumen shows compression of the true lumen of the proximal left common iliac artery (Fig. 3). The true lumen was stented with an 8-mm × 4-cm covered stent (Fluency, Bard Peripheral Vascular, Tempe, AZ) (Fig. 4).

Follow-up and Complications
The patient's claudication resolved after the stenting. In addition, during the 2 years since the stent placement, the false lumen of the dissection has nearly completely thrombosed.

Suggested Readings
Lopera J, Patino JH, Urbina C, et al: Endovascular treatment of complicated type-B aortic dissection with stent grafts: Midterm results. J Vasc Interv Radiol 14:195-203, 2003.

Vendantham S, Picus D, Sanchez LA, et al: Percutaneous management of ischemic complications in patients with type-B aortic dissection. J Vasc Interv Radiol 14:181-193, 2003.

Williams DM, Lee DY, Hamilton BH, et al: The dissected aorta: Percutaneous management of ischemic complications with endovascular stents and balloon fenestration. J Vasc Surg 23:241-253, 1996.

Case 69   139

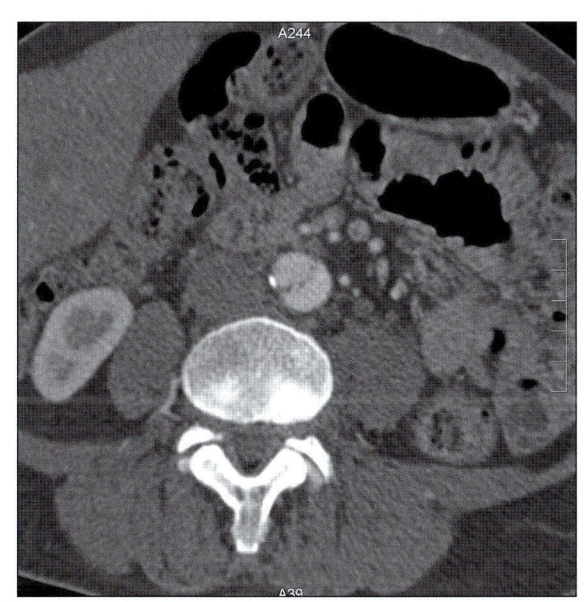

Figure 1. Contrast-enhanced CT shows an aortic dissection in the infrarenal abdominal aorta.

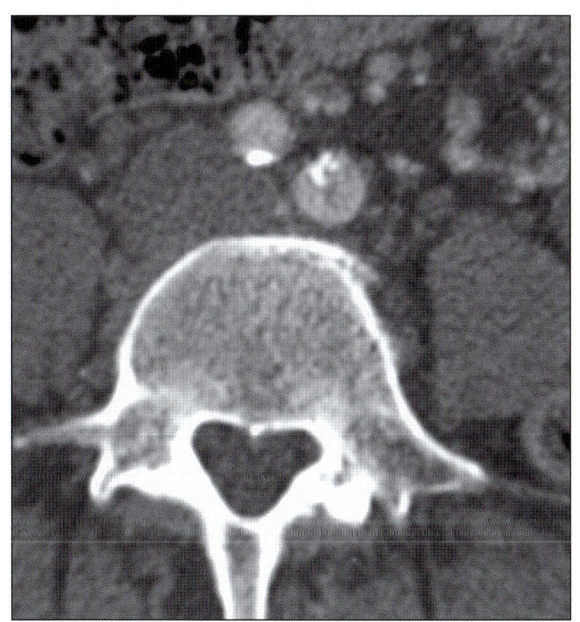

Figure 2. Slightly lower image shows the dissection flap extending into the left common iliac artery.

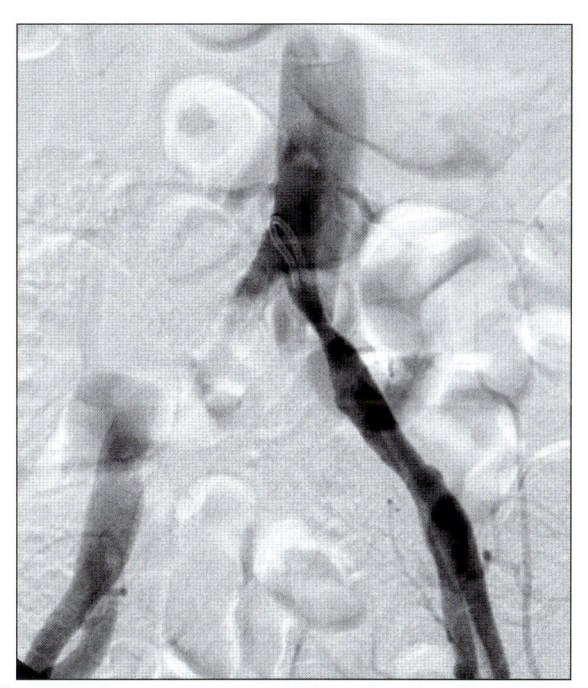

Figure 3. Pelvic arteriogram with the catheter in the true lumen shows narrowing of the true lumen of the left common iliac artery.

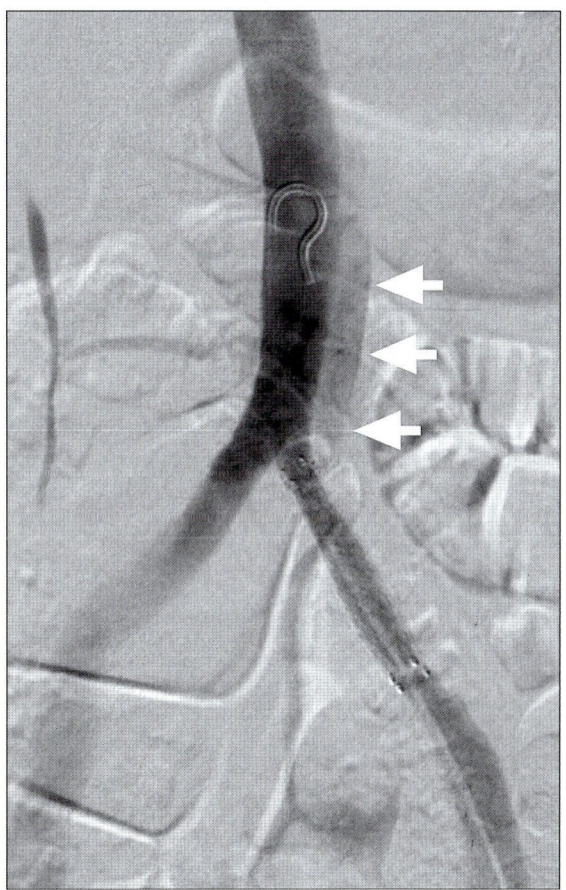

Figure 4. Follow-up pelvic arteriogram. A covered stent has been placed across the narrowed true lumen of the left common iliac artery. There is still filling of the false lumen *(arrows)*. Despite this, follow-up CT angiograms show subsequent thrombosis of the false lumen.

Case 70

DEMOGRAPHICS/CLINICAL HISTORY

A 71-year-old woman with a type B thoracic aortic dissection, undergoing computed tomography (CT) angiography, bypass graft placement, and nephrectomy.

DISCUSSION

History/Indications for Procedure
A 71-year-old woman has a type B aortic dissection and 5.5-cm thoracoabdominal aortic aneurysm. The patient also has poorly controlled hypertension despite taking five antihypertensive medications.

Procedure
Endograft for type B aortic dissection

Pre-procedure Imaging
CT angiogram demonstrates a type B aortic dissection extending from just distal to the left subclavian artery to the level of the renal arteries (Fig. 1). There is a 5.5-cm abdominal aortic aneurysm (Fig. 2).

Intraprocedural Findings
The patient underwent debranching of the abdominal aorta with bypass grafts to the celiac, superior mesenteric artery, and right renal arteries and left nephrectomy (Fig. 3). An endograft was placed from the origin of the left subclavian arteries to the common iliac arteries (Fig. 4).

Follow-up and Complications
Follow-up CT angiogram 1 month after endograft placement demonstrates thrombosis of the false lumen of the dissection. Her blood pressure improved and can be controlled with three medications.

Suggested Readings
Dake MD, Miller DC, Semba CP, et al: Transluminal placement of endovascular stent-grafts for the treatment of descending aortic aneurysms. N Engl J Med 331:1729-1734, 1994.

Kato N, Hirano T, Shimono T, et al: Treatment of chronic type aortic dissection with endovascular stent graft placement. Cardiovasc Intervent Radiol 23:60-62, 2000.

Lopera J, Patiño JH, Urbina C, et al: Endovascular treatment of complicated type-B aortic dissection with stent grafts: Midterm results. J Vasc Interv Radiol 14:195-203, 2003.

Won JY, Lee DY, Shim WH, et al: Elective endovascular treatment of descending thoracic aortic aneurysms and chronic dissections with stent-grafts. J Vasc Interv Radiol 12:575-582, 2001.

Case 70   141

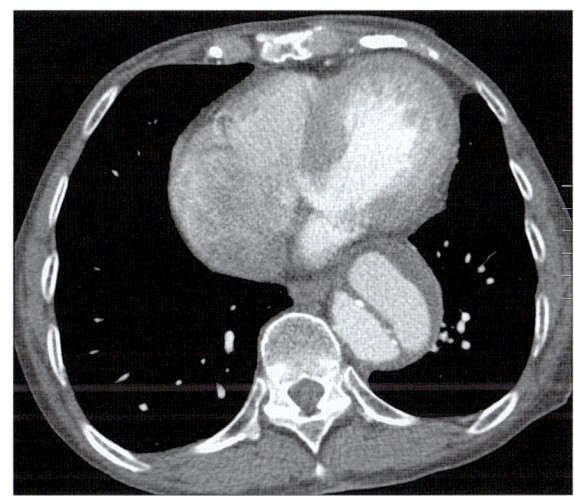

Figure 1. Single image from the CT angiogram demonstrates a chronic dissection in the descending thoracic aorta.

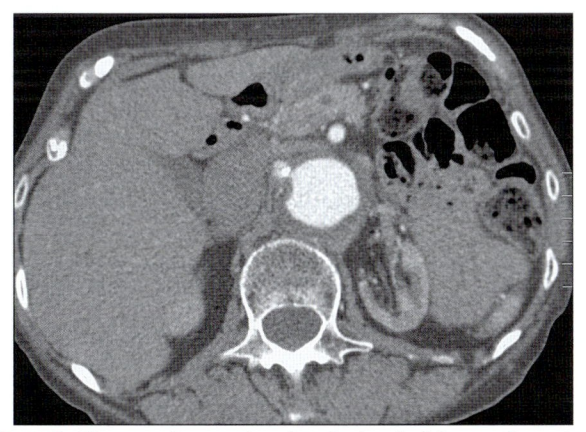

Figure 2. The aorta is aneurismal at the level of the renal arteries. The left kidney is small and hypoperfusing.

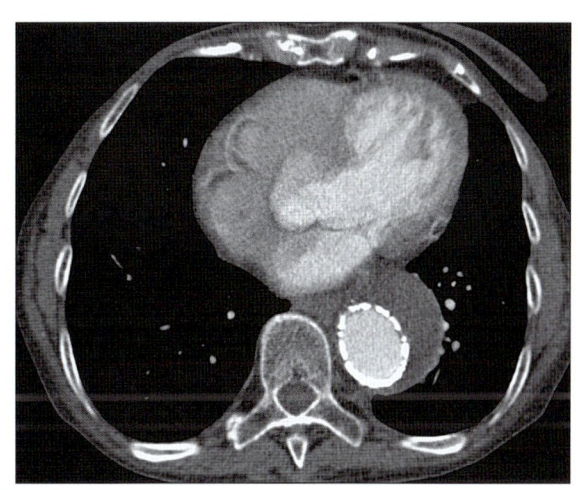

Figure 3. One month after endograft placement, the false lumen is thrombosed.

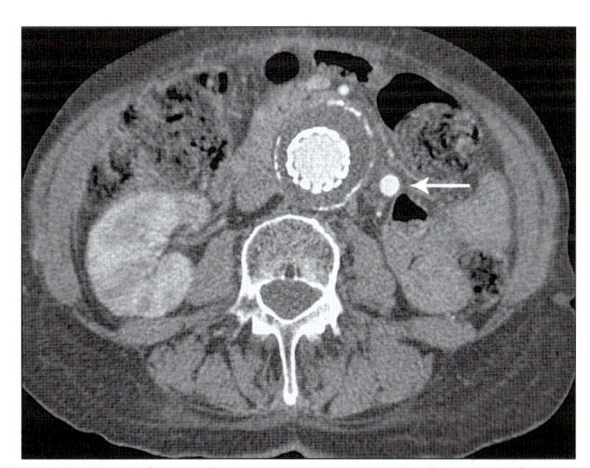

Figure 4. The infrarenal aneurysm was repaired, and perfusion to the right kidney was improved. A patent bypass graft is seen in the left retroperitoneum *(arrow)*.

Case 71

DEMOGRAPHICS/CLINICAL HISTORY
A 51-year-old man with type B aortic dissection.

DISCUSSION

History/Indications for Procedure
A 51-year-old man with a type B aortic dissection.

Procedure
Endovascular stent graft placement for type B aortic dissection

Pre-procedure Imaging
Contrast-enhanced CT of the chest shows a type B aortic dissection originating just distal to the origin of the left subclavian artery (Fig. 1); the proximal descending thoracic aorta is aneurysmal, measuring 5.1 cm in diameter. Thoracic aortogram shows filling of a dilated false lumen just distal to the origin of the left subclavian artery (Fig. 2).

Intraprocedural Findings
Before endograft placement, a right-to-left carotid-carotid bypass and a left carotid–to–subclavian artery bypass was performed with ligation of the proximal left common carotid and left subclavian arteries, in order to extend the stent-graft landing zone. Two overlapping 40-mm TAG (Gore, Flagstaff, AZ) thoracic stent-grafts were deployed across the proximal entry site of the dissection.

Follow-up and Complications
Follow-up CT 7 months after endograft placement shows thrombosis and near-complete resolution of the false lumen (Figs. 3 and 4).

Suggested Readings
Fattori R, Napoli G, Lovato L, et al: Descending thoracic aortic diseases: Stent-graft repair. Radiology 229:176-183, 2003.

Kato N, Hirano T, Shimono T, et al: Treatment of chronic type aortic dissection with endovascular stent graft placement. Cardiovasc Intervent Radiol 23:60-62, 2000.

Leurs LJ, Bell R, Degrieck Y, et al: Endovascular treatment of thoracic aortic diseases: Combined experience from the EUROSTAR and United Kingdom Thoracic Endograft registries. J Vasc Surg 40:670-679, 2004.

Lopera J, Patino JH, Urbina C, et al: Endovascular treatment of complicated type-B aortic dissection with stent grafts: Midterm results. J Vasc Interv Radiol 14:195-203, 2003.

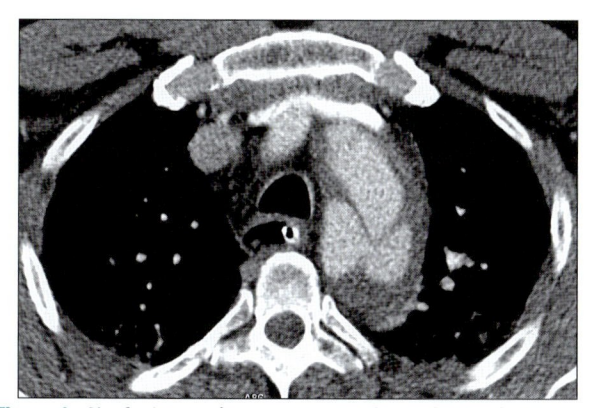

Figure 1. Single image from contrast-enhanced CT of the chest shows a complex dissection of the proximal descending thoracic aorta.

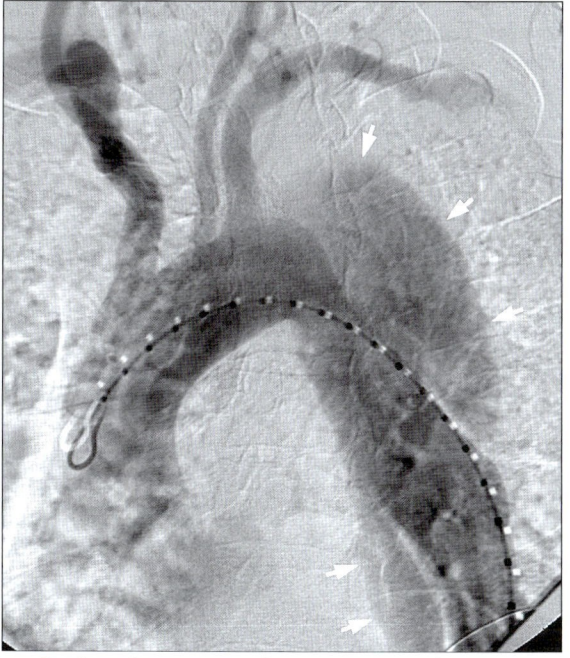

Figure 2. Thoracic aortogram shows narrowing of the true lumen and filling of a dilated false lumen (arrows) of the dissection.

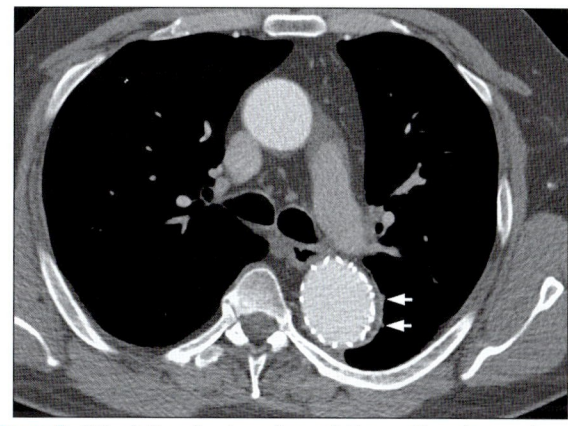

Figure 3. CT of the chest performed 7 months after endograft placement shows near-complete resolution of the false lumen (arrows).

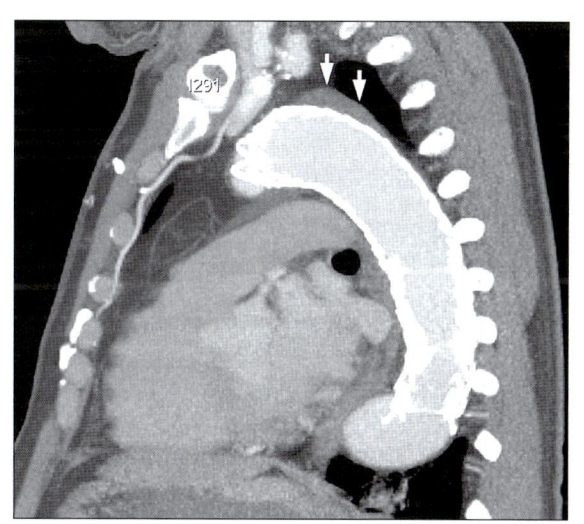

Figure 4. Sagital reconstructed image from CT performed 7 months after endograft placement shows thrombosis and near-complete resolution of the false lumen (arrows).

Case 72

DEMOGRAPHICS/CLINICAL HISTORY

A 68-year-old man involved in a high-speed motor vehicle collision at 20 years of age.

DISCUSSION

History/Indications for Procedure
A 68-year-old man involved in a high-speed motor vehicle collision at 20 years of age. He is currently asymptomatic.

Procedure
Endovascular repair of chronic thoracic aortic pseudoaneurysm

Pre-procedure Imaging
Contrast-enhanced CT of the chest shows irregularity of the wall of the proximal descending thoracic aorta, consistent with a post-traumatic aortic pseudoaneurysm (Fig. 1).

Intraprocedural Findings
Intraoperative thoracic aortogram shows a subtle double density and slight irregularity of the proximal descending thoracic aorta (Fig. 2). The pseudoaneurysm was treated with the placement of overlapping 34-mm × 10-cm and 34-mm × 15-cm (Excluder, Gore, Flagstaff, AZ) thoracic stent-grafts (Fig. 3).

Follow-up and Complications
The patient was discharged from the hospital the day after stent-graft placement. On follow-up imaging, the aortic pseudoaneurysm has nearly completely resolved (Fig. 4).

Suggested Readings
Hoffer EK, Forauer AR, Silas AM, et al: Endovascular stent-graft or open surgical repair for blunt thoracic aortic trauma: Systematic review. J Vasc Interv Radiol 19:1153–64, 2008.

McPherson SJ: Thoracic aortic and great vessel trauma and its management. Semin Interv Radiol 24:180–96, 2007.

Rousseau H, Dambrin C, Marcheix B, et al: Acute traumatic aortic rupture: A comparison of surgical and stent-graft repair. J Thorac Cardiovasc Surg 129:1050–55, 2005.

Case 72   145

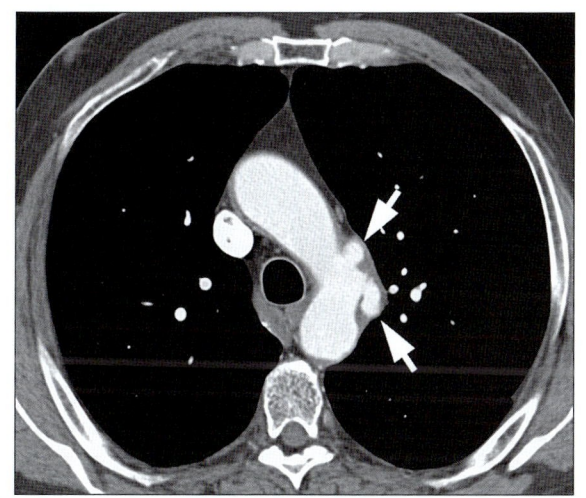

Figure 1. Contrast-enhanced CT of the chest shows two focal collections of contrast protruding from the lateral wall of the proximal descending thoracic aorta *(arrows)*. These are consistent with post-traumatic pseudoaneurysms.

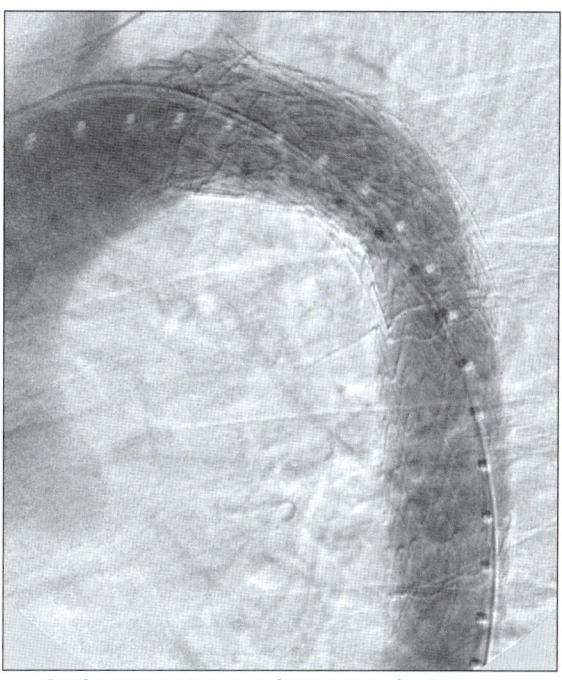

Figure 3. Thoracic aortogram after stent-graft placement shows occlusion of the thoracic aortic pseudoaneurysm. No endoleak is seen.

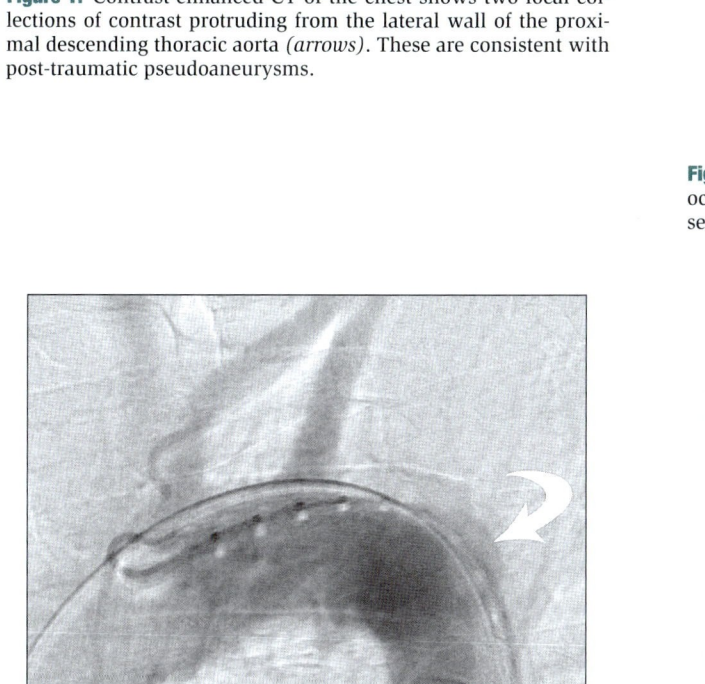

Figure 2. Intraoperative aortogram shows a subtle double density and irregularity of the proximal descending thoracic aorta *(curved arrow)*.

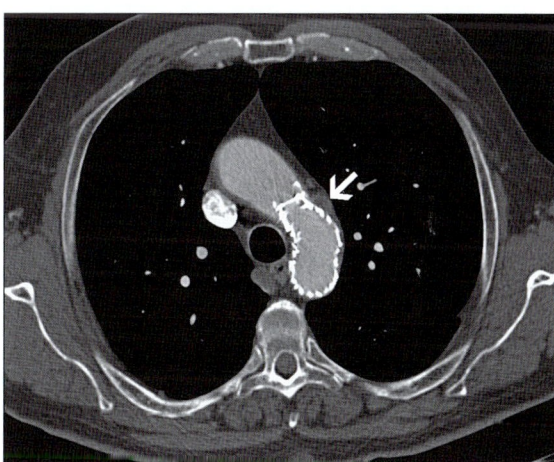

Figure 4. Follow-up contrast-enhanced thoracic CT 3 years after stent-graft placement shows near-complete resolution of the pseudoaneurysm *(arrow)*.

Case 73

DEMOGRAPHICS/CLINICAL HISTORY

A 75-year-old man with right-sided stroke and internal carotid artery (ICA) stenosis, undergoing angiography.

DISCUSSION

History/Indications for Procedure
This patient had a history of hypertension and diabetes and presented with a new right parietal infarct.

Procedure
Carotid artery stenting

Pre-procedure Imaging
Carotid Doppler shows a 60% to 99% stenosis of the right ICA. There is a 10% to 20% stenosis of the left ICA.

Intraprocedural Findings
There is an 80% stenosis at the origin of the right ICA (Fig. 1). The lesion was stented with a 6- to 8-mm × 30-mm Acculink stent while using an Accunet distal protection device (Abbot Vascular, Santa Clara, CA) (Figs. 2-4).

Follow-up and Complications
The patient was started on clopidogrel after the procedure and was discharged to a skilled nursing facility for stroke rehabilitation.

Suggested Readings

American College of Cardiology Foundation; American Society of Interventional and Therapeutic Neuroradiology; Society for Cardiovascular Angiography and Interventions; Society for Vascular Medicine and Biology; Society of Interventional Radiology; Bates ER, Babb JD, Casey DE Jr, et al: ACCF/SCAI/SVMB/SIR/ASITN 2007 clinical expert consensus document on carotid stenting: A report of the American College of Cardiology Foundation Task Force on Clinical Expert Consensus Documents (ACCF/SCAI/SVMB/SIR/ASITN Clinical Expert Consensus Document Committee on Carotid Stenting). J Am Coll Cardiol 49:126–170, 2007.

Gray WA, Yadav JS, Verta P, et al: The CAPTURE registry: Results of carotid stenting with embolic protection in the post approval setting. Catheter Cardiovasc Interv 69:341-348, 2007.

Macdonald S: The evidence for cerebral protection: An analysis and summary of the literature. Eur J Radiol 60:20-25, 2006.

Narins CR, Illig KA: Patient selection for carotid stenting versus endarterectomy: A systematic review. J Vasc Surg 44:661-672, 2006.

Case 73   147

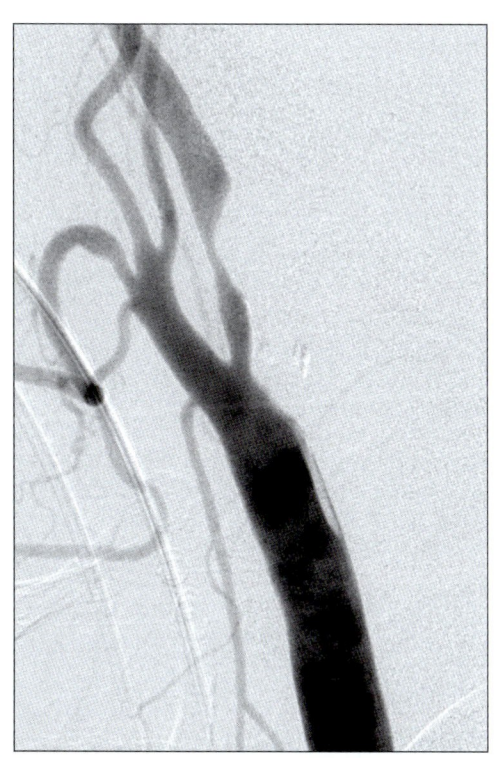

Figure 1. Lateral view of the carotid bifurcation shows an 80% stenosis at the origin of the ICA.

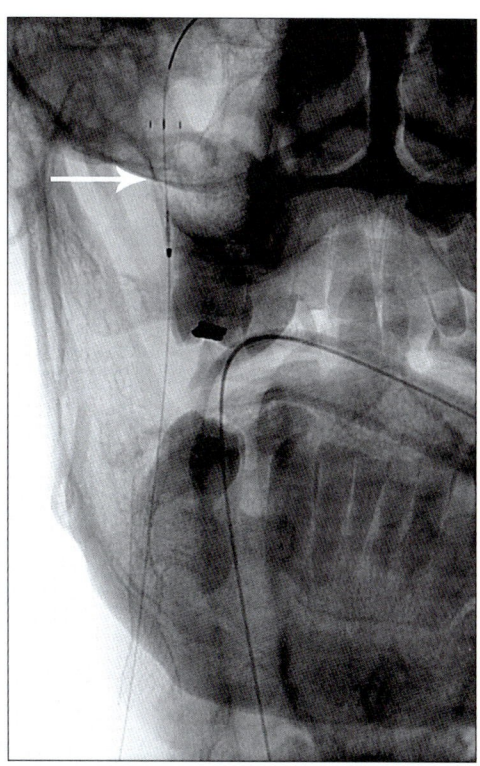

Figure 2. The Accunet distal protection device is in place *(arrow)*.

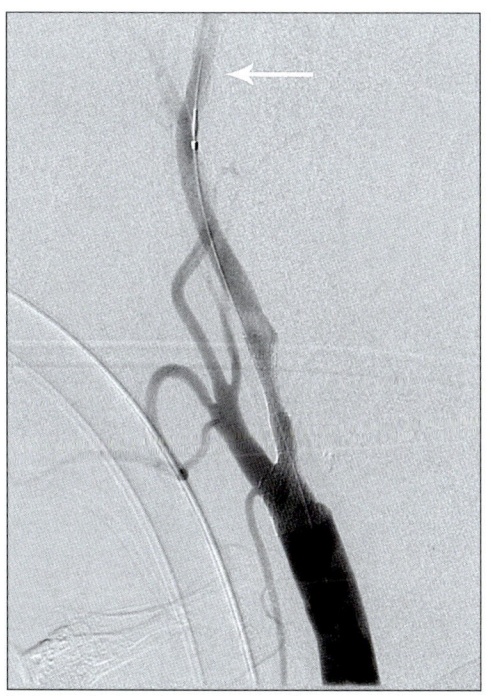

Figure 3. Lateral view immediately after stent placement shows significant residual stenosis. The Accunet appears free of debris *(arrow)*.

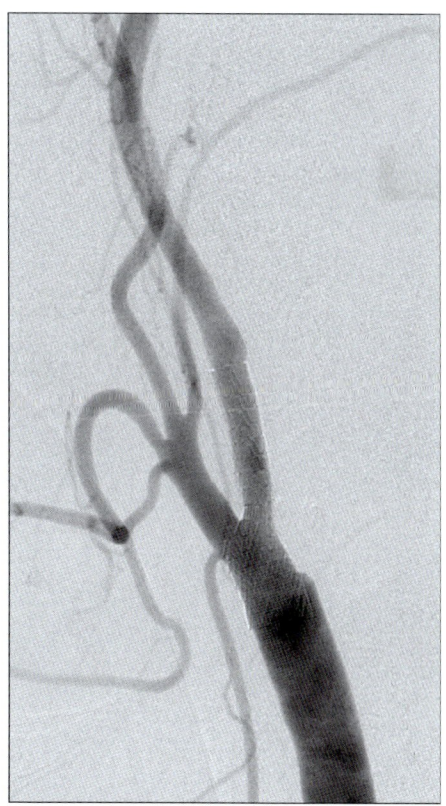

Figure 4. Lateral carotid angiogram after stent dilation shows significantly improved flow through the ICA. There also was improved right-sided intracranial circulation (not shown).

Case 74

DEMOGRAPHICS/CLINICAL HISTORY

A 56-year-old man with a history of prior left hemispheric stroke.

DISCUSSION

History/Indications for Procedure
A 56-year-old man with a history of prior left hemispheric stroke and right internal carotid artery stenosis.

Procedure
Placement of carotid stent

Pre-procedure Imaging
Carotid ultrasound shows 60% to 99% stenosis of the right internal carotid artery and occlusion of the left internal carotid artery. MRI confirms occlusion of the left internal carotid artery (Fig. 1), and diagnostic arteriogram shows impaired arterial supply to the left cerebral hemisphere through collaterals.

Intraprocedural Findings
There is an 80% stenosis of the proximal right internal carotid artery (Fig. 2). After placement of an embolic protection device, the stenosis was stented with a 6- to 8-mm × 40-mm Acculink (Abbot Vascular, Santa Clara, CA) stent (Fig. 3).

Follow-up and Complications
The patient did well until 2 years after stent placement, when he developed new symptoms of dizziness and transient left-sided visual loss. Repeat carotid arteriogram was performed showing the carotid artery stent to remain widely patent (Fig. 4).

Suggested Readings

Brahmanandam S, Ding EL, Conte MS, et al: Clinical results of carotid artery stenting compared with carotid endarterectomy. J Vasc Surg 47:343–49, 2008.

Connors JJ, Sacks D, Furlan AJ, et al: Training, competency, and credentialing standards for diagnostic cervicocerebral angiography, carotid stenting, and cerebrovascular intervention. J Vasc Interv Radiol 15:1347–56, 2004.

Macdonald S: The evidence for cerebral protection: An analysis and summary of the literature. Eur J Radiol 60:20–25, 2006.

Narins CR, Illig KA: Patient selection for carotid stenting versus endarterectomy: A systematic review. J Vasc Surg 44:661–672, 2006.

Case 74   149

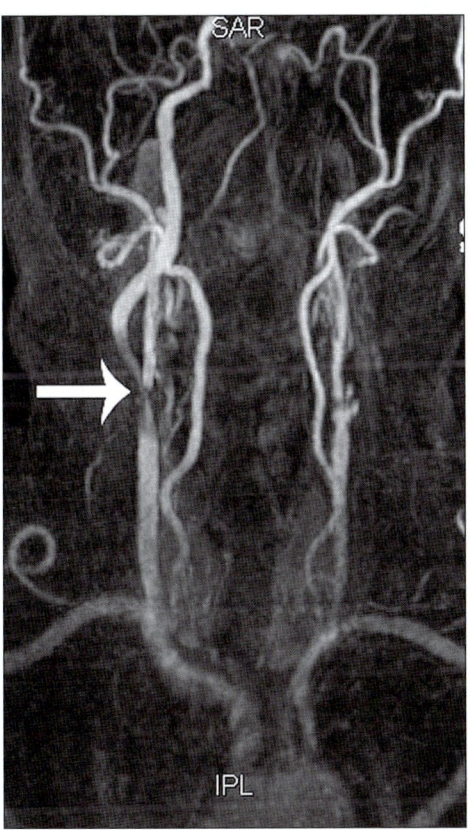

Figure 1. Coronal reformation from MR angiogram shows a high-grade stenosis at the origin of the right internal carotid artery *(arrow)*. The left internal carotid artery is occluded.

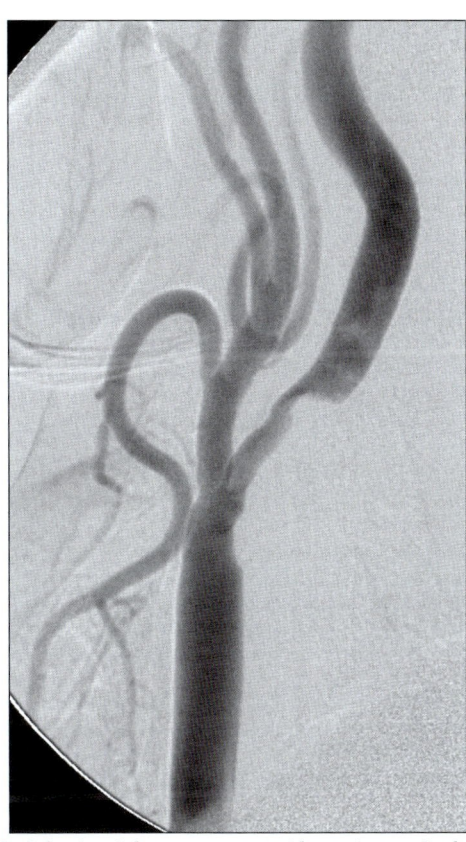

Figure 2. Selective right common carotid arteriogram in the lateral projection shows an 80% stenosis of the proximal right internal carotid artery.

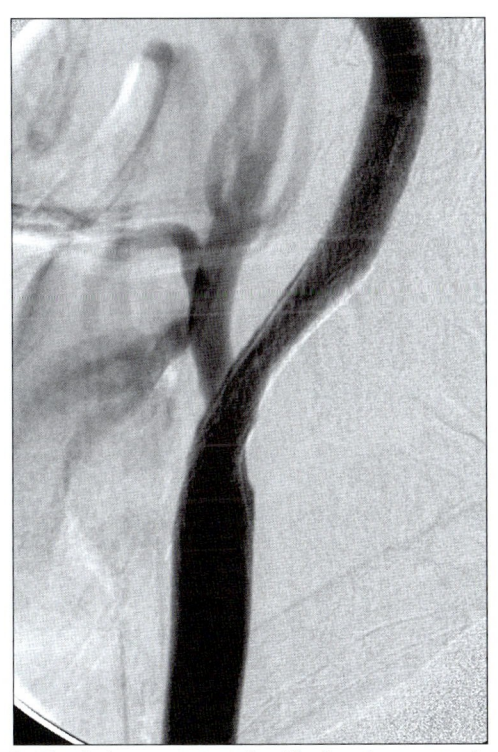

Figure 3. The lesion was treated with the placement of a 6- to 8-mm × 40-mm self-expanding stent.

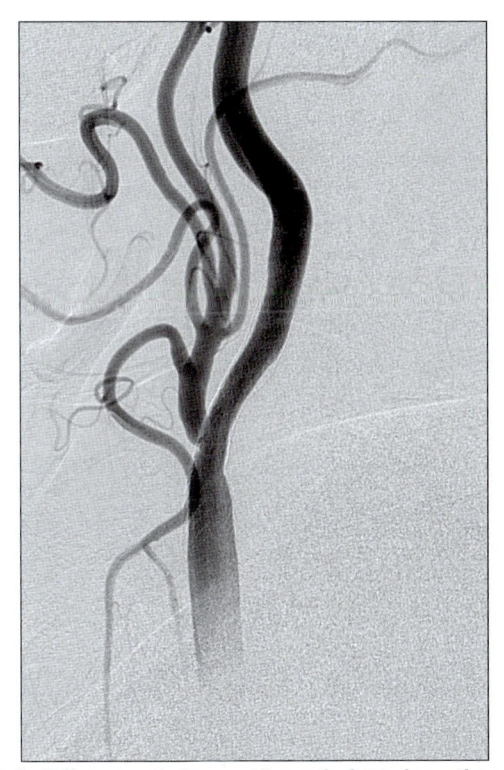

Figure 4. Follow-up arteriogram 18 months later shows the carotid artery stent to remain widely patent.

Case 75

DEMOGRAPHICS/CLINICAL HISTORY

A 49-year-old woman with recurrent carotid artery stenosis approximately 9 months after endarterectomy, undergoing arteriography.

DISCUSSION

History/Indications for Procedure
This patient had a history of hypertension and coronary artery disease and underwent right-sided carotid endarterectomy 9 months before presentation.

Procedure
Carotid artery stenting for recurrent stenosis after endarterectomy

Pre-procedure Imaging
MR angiography done at an outside hospital showed a 70% stenosis of the right internal carotid artery (ICA) (not shown).

Intraprocedural Findings
There is a 60% stenosis at the origin of the right ICA (Fig. 1). The lesion was stented using a 6- to 8-mm × 40-mm Acculink stent with the Accunet distal protection device (Abbot Vascular, Santa Clara, CA) (Figs. 2-4).

Follow-up and Complications
There was focal vasospasm at the level of the distal protection device at the end of the procedure (see Figs. 3 and 4). The patient was observed overnight, and discharged the following day on clopidogrel.

Suggested Readings

American College of Cardiology Foundation; American Society of Interventional and Therapeutic Neuroradiology; Society for Cardiovascular Angiography and Interventions; Society for Vascular Medicine and Biology; Society of Interventional Radiology; Bates ER, Babb JD, Casey DE Jr, et al: ACCF/SCAI/SVMB/SIR/ASITN 2007 clinical expert consensus document on carotid stenting: A report of the American College of Cardiology Foundation Task Force on Clinical Expert Consensus Documents (ACCF/SCAI/SVMB/SIR/ASITN Clinical Expert Consensus Document Committee on Carotid Stenting). J Am Coll Cardiol 49:126-170, 2007.

Gray WA, Yadav JS, Verta P, et al: The CAPTURE registry: Results of carotid stenting with embolic protection in the post approval setting. Catheter Cardiovasc Interv 69:341-348, 2007.

Macdonald S: The evidence for cerebral protection: An analysis and summary of the literature. Eur J Radiol 60:20-25, 2006.

Narins CR, Illig KA: Patient selection for carotid stenting versus endarterectomy: A systematic review. J Vasc Surg 44:661-672, 2006.

Case 75   151

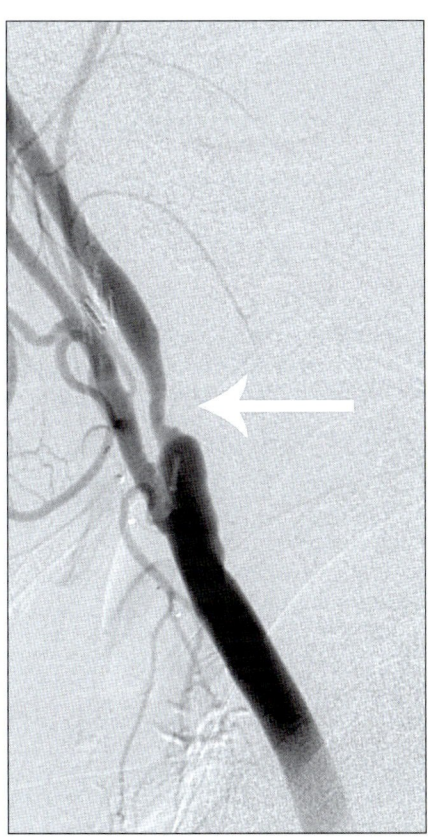

Figure 1. Lateral carotid arteriogram shows a 60% stenosis of the ICA adjacent to the site of prior endarterectomy *(arrow)*.

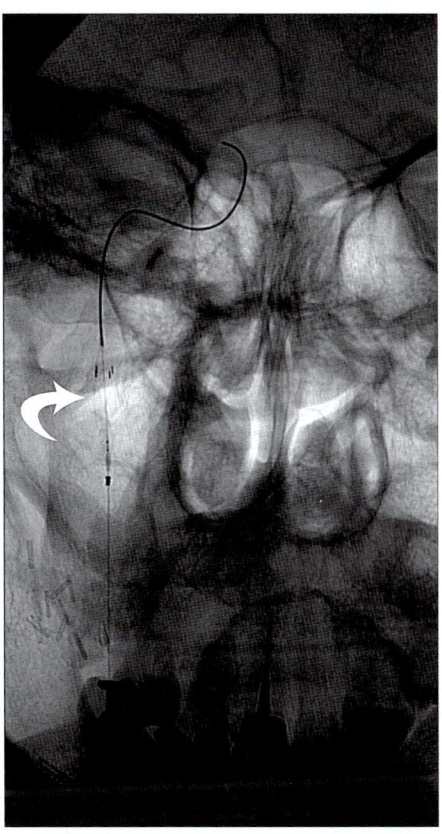

Figure 2. The Accunet distal protection device was deployed above the lesion *(arrow)*.

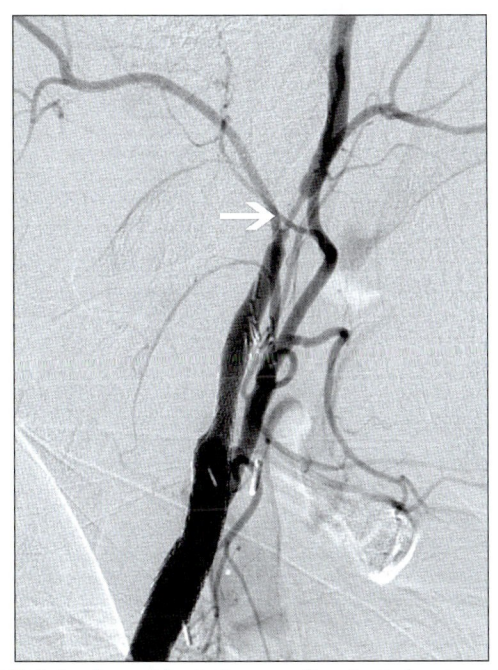

Figure 3. Lateral carotid arteriogram after stent placement shows only minimal narrowing at the level of the lesion. There is a focal stenosis of the ICA at the site of the distal protection device *(arrow)*. This is consistent with local vasospasm.

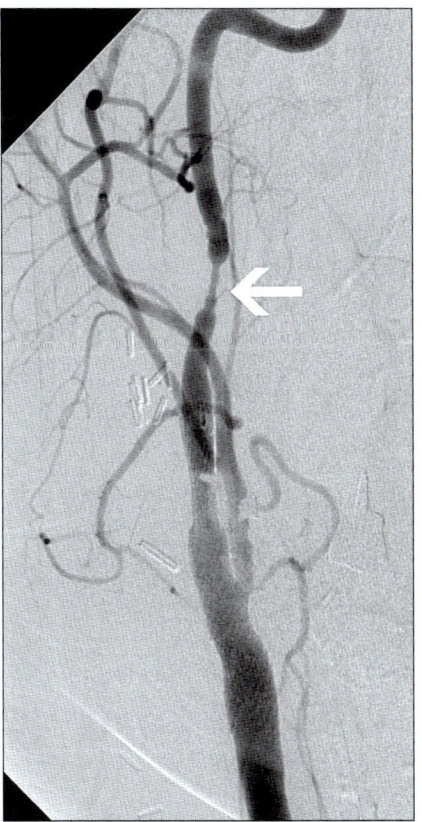

Figure 4. Anteroposterior carotid arteriogram after stent placement also shows focal arterial narrowing consistent with vasospasm *(arrow)*.

Case 76

DEMOGRAPHICS/CLINICAL HISTORY

A 39-year-old man with a history of polysubstance abuse who presents with right-sided weakness, undergoing angiography.

DISCUSSION

History/Indications for Procedure

A 38-year-old man with a history of polysubstance abuse initially presented with right-sided weakness. After diagnosing carotid dissection, the patient was treated with anticoagulation; 9 months later, he presents with recurrent symptoms.

Procedure

Carotid dissection

Pre-procedure Imaging

Magnetic resonance angiogram of the neck shows bilateral, short-segment dissections of the proximal internal carotid arteries.

Intraprocedural Findings

Cerebral angiogram shows a 60% stenosis of the proximal left internal carotid artery (Fig. 1), and a follow-up angiogram 9 months later shows significant worsening of the stenosis (Figs. 2 and 3). The dissection was treated with a 6- to 8-mm × 40-mm, self-expanding stent (Acculink, Abbot Vascular, Santa Clara, CA) (Fig. 4).

Follow-up and Complications

The patient was placed on aspirin and Plavix. He has required no further intervention during the year since the stent was placed.

Suggested Readings

Dziewas R, Konrad C, Dräger B, et al: Cervical artery dissection—clinical features, risk factors, therapy and outcome in 126 patients. J Neurol 250:1179-1184, 2003.

Edgell RC, Abou-Chebl A, Yadav JS: Endovascular management of spontaneous carotid artery dissection. J Vasc Surg 42:854-860, 2005.

Rubinstein SM, Peerdeman SM, van Tulder MW, et al: A systematic review of the risk factors for cervical artery dissection. Stroke 36:1575-1580, 2005.

Case 76   153

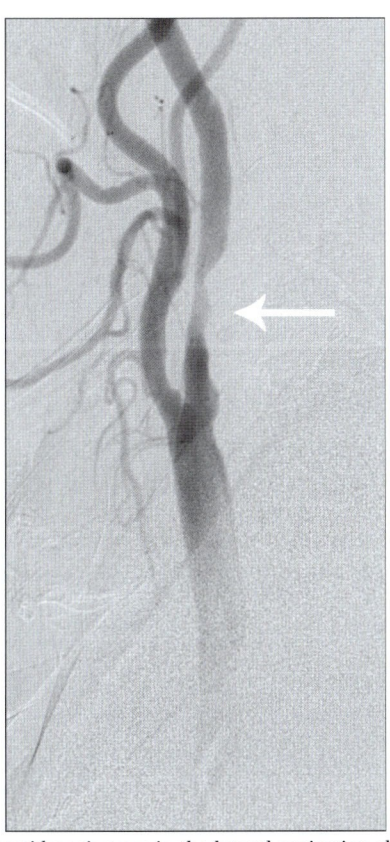

Figure 1. Carotid angiogram in the lateral projection shows a 60% stenosis of the proximal left internal carotid artery *(arrow)*.

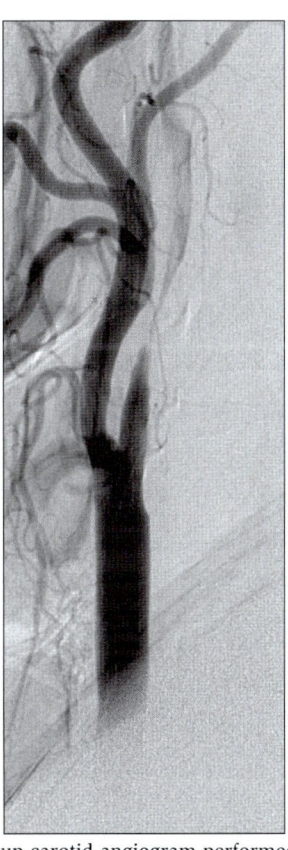

Figure 2. Follow-up carotid angiogram performed 9 months later, when the patient's symptoms returned, shows progression of the internal carotid stenosis. The lateral projection shows a smooth, high-grade stenosis of the proximal left internal carotid artery.

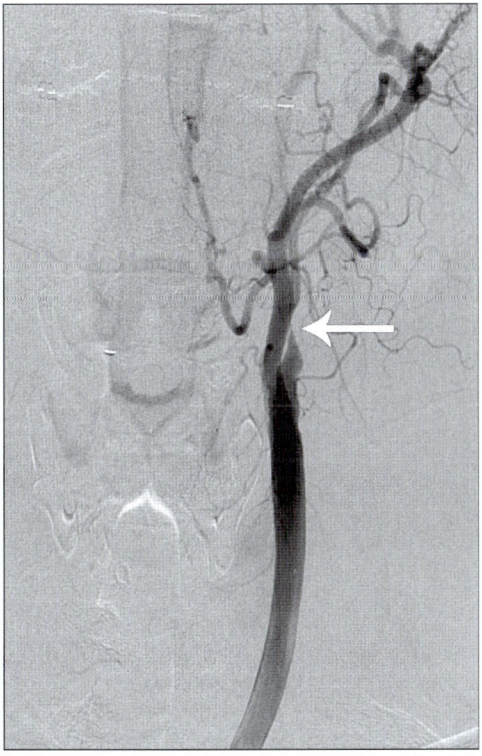

Figure 3. The flame-shaped dissection is well seen in the anteroposterior projection *(arrow)*.

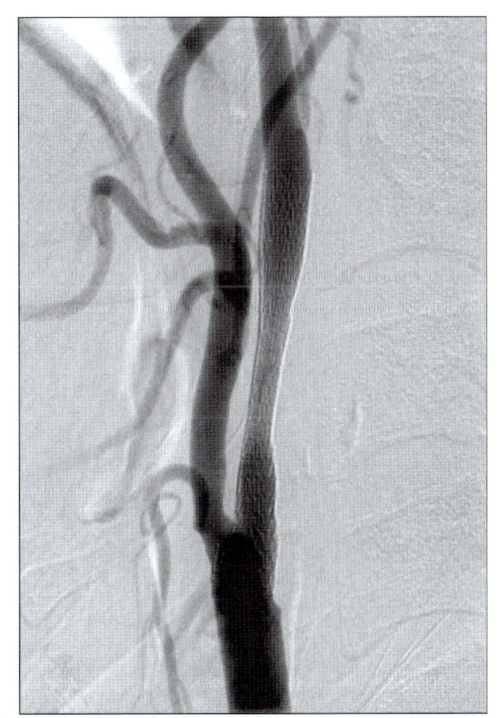

Figure 4. The carotid dissection was treated with the placement of a 6- to 8-mm × 40-mm, self-expanding stent.

Case 77

DEMOGRAPHICS/CLINICAL HISTORY

A 58-year-old woman with crescendo transient ischemic attacks (TIAs).

DISCUSSION

History/Indications for Procedure
A 58-year-old woman with intermittent episodes of right-hand numbness, weakness, and trouble speaking that have been increasing in frequency and duration.

Procedure
Endovascular management of internal carotid artery, dissecting aneurysm

Pre-procedure Imaging
MRI of the brain shows new, punctuate foci of restricted diffusion within the left parietal lobe, compatible with embolic infarcts. MR angiogram of the left carotid was normal.

Intraprocedural Findings
Carotid arteriogram shows irregularity of the left internal carotid artery, consistent with fibromuscular dysplasia, and a small dissecting aneurysm arising from the anterior wall of the internal carotid artery (Figs. 1 and 2). The diseased portion of the vessel was carefully crossed with a guidewire, and a 4.5-mm × 30-mm Neuroform stent (Boston Scientific, Natick, MA) was deployed across the dissecting aneurysm (Fig. 3).

Follow-up and Complications
The patient was started on clopidogrel, and her symptoms resolved following stent placement. Follow-up carotid arteriogram performed 2 years later shows no intrastent stenosis; the aneurysm is still visible but is stable in size (Figure 4).

Suggested Readings
Donas KP, Mayer D, Guber I, et al: Endovascular repair of extracranial carotid artery dissection: Current status and level of evidence. J Vasc Interv Radiol 19:1693-1698, 2008.

Kadkhodayan Y, Jeck DT, Moran CJ, et al: Angioplasty and stenting in carotid dissection with or without associated pseudoaneurysm. AJNR Am J Neuroradiol 26:2328-2335, 2005.

Liu AY, Paulsen RD, Marcellus ML, et al: Long-term outcomes after carotid stent placement treatment of carotid artery dissection. Neurosurgery 45:1368-1373, 1999.

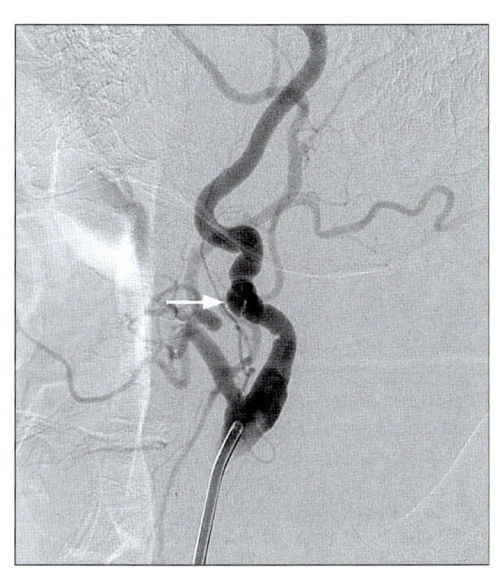

Figure 1. Left carotid arteriogram, lateral projection, shows an irregular segment of the internal carotid artery consistent with fibromuscular dysplasia. There is a small dissecting aneurysm arising from the anterior wall of the diseased artery *(arrow)*.

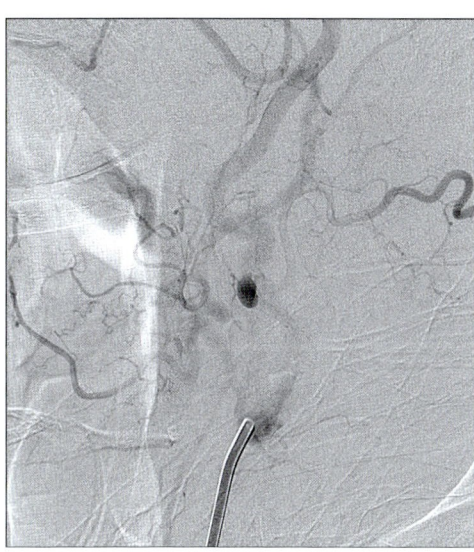

Figure 2. Delayed image from lateral left carotid arteriogram shows contrast retention within the dissecting aneurysm.

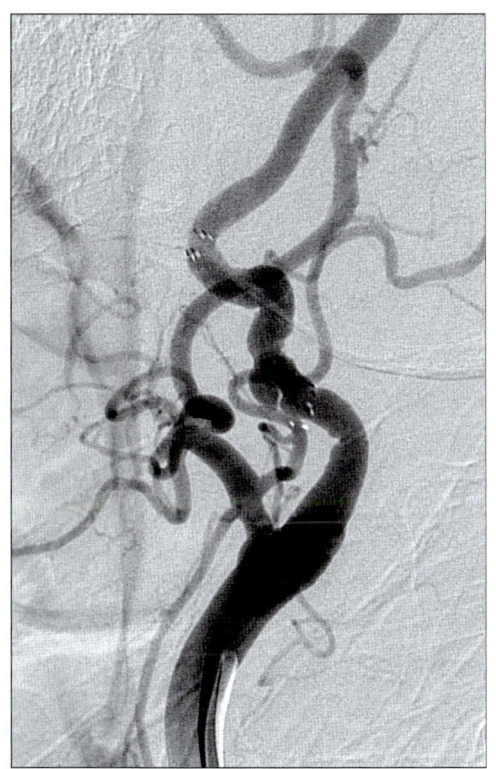

Figure 3. A 4.5-mm Neuroform stent has been placed across the aneurysm.

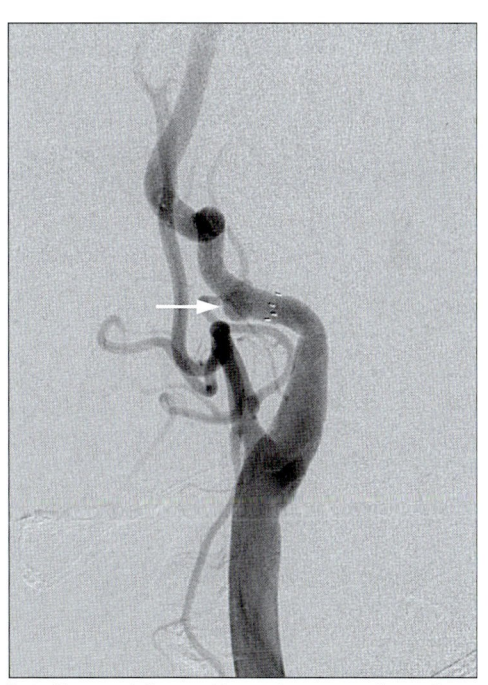

Figure 4. Follow-up left carotid arteriogram performed 2 years after stent placement shows a more regular appearance of the proximal left internal carotid artery. There is a small double density of contrast *(arrow)* resulting from the persistence of the small aneurysm. The aneurysm has remained stable in size, and the patient has remained asymptomatic.

Case 78

DEMOGRAPHICS/CLINICAL HISTORY

A 59-year-old man with a history of prior neck irradiation and hemorrhage from left carotid endarterectomy site, undergoing arteriography.

DISCUSSION

History/Indications for Procedure

A 59-year-old man with a history of modified radical neck dissection and radiation therapy for treatment of tonsillar carcinoma subsequently underwent carotid endarterectomy at an outside hospital for symptomatic carotid stenosis. Two months later, the patient presents with bleeding from the endarterectomy site.

Procedure

Internal carotid artery embolization

Pre-procedure Imaging

MR angiogram of the neck shows marked narrowing of the left internal carotid artery. A carotid arteriogram shows an irregular stenosis of the left internal carotid artery, just distal to the endarterectomy site, and filling of a 5-cm pseudoaneurysm arising from the distal endarterectomy site (Fig. 1).

Intraprocedural Findings

An occlusion balloon was inflated in the petrous portion of the left internal carotid artery for 20 minutes (Fig. 2). After the patient showed no neurologic changes with 20 minutes of test balloon occlusion, the left internal carotid artery was embolized with coils (Figs. 3 and 4).

Follow-up and Complications

The patient was closely monitored after the procedure and showed no neurologic effects from the embolization.

Suggested Readings

Chaloupka JC, Putman CM, Citardi MJ, et al: Endovascular therapy for the carotid blowout syndrome in head-and-neck surgical patients: Diagnostic and managerial considerations. AJNR Am J Neuroradiol 17:843, 1996.

Chang FC, Lirng JF, Luo CB, et al: Patients with head and neck cancers and associated postirradiated carotid blowout syndrome: Endovascular therapeutic methods and outcomes. J Vasc Surg 47:936, 2008.

Luo CB, Teng MM, Chang FC, et al: Radiation carotid blowout syndrome in nasopharyngeal carcinoma: Angiographic features and endovascular management. Otolaryngol Head Neck Surg 138:86, 2008.

Roh JL, Suh DC, Kim MR, et al: Endovascular management of carotid blowout syndrome in patients with head and neck cancers. Oral Oncol 44:844, 2008.

Case 78   157

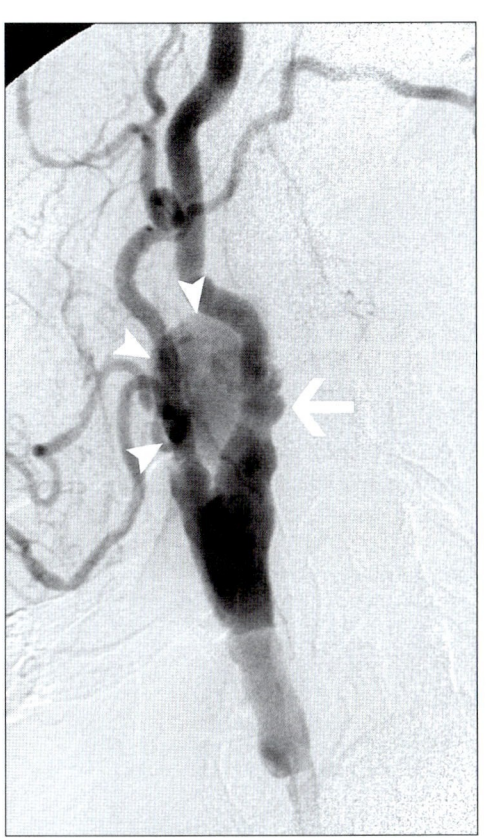

Figure 1. Left common carotid arteriogram shows irregularity of left common carotid artery, just distal to endarterectomy site *(arrow)*. There is also filling of 5-cm pseudoaneurysm *(arrowheads)*.

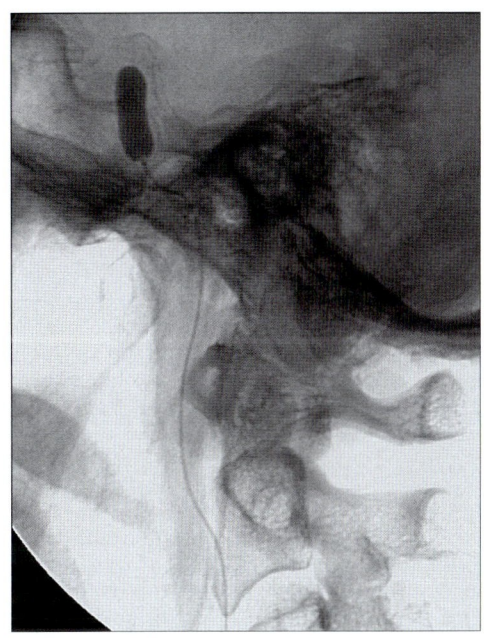

Figure 2. Occlusion balloon has been inflated in petrous portion of internal carotid artery.

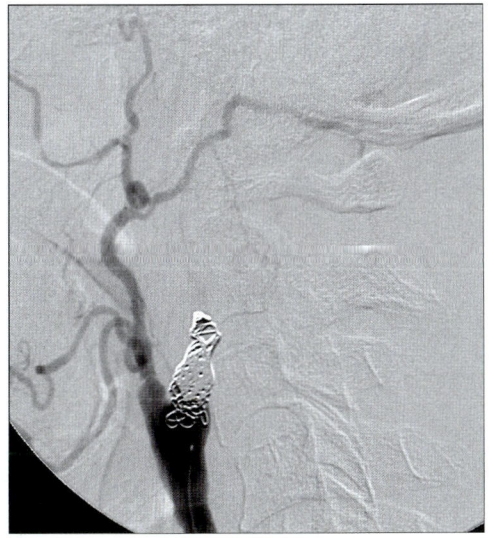

Figure 3. Follow-up arteriogram after embolization—lateral projection. Internal carotid artery has been completely occluded with coils.

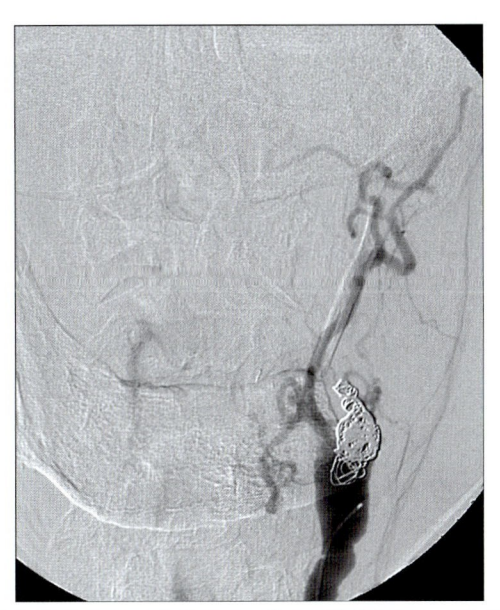

Figure 4. Follow-up arteriogram after embolization—AP projection. Internal carotid artery has been completely occluded with coils. There is continued filling of left external carotid artery.

Case 79

DEMOGRAPHICS/CLINICAL HISTORY

A 52-year-old man with unresectable oropharyngeal carcinoma and uncontrollable oropharyngeal hemorrhage, undergoing arteriography and arterial embolization.

DISCUSSION

History/Indications for Procedure
A 52-year-old man has unresectable oropharyngeal carcinoma, for which he is undergoing chemotherapy and radiation therapy. He presents with a new, massive oropharyngeal hemorrhage.

Procedure
Endovascular management of carotid blowout

Intraprocedural Findings
There is a pseudoaneurysm of the proximal left external carotid artery and irregularity of the left lingual artery (Figs. 1 and 2). The lingual artery was embolized with polyvinyl alcohol (PVA) microspheres, and the external carotid artery was embolized with coils (Fig. 3).

Follow-up and Complications
The patient stabilized after the embolization and was discharged from the hospital. He returned 3 weeks later with recurrent oropharyngeal bleeding, was placed on palliative care, and died shortly thereafter.

Suggested Readings
Cohen J, Rad I: Contemporary management of carotid blowout. Curr Opin Otolaryngol Head Neck Surg 12:110-115, 2004.
Kakizawa H, Toyota N, Naito A, Ito K: Endovascular therapy for management of oral hemorrhage in malignant head and neck tumors. Cardiovasc Intervent Radiol 28:722-729, 2005.
Turowski B, Zanella FE: Interventional neuroradiology of the head and neck. Neuroimaging Clin N Am 13:619-645, 2003.

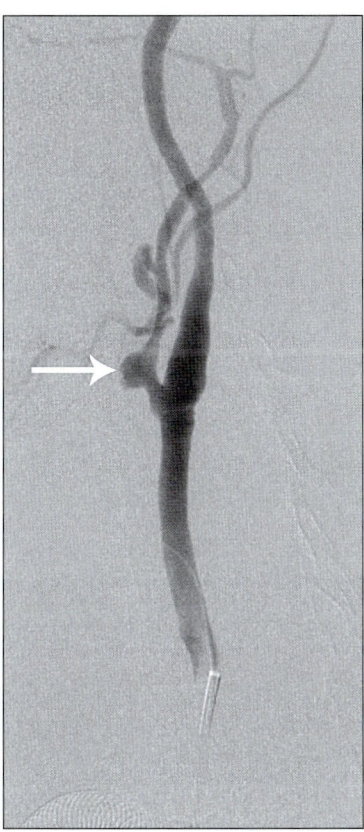

Figure 1. Left carotid arteriogram demonstrates an irregular pseudoaneurysm of the external carotid artery *(arrow)*.

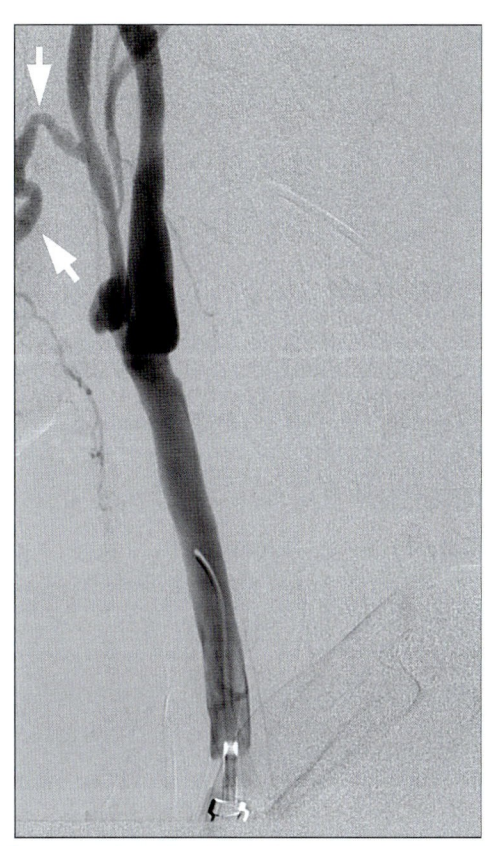

Figure 2. Slightly different obliquity shows the diffuse irregularity of the lingual artery *(arrows)*.

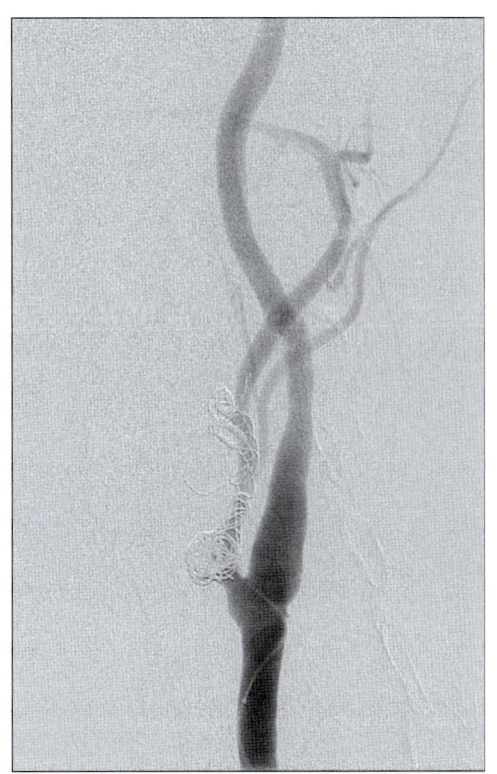

Figure 3. The lingual artery was embolized with PVA particles, and coils were placed from the origin of the lingual artery back, with packing of the pseudoaneurysm.

Case 80

DEMOGRAPHICS/CLINICAL HISTORY

An 11-year-old boy with a large juvenile nasal angiofibroma and epistaxis, undergoing magnetic resonance imaging (MRI) and angiography.

DISCUSSION

History/Indications for Procedure
An 11-year-old boy with a history of nosebleeds and a large nasopharyngeal mass.

Procedure
Embolization of juvenile nasal angiofibroma

Pre-procedure Imaging
Contrast-enhanced MRI demonstrates an extensive, enhancing soft tissue mass centered within the left nasal cavity (Fig. 1), consistent with a juvenile nasal angiofibroma.

Intraprocedural Findings
Left external carotid angiogram demonstrates a large vascular tumor with an arterial supply from the left internal maxillary artery and left ascending pharyngeal artery (Figs. 2 and 3). The tumor was embolized using a combination of polyvinyl alcohol particles and coils (Fig. 4).

Follow-up and Complications
The day after embolization, the patient underwent surgical resection of the mass. Since then, the patient has had no further episodes of epistaxis, and there has been no evidence of recurrence on fiberoptic sinonasal endoscopy.

Suggested Readings
Fagan JJ, Snyderman CH, Carrau RL, Janecka IP: Nasopharyngeal angiofibromas: Selecting a surgical approach. Head Neck 19:391-399, 1997.
Moulin G, Chagnaud C, Gras R, et al: Juvenile nasopharyngeal angiofibroma: Comparison of blood loss during removal in embolized group versus nonembolized group. Cardiovasc Intervent Radiol 18:158-161, 1995.
Scholtz AW, Appenroth E, Kammern-Jolly K, et al: Juvenile nasopharyngeal angiofibroma: Management and therapy. Laryngoscope 111(Pt 1):681-687, 2001.
Turowski B, Zanella FE: Interventional neuroradiology of the head and neck. Neuroimaging Clin N Am 13:619-645, 2003.
Valavanis A, Christoforidis G: Applications of interventional neuroradiology in the head and neck. Semin Roentgenol 35:72-83, 2000.

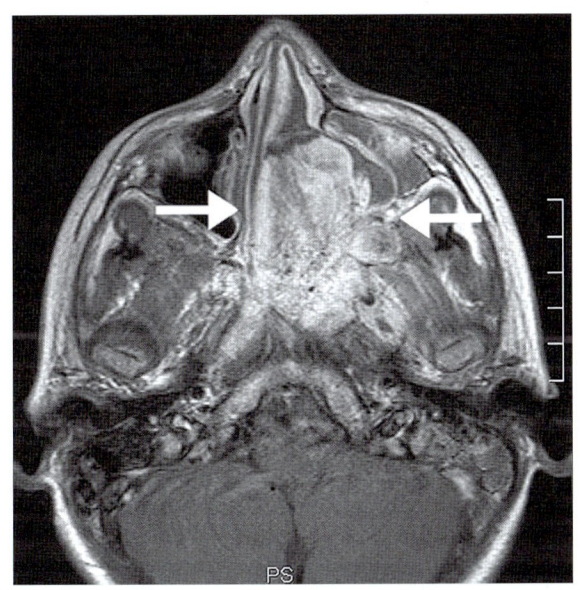

Figure 1. Postcontrast, axial, T1-weighted MR image through the nasopharynx demonstrates an extensive, enhancing soft tissue mass centered in the left nasal cavity with local invasion *(arrows)*. These findings are consistent with a juvenile nasal angiofibroma.

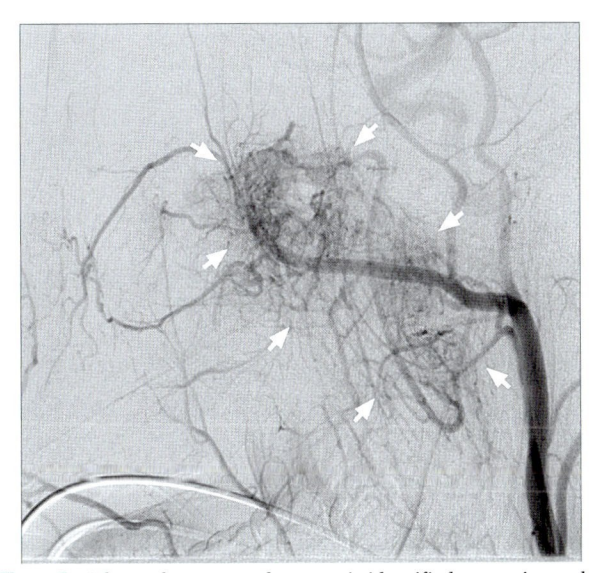

Figure 2. A large, hypervascular mass is identified on angiography of the left external carotid *(arrows)*.

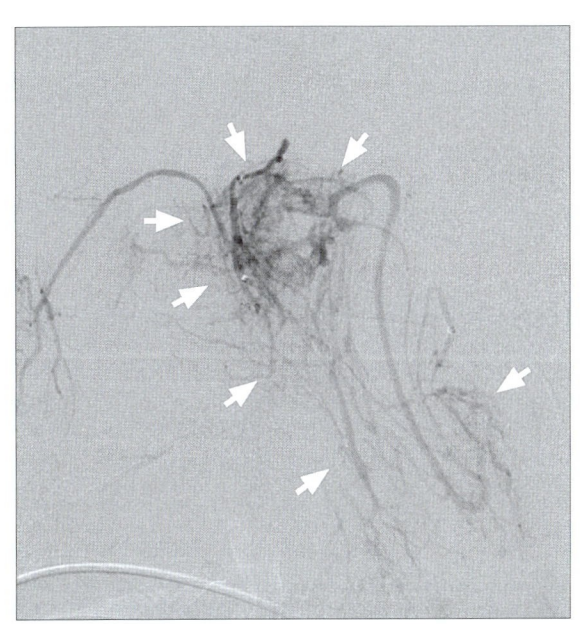

Figure 3. A microcatheter has been advanced into the distal left maxillary artery. Superselective angiogram demonstrates a portion of the mass supplied by the internal maxillary artery *(arrows)*.

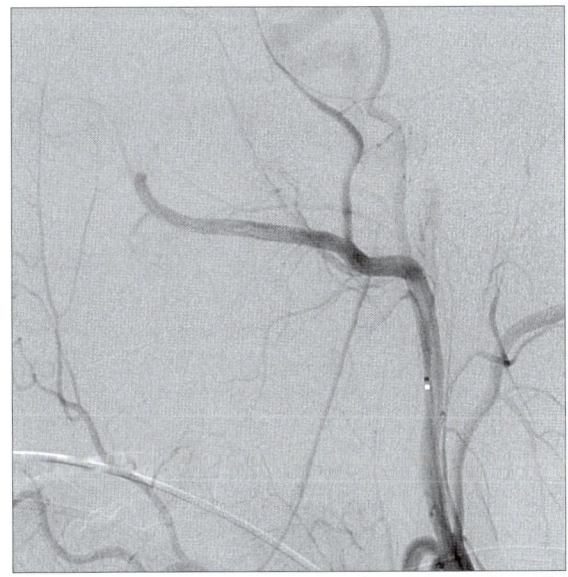

Figure 4. External carotid angiogram after embolization of the internal maxillary and ascending pharyngeal arteries shows no further filling of the tumor vasculature.

Case 81

DEMOGRAPHICS/CLINICAL HISTORY

A 75-year-old man with a hypervascular mass involving the right mandible, undergoing computed tomography (CT), angiography, and embolization.

DISCUSSION

History/Indications for Procedure
A 75-year-old man had a hypervascular mass involving the right mandible. The patient is undergoing preoperative embolization before resection of the mass.

Procedure
Embolization of mandibular mass

Pre-procedure Imaging
CT of the mandible demonstrates a 4.2-cm, multiloculated, expansile, lytic lesion in the right mandible (Fig. 1).

Intraprocedural Findings
External carotid angiogram demonstrates tumor blush within the right mandible, with supply from the right inferior alveolar artery (Fig. 2). The right inferior alveolar artery was embolized with polyvinyl alcohol particles (Fig. 3).

Follow-up and Complications
The patient underwent uncomplicated enucleation and curettage of the mandibular lesion. Pathologic examination determined the mass to be a myoepithelioma.

Suggested Readings
Liu DG, Ma XC, Li BM, Zhang JG: Clinical study of preoperative angiography and embolization of hypervascular neoplasms in the oral and maxillofacial region. Oral Surg Oral Med Oral Pathol Oral Radiol Endod 101:102-109, 2006.

Turowski B, Zanella FE: Interventional neuroradiology of the head and neck. Neuroimaging Clin N Am 13:619-645, 2003.

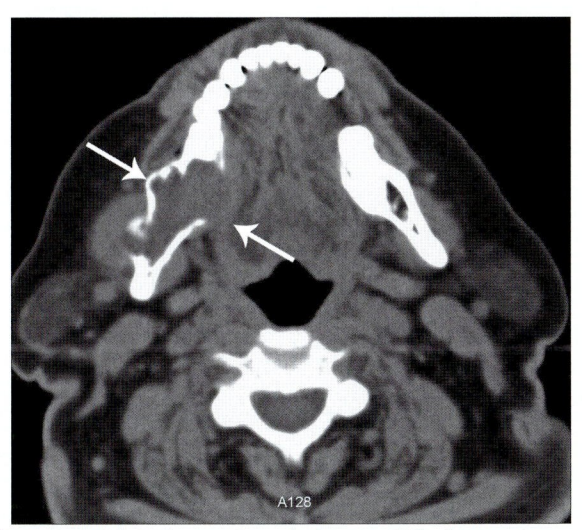

Figure 1. Axial CT image through the mandible demonstrates an expansile, lytic lesion in the mandible *(arrows)*, positioned just posterior to the first molar.

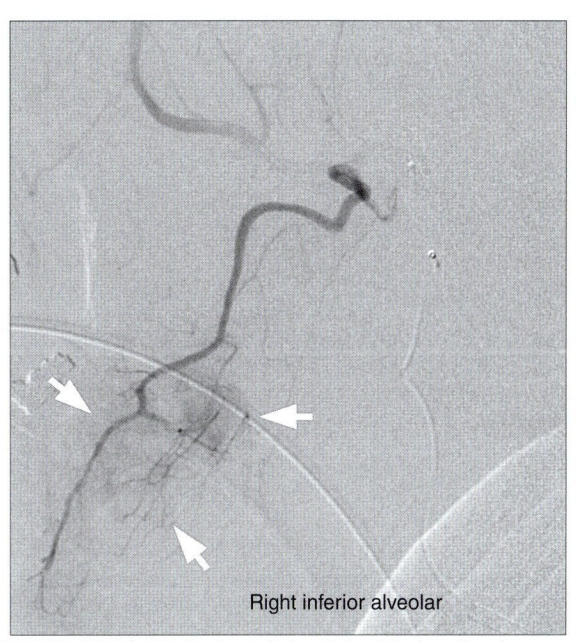

Figure 2. Selective injection of the right inferior alveolar artery demonstrates an abnormal blush in the right mandible *(arrows)*.

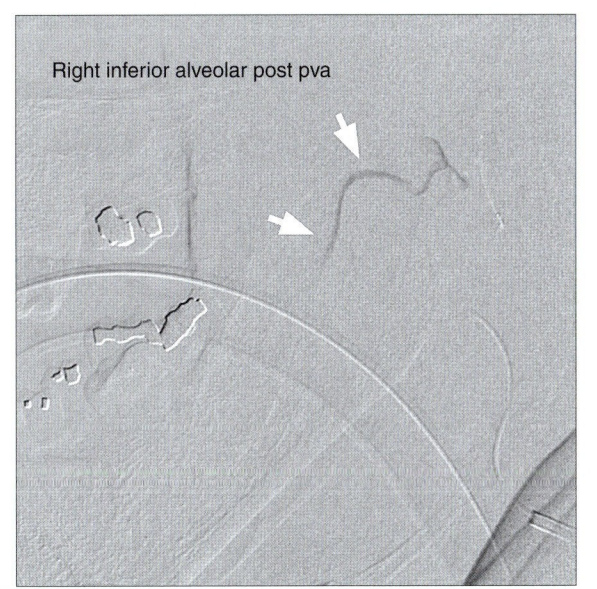

Figure 3. The right inferior alveolar artery was embolized to achieve stasis.

Case 82

DEMOGRAPHICS/CLINICAL HISTORY

A 71-year-old woman with prior left PCA stroke and vertebrobasilar insufficiency, undergoing arteriography.

DISCUSSION

History/Indications for Procedure
This patient presented with worsening vertigo and ataxia.

Procedure
Vertebral artery stenting

Pre-procedure Imaging
MRI of the head shows an old infarct in the left PICA and PCA territories. Diagnostic angiography reveals occlusion of the left vertebral artery and high-grade stenosis of the proximal right vertebral artery (Fig. 1).

Intraprocedural Findings
The lesion was predilated with a 2.25-mm balloon (Fig. 2) and stented with a 3.5-mm × 20-mm Wingspan Stent (Fig. 3).

Follow-up and Complications
The patient was placed on aspirin and clopidogrel to prevent stent thrombosis. The vertigo and ataxia resolved completely after stent placement.

Suggested Readings
Boulos AS, Levy EI, Bendok BR, et al: Evolution of neuroendovascular intervention: A review of advancement in device technology. Neurosurgery 54:438-453, 2004.

Moftakhar R, Turk AS, Niemann DB, et al: Effects of carotid or vertebrobasilar stent placement on cerebral perfusion and cognition. AJNR Am J Neuroradiol 26:1772-1780, 2005.

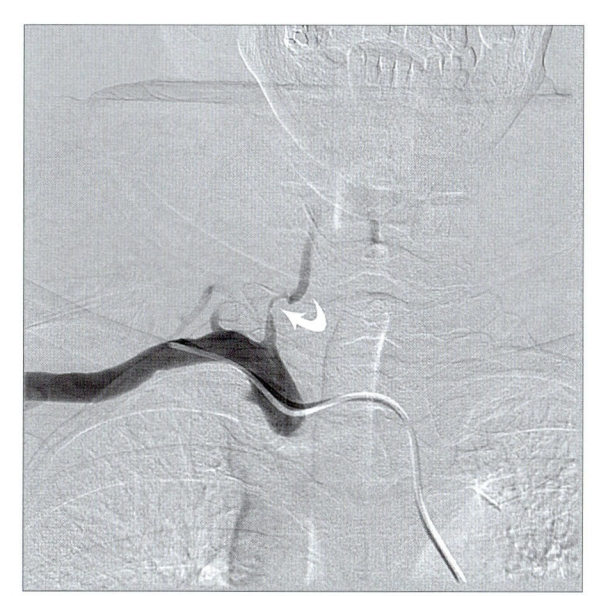

Figure 1. Diagnostic arteriogram shows a focal stenosis 1 cm from the origin of the right vertebral artery *(arrow)*.

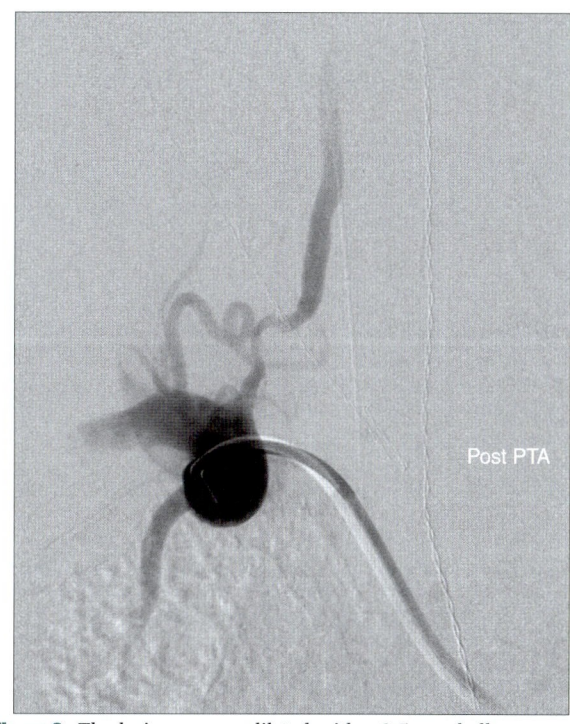

Figure 2. The lesion was predilated with a 2.5-mm balloon.

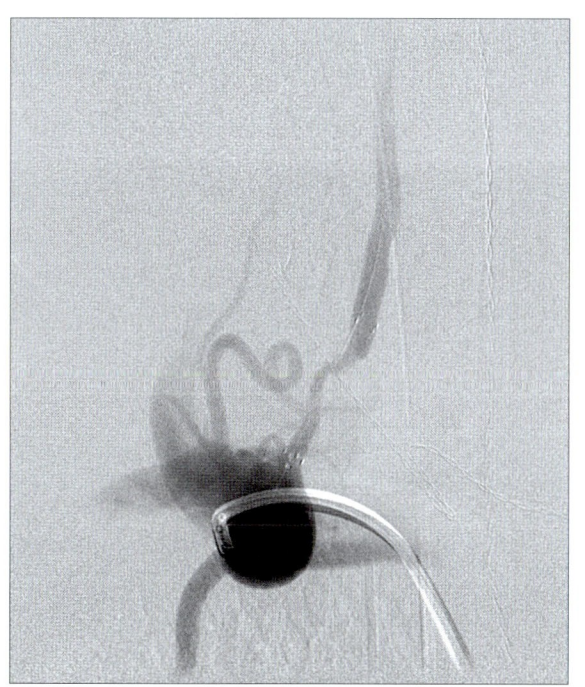

Figure 3. A 3.5- × 20-mm Wingspan stent was placed across the lesion. The patient's symptoms resolved after stenting.

Case 83

DEMOGRAPHICS/CLINICAL HISTORY

A 67-year-old woman with right hemispheric watershed stroke.

DISCUSSION

History/Indications for Procedure
A 67-year-old woman with right hemispheric watershed stroke.

Procedure
Intracranial stent placement

Pre-procedure Imaging
MRI shows abnormal signal intensity consistent with subacute infarcts in the right MCA/ACA territory; MR angiogram shows a stenosis of the supraclinoid internal carotid artery. Perfusion map shows delay time to peak and increased mean transit time in the right cerebral hemisphere.

Intraprocedural Findings
There is a 70% stenosis of the internal carotid artery extending from the ophthalmic segment to the level of the posterior communicating artery (Fig. 1). The lesion was angioplastied with a 2.5-mm balloon, and a 2.5-mm balloon expandable stent was placed for significant residual stenosis after angioplasty (Figs. 2, 3, and 4).

Follow-up and Complications
The patient was started on Plavix after stent placement. In the 2 years since stent placement, the patient had no further evidence of cerebral ischemia or stroke.

Suggested Readings
Intracranial angioplasty and stenting for cerebral atherosclerosis: A position statement of the American Society of Interventional and Therapeutic Neuroradiology, Society of Interventional Radiology, and the American Society of Neuroradiology. AJNR Am J Neuroradiol 26:2323-2327, 2005.

SSYLVIA Study Investigators: Stenting of symptomatic atherosclerotic lesions in the vertebral or intracranial arteries (SSYLVIA): Study results. Stroke 35:1388-1392, 2004.

Case 83   167

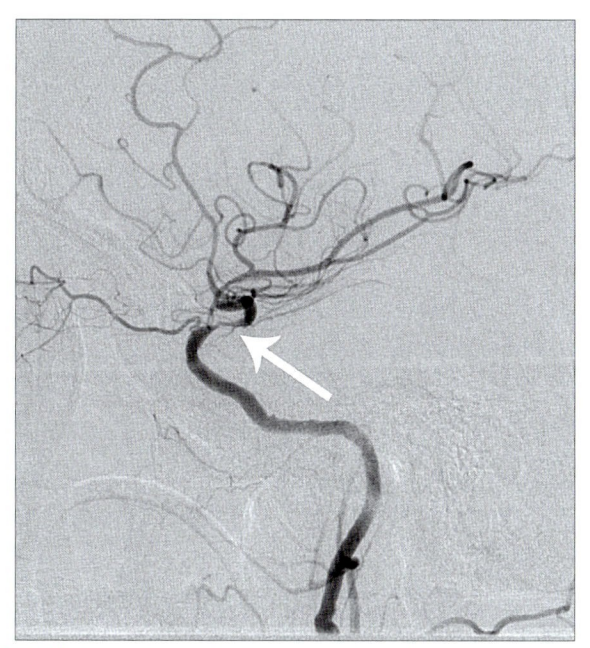

Figure 1. Internal carotid arteriogram, lateral projection shows a 70% stenosis of the supraclinoid internal carotid artery *(arrow)*.

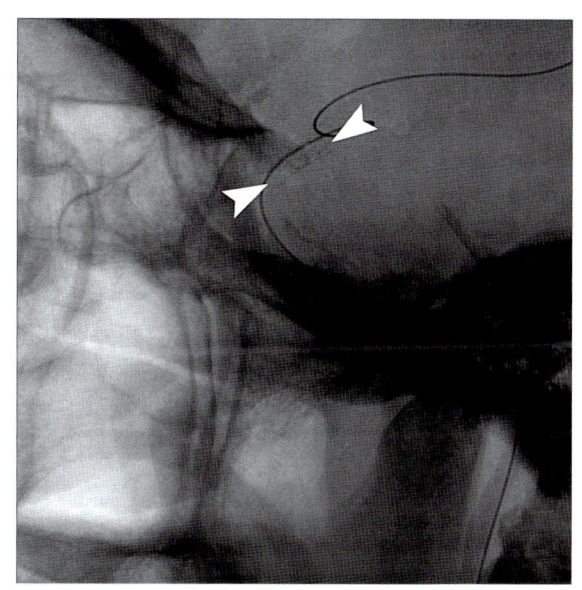

Figure 3. A 2.5-mm balloon expandable stent *(arrowheads)* was placed across the lesion.

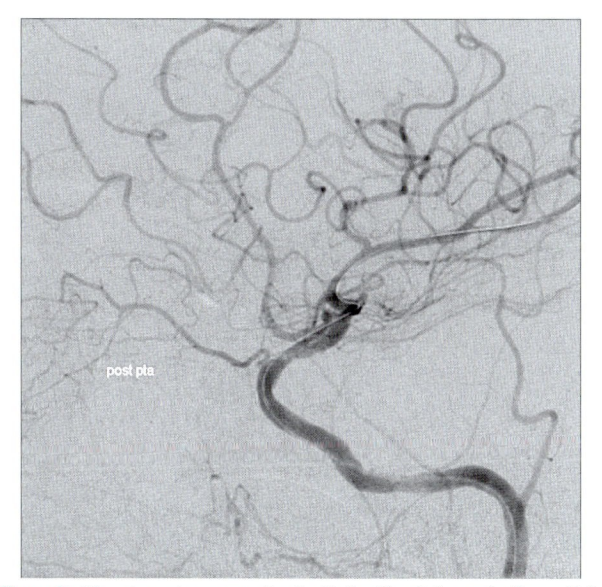

Figure 2. The stenosis was angioplastied with a 2.5-mm balloon. Follow-up injection shows a small dissection flap and >50% residual stenosis.

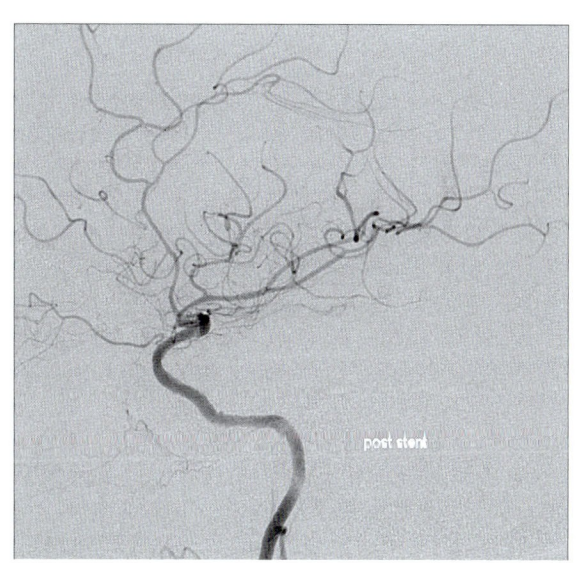

Figure 4. Follow-up arteriogram after stent placement shows a good angiographic result with no residual stenosis. There is improved perfusion to the right cerebral hemisphere.

Case 84

DEMOGRAPHICS/CLINICAL HISTORY

A 61-year-old woman with a right-sided watershed infarct, undergoing angiography.

DISCUSSION

History/Indications for Procedure
A 61-year-old woman who has a history of diabetes and hypertension presents with left upper extremity and bilateral lower extremity weakness.

Procedure
Intracranial angioplasty

Pre-procedure Imaging
Magnetic resonance imaging showed complete occlusion of the right internal carotid artery. Diagnostic arteriogram confirms occlusion of the right internal carotid artery, with reconstitution of the right anterior cerebral distribution through the anterior communicating artery; there is a focal, high-grade stenosis of the left A1 segment of the anterior cerebral artery (Fig. 1).

Intraprocedural Findings
The stenosis of the A1 segment of the left anterior cerebral artery was crossed with a 0.014-inch guidewire (Fig. 2), and the lesion was dilated with a 1.5-mm × 15-mm Maverick balloon (Boston Scientific, Natick, MA). After balloon angioplasty, there was improved flow through the anterior cerebral and anterior communicating arteries (Fig. 3).

Follow-up and Complications
The patient was started on clopidogrel after the procedure. In the subsequent 4 years, she has not had any further cerebrovascular accidents; follow-up angiograms confirmed that the stenosis has remained stable (Fig. 4).

Suggested Readings

Higashida RT, Meyers PM, Connors JJ 3rd, et al: Intracranial angioplasty and stenting for cerebral atherosclerosis: A position statement of the American Society of Interventional and Therapeutic Neuroradiology, Society of Interventional Radiology and the American Society of Neuroradiology. AJNR Am J Neuroradiol 26:2323-2327, 2005.

Kasner SE, Chimowitz MI, Lynn MJ, et al: Predictors of ischemic stroke in the territory of a symptomatic intracranial arterial stenosis. Circulation 113:555-563, 2006.

SSYLVIA Study Investigators: Stenting of Symptomatic Atherosclerotic Lesions in the Vertebral or Intracranial Arteries (SSYLVIA): Study results. Stroke 35:1388-1392, 2004.

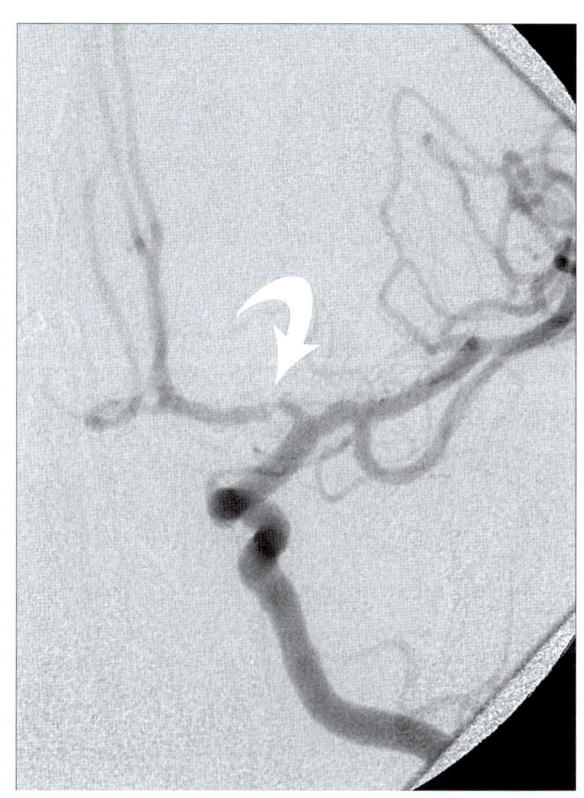

Figure 1. Anteroposterior arteriogram of the left internal carotid shows a focal, more than 90% stenosis of the A1 segment of the left anterior cerebral artery *(arrow)*.

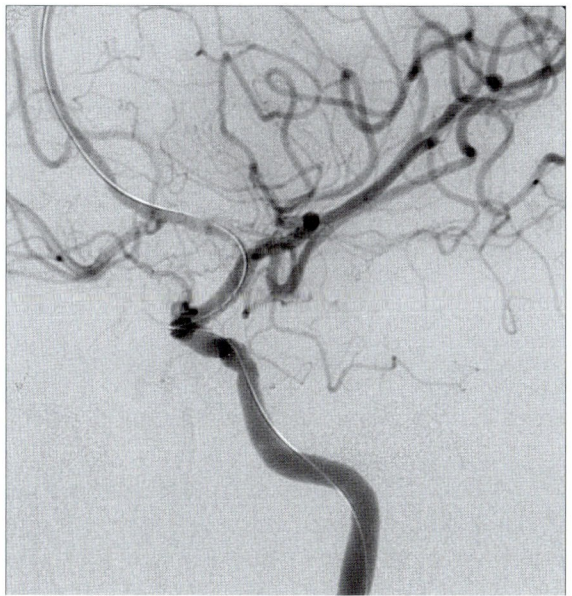

Figure 2. Oblique angiogram of the left internal carotid shows that a wire has been placed across the lesion in anticipation of angioplasty.

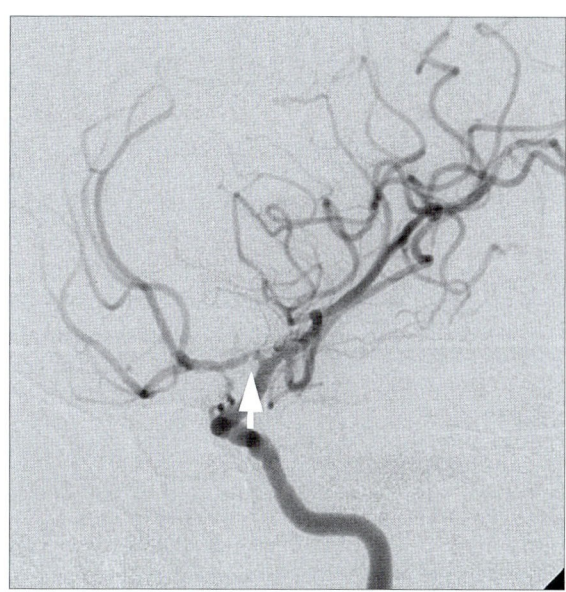

Figure 3. Oblique angiogram of the left internal carotid immediately after angioplasty shows improved flow through the anterior cerebral artery. There is mild residual narrowing *(arrow)*.

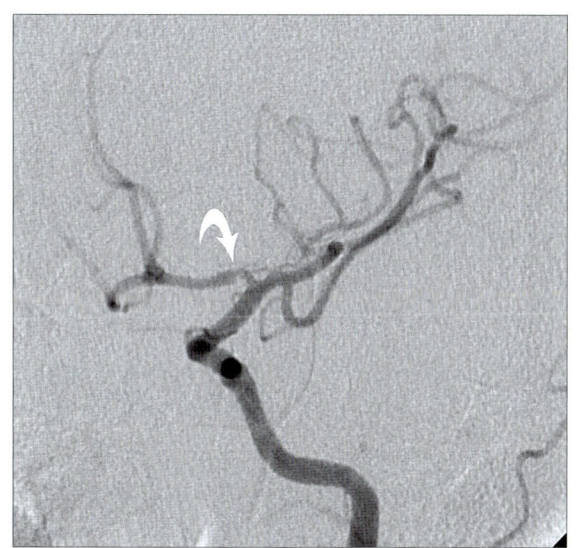

Figure 4. Oblique angiogram of the left internal carotid performed 7 months after the initial angioplasty shows a residual 50% stenosis of the proximal A1 segment of the anterior cerebral artery *(arrow)*. The patient has remained asymptomatic since the angioplasty.

Case 85

DEMOGRAPHICS/CLINICAL HISTORY

A 76-year-old woman with progressive left-hemispheric strokes.

DISCUSSION

History/Indications for Procedure
A 76-year-old woman with multiple medical problems and history of recent left cortical infarcts presents with worsening mental status.

Procedure
Middle cerebral artery angioplasty

Pre-procedure Imaging
MRI shows restricted diffusion in the left MCA distribution, involving the left-periventricular white matter. MRA shows a focal stenosis of the M1 segment of the left MCA (Fig. 1); perfusion-sensitive sequences show decreased cerebral blood flow, increased mean transit time, and increased time-to-peak throughout the left MCA distribution.

Intraprocedural Findings
There is a focal high-grade stenosis at the origin of the left middle cerebral artery, with delayed opacification of the entire left middle cerebral artery territory (Fig. 2). The lesion was crossed with a 0.014-inch guidewire; a 2-mm balloon was used for angioplasty (Fig. 3).

Follow-up and Complications
Follow-up arteriogram following angioplasty shows significant improved perfusion to the left cerebral hemisphere (Fig. 4). Follow-up MR perfusion study confirms the improved perfusion to the left cerebral hemisphere.

Suggested Readings

Cross DT III, Moran CJ, Derdeyn CP: Technique for intracranial balloon and stent-assisted angioplasty for atherosclerotic stenosis. Neuroimaging Clin N Am 17:365-380, 2007.

Ecker RD, Levy EI, Sauvageau E, et al: Current concepts in the management of intracranial atherosclerotic disease. Neurosurgery 59(5 Suppl 3):S210-S218, 2006.

Siddiq F, Vazquez G, Memon MZ, et al: Comparison of primary angioplasty with stent placement for treating symptomatic intracranial atherosclerotic diseases: A multicenter study. Stroke 39:2505-2510, 2008.

Taylor RA, Kasner SE: Treatment of intracranial arterial stenosis. Expert Rev Neurother 6:1685-1694, 2006.

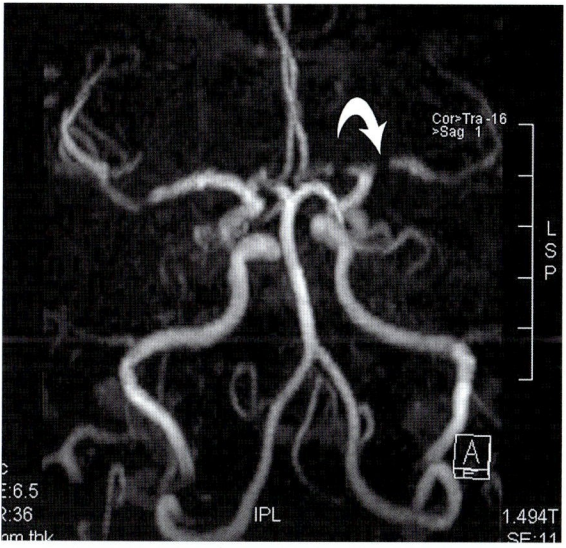

Figure 1. Reconstructed image from MR angiogram of the circle of Willis shows a focal, high-grade stenosis of the M1 segment of the middle cerebral artery *(curved arrow)*.

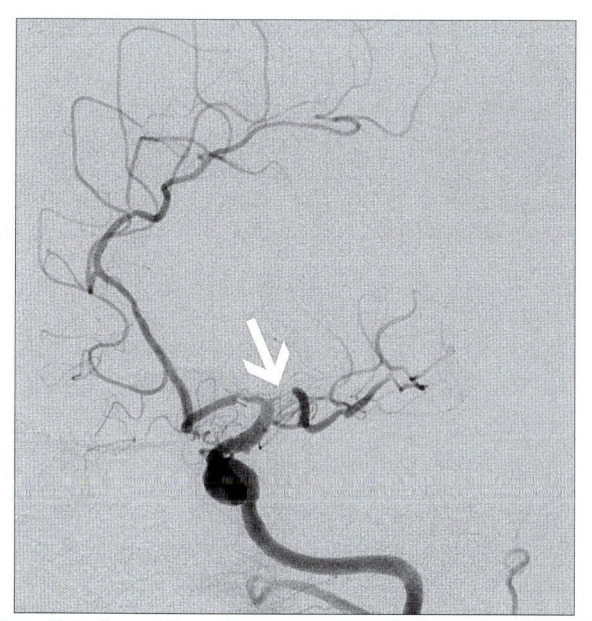

Figure 2. Left carotid arteriogram confirms the presence of a focal, high-grade stenosis at the origin of the middle cerebral artery *(arrow)*. There is delayed opacification of the distal branches in the middle cerebral artery territory.

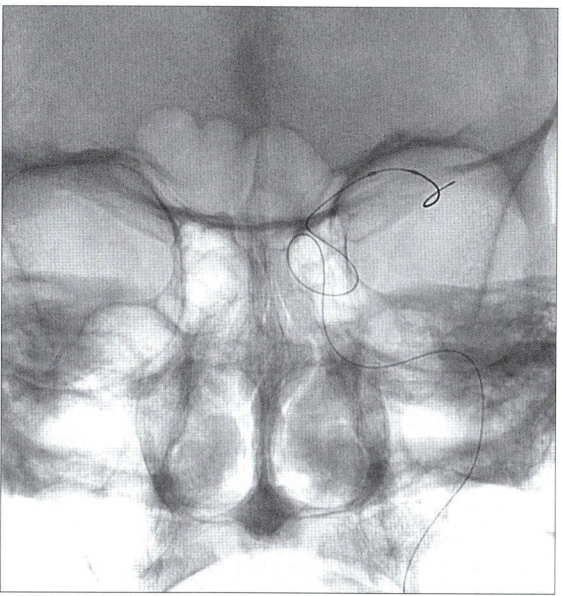

Figure 3. A 0.014-inch guidewire has been placed across the lesion. A 2-mm balloon is positioned across the stenosis.

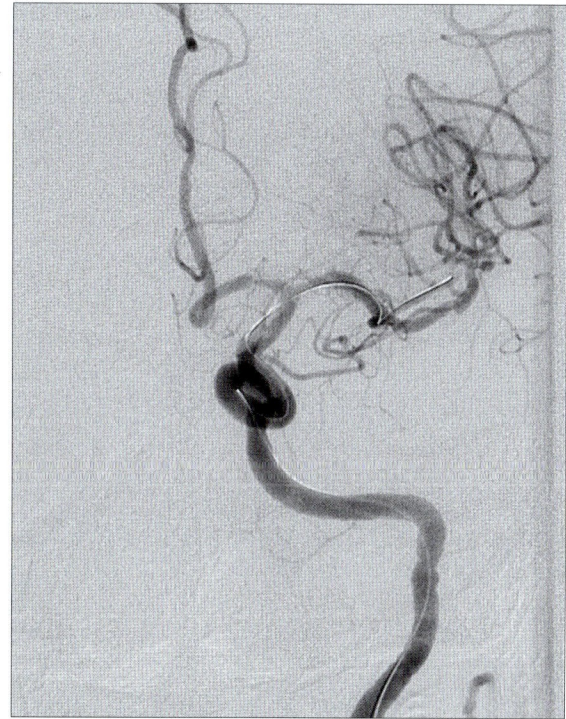

Figure 4. Follow-up arteriogram after angioplasty. There is mild residual narrowing at the site of the stenosis. There is no longer delay in the perfusion of the distal branches in the MCA vascular territory.

Case 86

DEMOGRAPHICS/CLINICAL HISTORY

A 65-year-old woman with a 4-day history of progressive expressive aphagia.

DISCUSSION

History/Indications for Procedure
A 65-year-old woman with a 4-day history of progressive expressive aphagia.

Procedure
Percutaneous angioplasty for middle cerebral artery stenosis

Pre-procedure Imaging
Unenhanced CT of the head shows low attenuation in the posterior left parietal lobe consistent with an acute to subacute infarct. MRI shows signal abnormalities in the left parietal lobe consistent with areas of acute infarction; perfusion MRI shows delayed perfusion of the left middle cerebral artery territory.

Intraprocedural Findings
Cerebral arteriogram shows a high-grade stenosis of the middle cerebral artery, just proximal to the bifurcation (Fig. 1). The stenosis was angioplastied with a 1.5-mm balloon; follow-up angiogram following angioplasty showed 50% residual stenosis (Fig. 2) but with markedly improved flow to the distal MCA territory.

Follow-up and Complications
The patient's expressive aphasia improved during her hospital stay and in follow-up. She underwent a follow-up arteriogram 1 year after angioplasty that showed only mild residual narrowing of the MCA at the site of prior angioplasty (Fig. 3).

Suggested Readings

Ecker RD, Levy EI, Sauvageau E, et al: Current concepts in the management of intracranial atherosclerotic disease. Neurosurgery 62:1425-1433, 2008.

Marks MP, Marcellus ML, Do HM, et al: Intracranial angioplasty without stenting for symptomatic atherosclerotic stenosis: Long-term follow-up. AJNR Am J Neuroradiol 26:525-530, 2005.

Siddiq F, Vazquez G, Memon MZ, et al: Comparison of primary angioplasty with stent placement for treating symptomatic intracranial atherosclerotic diseases: A multicenter study. Stroke 39:2505-2510, 2008.

Wojak JC, Dunlap DC, Hargrave KR, et al: Intracranial angioplasty and stenting: Long-term results from a single center. AJNR Am J Neuroradiology 27:1882-1892, 2006.

Case 86   173

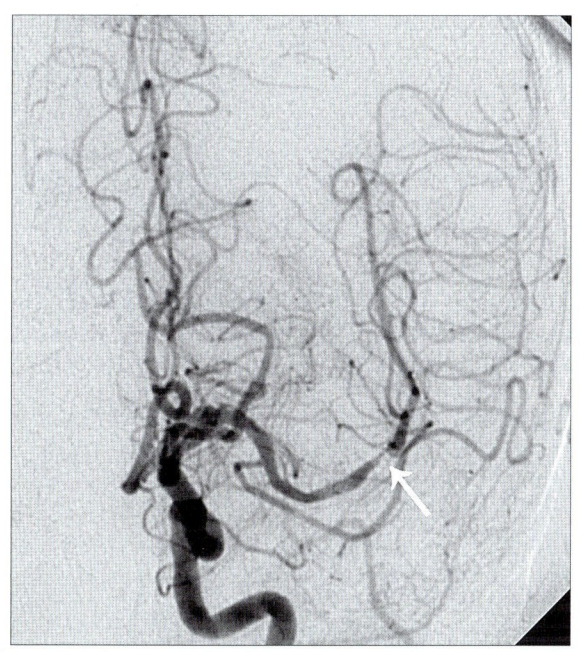

Figure 1. Left common carotid arteriogram shows a focal, high-grade stenosis of the distal M1 segment of the middle cerebral artery (arrow).

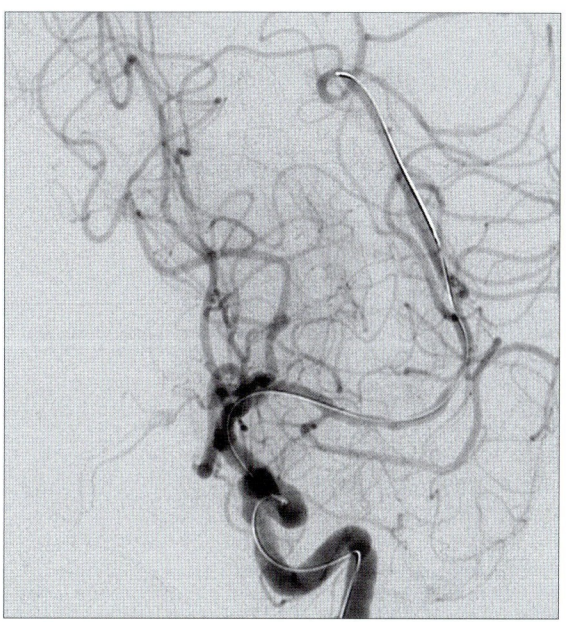

Figure 2. Follow-up arteriogram after balloon angioplasty shows significant residual stenosis. Despite this appearance, there was improved flow to the peripheral branches, and no further angioplasty was performed.

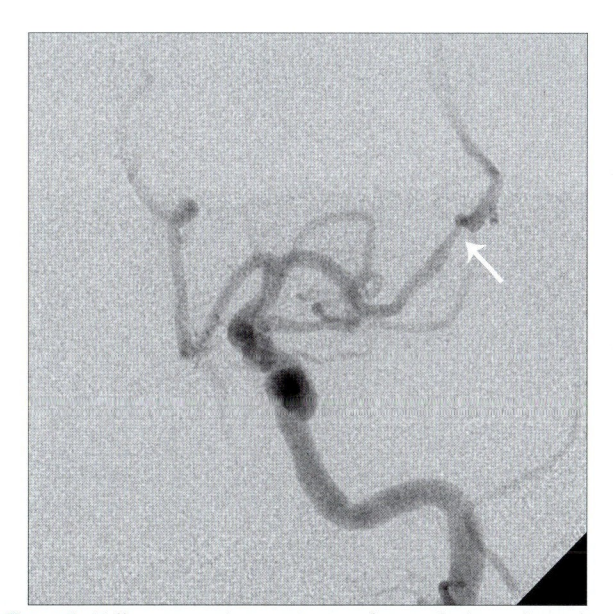

Figure 3. Follow-up angiogram 1 year after angioplasty shows improved caliber at the site of angioplasty (arrow). There is now only a mild narrowing at this location.

Case 87

DEMOGRAPHICS/CLINICAL HISTORY

A 69-year-old woman with a history of atrial fibrillation and new left-sided weakness, undergoing arteriography.

DISCUSSION

History/Indications for Procedure
A 69-year-old woman with a 3-hour history of left-sided weakness.

Procedure
Endovascular stroke management

Pre-procedure Imaging
Unenhanced CT scan of the head (not shown) showed new hypodensity in the right frontoparietal region. No intracranial hemorrhage was present.

Intraprocedural Findings
A selective right carotid arteriogram shows complete occlusion of the right middle cerebral artery just distal to its origin (Fig. 1). Flow was restored after mechanical thrombectomy using the Merci Retriever (Concentric Medical, Mountain View, CA) (Figs. 2-4).

Follow-up and Complications
The patient continued to have worsening edema and mass effect on follow-up CT scans. The stroke evolved into a hemorrhagic stroke 2 days after the thrombectomy; the patient died shortly thereafter.

Suggested Readings

Adams HP Jr, Adams RJ, Brott T, et al: Stroke Council of the American Stroke Association: Guidelines for the early management of patients with ischemic stroke: A scientific statement from the Stroke Council of the American Stroke Association. Stroke 34:1056-1083, 2003.

Katz JM, Gobin YP, Segal AZ, et al: Mechanical embolectomy. Neurosurg Clin North Am 16:463-474, 2005.

Smith WS, Sung G, Starkman S, et al: MERCI Trial Investigators: Safety and efficacy of mechanical embolectomy in acute ischemic stroke: Results of the MERCI trial. Stroke 36:1432-1440, 2005.

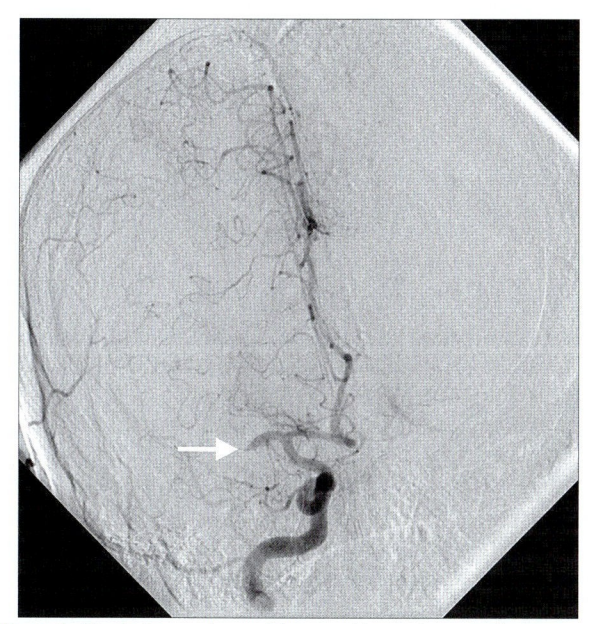

Figure 1. Single image from right carotid arteriogram shows complete occlusion of the M1 segment of the right middle cerebral artery *(arrow)*.

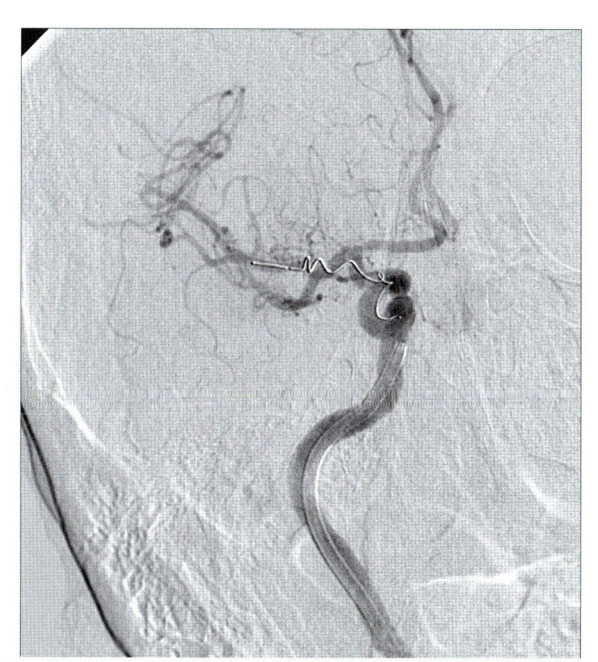

Figure 2. A guiding sheath has been advanced into the distal internal carotid artery, and the Merci Retriever has been deployed into the clot.

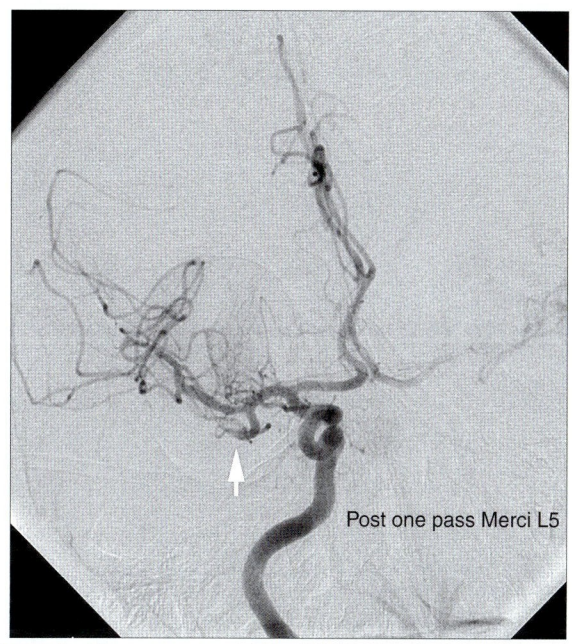

Figure 3. After one pass with the Merci Retriever, there is complete restoration of flow to the M1 segment and its superior division. There is continued poor perfusion to the inferior division *(arrow)*.

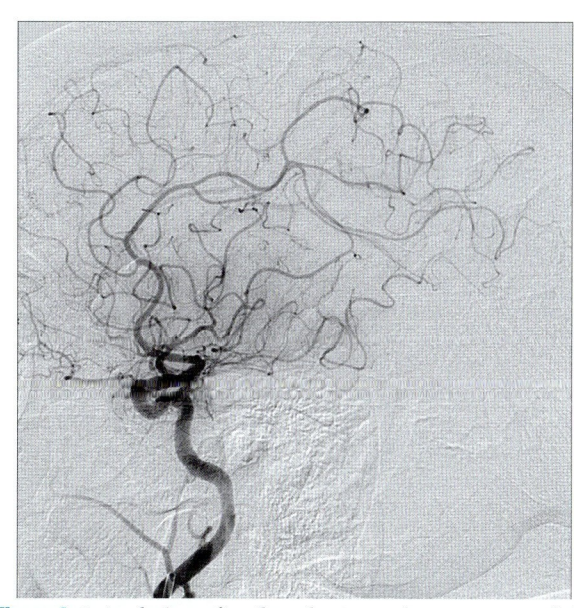

Figure 4. Lateral view after thrombectomy shows patency of the middle cerebral artery.

Case 88

DEMOGRAPHICS/CLINICAL HISTORY

A 76-year-old man with acute onset of lethargy and slurring of speech.

DISCUSSION

History/Indications for Procedure
A 76-year-old man with acute onset of lethargy and slurring of speech.

Procedure
Endovascular management of basilar artery thrombosis

Pre-procedure Imaging
Cerebral arteriogram performed 4 days earlier shows occlusion of the right vertebral artery and high-grade stenosis of the distal left vertebral artery (Fig. 1). MR angiogram at the time of onset of symptoms shows absence of flow within the left vertebral and basilar arteries (Fig. 2).

Intraprocedural Findings
Cerebral arteriogram shows occlusion of the basilar artery and left vertebral artery (Fig. 3). Flow was restored in the basilar and vertebral arteries with the intra-arterial administration of a total of 7 mg tPa, infused over 45 minutes (Fig. 4); the vertebral artery stenosis was then treated with the placement of a 3-mm balloon expandable stent (Velocity, Cordis, Miami Lakes, FL).

Follow-up and Complications
After the procedure, the patient was started on a platelet inhibitor (Clopidogrel), and his mental status returned to normal. The patient has had no recurrence of symptoms in the year since the procedure.

Suggested Readings

Arnold M, Nedeltchev K, Schroth G, et al: Clinical and radiological predictors of recanalisation and outcome of 40 patients with acute basilar artery occlusion treated with intra-arterial thrombolysis. J Neurol Neurosurg Psychiatry 75:811-812, 2004.

Brandt T: Diagnosis and thrombolytic therapy of acute basilar artery occlusion: A review. Clin Exp Hypertens 24:611-622, 2002.

Smith WS: Intra-arterial thrombolytic therapy for acute basilar occlusion: Pro. Stroke 38:701-703, 2007.

Case 88   177

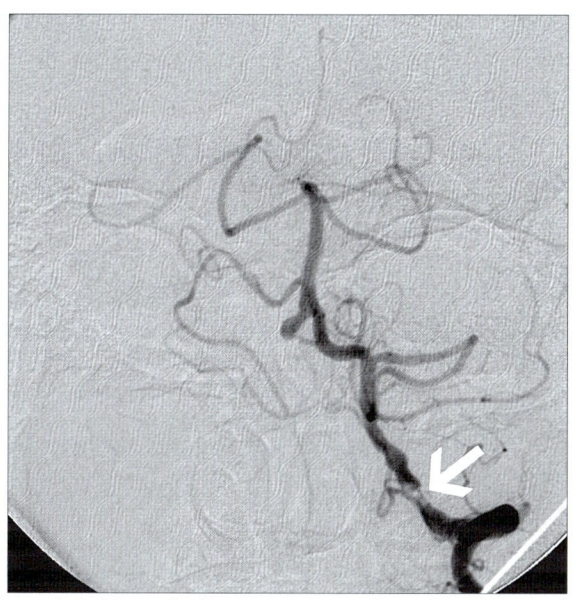

Figure 1. Left vertebral arteriogram performed 4 days earlier shows a focal, high-grade stenosis of the distal left vertebral artery *(arrow)*. The right vertebral artery is occluded.

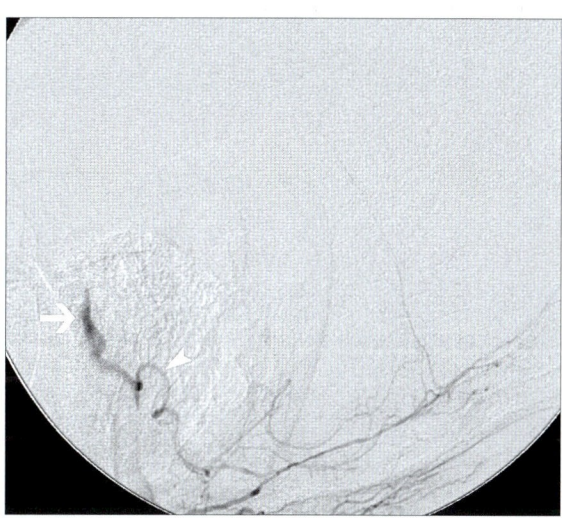

Figure 3. Left vertebral arteriogram in the lateral projection shows absence of flow in the left vertebral artery. A short segment of the thrombosed basilar artery *(arrow)* is opacified through a small collateral *(arrowhead)*.

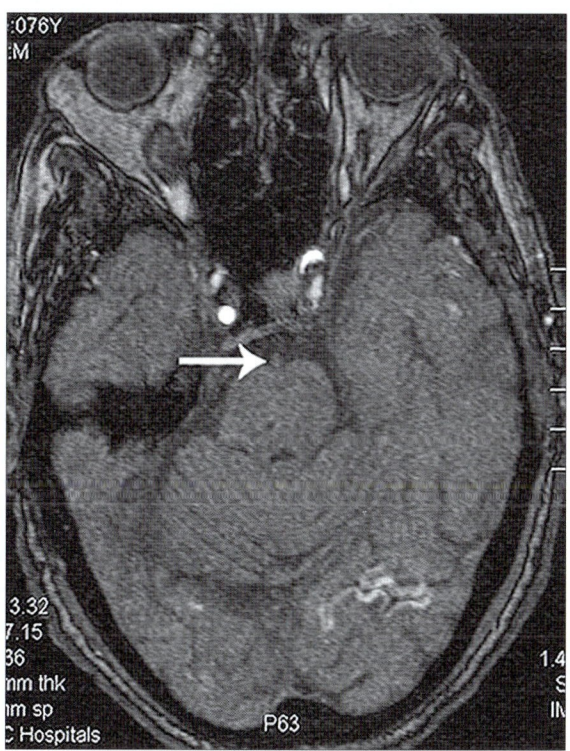

Figure 2. Post-contrast MR image shows occlusion of the basilar artery *(arrow)*.

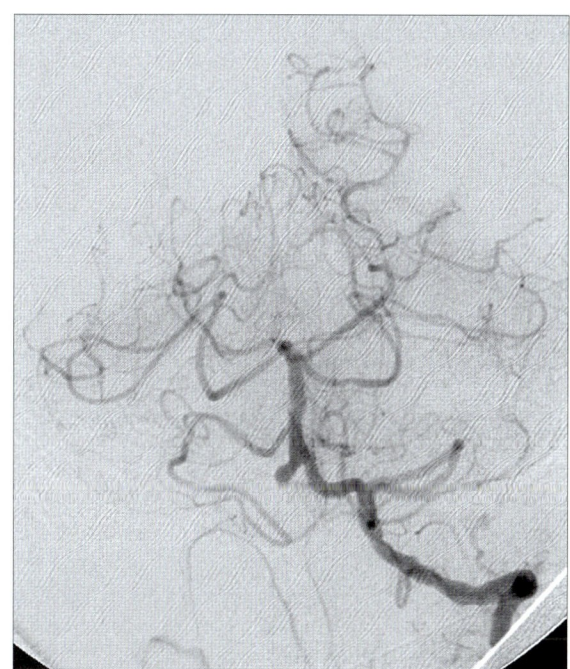

Figure 4. Final arteriogram. Flow has been restored through the left vertebral and basilar arteries. No residual thrombus is identified. The left vertebral artery stenosis has been successfully treated with the placement of a 3-mm balloon expandable stent.

Case 89

DEMOGRAPHICS/CLINICAL HISTORY

A 43-year-old man with headache, undergoing computed tomography (CT), ultrasonography, and embolization.

DISCUSSION

History/Indications for Procedure
A 43-year-old man presented with headache.

Procedure
Diagnosis and management of subarachnoid hemorrhage

Pre-procedure Imaging
Non-enhanced CT of the head shows a subarachnoid hemorrhage within the cortical sulci of the anterior frontal lobes (Fig. 1).

Intraprocedural Findings
A 6-mm aneurysm arises from the anterior communicating artery (Fig. 2). The aneurysm was treated by coil embolization (Fig. 3).

Follow-up and Complications
After embolization, the patient had signs of cerebral salt-wasting syndrome, which was treated with a hypertonic saline drip. The patient also had mild vasospasm seen on transcranial Doppler that resolved with intravenous fluids and hypertonic saline.

Suggested Readings
Chappell ET, Moure FC, Good MC: Comparison of computed tomographic angiography with digital subtraction angiography in the diagnosis of cerebral aneurysms: A meta-analysis. Neurosurgery 52:624-631, 2003.

Molyneux A, Kerr R, Stratton I, et al, for the International Subarachnoid Aneurysm Trial (ISAT) Collaborative Group: International Subarachnoid Aneurysm Trial (ISAT) of neurosurgical clipping versus endovascular coiling in 2143 patients with ruptured intracranial aneurysms: A randomised trial. Lancet 360:1267-1274, 2002.

Case 89   179

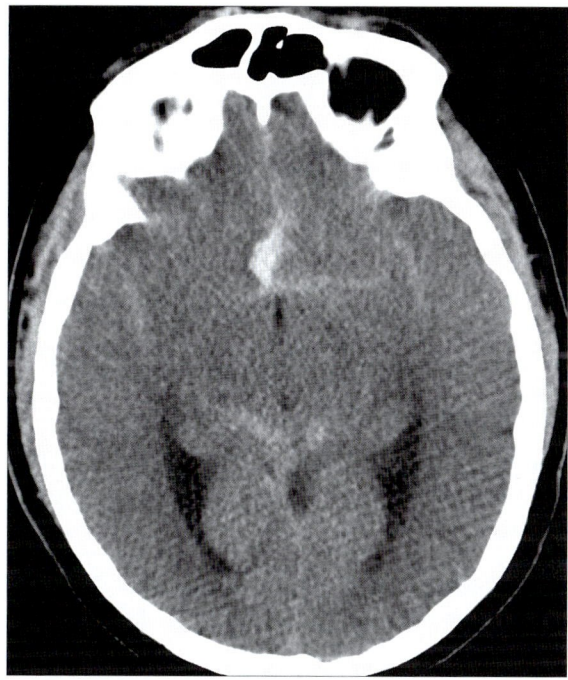

Figure 1. Single image from an axial CT study of the head. No contrast was administered. There is high-density fluid in the cortical sulci of the frontal lobes.

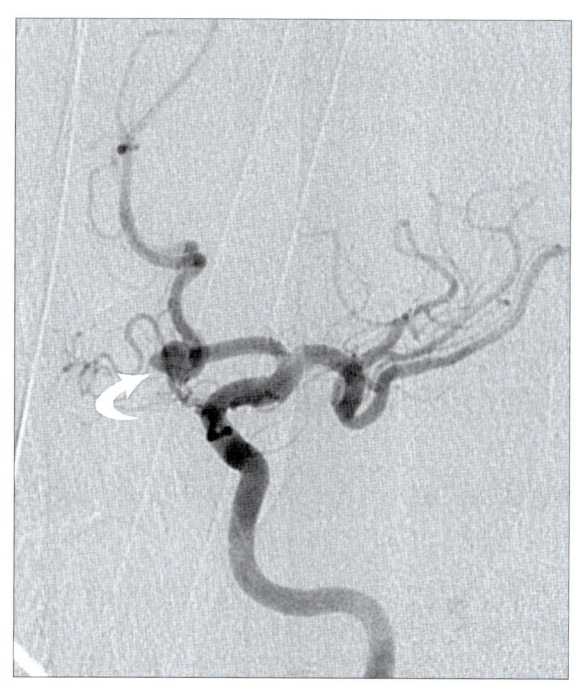

Figure 2. Diagnostic cerebral arteriogram shows an aneurysm arising from the anterior communicating artery *(arrow)*.

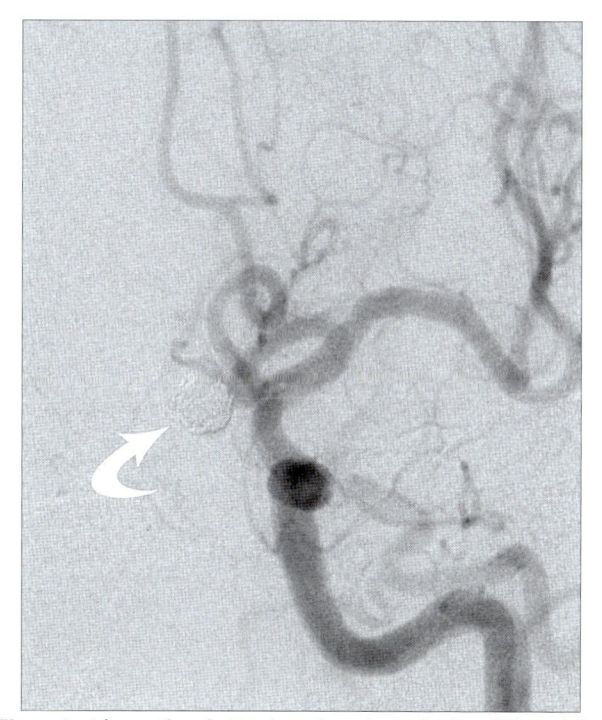

Figure 3. After coil embolization, there is no further filling of the aneurysm *(arrow)*.

Case 90

DEMOGRAPHICS/CLINICAL HISTORY

A 52-year-old man with subarachnoid hemorrhage.

DISCUSSION

History/Indications for Procedure
A 52-year-old man with subarachnoid hemorrhage.

Procedure
Endovascular treatment of intracranial aneurysm

Pre-procedure Imaging
Unenhanced CT of the head shows increased density in the sylvian fissures and cortical sulci bilaterally, consistent with diffuse subarachnoid hemorrhage (Fig. 1).

Intraprocedural Findings
There is a 7-mm × 5-mm aneurysm located at the origin of the left posterior communicating artery (Fig. 2). The artery was embolized with GDC coils (Figs. 3 and 4).

Follow-up and Complications
The patient did well after the embolization and has shown no evidence of aneurysm recurrence.

Suggested Readings
Molyneux A, Kerr R, Stratton I, et al: International Subarachnoid Aneurysm Trial (ISAT) of neurosurgical clipping versus endovascular coiling in 2143 patients with ruptured intracranial aneurysms: A radomised trial. Lancet 360:1267-1274, 2002.

van Gijn J, Rinkel GJ: Subrachnoid haemorrhage: Diagnosis, causes and management. Brain 124:249-278, 2001.

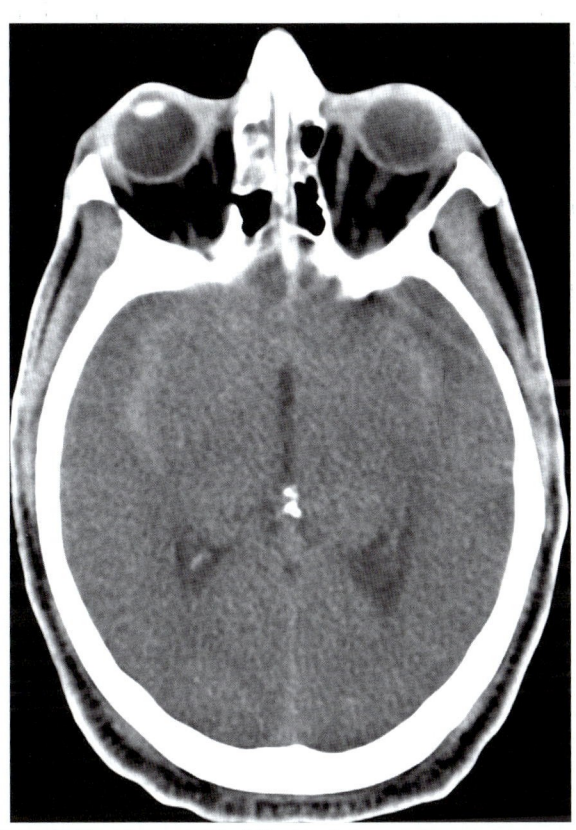

Figure 1. Unenhanced CT of the head shows abnormal increased density in the sylvian fissures bilaterally, consistent with diffuse subarachnoid hemorrhage.

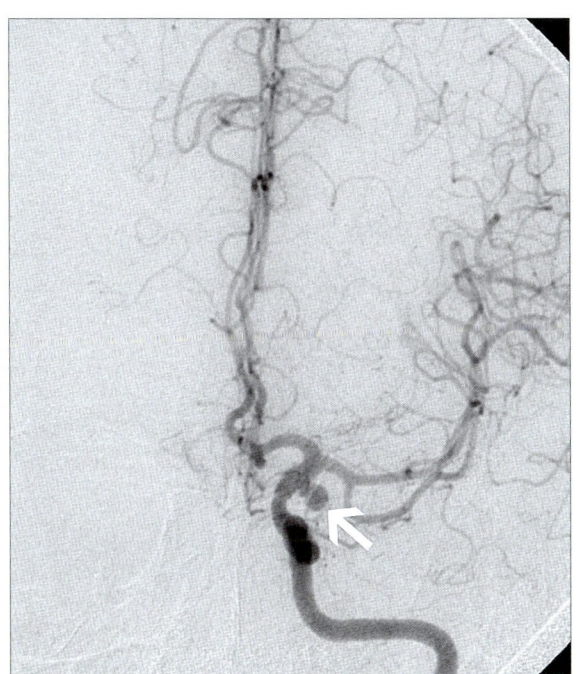

Figure 2. Left internal carotid arteriogram, AP projection, shows a 7- × 5-mm aneurysm arising from the origin of the left posterior communicating artery *(arrow)*.

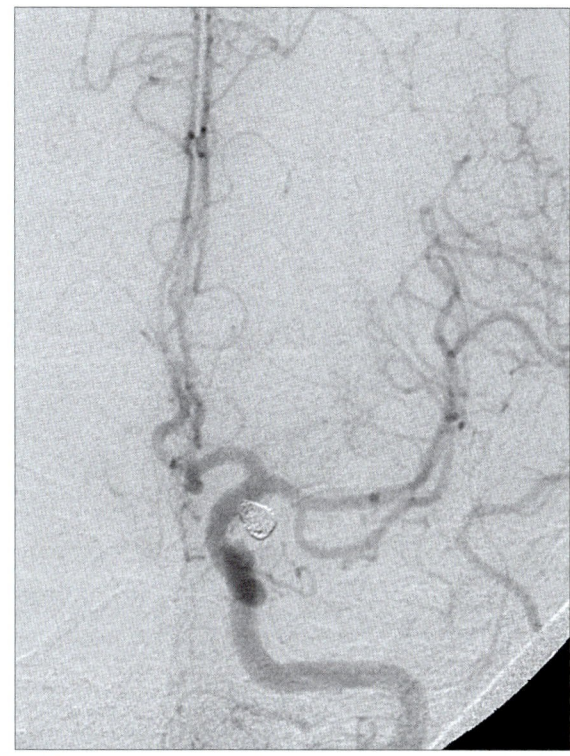

Figure 3. Left internal carotid arteriogram, AP projection, following embolization shows complete occlusion of the aneurysm by coils.

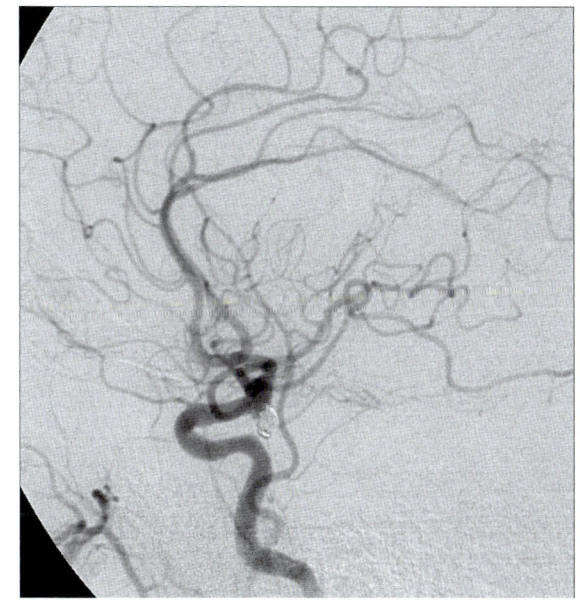

Figure 4. Left internal carotid arteriogram, lateral projection, following embolization also shows complete occlusion of the aneurysm.

Case 91

DEMOGRAPHICS/CLINICAL HISTORY

A 50-year-old woman with a history of hemorrhagic hereditary telangiectasia (HHT) and severe epistaxis.

DISCUSSION

History/Indications for Procedure
A 50-year-old woman with a history of HHT and severe epistaxis underwent ligation of bilateral anterior ethmoid arteries and nasal packing with significant hemorrhage on removal of nasal packing.

Procedure
Embolization for epistaxis secondary to HHT

Intraprocedural Findings
There is extensive hyperemia of the anterior nasal mucosa supplied by the internal maxillary and facial arteries bilaterally (Figs. 1 to 4). Bilateral internal maxillary arteries and distal facial arteries were embolized with particles of polyvinyl alcohol.

Follow-up and Complications
The nasal packing was removed immediately after the procedure. The patient had no further epistaxis following the embolization.

Suggested Readings
Elden L, Montanera W, Terbrugge K, et al: Angiographic embolization for the treatment of epistaxis: A review of 108 cases. Otolaryngol Head Neck Surg 111:44-50, 1994.

Mahavedia A, Murphy K, Obray R, Gailloud P: Embolization for intractable epistaxis. Tech Vasc Interv Radiol 8:134-138, 2005.

Oguni T, Korogi Y, Yasunaga T, et al: Superselective embolization for intractable idiopathic epistaxis. Br J Radiol 73:1148-1153, 2000.

Sokoloff J, Waskom T, McDonald D, et al: Therapeutic percutaneous embolizationin intractable epistaxis. Radiology 111:285-287, 1974.

Strother CM, Newton TH: Percutaneous embolization to control epistaxis in Rendu-Osler-Weber disease. Arch Otolaryngol 102:58-60, 1976.

Case 91   183

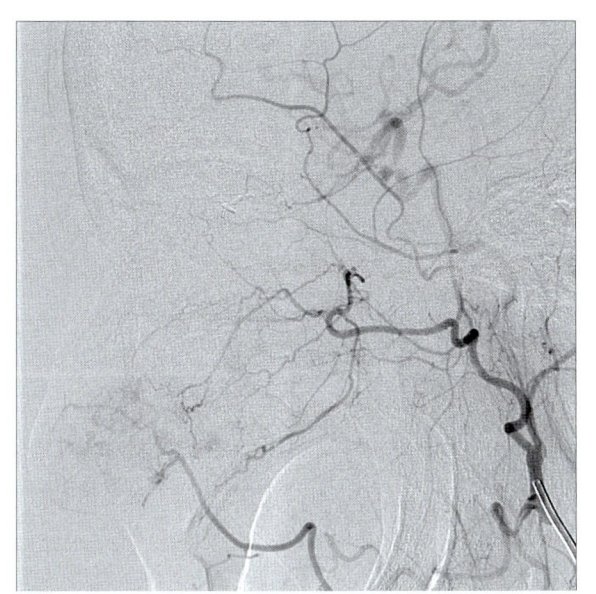

Figure 1. Lateral angiogram, right external carotid artery injection. There is diffuse hypervascularity of the nasal mucosa from both the facial and internal maxillary arteries.

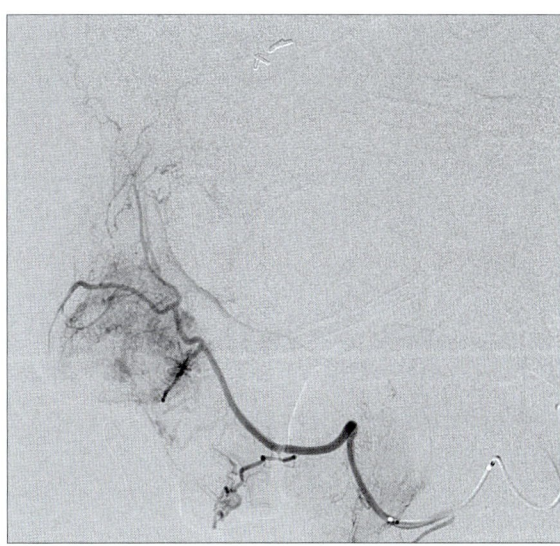

Figure 3. Selective injection of the right facial artery shows marked hypervascularity of the nasal mucosa. There is also a tangle of prominent vessels within the upper lip, supplied by the facial artery.

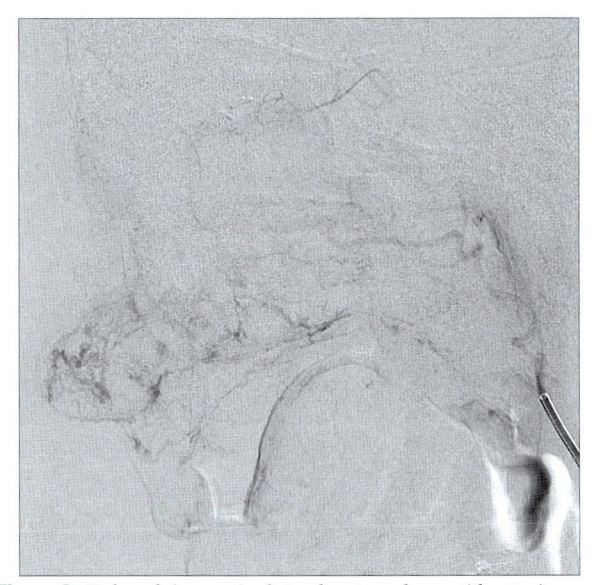

Figure 2. Delayed image in lateral external carotid arteriogram shows filling of multiple prominent veins within the nasal mucosa.

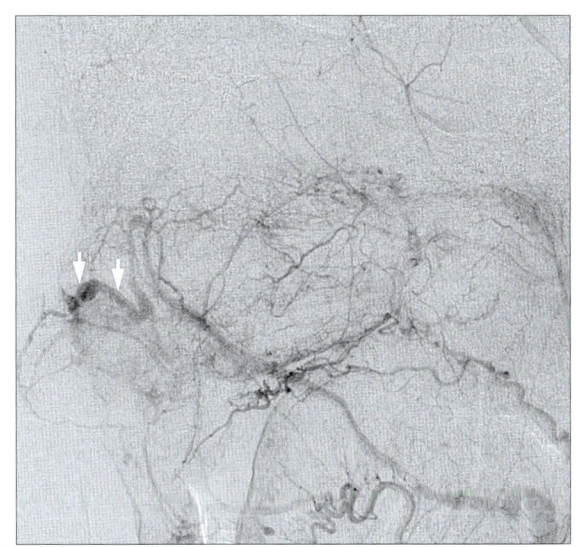

Figure 4. Lateral angiogram of the left external carotid also shows diffuse hypervascularity of the nasal mucosa, as well as an early, prominent draining vein *(arrows)*.

Case 92

DEMOGRAPHICS/CLINICAL HISTORY

A 57-year-old man with uncontrollable epistaxis, undergoing catheterization and embolization.

DISCUSSION

History/Indications for Procedure
A 57-year-old man fell from a tractor 3 days before presentation. After the fall, the patient developed minor nasal bleeding that has become brisk and persistent, despite packing.

Procedure
Endovascular management of epistaxis

Intraprocedural Findings
Bilateral external carotid arteries were selectively catheterized, and no pseudoaneurysm or active extravasation was seen (Fig. 1). Bilateral internal maxillary arteries were embolized with 500- to 700-μm calibrated microspheres (Figs. 2 and 3).

Follow-up and Complications
The patient's hemoglobin levels remained stable after the embolization. The nasal packing was removed without any additional hemorrhage.

Suggested Readings
Elden L, Montanera W, Terbrugge K, et al: Angiographic embolization for the treatment of epistaxis: A review of 108 cases. Otolaryngol Head Neck Surg 111:44-50, 1994.

Narducci CA, Willing SJ, Sillers MJ: Angiographic embolization for epistaxis: A review of 114 cases. Laryngoscope 108:615-619, 1998.

Case 92   185

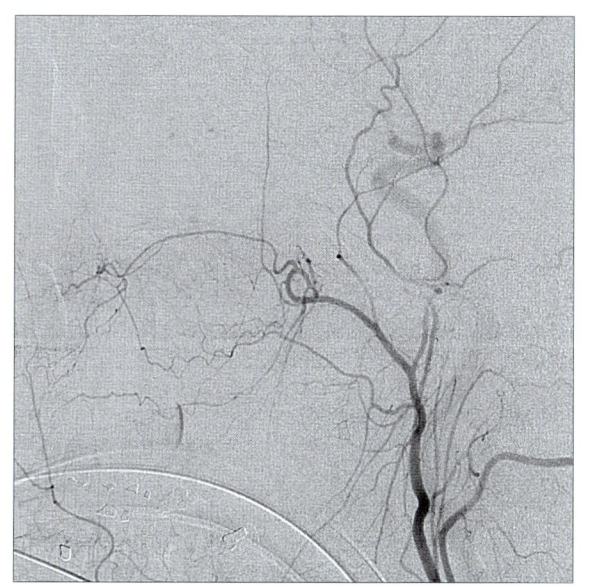

Figure 1. Left external carotid angiogram is normal. No pseudoaneurysm or active extravasation is seen.

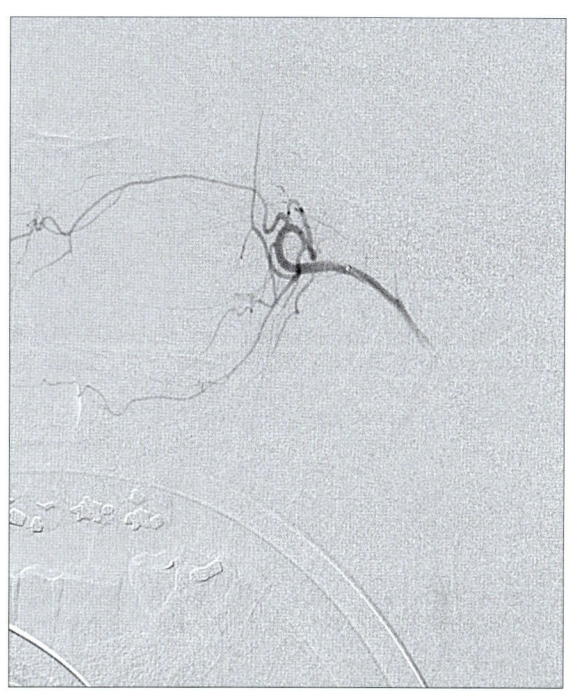

Figure 2. A microcatheter is advanced into the distal internal maxillary artery.

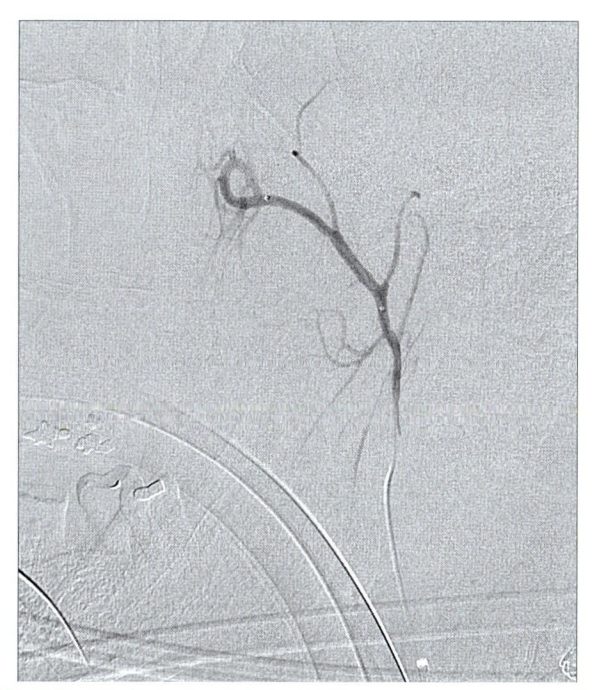

Figure 3. The distal internal maxillary artery was embolized with calibrated microspheres.

Case 93

DEMOGRAPHICS/CLINICAL HISTORY

A 29-year-old man involved in a motorcycle accident, undergoing arteriography.

DISCUSSION

History/Indications for Procedure
This patient presented with persistent epistaxis.

Procedure
External carotid artery embolization in trauma

Pre-procedure Imaging
Maxillofacial CT scan showed multiple complex maxillofacial fractures (not shown). High-density fluid filled the paranasal sinuses.

Intraprocedural Findings
Selective injection of the right external carotid artery shows filling of a 10-mm × 15-mm pseudoaneurysm arising from the distal infraorbital artery (Figs. 1 and 2). The right infraorbital artery was embolized with coils (Fig. 3).

Follow-up and Complications
The patient had no further epistaxis after the embolization.

Suggested Readings
Smith TP: Embolization in the external carotid artery. J Vasc Interv Radiol 17:1897-1913, 2006.

Case 93   187

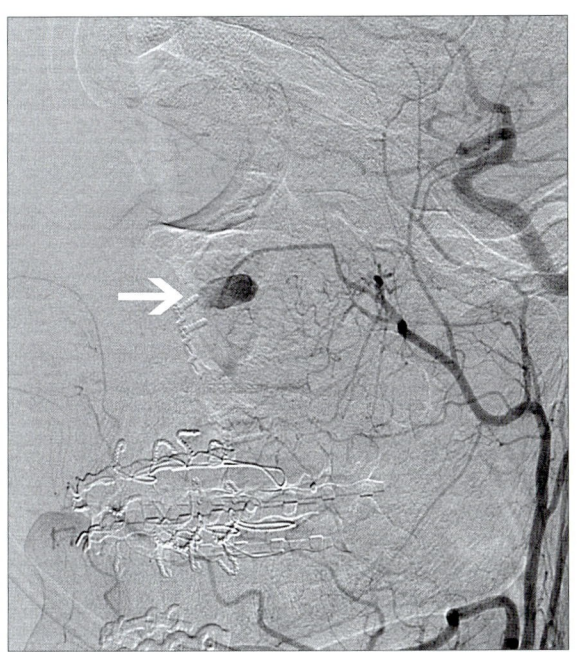

Figure 1. Single lateral image from common carotid arteriogram shows filling of a pseudoaneurysm adjacent to the distal internal maxillary artery *(arrow)*.

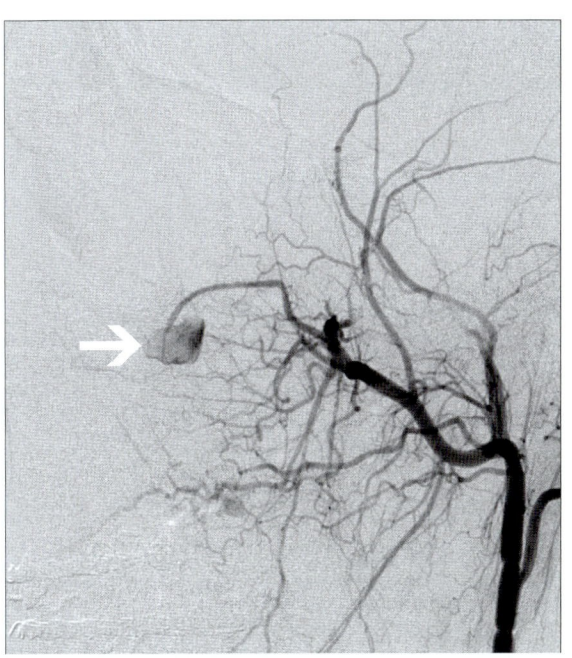

Figure 2. Selective external carotid injection shows the pseudoaneurysm *(arrow)*. Subselective catheter injection revealed the pseudoaneurysm arising from the distal infraorbital artery.

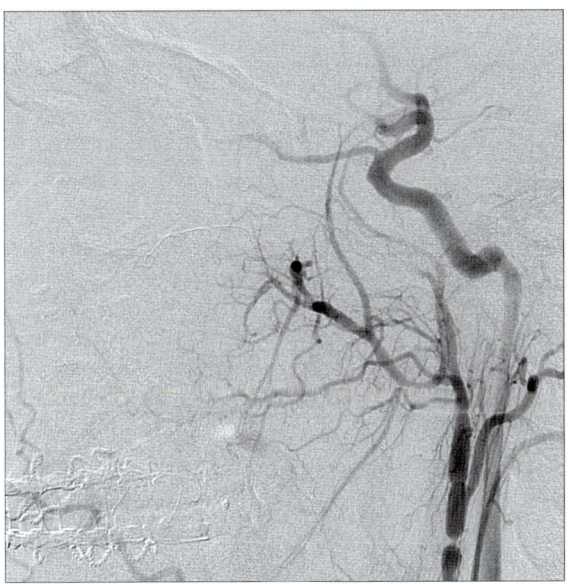

Figure 3. Single lateral image from common carotid arteriogram after coil embolization of the infraorbital artery. The pseudoaneurysm no longer fills.

Case 94

DEMOGRAPHICS/CLINICAL HISTORY

A 37-year-old man who was struck in the face by a metal fan blade, undergoing computed tomography (CT) and arterial embolization.

DISCUSSION

History/Indications for Procedure
A 37-year-old man was struck in the face by a metal fan blade. The patient developed significant epistaxis that persisted despite nasal packing.

Procedure
External carotid artery embolization in the trauma setting

Pre-procedure Imaging
Unenhanced CT scan through the face demonstrates extensive maxillofacial fractures and hemorrhage within the maxillary sinuses (Fig. 1).

Intraprocedural Findings
The left sphenopalatine artery is occluded just distal to its origin (Figs. 2 and 3). The sphenopalatine artery was catheterized with a microcatheter and embolized with 150 to 250 μm polyvinyl alcohol microspheres.

Follow-up and Complications
The patient's hemoglobin levels remained stable after embolization, and the packing was removed without evidence of further hemorrhage (Fig. 4). The patient has since undergone several operations to repair the complex facial fractures.

Suggested Readings
Ray CE Jr, Spalding SC, et al: State of the art: Noninvasive imaging and management of neurovascular trauma. World J Emerg Surg 2:1-21, 2007.

Smith TP: Embolization in the external carotid artery. J Vasc Interv Radiol 17:1897-1913, 2006.

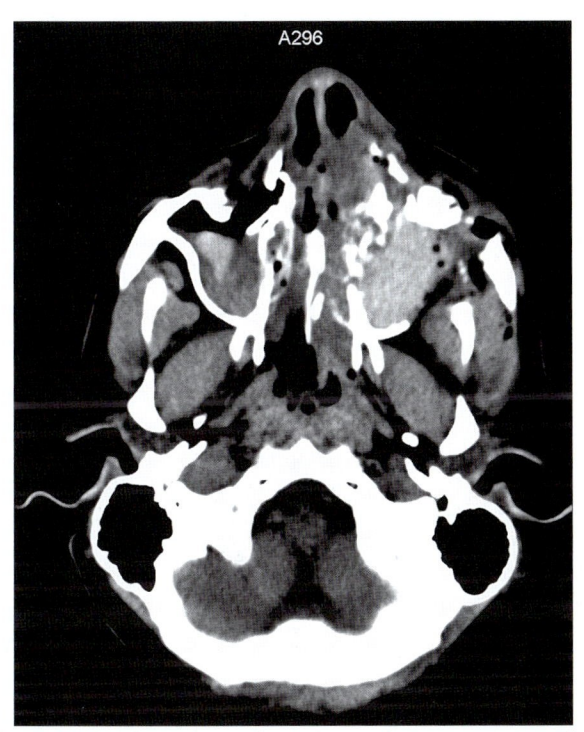

Figure 1. Unenhanced, axial CT image demonstrates complex maxillofacial fractures. There is hemorrhage in both maxillary sinuses.

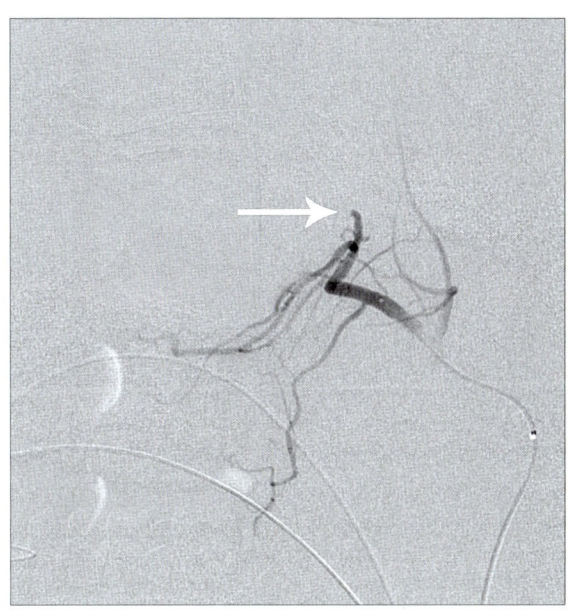

Figure 3. Selective injection of the distal left internal maxillary artery also shows the abrupt occlusion of the proximal left sphenopalatine artery *(arrow)*.

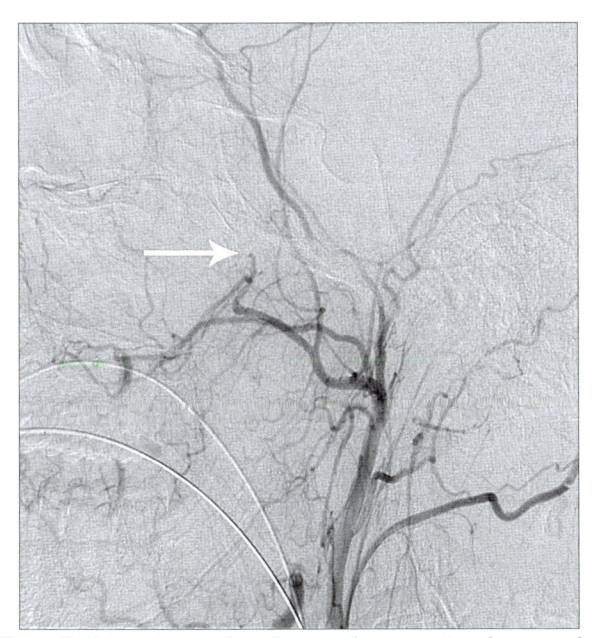

Figure 2. External carotid angiogram demonstrates abrupt occlusion of the left sphenopalatine artery *(arrow)*.

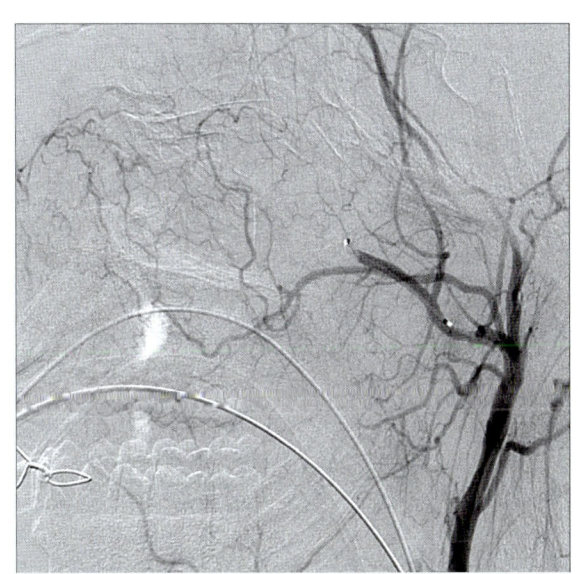

Figure 4. External carotid angiogram after embolization shows that there is stasis of flow in the left internal maxillary artery.

Case 95

DEMOGRAPHICS/CLINICAL HISTORY

An 86-year-old woman with a pulsatile mass of the right face and neck, undergoing ultrasonography and arteriography.

DISCUSSION

History/Indications for Procedure
An 86-year-old woman has a pulsatile mass of the right face and neck. The patient has had no known trauma to this region.

Procedure
Stent placement for external carotid pseudoaneurysm

Pre-procedure Imaging
Angiography performed at an outside institution showed a pseudoaneurysm arising from the right external carotid artery. Doppler ultrasound confirms the presence of a large pseudoaneurysm arising from the external carotid artery (Fig. 1).

Intraprocedural Findings
A 3.8-cm pseudoaneurysm arises from the right external carotid artery, just distal to the origin of the facial artery (Fig. 2). The aneurysm was treated with the placement of a 4-mm × 19-mm Jomed covered stent (Jomed International AB, Helsingborg, Sweden) (Fig. 3).

Follow-up and Complications
The pseudoaneurysm was excluded on angiography performed after stent placement (Fig. 4). Follow-up ultrasound scans have shown no recurrence.

Suggested Readings
Ray CE Jr, Spalding SC, Cothren CC, et al: State of the art: Noninvasive imaging and management of neurovascular trauma. World J Emerg Surg 2:1-21, 2007.
Smith TP: Embolization in the external carotid artery. J Vasc Interv Radiol 17:1897-1913, 2006.

Case 95   191

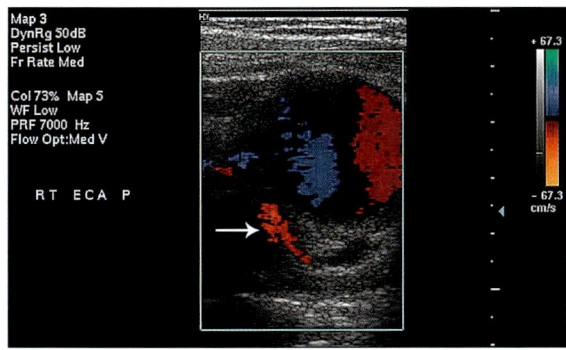

Figure 1. Color Doppler ultrasound shows a large pseudoaneurysm with the characteristic yin-yang flow pattern. The neck of the pseudoaneurysm communicates with the external carotid artery *(arrow)*.

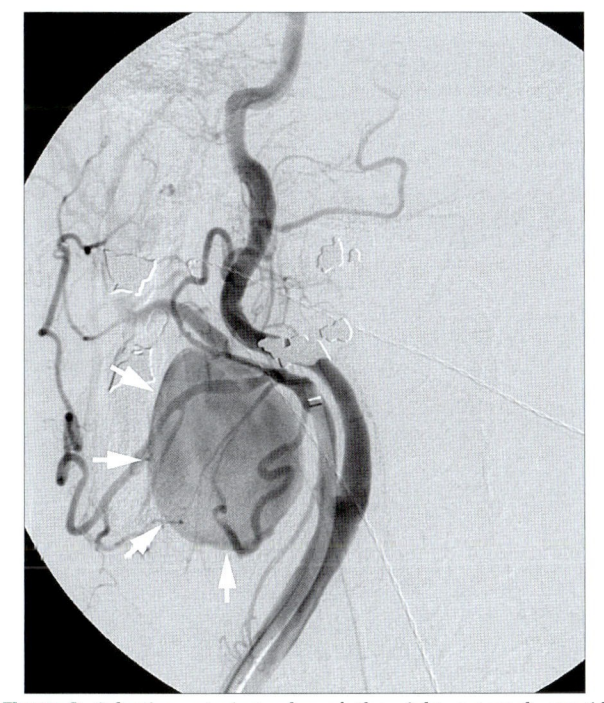

Figure 2. Selective arteriography of the right external carotid shows filling of the large pseudoaneurysm *(arrows)*.

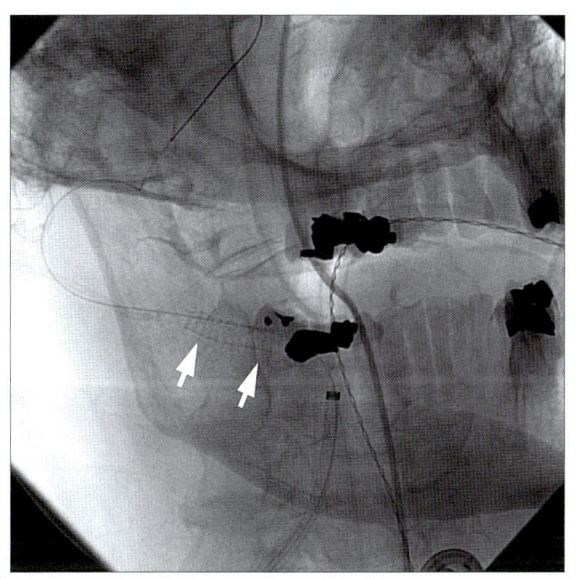

Figure 3. A covered stent has been placed across the neck of the pseudoaneurysm *(arrows)*.

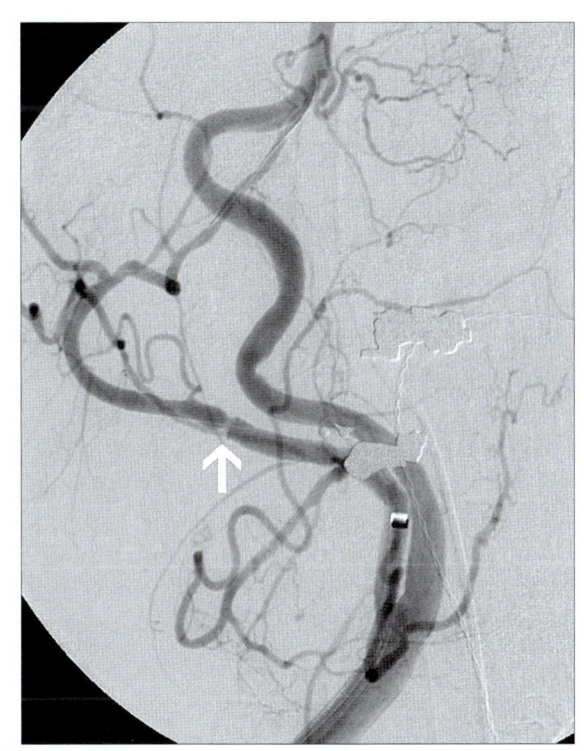

Figure 4. A follow-up arteriogram after placement of a covered stent shows successful exclusion of the pseudoaneurysm. Vasospasm can be seen adjacent to the distal edge of the stent *(arrow)*.

Case 96

DEMOGRAPHICS/CLINICAL HISTORY

A 17-year-old girl with a history of cystic fibrosis and hemoptysis, undergoing radiography and bronchial artery embolization.

DISCUSSION

History/Indications for Procedure
A 17-year-old girl has a history of cystic fibrosis and hemoptysis. She reports feeling dizzy, and she has chest pain localized to the right middle lobe anteriorly.

Procedure
Bronchial artery embolization

Pre-procedure Imaging
The chest radiograph shows diffuse peribronchial thickening, bronchiectasis, and cystic dilatation. There was no focal opacity to suggest the source of pulmonary hemorrhage.

Intraprocedural Findings
The right bronchial artery is hypertrophied and supplies a large area of abnormal hyperemia in the right middle and upper lung fields (Figs. 1 and 2). The right bronchial artery was embolized with 300- to 500-µm calibrated microspheres (Fig. 3).

Follow-up and Complications
The hemoptysis resolved after bronchial artery embolization, although the patient did continue to have mild chest discomfort the day after the procedure.

Suggested Readings
Burke C, et al: Bronchial artery embolization. Semin Intervent Radiol 21:43-48, 2004.
Cohen AM, Doershuk CF, Stern RC: Bronchial artery embolization to control hemoptysis in cystic fibrosis. Radiology 175:401-405, 1990.
Mal H, Rullon I, Mellot F, et al: Immediate and long-term results of bronchial artery embolization for life-threatening hemoptysis. Chest 115:996-1001, 1999.

Case 96   193

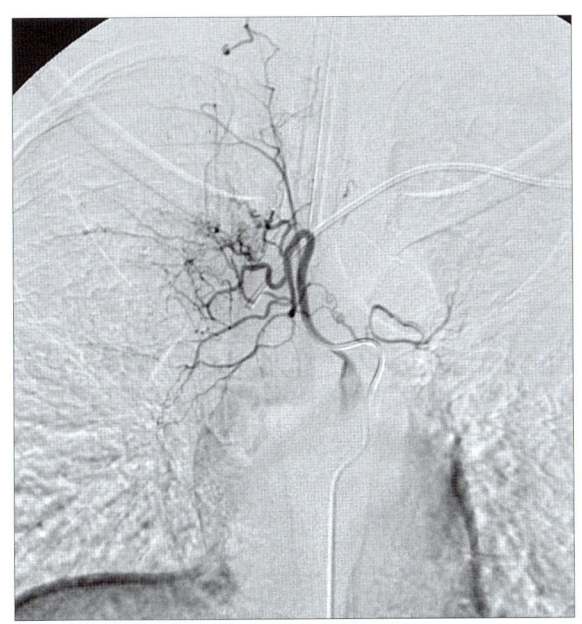

Figure 1. The right bronchial artery is hypertrophied.

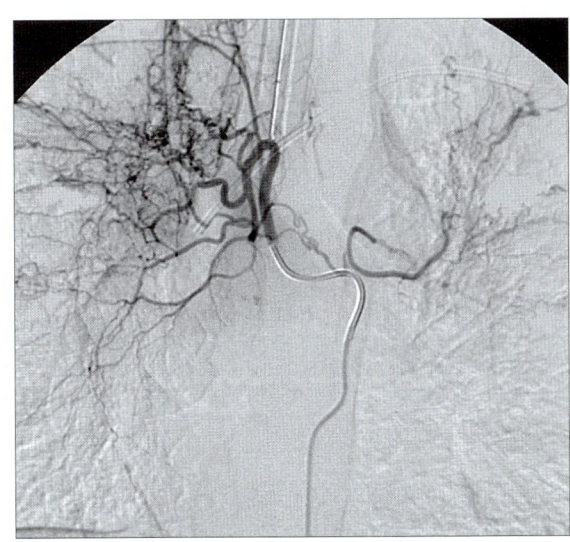

Figure 2. Slightly later image during bronchial artery injection demonstrates a large area of hyperemia with abnormal vessels in the right middle and upper lung fields. There is collateral communication across the mediastinum opacifying the left bronchial artery.

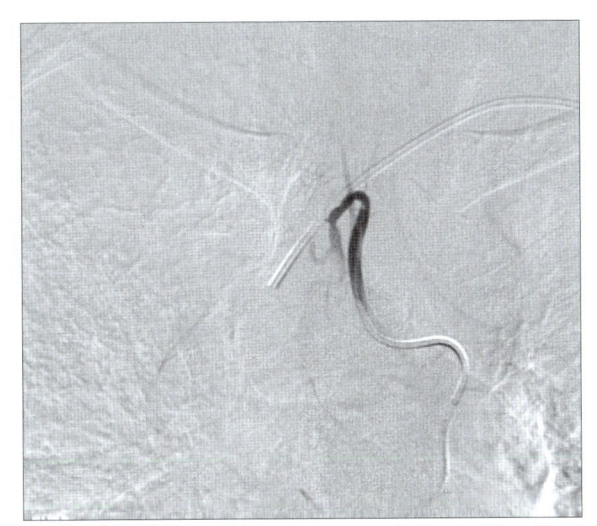

Figure 3. The right bronchial artery was embolized with calibrated microspheres until stasis.

Case 97

DEMOGRAPHICS/CLINICAL HISTORY

A 43-year-old man with hemoptysis, undergoing computed tomography (CT) and angiography.

DISCUSSION

History/Indications for Procedure
A 43-year-old man with a history of *Mycobacterium avium* complex (MAC) lung disease presented with hemoptysis. The patient reported three episodes of hemoptysis, and during each episode he coughed up 0.5 to 1 cup of blood.

Procedure
Bronchial artery embolization

Pre-procedure Imaging
CT of the chest shows an 8.7-cm × 7.3-cm cavitary mass in the right lung apex (Fig. 1). The bilateral, diffuse, nodular opacities are consistent with the patient's history of MAC lung disease.

Intraprocedural Findings
The right bronchial and supreme intercostal artery is hypertrophied and supplies a large area of hyperemia in the right upper lung field (Figs. 2 and 3). This artery was embolized with 300- to 500-μm and 500- to 700-μm calibrated microspheres (Embospheres, BioSphere Medical Inc., Rockland, MA) (Fig. 4).

Follow-up and Complications
The patient has had no further episodes of hemoptysis since the embolization.

Suggested Readings
Kato A, Kudo S, Matsumoto K, et al: Bronchial artery embolization for hemoptysis due to benign diseases: Immediate and long term results. Cardiovasc Intervent Radiol 23:351-357, 2000.

Pelage JP: Bronchial artery embolization: Anatomy and technique. Tech Vasc Intervent Radiol 10:274-275, 2007.

Serasli E, Kalpakidis V, Iatrou K, et al: Percutaneous bronchial artery embolization in the management of massive hemoptysis in chronic lung disease. Immediate and long-term outcomes. Intervent Angiol 27:319-328, 2008.

Case 97   195

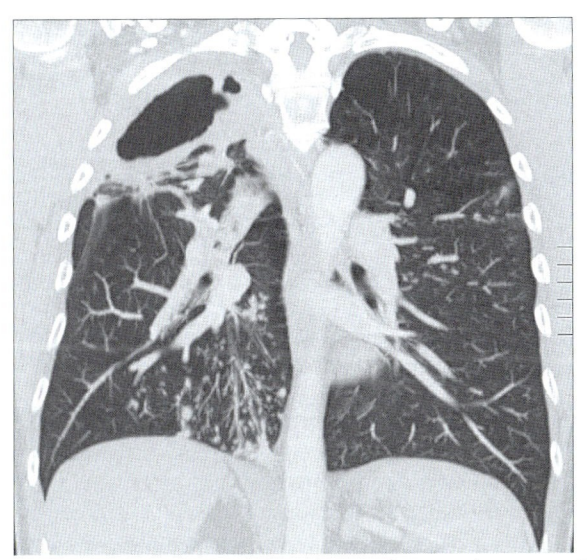

Figure 1. Coronal CT of the chest shows a large cavitary mass in the right lung apex. Multiple nodular opacities are most prominent in the medial right lung base and left perihilar region.

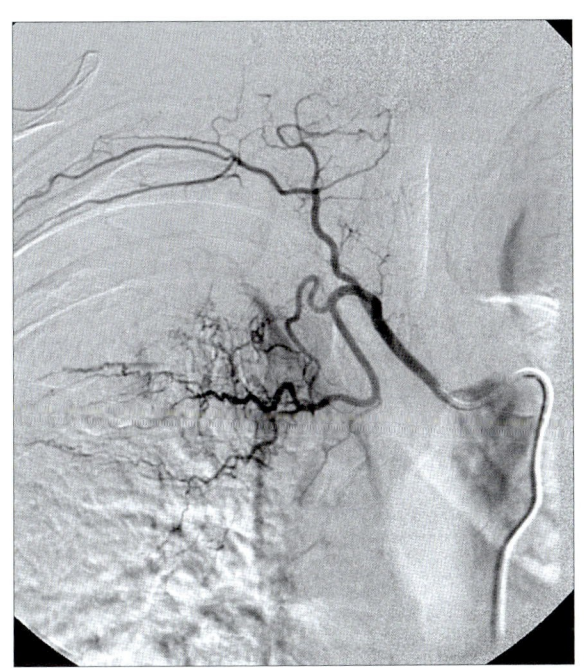

Figure 2. Arteriography shows a common origin of the right bronchial artery and right supreme intercostal artery. The right bronchial artery supplies a region of diffuse hyperemia in the right perihilar region.

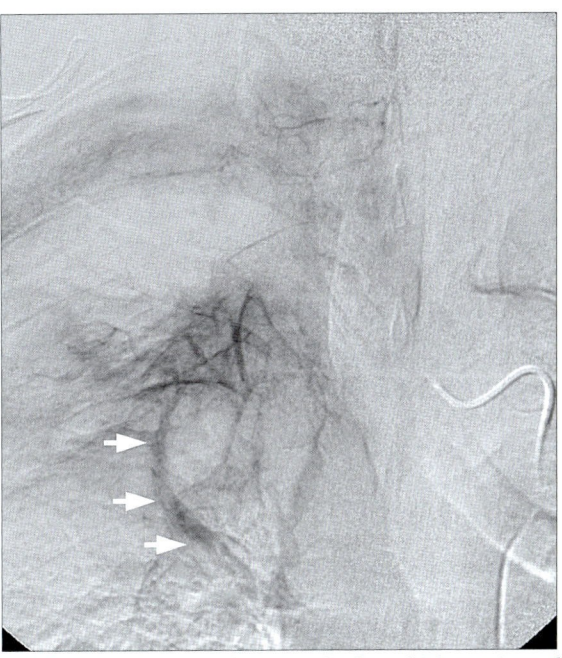

Figure 3. Delayed image during right bronchial arteriography shows prominent shunting to the right superior pulmonary vein *(arrows)*.

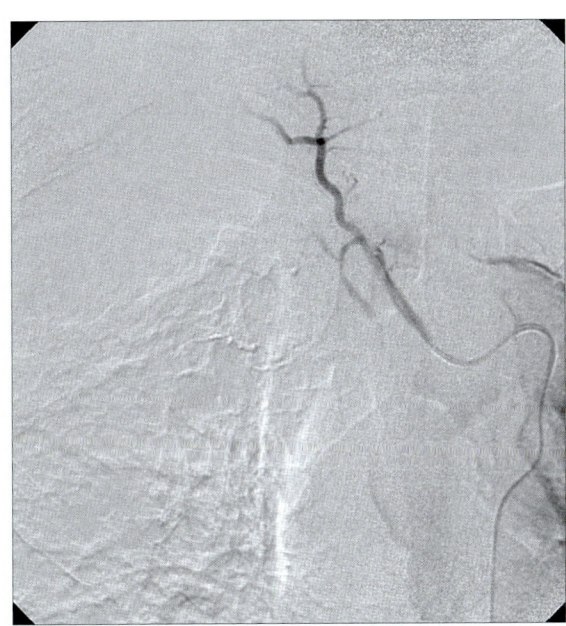

Figure 4. The follow-up angiogram after embolization shows minimal flow within the right bronchial artery. The zone of hyperemia is no longer seen, and there is reduced flow in the right supreme intercostal artery.

Case 98

DEMOGRAPHICS/CLINICAL HISTORY

A 53-year-old woman with sarcoidosis and left upper lobe aspergilloma.

DISCUSSION

History/Indications for Procedure
A 53-year-old woman with stage IV sarcoidosis and left upper lobe mycetoma. The patient has had recent episodes of severe hemoptysis.

Procedure
Bronchial artery embolization for invasive pulmonary aspergillosis

Pre-procedure Imaging
CT of the chest shows a 5-cm × 6.5-cm soft-tissue mass in the left upper lobe consistent with an aspergilloma (Fig. 1). In addition, there is severe underlying pulmonary parenchymal disease secondary to the patient's underlying pulmonary sarcoidosis.

Intraprocedural Findings
There is marked hyperemia in the left upper lobe, supplied predominantly by a branch of the thyrocervical trunk (Fig. 2). The thyrocervical trunk was catheterized with a 3-French microcatheter and embolized with 355- to 500-μm polyvinyl alcohol particles (Fig. 3).

Follow-up and Complications
After the embolization, the patient underwent CT-guided intra-cavitary injection of amphotericin (Fig. 4). The patient had no further hemoptysis following the treatment; 2 months later she underwent uncomplicated wedge resection of the fungal ball.

Suggested Readings

Corr P: Management of severe hemoptysis from pulmonary aspergilloma using endovascular embolization. Cardiovasc Intervent Radiol 29:807-810, 2006.

Keller FS, Rosch J, Loflin TG, et al: Nonbronchial systemic collateral arteries: Significance in percutaneous embolotherapy for hemoptysis. Radiology 164:687-692, 1987.

Lee KS, Kim HT, Kim YH, et al: Treatment of hemoptysis in patients with cavitary aspergilloma of the lung: Value of percutaneous instillation of amphotericin B. AJR Am J Roentgenol 161:727-731, 1993.

Shapiro MJ, Albelda SM, Mayock RL, et al: Severe hemoptysis associated with pulmonary aspergilloma: Percutaneous intracavitary treatment. Chest 94:1225-1231, 1988.

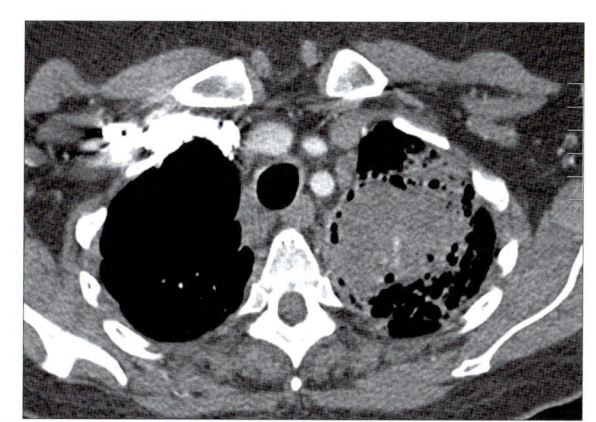

Figure 1. Contrast-enhanced CT of the chest shows a 5- × 6.5-cm soft-tissue mass in the left lung apex consistent with the patient's known mycetoma.

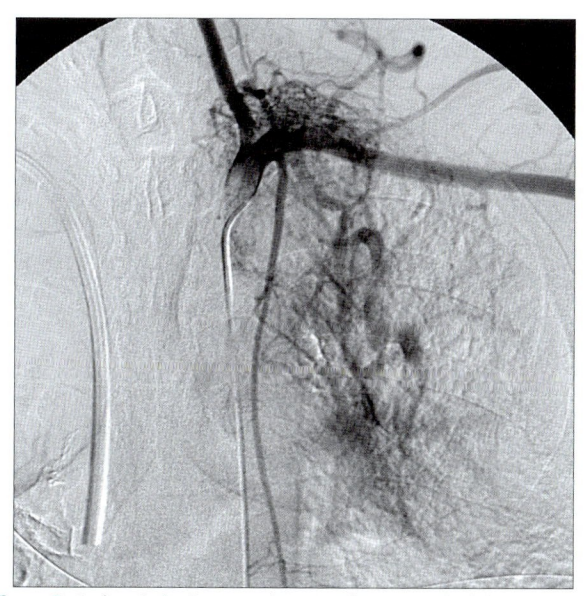

Figure 2. Left subclavian arteriogram shows marked hypervascularity in the left lung apex, supplied predominantly by a branch of the thyrocervical trunk.

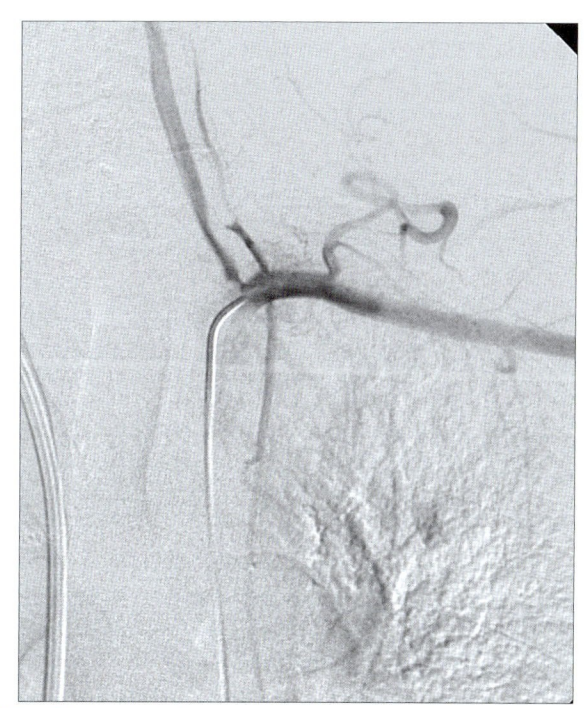

Figure 3. Post-embolization arteriogram. The thyrocervical trunk has been embolized. The previously identified hypervascularity is no longer seen.

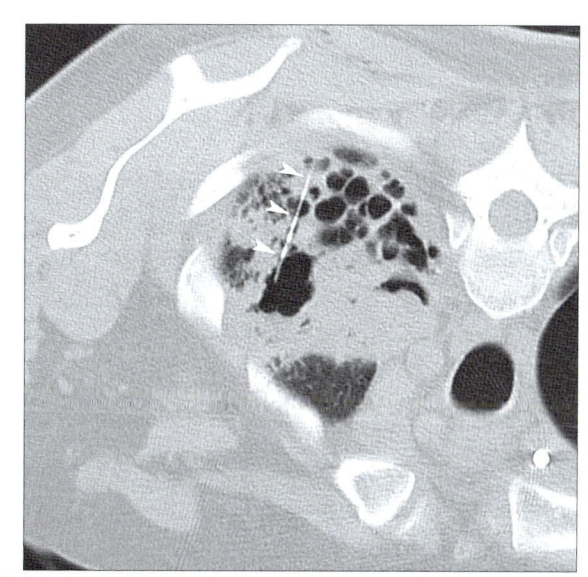

Figure 4. Using CT-guidance, a 25-gauge needle was inserted into the mycetoma *(arrowheads)*. Once the needle was within the center of the fungal ball, the amphotericin was slowly injected.

Case 99

DEMOGRAPHICS/CLINICAL HISTORY

A 42-year-old man with cystic fibrosis and hemoptysis, undergoing computed tomography (CT) and arteriography.

DISCUSSION

History/Indications for Procedure
A 42-year-old man, who has cystic fibrosis that was diagnosed when he was 17 years old, presents with recurrent hemoptysis. He has undergone numerous prior bronchial artery embolizations.

Procedure
Bronchial artery embolization

Pre-procedure Imaging
Contrast-enhanced CT of the chest shows a massively enlarged right bronchial artery and multiple enhancing vessels in the mediastinum (Fig. 1). An enlarged right inferior phrenic artery is also identified.

Intraprocedural Findings
The right bronchial artery is massively enlarged and supplies an abnormal area of hypervascularity in the right middle and upper lung field (Figs. 2 and 3). The right bronchial artery was embolized with 300- to 500-μm polyvinyl alcohol (PVA) microspheres until stasis was achieved. The right inferior phrenic artery was catheterized and found to be a source of collateral supply to an area of hyperemia in the right hilar region (Fig. 4); this artery also was embolized with 300- to 500-μm PVA microspheres.

Follow-up and Complications
The patient became hyponatremic after the embolization, a reaction probably related to the syndrome of inappropriate antidiuretic hormone secretion (SIADH) resulting from the acute lung injury. This resolved with conservative management, and the patient has had no further hemoptysis.

Suggested Readings
Burke CT, Mauro MA: Bronchial artery embolization. Semin Intervent Radiol 21:43-48, 2004.
Pelage JP: Bronchial artery embolization: Anatomy and technique. Tech Vasc Intervent Radiol 10:274-275, 2007.
Yoon W, Kim JK, Kim YH, et al: Bronchial and nonbronchial systemic artery embolization for life-threatening hemoptysis: A comprehensive review. Radiographics 22:1395-1409, 2002.

Case 99   199

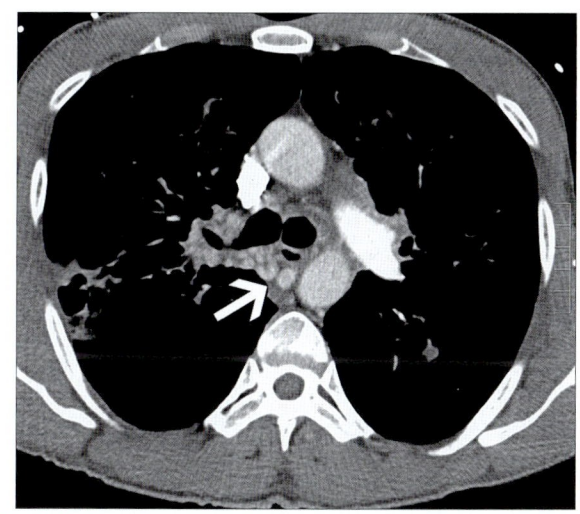

Figure 1. Contrast-enhanced CT shows multiple, enlarged, enhancing vessels in the mediastinum and right hilum. The right bronchial artery is massively hypertrophied *(arrow)*.

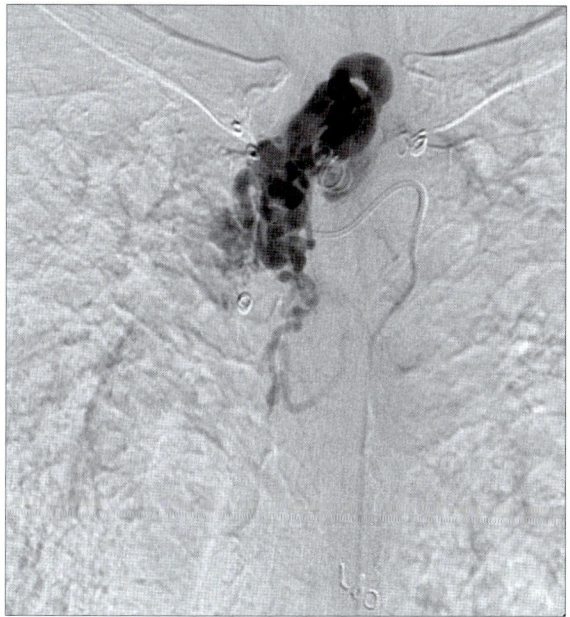

Figure 2. Selective injection of the right bronchial artery shows massive hypertrophy and tortuosity of the right bronchial artery.

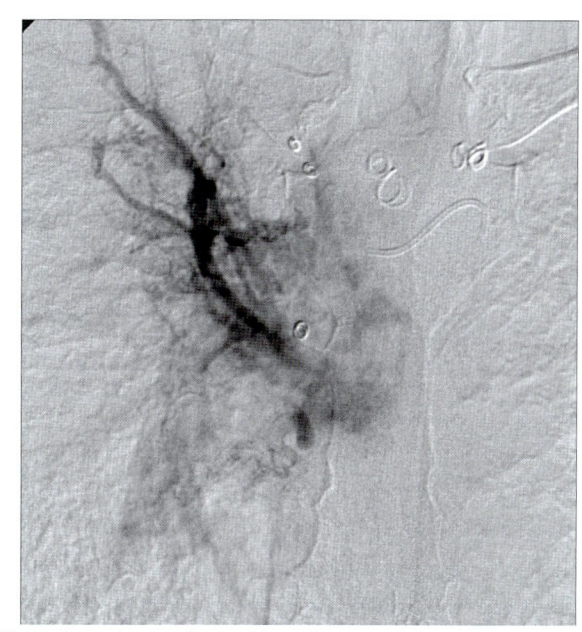

Figure 3. An image obtained later during right bronchial artery injection shows hyperemia in the right middle and upper lung field, with prominent shunting into the right superior pulmonary vein.

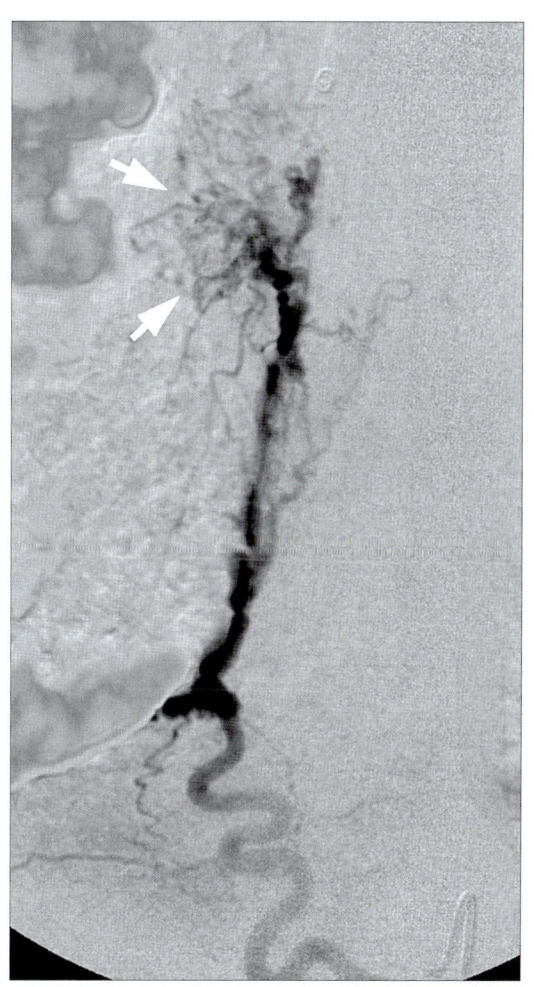

Figure 4. Selective injection shows the right inferior phrenic artery, which provides collateral supply to an area of hyperemia in the right hilar region *(arrows)*.

Case 100

DEMOGRAPHICS/CLINICAL HISTORY

A 28-year-old woman with cystic fibrosis, undergoing aortography.

DISCUSSION

History/Indications for Procedure
This patient with cystic fibrosis has had worsening hemoptysis for 6 days.

Procedure
Bronchial artery embolization

Intraprocedural Findings
An aortogram shows hypertrophied right and left bronchial arteries supplying regions of pulmonary hyperemia (Figs. 1 and 2). The bronchial arteries were embolized with 300- to 500-μm polyvinyl alcohol particles (Fig. 3).

Follow-up and Complications
The hemoptysis resolved after the embolization. The patient presented with hemoptysis again 14 months later and underwent repeat bronchial artery embolization.

Suggested Readings
Burke C, et al: Bronchial artery embolization. Semin Intervent Radiol 21:43-48, 2004.

Cohen AM, Doershuk CF, Stern RC: Bronchial artery embolization to control hemoptysis in cystic fibrosis. Radiology 175:401-405, 1990.

Mal H, Rullon I, Mellot F, et al: Immediate and long term results of bronchial artery embolization for life threatening hemoptysis. Chest 115:996-1001, 1999.

Case 100   201

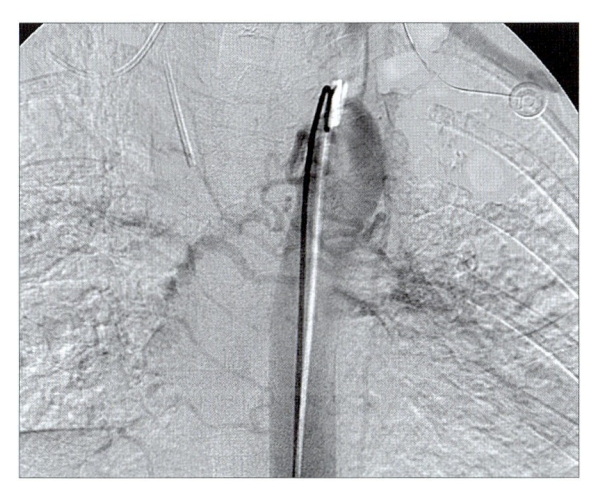

Figure 1. Aortogram shows hypertrophied right and left bronchial arteries.

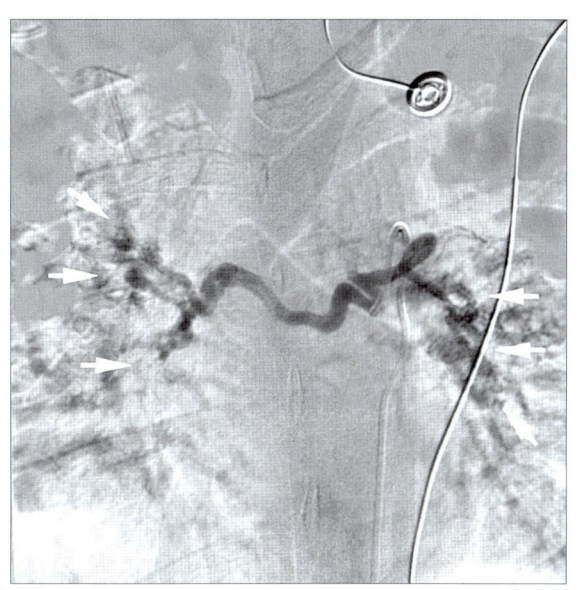

Figure 2. Selective catheterization of a common trunk of the right and left bronchial arteries. The bronchial arteries supply areas of hyperemia in the perihilar regions bilaterally *(arrows)*.

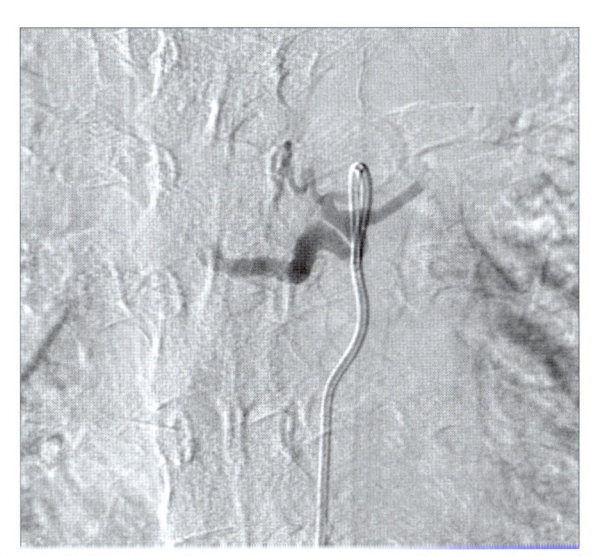

Figure 3. The bronchial arteries were embolized to stasis with polyvinyl alcohol particles.

Case 101

DEMOGRAPHICS/CLINICAL HISTORY

A 43-year-old man with primary ciliary dyskinesia and hemoptysis.

DISCUSSION

History/Indications for Procedure
A 43-year-old man with a history of primary ciliary dyskinesia. He has been having small-volume hemoptysis that has been increasing over the past several weeks.

Procedure
Bronchial artery embolization

Pre-procedure Imaging
CT of the chest performed 4 months earlier shows bilateral apical bronchiectasis (Fig. 1). In addition, ground-glass and nodular opacities are seen throughout both lung fields.

Intraprocedural Findings
The right external iliac artery is occluded, and the right internal iliac artery is hypertrophied (Fig. 2). The right bronchial artery is hypertrophied and supplies an area of hyperemia in the right lung apex; the right bronchial artery was embolized with 500-μm to 700-μm calibrated microspheres (Figs. 3,4).

Follow-up and Complications
The patient's hemoptysis resolved following the embolization.

Suggested Readings
Burke CT, Mauro MA: Bronchial artery embolization. Sem Intervent Radiol 21:43-48, 2004.
Pelage JP: Bronchial artery embolization: Anatomy and technique. Tech Vasc Intervent Radiol 10:274-275, 2007.
Yoon W, Kim JK, Kim YH, et al: Bronchial and nonbronchial systemic artery embolization for life-threatening hemoptysis: A comprehensive review. Radiographics 22:1395-1409, 2002.

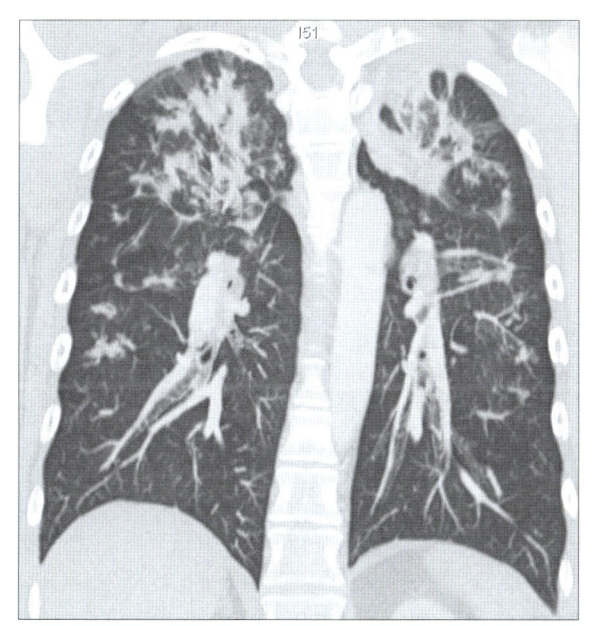

Figure 1. Coronal image from contrast-enhanced CT performed 4 months prior to presentation shows bilateral upper lobe bronchiectasis. Scattered nodular opacities are also seen.

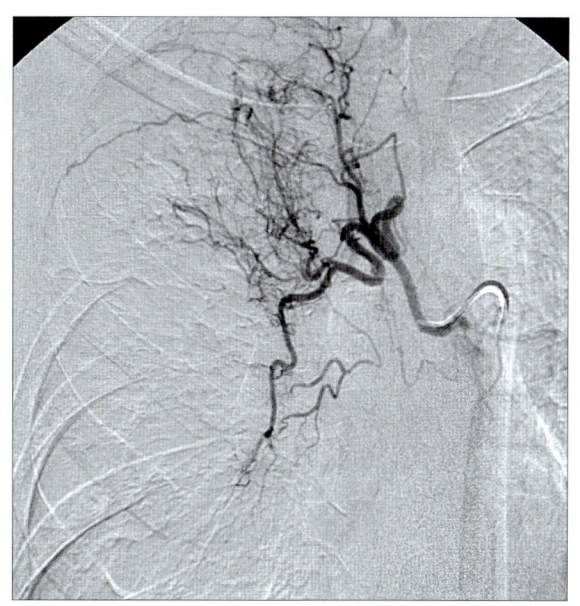

Figure 3. Selective injection of the right bronchial artery. There is a combined bronchial-intercostal trunk that is enlarged. Diffuse hyperemia is seen throughout the right upper lobe.

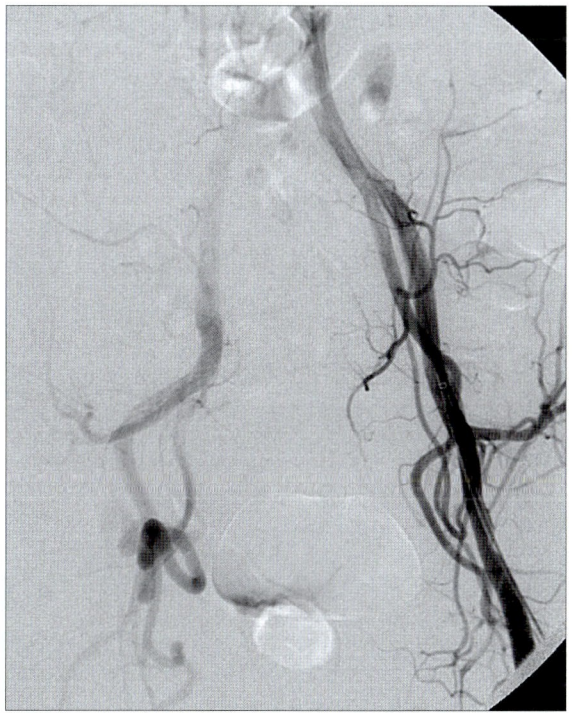

Figure 2. Pelvic arteriogram shows complete occlusion of the right external iliac artery. There is diffuse enlargement of the right internal iliac artery that reconstituted the right common femoral artery. On further questioning, the patient stated that he had undergone an angiogram when he was an infant.

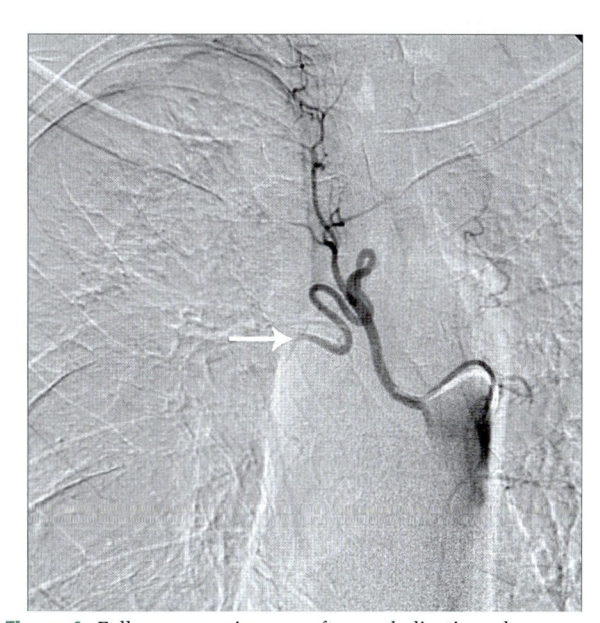

Figure 4. Follow-up angiogram after embolization shows continued flow within the supreme intercostal artery. The right bronchial artery is occluded *(arrow)* and the hyperemic changes are no longer present.

Case 102

DEMOGRAPHICS/CLINICAL HISTORY

A 56-year-old woman with symptomatic angiomyolipoma of the right kidney, undergoing MRI.

DISCUSSION

History/Indications for Procedure
Embolization was indicated for this patient with right flank pain.

Procedure
Embolization of renal angiomyolipoma

Pre-procedure Imaging
Contrast-enhanced MRI shows a 4.4-cm × 4.7-cm fat-containing mass arising from the lower pole of the right kidney (Figs. 1 and 2).

Intraprocedural Findings
Selective angiogram shows a hypervascular mass projecting from the lower pole of the right kidney (Fig. 3).

Follow-up and Complications
MRI obtained 3 months after the embolization shows decreased enhancement of the solid portion of the mass, and the mass has reduced in size to 3.6-cm × 3.8-cm (Fig. 4). The patient's symptoms also had resolved.

Suggested Readings
Han YM, Kim JK, Roh BS, et al: Renal angiomyolipoma: Selective arterial embolization—effectiveness and changes in angiomyogenic components in long-term follow-up. Radiology 204:65-70, 1997.

Kothary N, Soulen MC, Clark TW, et al: Renal angiomyolipoma: Long-term results after arterial embolization. J Vasc Intervent Radiol 16: 45-50, 2005.

Rimon U, Duvdevani M, Garniek A, et al: Ethanol and polyvinyl alcohol mixture for transcatheter embolization of renal angiomyolipoma. AJR Am J Roentgenol 187:762-768, 2006.

Case 102   205

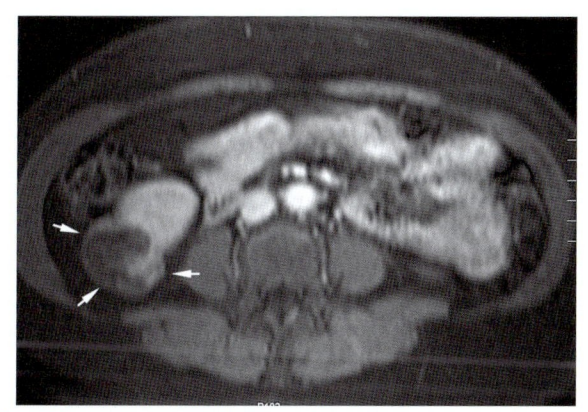

Figure 1. Axial postgadolinium T1-weighted fat-saturated image shows an exophytic, predominantly fat-containing mass off the posterior right kidney *(arrowheads)*.

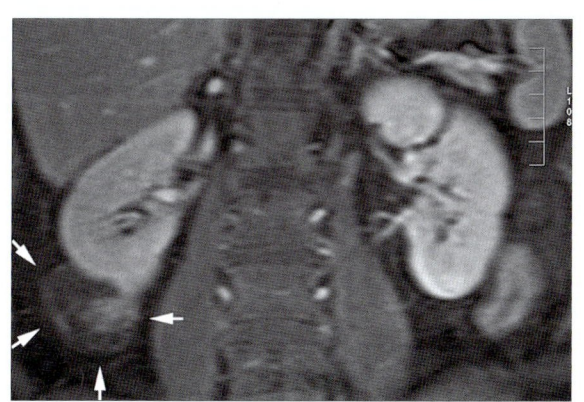

Figure 2. Coronal postgadolinium T1-weighted fat-saturated image shows an exophytic, predominantly fat-containing mass arising off the inferior aspect of the right kidney *(arrowheads)*.

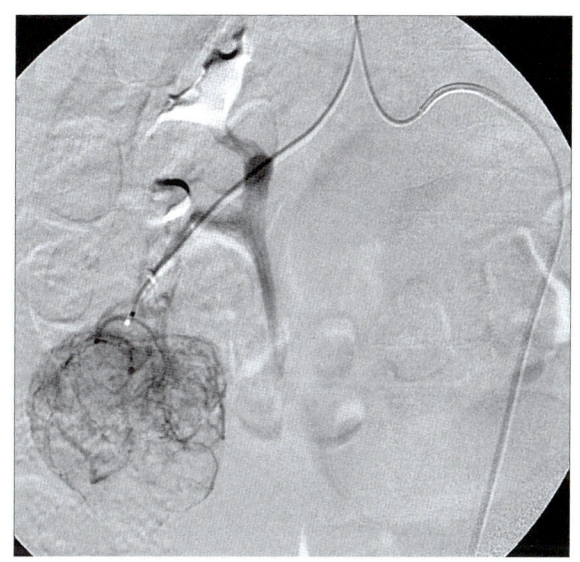

Figure 3. Superselective angiography shows the hypervascular nature of most of the mass. The mass was embolized with ethanol.

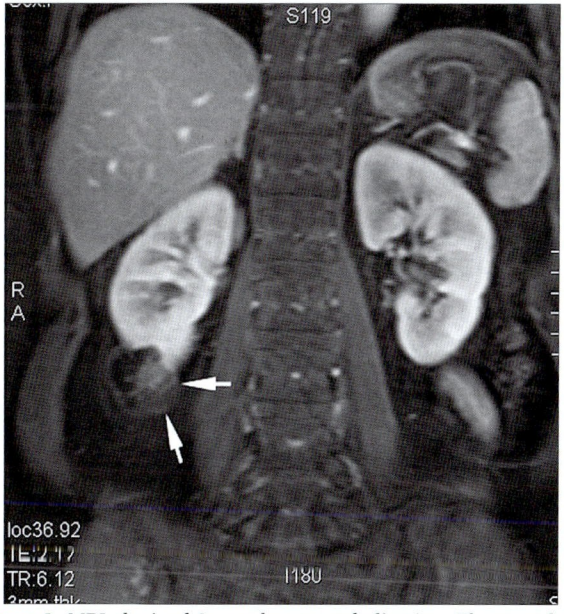

Figure 4. MRI obtained 3 months postembolization. The mass has decreased in size, but some enhancement remains within the solid portion of the mass *(arrowheads)*.

Case 103

DEMOGRAPHICS/CLINICAL HISTORY

A 74-year-old man with hematuria after ureteral stent placement, undergoing arteriography.

DISCUSSION

History/Indications for Procedure
A 74-year-old man with a history of bladder carcinoma developed a large amount of hematuria after antegrade ureteral stent placement.

Procedure
Embolotherapy for iatrogenic renal arteriovenous fistula

Intraprocedural Findings
Left renal arteriogram shows a renal arteriovenous fistula in the parenchyma of the middle of the left kidney (Figs. 1 and 2). The feeding artery was selectively catheterized and embolized with two 3-mm (0.018-inch) coils (Figs. 3 and 4).

Follow-up and Complications
The hematuria slowed significantly after the embolization, and the patient was discharged to home the next morning. The patient was evaluated 1 week later; his urine had cleared, and he was asymptomatic.

Suggested Readings

Chatziioannou A, Brountzos E, Primetis E, et al: Effects of superselective embolization for renal vascular injuries on renal parenchyma and function. Eur J Vasc Endovasc Surg 28:201-206, 2004.

Giavroglou CE, Farmakis TM, Kiskinis D: Idiopathic renal arteriovenous fistula treated by transcatheter embolization. Acta Radiol 46:368-370, 2005.

Sofocleous CT, Hinrichs C, Hubbi B, et al: Angiographic findings and embolotherapy in renal arterial trauma. Cardiovasc Intervent Radiol 28:39-47, 2005.

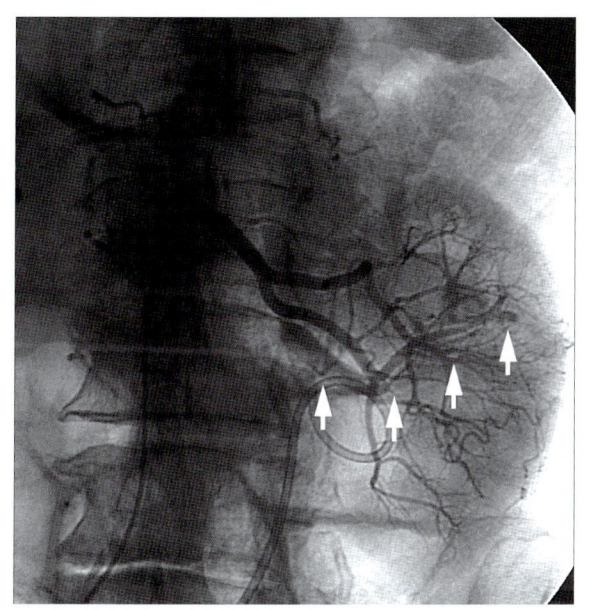

Figure 1. Arterial phase of the left renal arteriogram shows early opacification of the left renal vein (*arrows*).

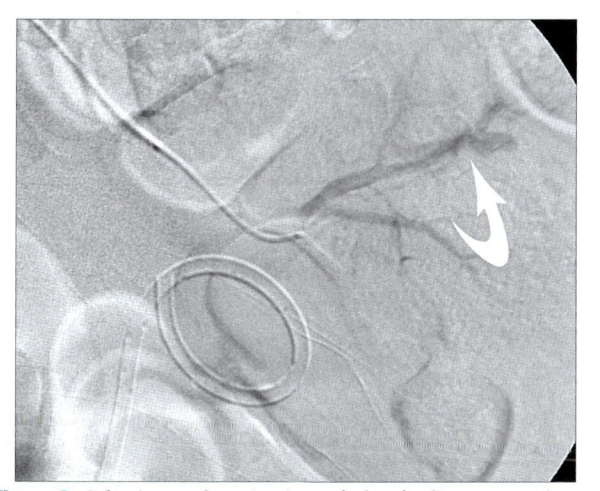

Figure 2. Selective catheterization of the feeding artery better delineates the arteriovenous fistula (*arrow*).

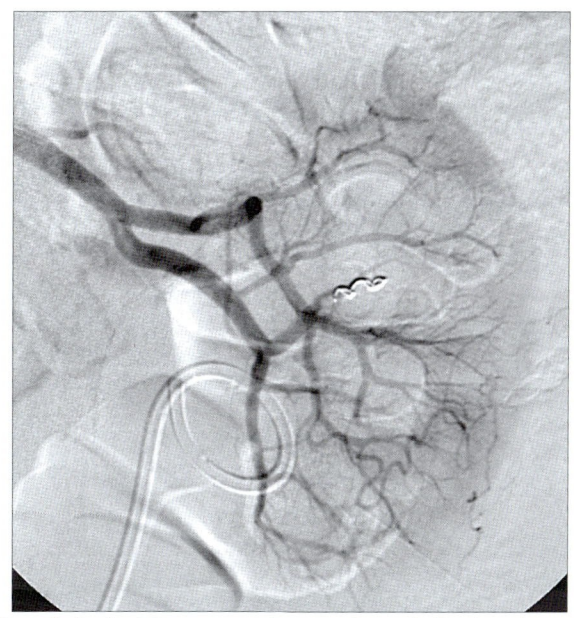

Figure 3. In the follow-up arteriogram after embolization, the arteriovenous fistula is no longer seen.

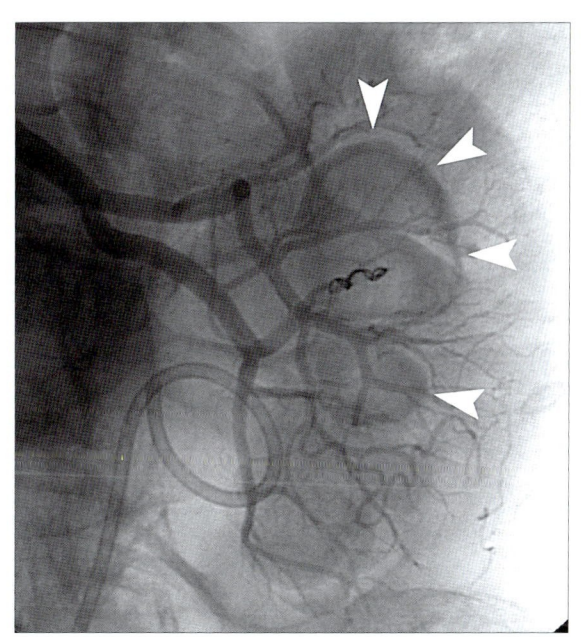

Figure 4. Unsubtracted image from postembolization arteriography shows severe hydronephrosis with large filling defects in the renal collecting system, which is consistent with a clot (*arrowheads*).

Case 104

DEMOGRAPHICS/CLINICAL HISTORY

A 16-year-old girl who fell off a horse and lacerated the left kidney, undergoing arteriography and computed tomography (CT).

DISCUSSION

History/Indications for Procedure
A 16-year-old girl fractured her left kidney after falling off a horse. The patient is a Jehovah's Witness and refused blood products, despite continued hemorrhage and dropping hemoglobin levels.

Procedure
Renal artery embolization in trauma

Pre-procedure Imaging
Outside CT showed a large laceration through the lower pole of the left kidney, with a large perinephric hematoma.

Intraprocedural Findings
Selective left renal arteriogram shows no perfusion of the lower pole of the kidney without active extravasation (Figs. 1 and 2). The inferior branches of the anterior and posterior segmental arteries were selectively catheterized and embolized with coils (Fig. 3).

Follow-up and Complications
The patient's hemoglobin levels stabilized after the embolization, and the hematuria cleared after 1 week. Follow-up CT showed atrophy of the embolized lower pole and resolution of the perinephric hematoma (Fig. 4).

Suggested Readings
Hagiwara A, Sakaki S, Goto H, et al: The role of interventional radiology in the management of blunt renal injury: A practical protocol. J Trauma 51:526-531, 2001.

Sofocleous CT, Hinrichs C, Hubbi B, et al: Angiographic findings and embolotherapy in renal arterial trauma. Cardiovasc Intervent Radiol 28:39-47, 2005.

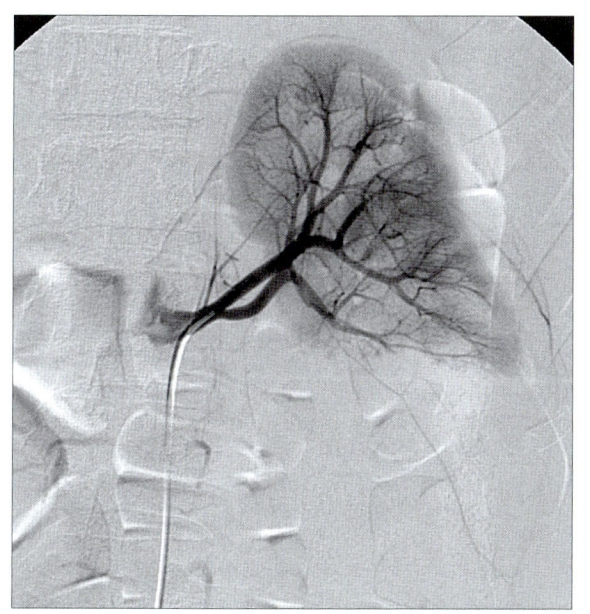

Figure 1. Left renal arteriogram shows a lack of perfusion to the lower pole of the left kidney that is consistent with the known renal laceration.

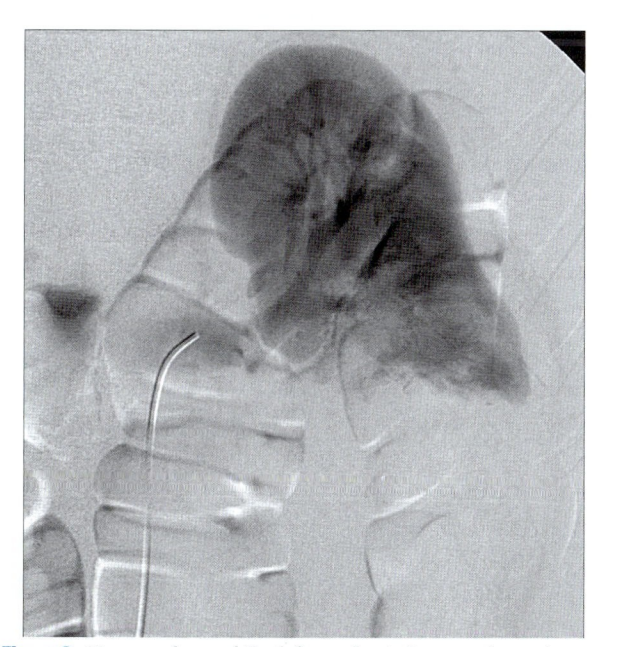

Figure 2. Venous phase of the left renal arteriogram shows irregular contrast accumulation along the fractured surface of the kidney, but no frank extravasation.

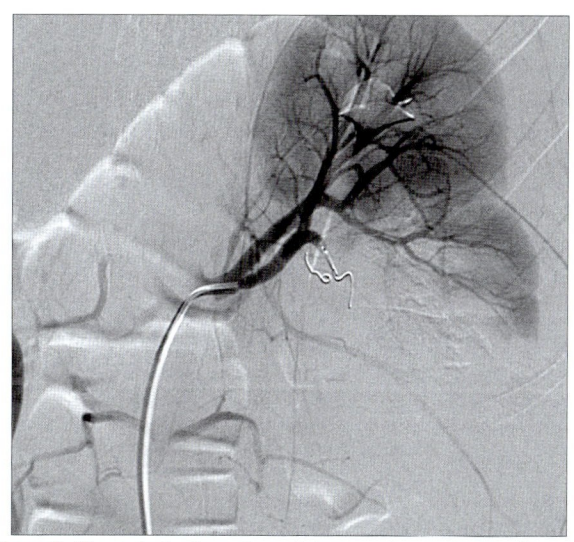

Figure 3. The inferior branches of the anterior and posterior segmental arteries were embolized with coils. The perfusion of the upper and middle portions of the left kidney is preserved.

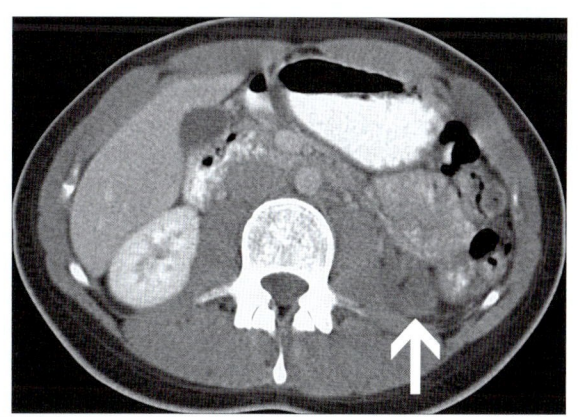

Figure 4. Follow-up CT 3 months after the embolization shows a nonperfused lower pole remnant *(arrow)*. The perinephric hematoma has resolved.

Case 105

DEMOGRAPHICS/CLINICAL HISTORY

A 38-year-old man with autosomal dominant polycystic kidney disease (ADPCK) presents with hematuria and right lower quadrant pain.

DISCUSSION

History/Indications for Procedure
A 38-year-old man with ADPCK disease presents with hematuria and right lower quadrant pain. The patient's hematocrit has fallen from 38% to 26% over the past 30 hours.

Procedure
Selective embolization for hemorrhagic cyst in a patient with polycystic kidney disease

Pre-procedure Imaging
Non-contrast CT of the abdomen shows changes characteristic of ADPCK disease. There are new areas of hyperdensity within several of the cysts on the right, consistent with intracyst hemorrhage, and new right retroperitoneal hemorrhage (Fig. 1).

Intraprocedural Findings
Right renal arteriogram shows diffuse distortion of the intrarenal arteries, consistent with mass effect from the numerous renal cysts (Fig. 2). Two small pseudoaneurysms were identified within distal branches in the lower pole of the right kidney; the offending artery was selectively catheterized and embolized with 300-µm to 500-µm calibrated microspheres followed by coils (Fig. 3).

Follow-up and Complications
Follow-up arteriogram after embolization shows no further arterial supply to the lower pole of the right kidney. The patient's hemoglobin levels remained stable following the procedure; he was managed for post-embolization pain for the next 24 hours and discharged home the following day.

Suggested Readings

Pappas P, Leonardou P, Papadoukakis S, et al: Urgent superselective segmental renal artery embolization in the treatment of life-threatening renal hemorrhage. Urol Int 77:34-41, 2006.

Poulakis V, Rerakis N, Becht E, et al: Treatment of renal-vascular injury by transcatheter embolization: Immediate and long-term effects on renal function. J Endourol 20:405-409, 2006.

Sofocleous CT, Hinrichs C, Hubbi B, et al: Angiographic findings and embolotherapy in renal arterial trauma. Cardiovasc Intervent Radiol 28:39-47, 2005.

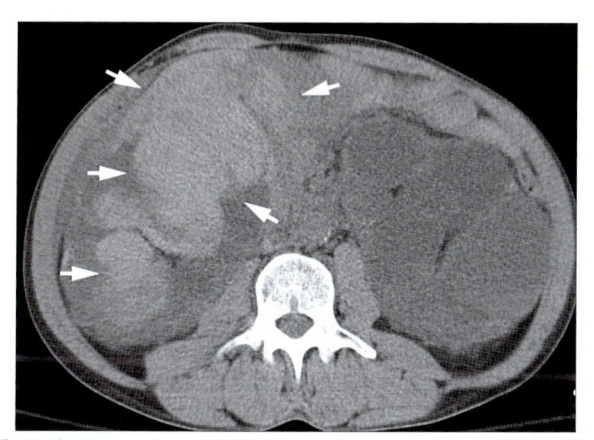

Figure 1. Noncontrast CT shows numerous renal cysts bilaterally. Hemorrhage is present within several of the lower pole cysts on the right and extends into the anterior pararenal space *(arrows)*.

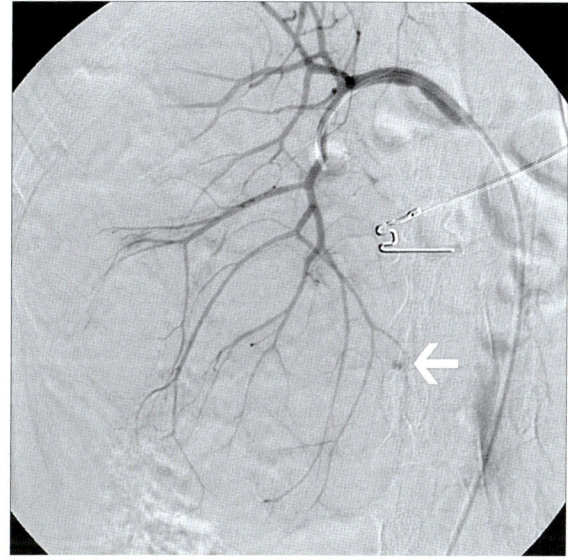

Figure 2. Selective injection of a lower pole branch of the right renal artery shows distortion of the intrarenal arterial branches from mass effect of the renal cysts. There is filling of a small pseudoaneurysm supplied by a small branch of the lower pole renal artery *(arrow)*.

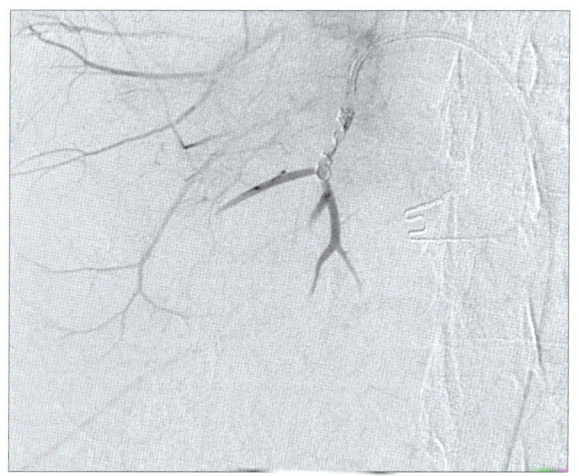

Figure 3. Post-embolization arteriogram shows minimal flow to the lower pole branch of the right renal artery.

Case 106

DEMOGRAPHICS/CLINICAL HISTORY

A 50-year-old man with urine leak after resection of large abdominal gastrointestinal stromal tumor, undergoing CT and arteriography.

DISCUSSION

History/Indications for Procedure
A 50-year-old man presented with urine leak after resection of large abdominal gastrointestinal stromal tumor. The ureter was removed as part of the resection; however, the kidney was not involved and did not appear functional at surgery and so was left in place.

Procedure
Transarterial ablation of the kidney

Pre-procedure Imaging
A contrast-enhanced CT scan before the mass resection shows a large mass that occupies nearly the entire right side of the abdomen (Fig. 1). The mass displaces the right kidney, but does not appear to involve the right kidney.

Intraprocedural Findings
The right renal arteriogram was normal (Fig. 2). An 8.5-mm occlusion balloon was inflated in the main right renal artery, and the right renal artery was embolized with alcohol (Figs. 3 and 4).

Follow-up and Complications
The output from the surgical drain decreased significantly after the procedure and was removed 2 weeks after the embolization. The patient had no further evidence for urine leak.

Suggested Readings
DeBaere T, Lagrange C, Kuoch V, et al: Transcatheter ethanol renal ablation in 20 patients with persistent urine leaks: An alternative to surgical nephrectomy. J Urol 164:1148, 2000.

Ebisuno S, Aoshi H, Ohkawa T: Nephrectomy in situ: Treatment of ureteral fistula due to progressive malignancy. Urol Radiol 11:102, 1989.

Case 106   213

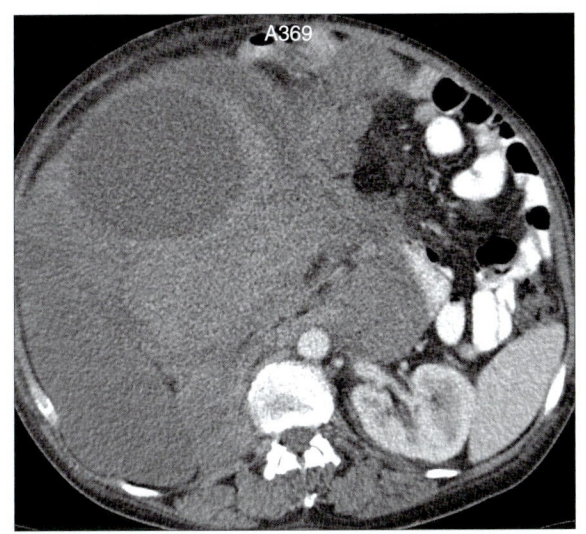

Figure 1. Contrast-enhanced CT scan shows large, heterogeneous mass occupying much of the right side of the abdomen.

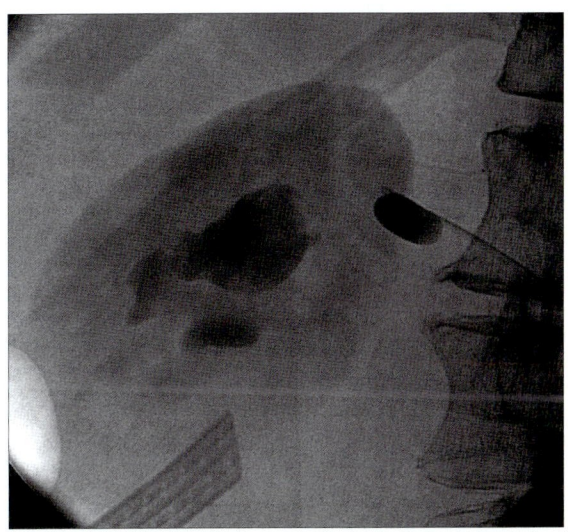

Figure 3. An 8.5-mm occlusion balloon has been inflated in the main right renal artery. Note the excretion of contrast material into a dilated renal collecting system.

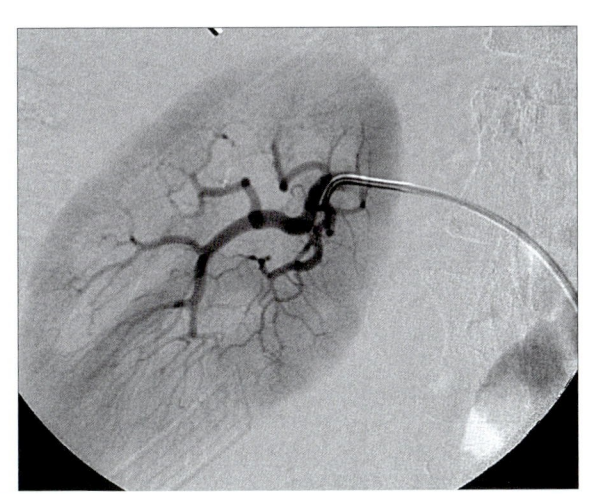

Figure 2. Selective right renal arteriogram shows right renal artery and branches are normal.

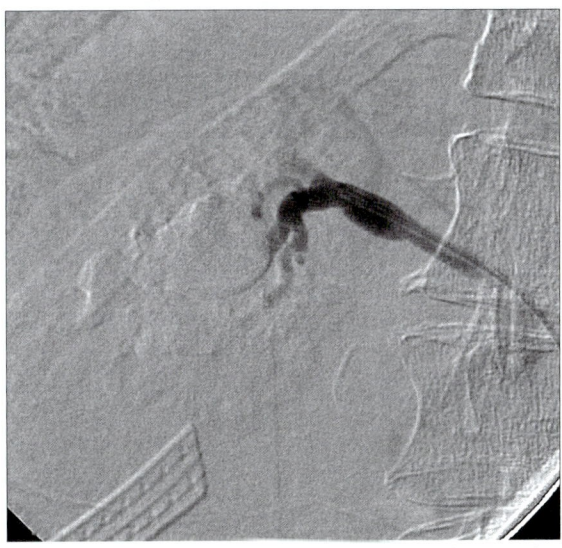

Figure 4. Follow-up arteriogram after alcohol embolization shows that intrarenal branches no longer fill.

Case 107

DEMOGRAPHICS/CLINICAL HISTORY

A 43-year-old man with a history of chronic pancreatitis and massive upper gastrointestinal hemorrhage, undergoing endoscopy, computed tomography (CT), angiography, and embolization.

DISCUSSION

History/Indications for Procedure
A 43-year-old man with a history of chronic pancreatitis presents with abdominal pain and hematemesis. A gastric ulcer was identified at endoscopy; the ulcer was injected with epinephrine, and a metallic clip was placed.

Procedure
Acute upper gastrointestinal hemorrhage

Pre-procedure Imaging
Contrast-enhanced CT performed 5 days before presentation demonstrated a small atrophic pancreas with many calcifications in the pancreatic tail. There is a small hyperdense fluid collection adjacent to the pancreatic tail and distal splenic artery (Fig. 1).

Intraprocedural Findings
There is active extravasation from the distal splenic artery, with free flow of contrast into the gastric lumen (Figs. 2 and 3). The splenic artery was embolized with coils (Fig. 4).

Follow-up and Complications
The patient stabilized immediately after embolization. He was discharged from the hospital 4 days later with no further evidence of bleeding.

Suggested Readings
Frisoli JK, Sze DY, Kee S: Transcatheter embolization for the treatment of upper gastrointestinal bleeding. Tech Vasc Intervent Radiol 7:136-142, 2005.

Nicholson AA, Patel J, McPherson S, et al: Endovascular treatment of pancreatitis associated visceral aneurysms and a suggested classification with therapeutic implications. J Vasc Intervent Radiol 17:1279-1285, 2006.

Schenker MP, Duszak R Jr, Soulen MC, et al: Upper gastrointestinal hemorrhage and transcatheter embolotherapy: Clinical and technical factors impacting on success and survival. J Vasc Intervent Radiol 12:1263-1271, 2001.

Case 107   215

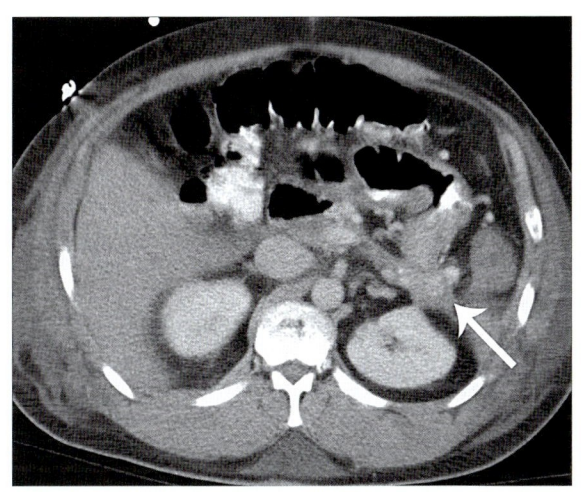

Figure 1. Contrast-enhanced CT demonstrates a small hyperdense fluid collection *(arrow)* adjacent to the tail of the pancreas.

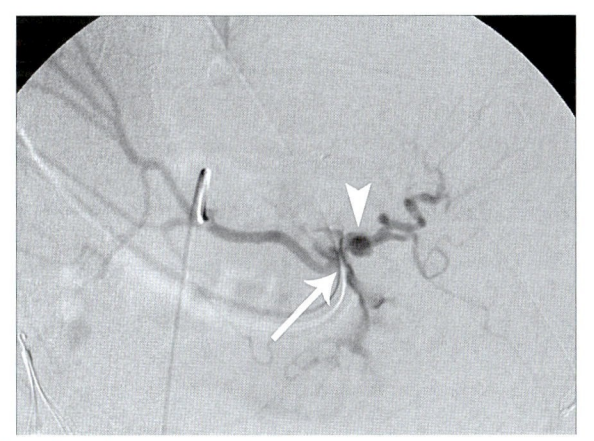

Figure 2. Celiac angiogram demonstrates active extravasation from the distal splenic artery *(arrow)*. A small aneurysm *(arrowhead)* of the splenic artery is just distal to the site of injury.

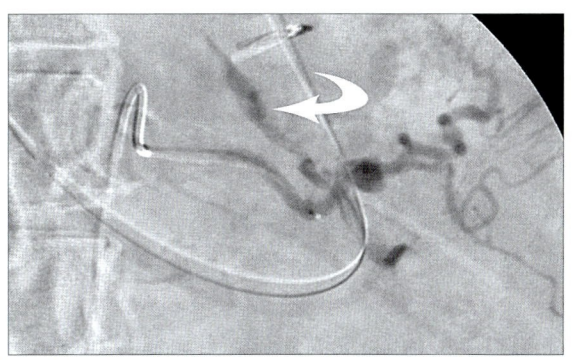

Figure 3. A 3-French microcatheter was advanced to the site of hemorrhage. A portion of the extravasated contrast passed into the gastric lumen *(arrow)*.

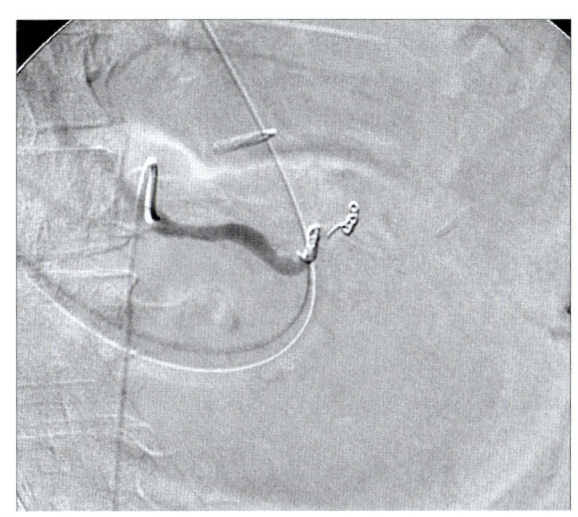

Figure 4. The splenic artery was embolized with coils placed across the site of injury.

Case 108

DEMOGRAPHICS/CLINICAL HISTORY

An 87-year-old woman with new-onset hematemesis, undergoing endoscopy and angiography in the endovascular management of gastrointestinal hemorrhage.

DISCUSSION

History/Indications for Procedure
An 87-year-old woman has new-onset hematemesis. In the emergency department, she was tachycardic and hypotensive.

Procedure
Acute upper gastrointestinal hemorrhage

Pre-procedure Imaging
Upper endoscopy demonstrated active bleeding from a duodenal ulcer. Despite the placement of a clip across the hemorrhaging vessel, the patient continued to bleed (Fig. 1).

Intraprocedural Findings
Selective angiogram of the gastroduodenal artery demonstrated active extravasation into the duodenum (Fig. 2). The gastroduodenal artery was embolized with coils (Fig. 3).

Follow-up and Complications
The patient's vital signs and hematocrit stabilized after the embolization, and she had no further evidence of bleeding (Fig. 4). However, after she was transferred to the floor, she developed an acute pulmonary embolus and was eventually discharged from the hospital for comfort care.

Suggested Readings
Defreyne L, Vanlangenhove P, De Vos M, et al: Embolization as a first approach with endoscopically unmanageable acute non-variceal gastrointestinal hemorrhage. Radiology 218:739-748, 2001.

Frisoli JK, Sze DY, Kee S: Transcatheter embolization for the treatment of upper gastrointestinal bleeding. Tech Vasc Intervent Radiol 7:136-142, 2005.

Lang EK: Transcatheter embolization in the management of hemorrhage from duodenal ulcer: Long-term results and complications. Radiology 182:703-707, 1992.

Schenker MP, Duszak R Jr, Soulen MC, et al: Upper gastrointestinal hemorrhage and transcatheter embolotherapy: Clinical and technical factors impacting on success and survival. J Vasc Intervent Radiol 12:1263-1271, 2001.

Case 108   217

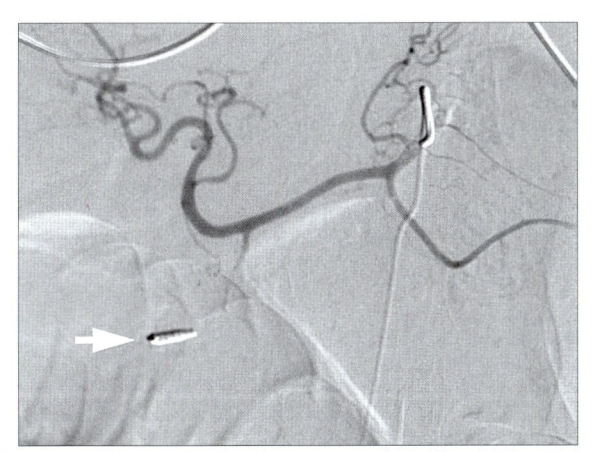

Figure 1. Celiac arteriogram demonstrates little flow in the gastroduodenal artery, and no active extravasation was seen. The clip was placed endoscopically *(arrow)*.

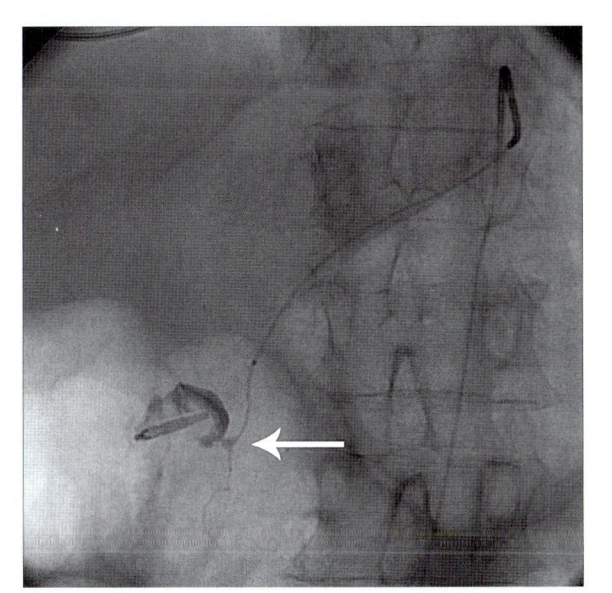

Figure 2. Selective injection of the gastroduodenal artery demonstrates a large amount of active extravasation *(arrow)* into the second portion of the duodenum.

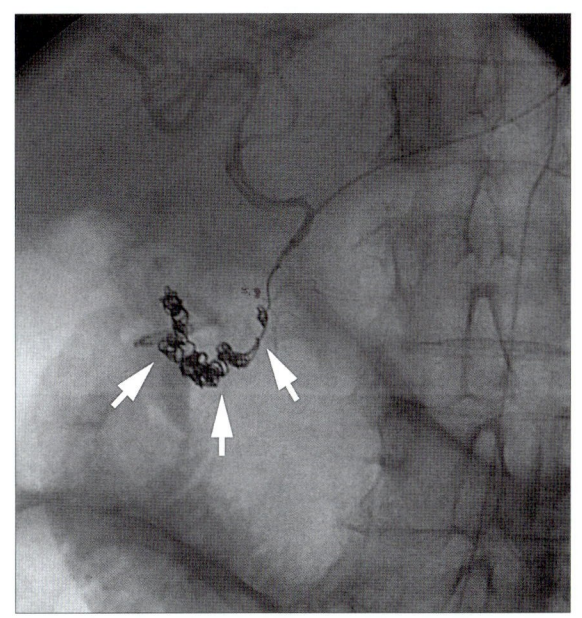

Figure 3. The point of extravasation and the gastroduodenal artery were embolized with coils *(arrows)*.

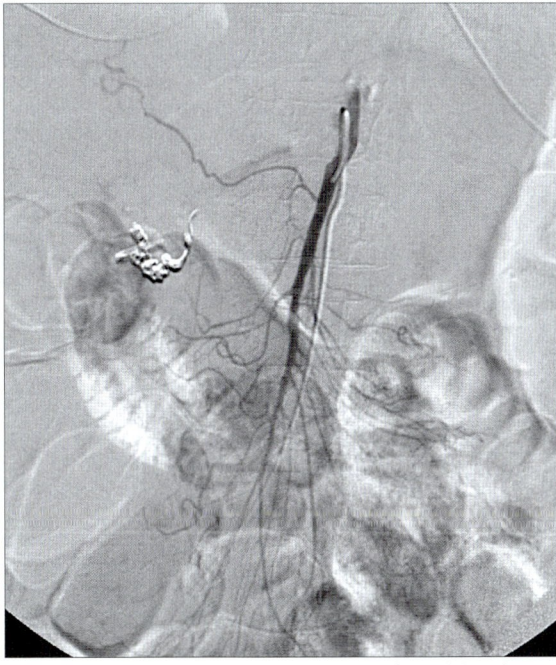

Figure 4. Superior mesenteric arteriogram confirmed that there was no further hemorrhage through the pancreatoduodenal arcade.

Case 109

DEMOGRAPHICS/CLINICAL HISTORY

A 71-year-old woman with melena, undergoing arteriography and nuclear medicine.

DISCUSSION

History/Indications for Procedure

For a 71-year-old woman with melena, upper and lower endoscopy and capsule endoscopy failed to identify a source of hemorrhage.

Procedure

Management of gastrointestinal hemorrhage

Pre-procedure Imaging

The initial superior mesenteric arteriogram was normal, and intra-arterial tissue plasminogen activator (tPA) and intravenous heparin were administered. A nuclear medicine scan of tagged red blood cells shows radiotracer accumulation in the left upper quadrant (Fig. 1).

Intraprocedural Findings

A celiac arteriogram shows active extravasation from a branch of the left gastric artery (Fig. 2). The left gastric artery was selectively catheterized with a 3-French microcatheter and embolized with 355-μm to 500-μm polyvinyl alcohol (PVA) microspheres (Fig. 3).

Follow-up and Complications

The patient's hemoglobin levels remained stable after the procedure, and the melena resolved. The patient has not returned during the 5 years since the procedure for recurrent gastrointestinal bleeding.

Suggested Readings

Johnston C, Tuite D, Pritchard R, et al: Use of provocative angiography to localize site in recurrent gastrointestinal bleeding. Cardiovasc Intervent Radiol 30:1042-1046, 2007.

Malden ES, Hicks ME, Royal HD, et al: Recurrent gastrointestinal bleeding: Use of thrombolysis with anticoagulation in diagnosis. Radiology 207:147-151, 1998.

Ryan JM, Key SM, Dumbleton SA, Smith TP: Nonlocalized lower gastrointestinal bleeding: Provocative bleeding studies with intraarterial tPA, heparin, and tolazoline. J Vasc Intervent Radiol 12:1273-1277, 2001.

Case 109 219

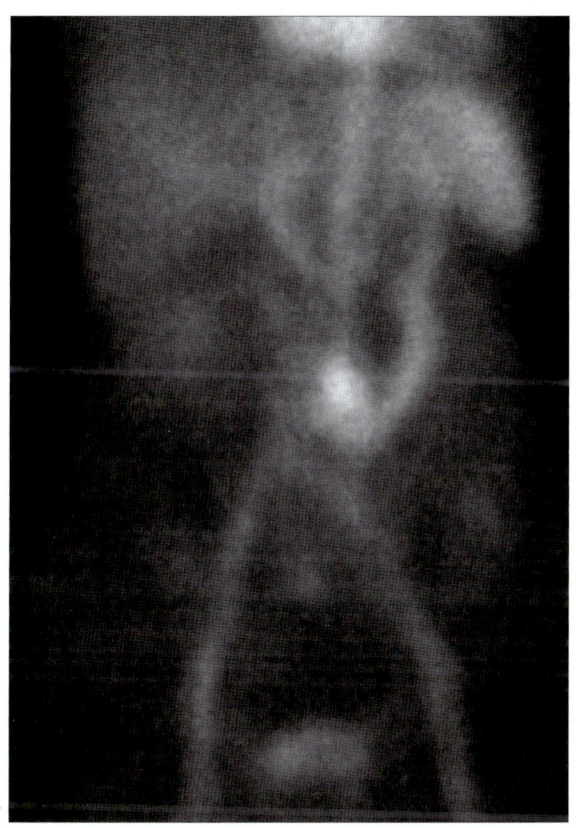

Figure 1. Nuclear medicine scan of tagged red blood cells shows radiotracer accumulation in the left upper quadrant and middle abdomen.

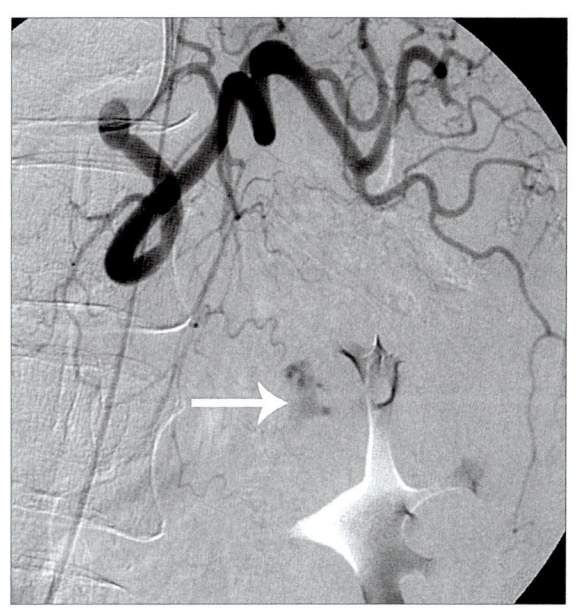

Figure 2. The celiac arteriogram shows active contrast extravasation from a small branch of the left gastric artery (arrow).

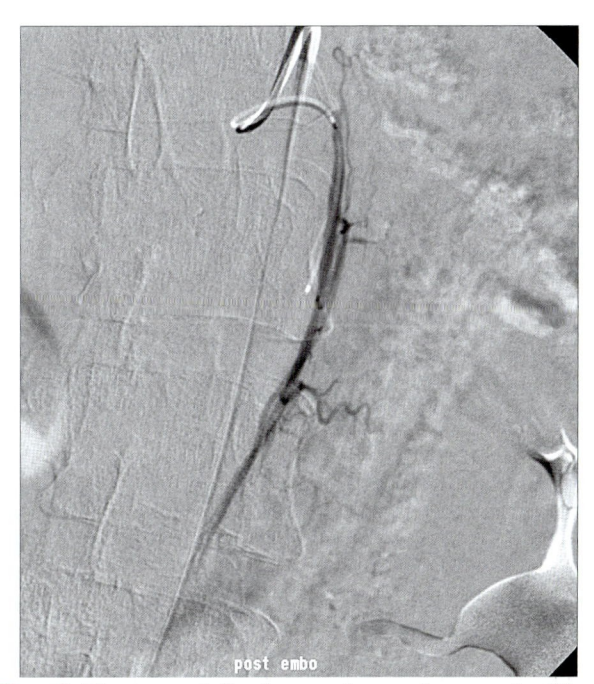

Figure 3. The post-embolization arteriogram shows stasis of flow in the left gastric artery, and contrast extravasation is no longer seen.

Case 110

DEMOGRAPHICS/CLINICAL HISTORY

A 56-year-old woman with hemobilia.

DISCUSSION

History/Indications for Procedure
A 56-year-old woman who became acutely hypotensive with pulsitile hemorrhage from the common bile duct during endoscopic removal of a biliary stent. The stent was placed during a recent open cholecystemomy at an outside hospital.

Procedure
Endovascular management for massive hemobilia secondary to hepatic artery pseudoaneurysm

Pre-procedure Imaging
Contrast-enhanced CT shows a complex, enhancing mass in the porta hepatis consistent with a large pseudoaneurysm (Fig. 1).

Intraprocedural Findings
There is a large pseudoaneurysm arising from an accessory right hepatic artery (Fig. 2). A 3-French microcatheter was advanced to the level of the pseudoaneurysm (Fig. 3), and the accessory right hepatic artery was embolized with coils (Fig. 4).

Follow-up and Complications
The hemorrhage stopped after the embolization. The patient's hemoglobin levels remained stable, and she was discharged from the hospital 5 days after the procedure.

Suggested Readings
Christensen T, Matsuoka L, Heestand G, et al: Iatrogenic pseudoaneurysms of the extrahepatic arterial vascularture: Management and outcome. HPB (Oxford) 8:458-464, 2006.

Okazaki M, Ono H, Higashihara H, et al: Angiographic management of massive hemobilia due to iatrogenic trauma. Gastrointest Radiol 16:205-304, 1991.

Strivastava DN, Sharma S, Pal S, et al: Transcatheter arterial embolization in the management of hemobilia. Abdom Imaging 31:439-448, 2006.

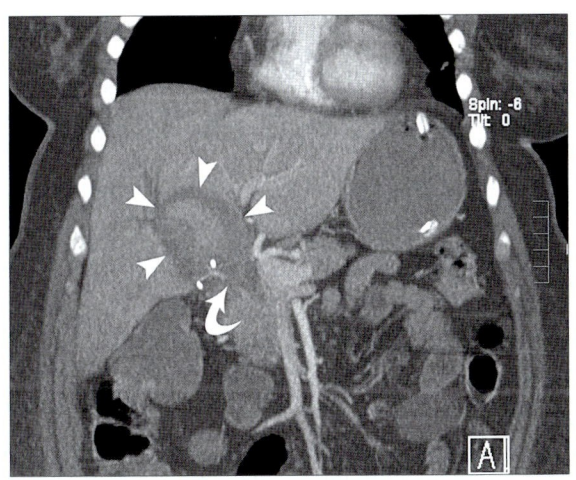

Figure 1. Contrast-enhanced CT of the abdomen, coronal reconstruction. There is a large, mixed-attenuation mass in the porta hepatis *(arrowheads)*, consistent with a pseudoaneurysm. The pseudoaneurysm is supplied by a small accessory hepatic artery *(curved arrow)* arising from the superior mesenteric artery.

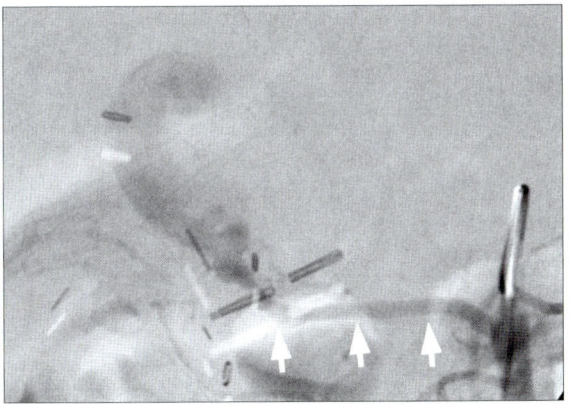

Figure 2. Superior mesenteric arteriogram shows opacification of the pseudoaneurysm that is supplied by an accessory hepatic artery *(arrows)*.

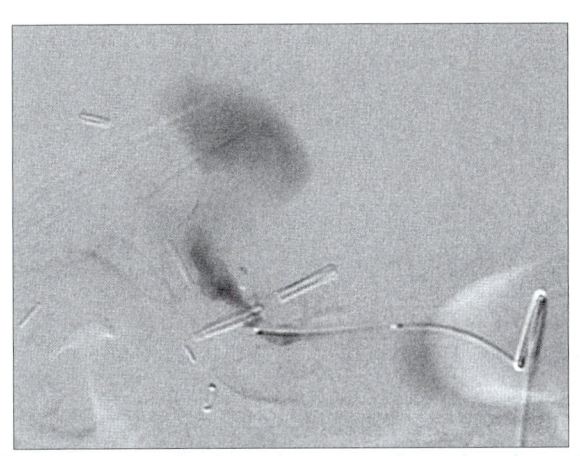

Figure 3. A 3-French microcatheter was advanced to the neck of the pseudoaneurysm.

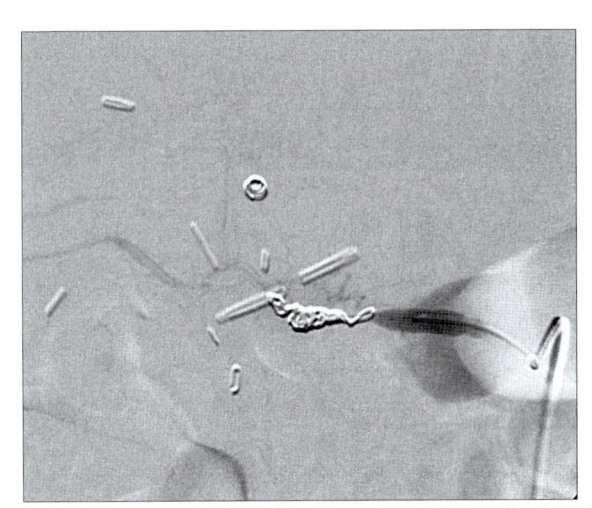

Figure 4. The accessory right hepatic artery was embolized with coils. There is no longer opacification of the pseudoaneurysm.

Case 111

DEMOGRAPHICS/CLINICAL HISTORY

A 48-year-old man with recurrent lower gastrointestinal bleeding, undergoing nuclear medicine scan, embolization, and angiography.

DISCUSSION

History/Indications for Procedure
A 48-year-old man has recurrent lower gastrointestinal bleeding. The patient has bright red blood per rectum and is diaphoretic and tachycardic in the emergency department.

Procedure
Lower gastrointestinal bleeding

Pre-procedure Imaging
Nuclear medicine ^{99m}Tc-tagged red blood cell scan demonstrated active hemorrhage in the ascending colon.

Intraprocedural Findings
The result of the initial selective superior mesenteric injection was negative (Fig. 1). Intra-arterial tissue plasminogen activator (tPA, 4 mg) was given, and the site of hemorrhage was identified and embolized with a microcoil (Figs. 2 to 4).

Follow-up and Complications
The patient's blood pressure stabilized immediately after embolization, his hemoglobin level remained stable, and there was no further evidence of bleeding. He was discharged from the hospital 2 days after admission.

Suggested Readings

Bandi R, Shetty PC, Sharma RP, et al: Superselective arterial embolization for the treatment of lower gastrointestinal hemorrhage. J Vasc Intervent Radiol 12:1399-1405, 2001.

Evangelista PT, Hallisey MJ: Transcatheter embolization for acute lower gastrointestinal hemorrhage. J Vasc Intervent Radiol 11: 601-606, 2000.

Funaki B, Kostelic JK, Lorenz J, et al: Superselective microcoil embolization of colonic hemorrhage. AJR Am J Roentgenol 177:829-836, 2001.

Ryan JM, Key SM, Dumbleton SA, Smith TP: Nonlocalized lower gastrointestinal bleeding: Provocative bleeding studies with intra-arterial tPA, heparin, and tolazoline. J Vasc Intervent Radiol 12: 1273-1277, 2001.

Case 111   223

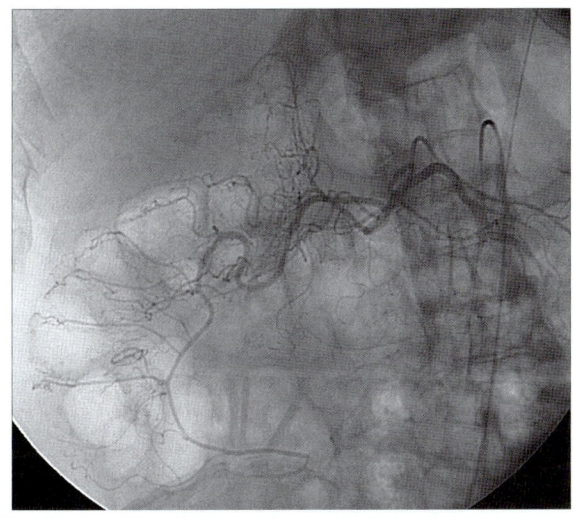

Figure 1. Unsubtracted image from selective superior mesenteric artery injection. There is no active extravasation.

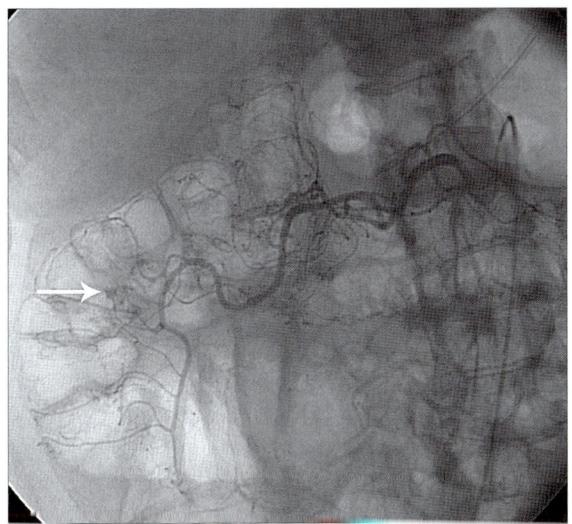

Figure 2. Repeat superior mesenteric artery arteriogram 18 minutes after the intra-arterial administration of 4 mg of tPA demonstrates active extravasation into the bowel lumen near the hepatic flexure (*arrow*).

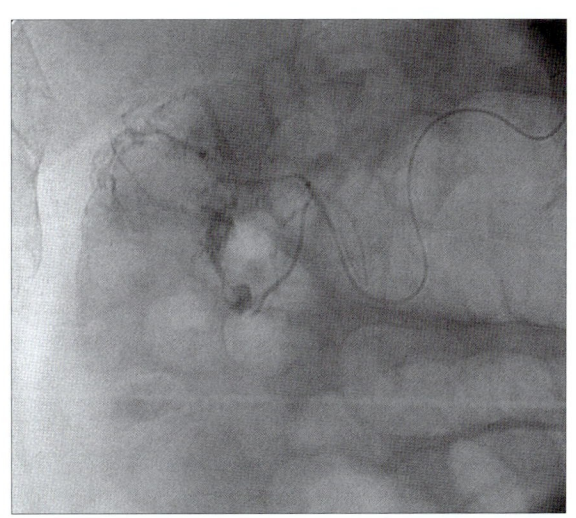

Figure 3. A microcatheter was used to selectively catheterize the middle colic artery and was advanced as close to the site of extravasation as possible.

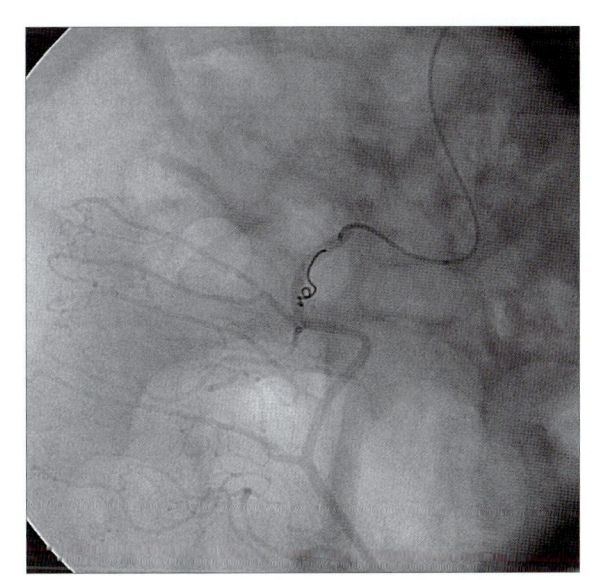

Figure 4. A vasa recta branch was embolized with a single 0.018-inch coil. No further extravasation was seen on the follow-up angiogram.

Case 112

DEMOGRAPHICS/CLINICAL HISTORY

An 85-year-old man with a history of atrial fibrillation presents with acute lower gastrointestinal hemorrhage.

DISCUSSION

History/Indications for Procedure
An 85-year-old man with a history of atrial fibrillation presents with hematochezia and hypotension.

Procedure
Superselective embolization for acute lower gastrointestinal hemorrhage

Pre-procedure Imaging
Nuclear medicine tagged red blood cell scan shows radiotracer accumulation in the right upper quadrant consistent with active lower gastrointestinal bleed originating from the ascending colon (Fig. 1).

Intraprocedural Findings
There is a focus of contrast extravasation within the lumen of the mid-ascending colon (Figs. 2 and 3). The offending vasa recta branch was selectively catheterized and embolized with a single 2-mm × 3-mm coil (Fig. 4).

Follow-up and Complications
The patient's blood pressure normalized at the completion of the procedure. He had no further episodes of bleeding; colonoscopy was performed 2 days later, confirming diverticulosis as the etiology of the bleeding.

Suggested Readings
Darcy M: Treatment of lower gastrointestinal bleeding: Vasopressin infusion versus embolization. J Vasc Intervent Radiol 14:535-543, 2003.

Funaki B, Kostelic JK, Lorenz J, et al: Superselective microcoil embolization of colonic hemorrhage. AJR Am J Roentgenol 177: 829-836, 2001.

Kuo WT, Lee DE, Saad WE, et al: Superselective microcoil embolization for the treatment of lower gastrointestinal hemorrhage. J Vasc Intervent Radiol 14:1503-1509, 2003.

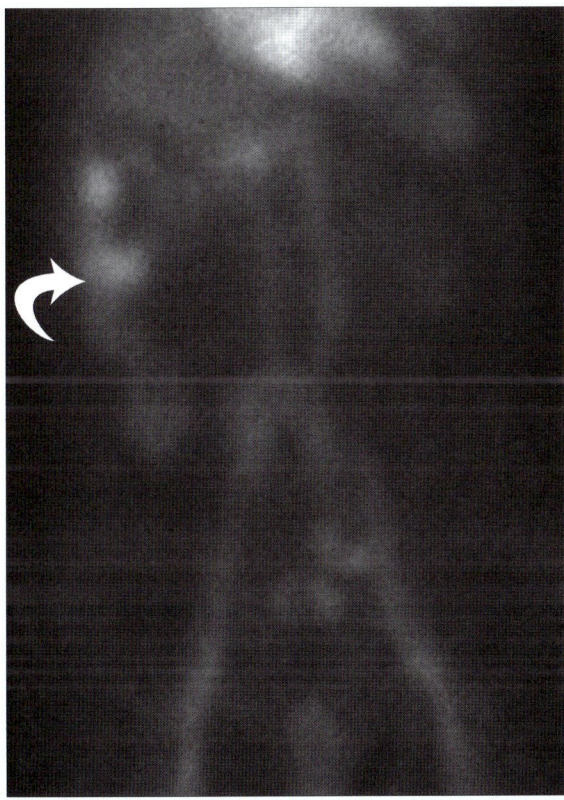

Figure 1. Single image from nuclear medicine tagged red blood cell scan shows radiotracer accumulation in the right upper quadrant *(curved arrow)*. This corresponds to a site of active hemorrhage in the ascending colon.

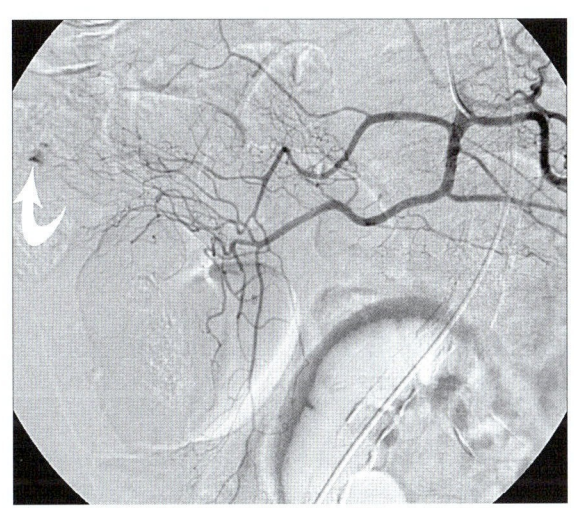

Figure 3. Single image from superior mesenteric arteriogram. The catheter has been advanced to the origin of the right colic artery. Contrast extravasation is again seen in the mid-ascending colon *(curved arrow)*.

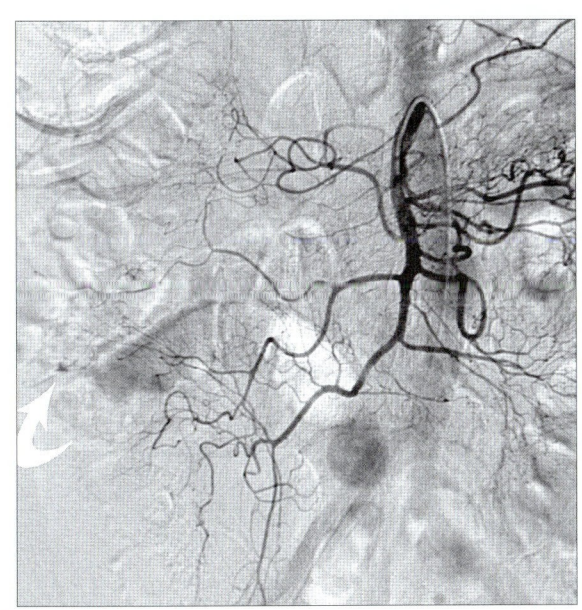

Figure 2. Single image from superior mesenteric arteriogram, arterial phase, shows a focus of contrast extravasation in the mid-ascending colon *(curved arrow)*.

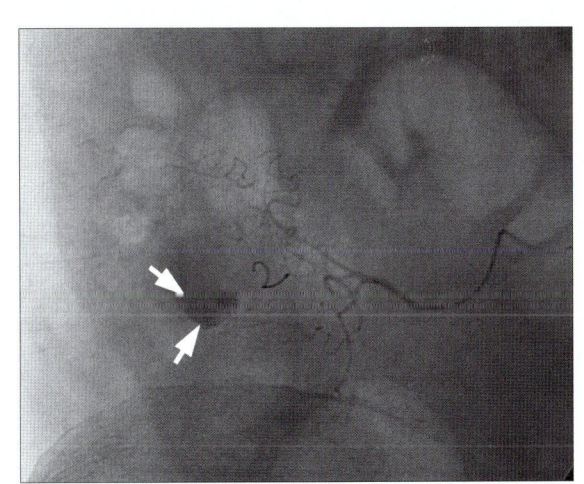

Figure 4. Follow-up unsubtracted image after coil embolization shows no further extravasation. There is accumulation of contrast in the bowel lumen *(arrows)* from earlier contrast injections.

Case 113

DEMOGRAPHICS/CLINICAL HISTORY

A 57-year-old man with recurrent lower gastrointestinal hemorrhage, undergoing nuclear medicine imaging and angiography.

DISCUSSION

History/Indications for Procedure

A 57-year-old man has a history of diverticulosis and new, bright red blood per rectum. The patient has undergone prior right colectomy for a cecal polyp.

Procedure

Endovascular management of lower gastrointestinal hemorrhage

Pre-procedure Imaging

Nuclear medicine tagged red blood cell bleeding study of the gastrointestinal tract shows radiotracer accumulation in the right upper quadrant corresponding to the hepatic flexure and proximal transverse colon (Fig. 1).

Intraprocedural Findings

Contrast extravasation into the bowel lumen was identified and found to arise from a straight artery (i.e., arteriae rectae) of the hepatic flexure of the colon (Figs. 2 and 3). The offending artery was embolized with two 0.018-inch, 5-mm straight coils (Fig. 4).

Follow-up and Complications

The patient had no further evidence of hemorrhage. The day after embolization, the patient developed abdominal pain, and colonoscopy showed a focal area of ischemic colitis. He was managed conservatively, and no further intervention was required.

Suggested Readings

Bandi R, Shetty PC, Sharma RP, et al: Superselective arterial embolization for the treatment of lower gastrointestinal hemorrhage. J Vasc Intervent Radiol 12:1399-1405, 2001.

Darcy M: Treatment of lower gastrointestinal bleeding: Vasopressin versus embolization. J Vasc Intervent Radiol 14:535-543, 2003.

Tew K, Davies RP, Jadun CK, Kew J: MDCT of acute lower gastrointestinal bleeding. AJR AM J Roentgenol 182:427-430, 2004.

Zuckerman DA, Bocchini TP, Birnbaum EH: Massive hemorrhage in the lower gastrointestinal tract in adults: Diagnostic imaging and intervention. AJR Am J Roentgenol 161:703-711, 1993.

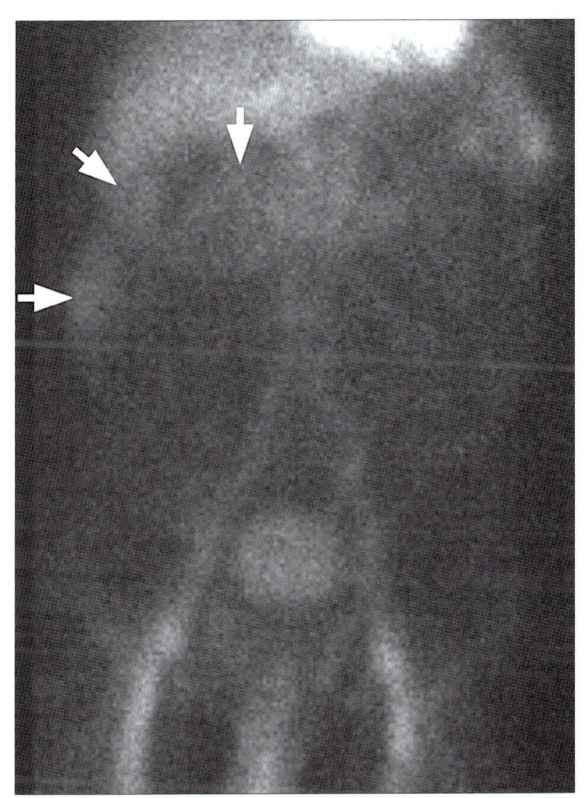

Figure 1. Single image from nuclear medicine tagged red blood cell bleeding scan shows radiotracer accumulation in the hepatic flexure and proximal transverse colon (arrows).

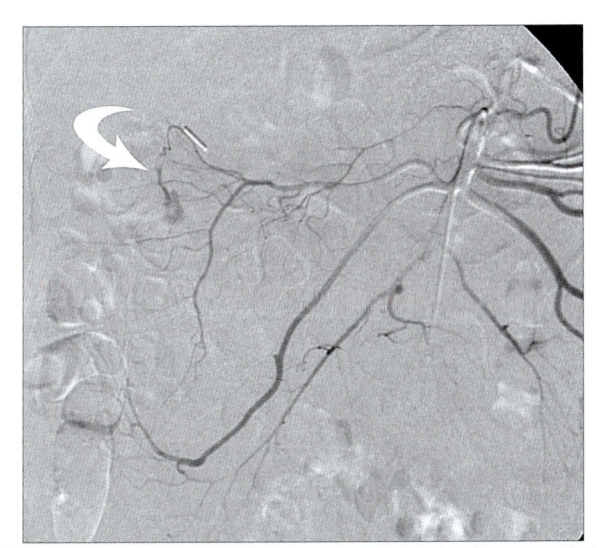

Figure 2. There is a focus of contrast extravasation from a straight artery off the marginal artery and bleeding into the hepatic flexure (arrow).

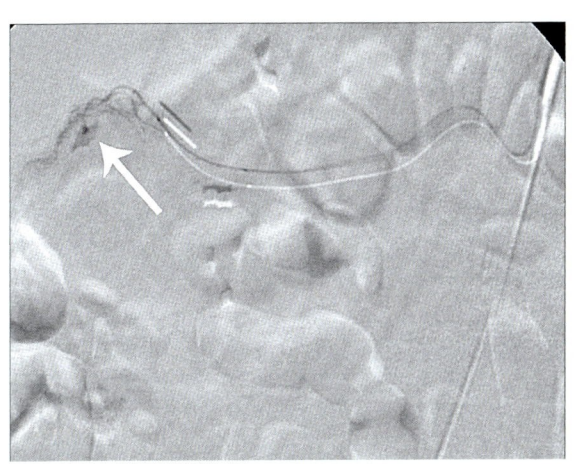

Figure 3. The straight artery was selectively catheterized with a 2.3-French microcatheter. The contrast extravasation is confirmed on this superselective injection (arrow).

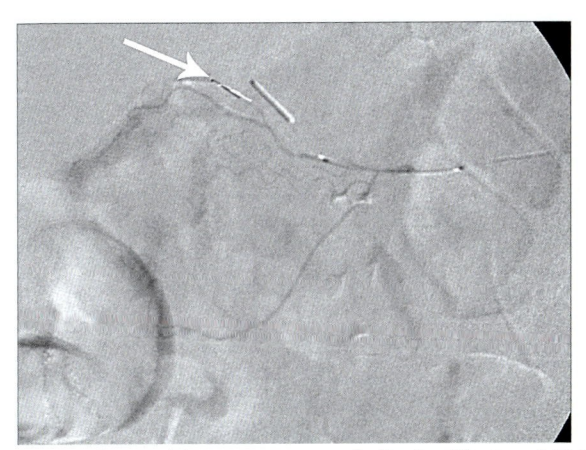

Figure 4. The straight artery was embolized with two 0.018-inch straight coils (arrow). No further bleeding was seen on the postembolization angiogram.

Case 114

DEMOGRAPHICS/CLINICAL HISTORY

A 74-year-old woman with bright red blood per rectum, undergoing angiography.

DISCUSSION

History/Indications for Procedure
A 74-year-old woman had bright red blood per rectum. After admission into the hospital, the patient continued to have bright red blood per rectum requiring multiple transfusions; a colonoscopy revealed colonic diverticulosis but no active hemorrhage.

Procedure
Management of acute lower gastrointestinal hemorrhage

Pre-procedure Imaging
On the second hospital day, a nuclear medicine radiotracer-tagged red blood cell bleeding study of the gastrointestinal tract revealed radiotracer accumulation in the right lower quadrant, suggesting active hemorrhage in the region of the cecum or ascending colon.

Intraprocedural Findings
Superior mesenteric angiogram identified a focus of contrast extravasation within the middle of the ascending colon (Figs. 1 and 2). A straight artery (i.e., arteriae rectae) off the marginal artery was selectively catheterized with a 2.3-French microcatheter (Fig. 3), and the bleeding vessel was embolized with two 0.018-inch straight coils (Fig. 4).

Follow-up and Complications
The patient had no further evidence of gastrointestinal hemorrhage after the embolization and was discharged to home 1 week later. Her hospital course was complicated by a non-ST-elevation myocardial infarction, which was diagnosed at the time of admission.

Suggested Readings

Bandi R, Shetty PC, Sharma RP, et al: Superselective arterial embolization for the treatment of lower gastrointestinal hemorrhage. J Vasc Intervent Radiol 12:1399-1405, 2001.

Kuo WT, Lee DE, Saad WE, et al: Superselective microcoil embolization for the treatment of lower gastrointestinal hemorrhage. J Vasc Intervent Radiol 14:1503-1509, 2003.

Evangelista PT, Hallisey MJ: Transcatheter embolization for acute lower gastrointestinal hemorrhage. J Vasc Intervent Radiol 11:601-606, 2000.

Millward SF: ACR appropriateness criteria on treatment of acute non-variceal gastrointestinal tract bleeding. J Am Coll Radiol 5:550-554, 2008.

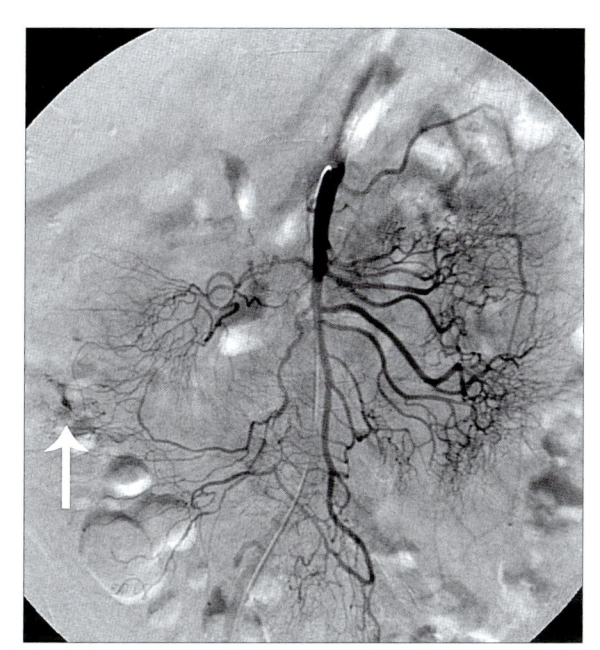

Figure 1. Selective superior mesenteric arteriogram shows a focus of active contrast extravasation in the middle of the ascending colon (arrow).

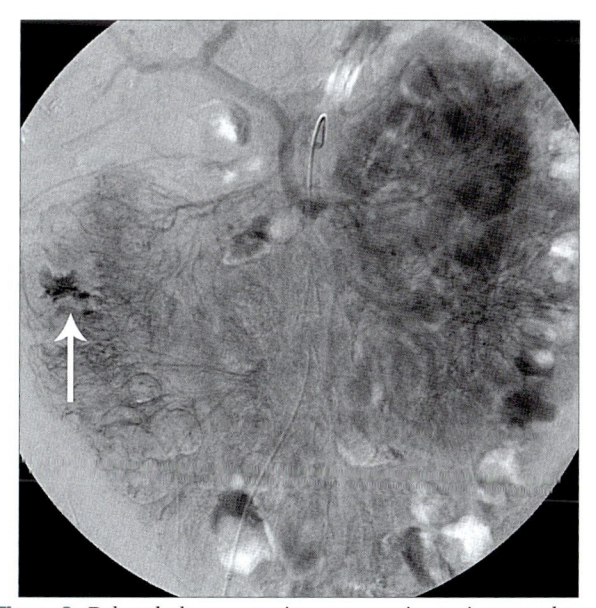

Figure 2. Delayed-phase superior mesenteric angiogram shows pooling of contrast in the lumen of the ascending colon (arrow).

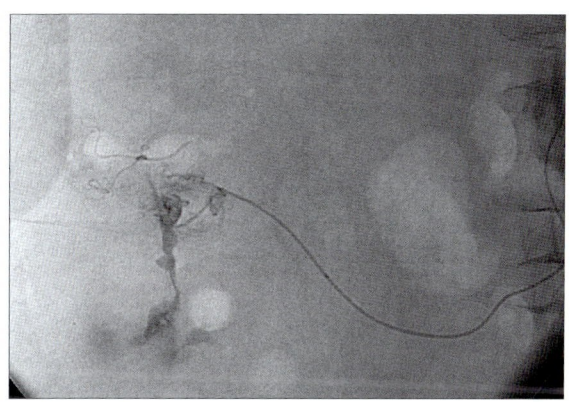

Figure 3. A 2.3-French microcatheter has been used to selectively catheterize a straight artery off the marginal artery. There is brisk extravasation into the bowel lumen.

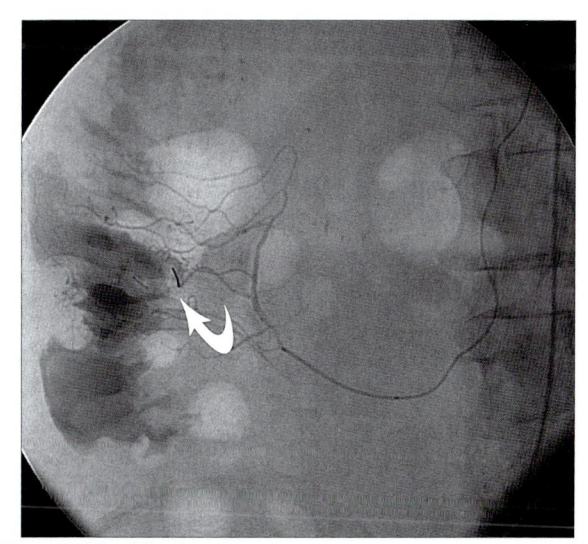

Figure 4. The bleeding straight artery was embolized with two 0.018-inch straight coils (arrow).

Case 115

DEMOGRAPHICS/CLINICAL HISTORY

A 68-year-old woman with an acute lower gastrointestinal bleed.

DISCUSSION

History/Indications for Procedure
A 68-year-old woman with multiple medical problems was admitted to the hospital for management of a nonhealing foot ulcer. While in the hospital, she developed an acute lower gastrointestinal bleed.

Procedure
Superselective embolization for lower gastrointestinal hemorrhage

Pre-procedure Imaging
Nuclear medicine tagged red blood cell scan shows radiotracer accumulation in the right lower quadrant, consistent with active hemorrhage in the region of the cecum (Fig. 1).

Intraprocedural Findings
There is a small focus of contrast extravasation in the cecum (Fig. 2). A 3-French microcatheter was advanced to the vasa recta of the cecum (Fig. 3), as close to the site of hemorrhage as possible, and vasa recta branch was embolized with coils (Fig. 4).

Follow-up and Complications
The bleeding immediately stopped after the embolization, and the patient has had no recurrence of bleeding.

Suggested Readings
Bandi R, Shetty PC, Sharma RP, et al. Superselective arterial embolization for the treatment of lower gastrointestinal hemorrhage. J Vasc Intervent Radiol 12:1399-1405, 2001.

Kickuth R, Rattunde H, Gschossmann J, et al. Acute lower gastrointestinal hemorrhage: Minimally invasive management with microcatheter embolization. J Vasc Intervent Radiol 19:1289-1296, 2008.

Kuo WT, Lee DE, Saad WE, et al: Superselective microcoil embolization for the treatment of lower gastrointestinal hemorrhage. J Vasc Intervent Radiol 14:1503-1509, 2003.

Case 115   231

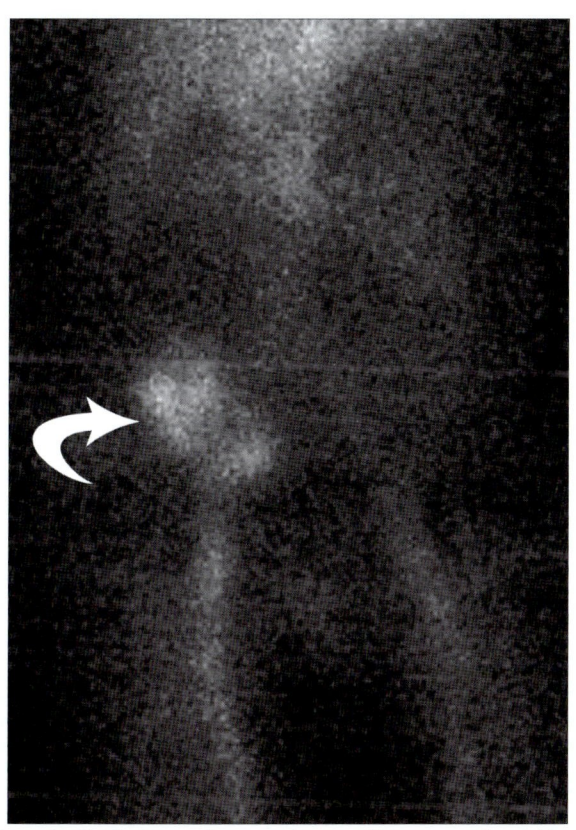

Figure 1. Single image from nuclear medicine tagged red blood cell scan shows radiotracer accumulation in the right lower quadrant (curved arrow).

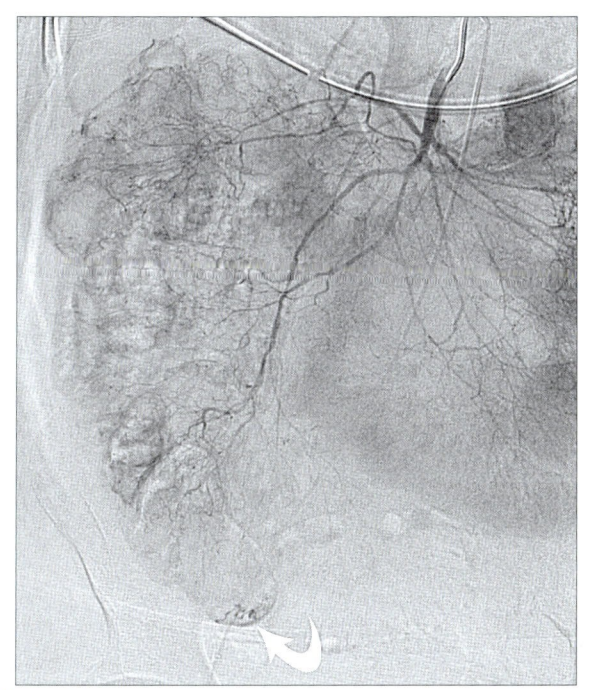

Figure 2. Superior mesenteric arteriogram shows abnormal contrast accumulation in the tip of the cecum (curved arrow).

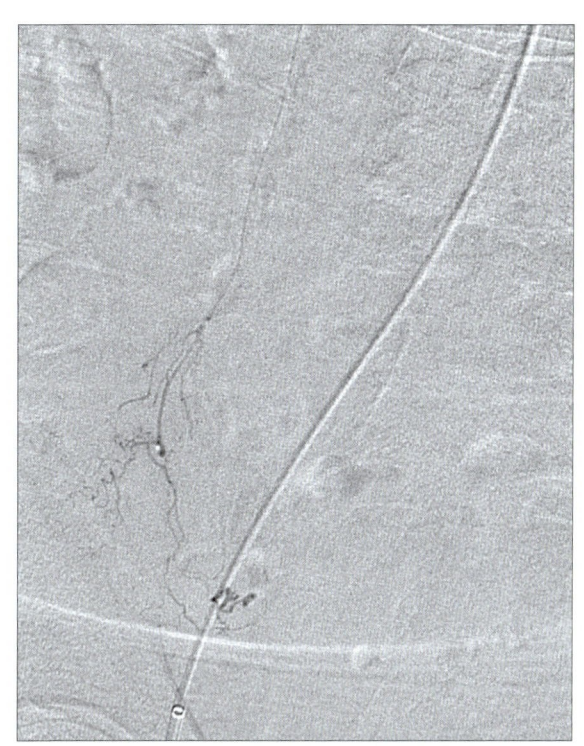

Figure 3. The microcatheter was advanced to the origin of the offending vessel. The catheter could not be advanced closer to the site of hemorrhage because of the acute angle of the origin of the vessel and the small size of the artery.

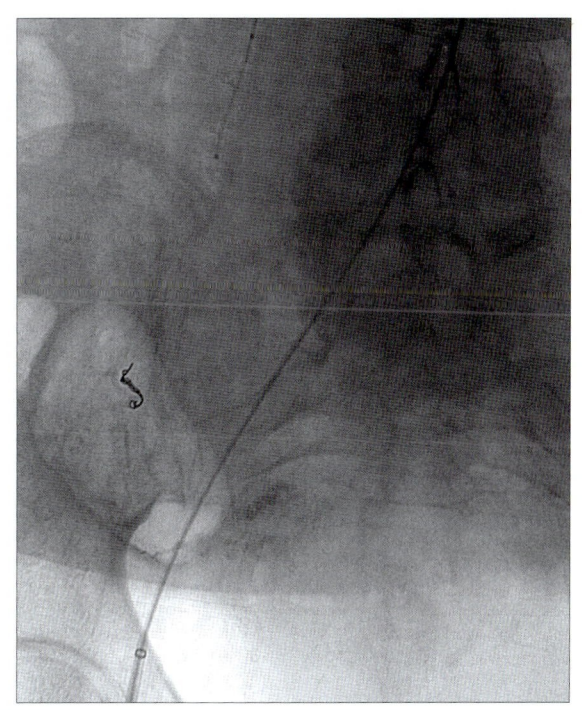

Figure 4. The origin of the vasa recta branch was embolized with coils. No further extravasation was seen on follow-up contrast injection.

Case 116

DEMOGRAPHICS/CLINICAL HISTORY

A 27-year-old man with a high-flow arteriovenous malformation (AVM) on the right forearm, undergoing arteriography.

DISCUSSION

History/Indications for Procedure
The AVM on the right forearm of this patient has been palpable for approximately 6 years. The mass has been enlarging, and the patient has been experiencing increasing pain over the past several months.

Procedure
Embolization of forearm arteriovenous malformation

Pre-procedure Imaging
MRI showed a high-flow vascular malformation in the superficial soft tissues of the dorsal right forearm (not shown). The lesion involved several extensor muscle bellies and the posterior interosseous nerve.

Intraprocedural Findings
An arteriogram shows the AVM to be supplied by branches of the radial and the ulnar arteries (Fig. 1). The lesion was nearly completely embolized with n-butyl cyanoacrylate (Trufil; Cordis, Miami Lakes, FL) (Figs. 2-4).

Follow-up and Complications
Three days after embolization, the patient underwent surgical resection. The lesion was completely resected; there is no evidence of recurrence 3 years after resection.

Suggested Readings
Osuga K, Hori S, Kitayoshi H, et al: Embolization of high flow arteriovenous malformations: Experience with use of superabsorbent polymer microspheres. J Vasc Intervent Radiol 13:1125-1133, 2002.

White RI Jr, Pollak J, Persing J, et al: Long-term outcome of embolotherapy and surgery for high-flow extremity arteriovenous malformations. J Vasc Intervent Radiol 11:1285-1295, 2000.

Yakes WF, Haas DK, Parker SH, et al: Symptomatic vascular malformations: Ethanol embolotherapy. Radiology 170:1059-1066, 1989.

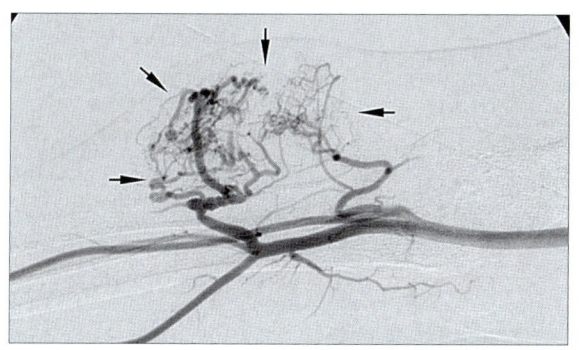

Figure 1. Right upper extremity arteriogram shows a high-flow AVM on the dorsum of the right forearm. The nidus of the AVM *(arrows)* is supplied by branches of the radial and ulnar arteries.

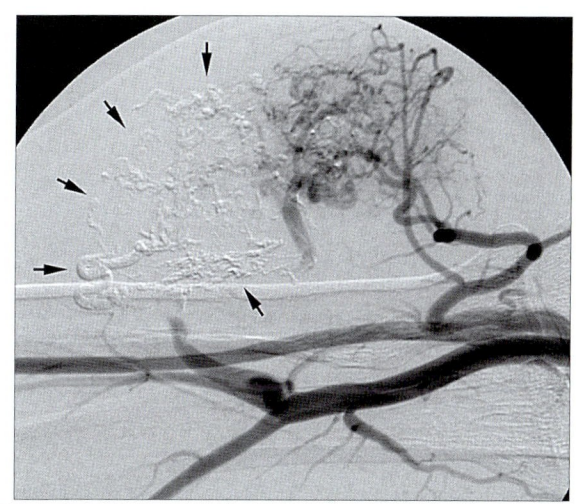

Figure 3. Follow-up arteriogram during embolization shows occlusion of approximately 50% of the AVM with n-butyl cyanoacrylate *(arrows)*.

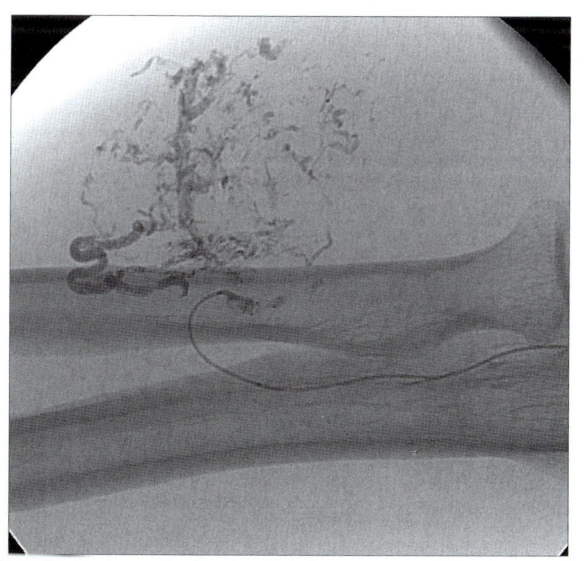

Figure 2. During embolization, it is important to occlude the nidus of the malformation. In this case, n-butyl cyanoacrylate was the embolic agent used to occlude the nidus of the AVM.

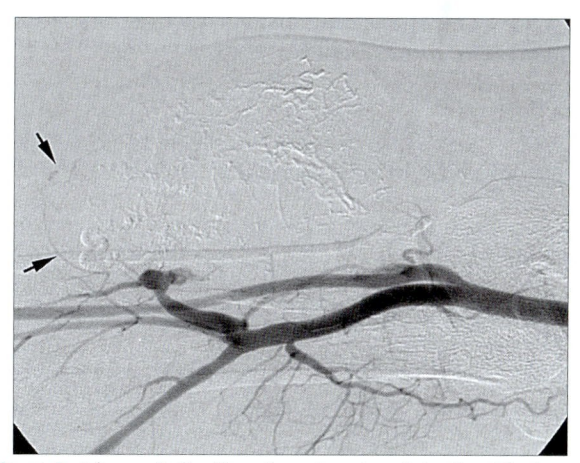

Figure 4. After embolization, there is only minimal residual arterial supply to the lesion *(arrows)*. The patient went on to surgical resection 3 days after the embolization procedure.

Case 117

DEMOGRAPHICS/CLINICAL HISTORY

A 35-year-old man with a large right shoulder AVM, undergoing MRI and angiography.

DISCUSSION

History/Indications for Procedure
This patient has had a large right shoulder AVM since childhood. The malformation began to enlarge 5 to 6 years before presentation and causes occasional symptoms of shoulder swelling and pain (Fig. 1).

Procedure
Management of large, high-flow shoulder arteriovenous malformation (AVM)

Pre-procedure Imaging
Contrast-enhanced MRI shows a large vascular malformation throughout the subcutaneous tissues and deltoid musculature of the right shoulder (Fig. 2). Prominent flow voids and enlargement of the subclavian vein also are noted.

Intraprocedural Findings
A right upper extremity angiogram shows a large vascular malformation in the right shoulder with prominent arteriovenous shunting and dilation of the brachial and subclavian veins (Fig. 3). The lesion was partially embolized with n-butyl cyanoacrylate (Fig. 4).

Follow-up and Complications
The patient has undergone multiple embolization procedures, and has not yet developed any complications related to the embolizations. The lesion has decreased in size, and the symptoms have been controlled.

Suggested Readings
Osuga K, Hori S, Kitayoshi H, et al: Embolization of high flow arteriovenous malformations: Experience with use of superabsorbent polymer microspheres. J Vasc Intervent Radiol 13:1125-1133, 2002.

White RI Jr, Pollak J, Persing J, et al: Long-term outcome of embolotherapy and surgery for high-flow extremity arteriovenous malformations. J Vasc Intervent Radiol 11:1285-1295, 2000.

Yakes WF, Haas DK, Parker SH, et al: Symptomatic vascular malformations: Ethanol embolotherapy. Radiology 170:1059-1066, 1989.

Case 117   235

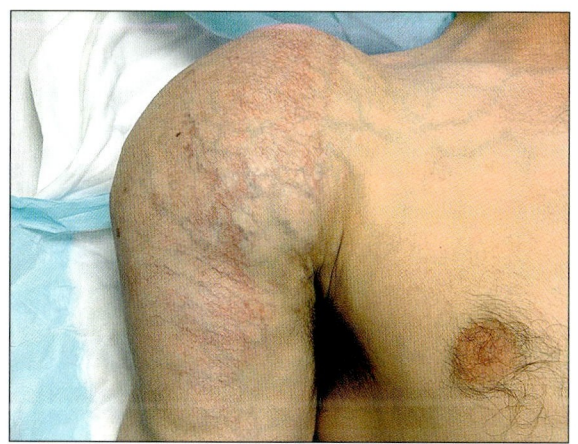

Figure 1. Photograph of the patient's shoulder shows enlargement, erythema, and multiple dilated veins.

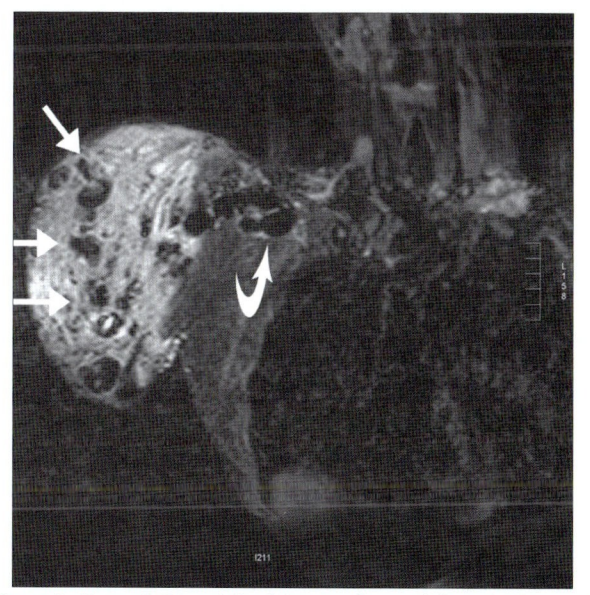

Figure 2. Coronal T2-weighted image shows diffuse high signal throughout the soft tissues and musculature of the right shoulder consistent with a large vascular malformation. There are prominent vessels within the malformation *(straight arrows)* and dilation of the draining axillary vein *(curved arrow)*.

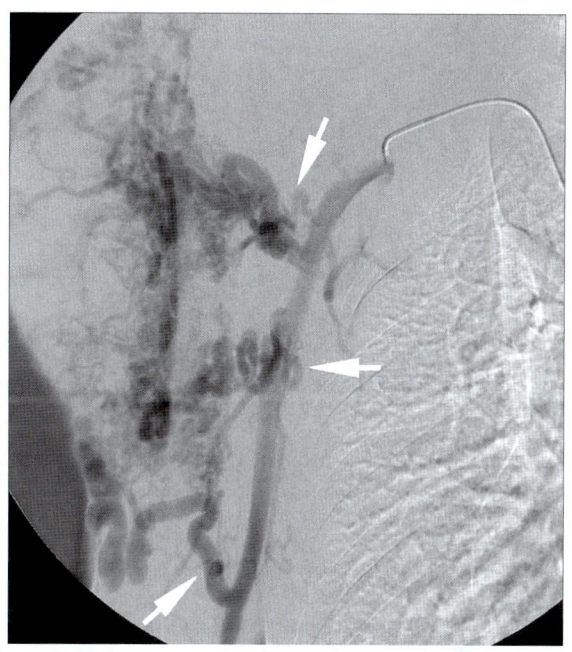

Figure 3. Right upper-extremity angiogram shows large right shoulder AVM. Arterial supply is from multiple branches of the axillary and brachial arteries, including hypertrophied circumflex humeral and deep brachial branches *(arrows)*.

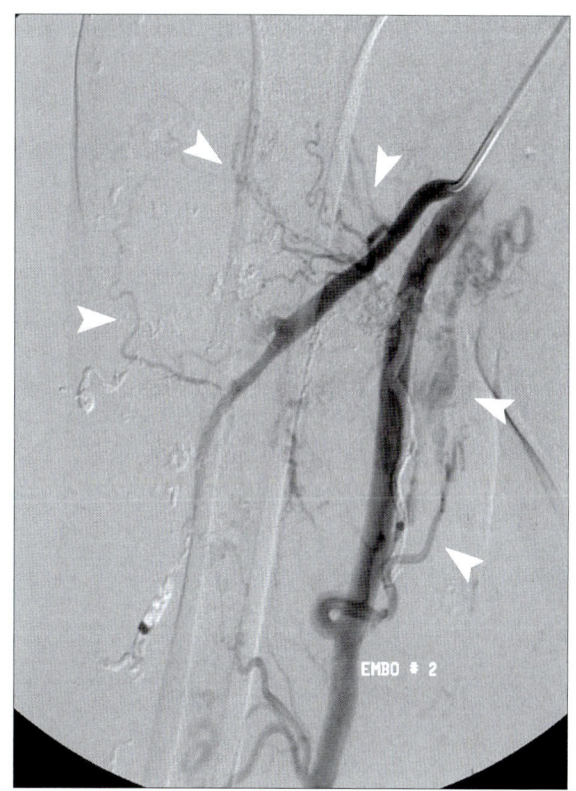

Figure 4. After embolization with n-butyl cyanoacrylate, there is marked reduction in flow with only small residual arterial feeders present *(arrowheads)*.

Case 118

DEMOGRAPHICS/CLINICAL HISTORY

A 36-year-old man with a large pelvic arteriovenous malformation (AVM).

DISCUSSION

History/Indications for Procedure
A 36-year-old man with large pelvic AVM. He is currently asymptomatic and has undergone a single prior embolization procedure at an outside hospital.

Procedure
Embolization of large pelvic arteriovenous malformation

Pre-procedure Imaging
Contrast-enhanced CT shows an extensive pelvic AVM with numerous large draining veins (not shown).

Intraprocedural Findings
There is an extremely large pelvic AVM supplied predominantly by a hypertrophied right internal iliac artery with some contribution from the left internal iliac artery (Figs. 1 and 2). Multiple branches within the nidus of the malformation were selectively catheterized with a microcatheter and embolized with n-butyl cyanoacrylate (Fig. 3).

Follow-up and Complications
The patient had no complications from the embolization procedure. He has returned for numerous additional embolization procedures in the 5 years since his initial presentation; despite these procedures, there continues to be some flow within the nidus (Fig. 4).

Suggested Readings
Osuga K, Hori S, Kitayoshi H, et al: Embolization of high flow arteriovenous malformations: Experience with use of superabsorbent polymer microspheres. J Vasc Intervent Radiol 13:1125-1133, 2002.

Tan KT, Simons ME, Rajan DK, Terbrugge K: Peripheral high-flow arteriovenous vascular malformations: A single-center experience. J Vasc Intervent Radiol 15:1071-1080, 2004.

White RI Jr, Pollak J, Persing J, et al: Long-term outcome of embolotherapy and surgery for high-flow extremity arteriovenous malformations. J Vasc Intervent Radio 11:1285-1295, 2000.

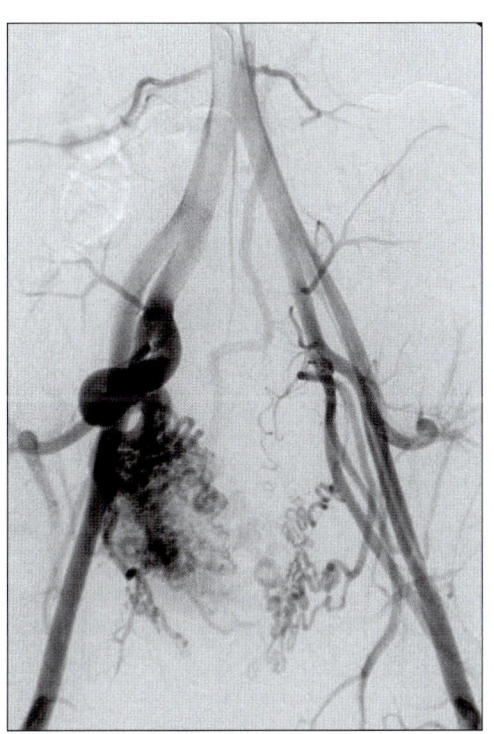

Figure 1. Pelvic arteriogram, arterial phase, shows marked hypertrophy of the right internal iliac artery. There are multiple enlarged feeders to the pelvic AVM from the internal iliac arteries bilaterally.

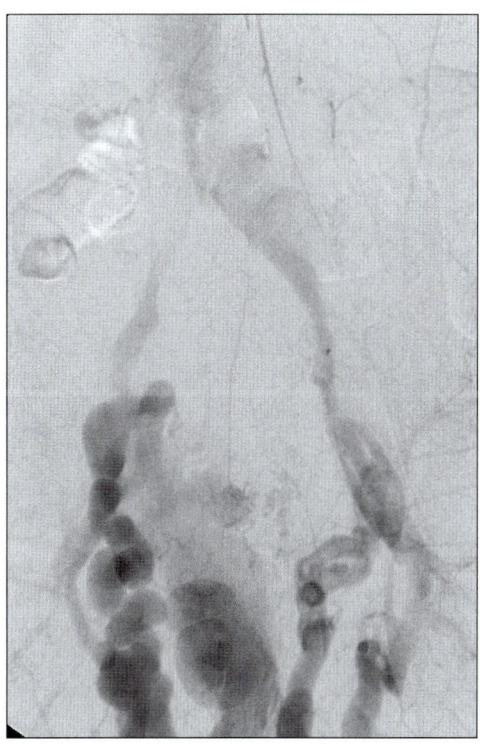

Figure 2. Pelvic arteriogram, venous phase, shows massively dilated pelvic veins.

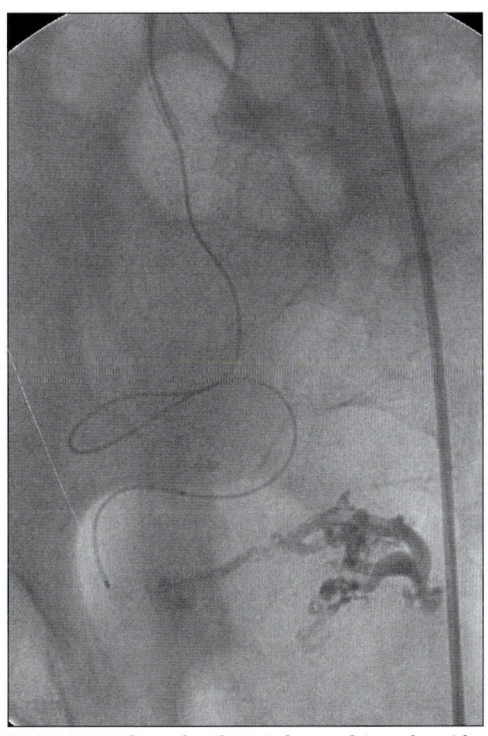

Figure 3. A microcatheter has been advanced into the nidus of the AVM. A cast of glue is occluding a portion of the nidus.

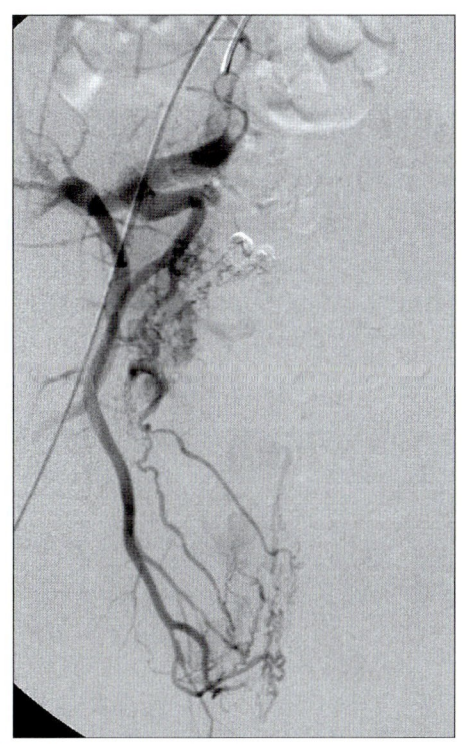

Figure 4. Follow-up arteriogram 3.5 years after the initial embolization shows significant reduction in arterial supply from the right internal iliac artery. There is continued abnormal vascularity along the lateral aspect of the malformation; repeat embolization was performed.

Case 119

DEMOGRAPHICS/CLINICAL HISTORY

A 37-year-old woman with a painful mass in the right hand, undergoing magnetic resonance imaging (MRI), arteriography, catheterization, and embolization.

DISCUSSION

History/Indications for Procedure
A 37-year-old woman has a painful mass of the right hand along the thenar eminence. The fingertips of the right hand are slightly cool and blue, with delayed capillary refill.

Procedure
Arteriovenous malformation in the hand

Pre-procedure Imaging
Contrast-enhanced MRI demonstrates a mass of the right hand that is located deep to the thenar muscles and extends to the superficial surface of the thenar eminence more medially (Fig. 1). The mass has increased T2-weighted signal with many internal flow voids, which is consistent with an arteriovenous malformation.

Intraprocedural Findings
Arteriogram of the right hand shows that the arteriovenous malformation is supplied from the distal radial artery (Fig. 2). A microcatheter was advanced into the nidus of the mass, and embolization was performed using n-butyl cyanoacrylate (Fig. 3).

Follow-up and Complications
The patient underwent two embolization procedures; after the second, she developed severe pain, likely due to inflammation and arterial steal (Fig. 4). She recovered uneventfully, and the malformation remained stable over the next 3 years.

Suggested Readings
Numan F, Omeroglu A, Kara B, et al: Embolization of peripheral vascular malformations with ethylene vinyl alcohol copolymer (Onyx). J Vasc Intervent Radiol 15:939-946, 2004.

Osuga K, Hori S, Kitayoshi H, et al: Embolization of high flow arteriovenous malformations: Experience with use of superabsorbent polymer microspheres. J Vasc Intervent Radiol 13:1125-1133, 2002.

White RI Jr, Pollak J, Persing J, et al: Long-term outcome of embolotherapy and surgery for high-flow extremity arteriovenous malformations. J Vasc Intervent Radiol 11:1285-1295, 2000.

Yakes WF, Haas DK, Parker SH, et al: Symptomatic vascular malformations: Ethanol embolotherapy. Radiology 170:1059-1066, 1989.

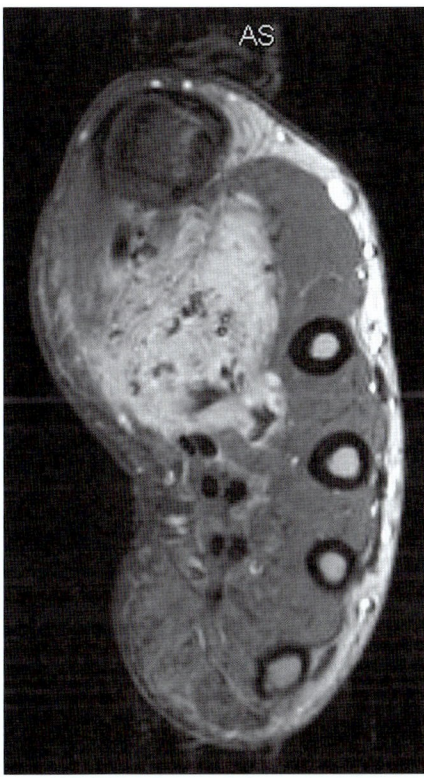

Figure 1. T2-weighted MR image of the hand demonstrates diffuse high signal intensity throughout the musculature of the lateral aspect of the right hand. The mass involves most of the thenar muscles.

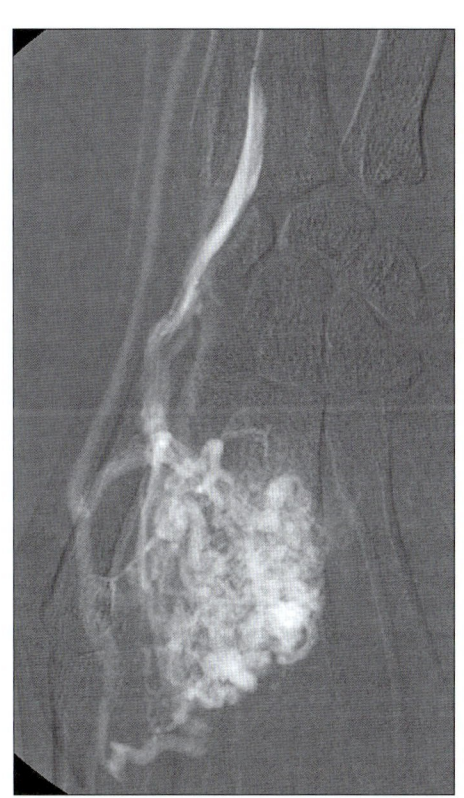

Figure 2. Arteriogram of the right upper extremity demonstrates a large arteriovenous malformation supplied by the distal radial artery.

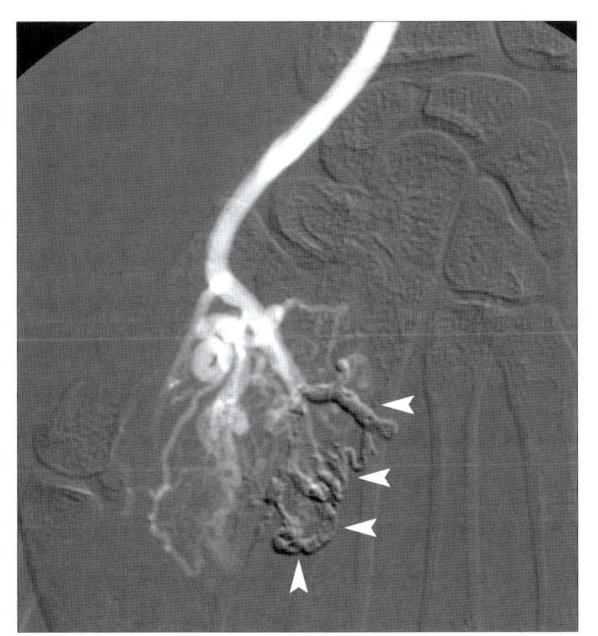

Figure 3. The lesion was embolized with *n*-butyl cyanoacrylate *(arrowheads)*. Because of the size of the lesion, embolization was staged, and the patient was brought back at a later date to complete the occlusion.

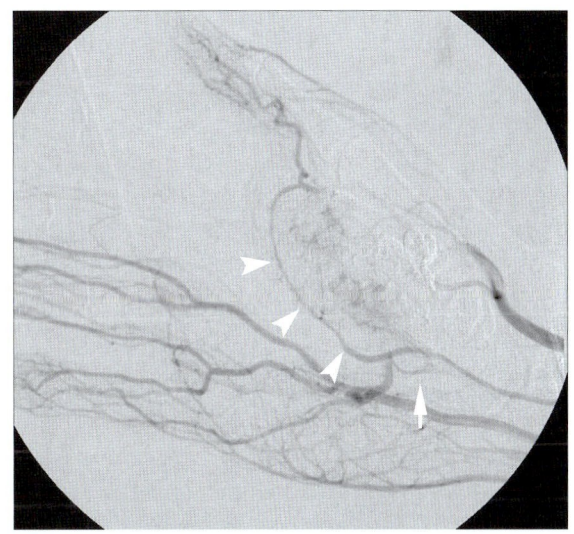

Figure 4. Soon after the second embolization procedure, the patient complained of severe pain. Angiogram of the right upper extremity demonstrates recruitment of blood supply from the ulnar artery *(arrow)* and interosseus artery *(arrowheads)*. Notice the lack of perfusion to the index and middle fingers.

Case 120

DEMOGRAPHICS/CLINICAL HISTORY

A 22-year-old woman with recurrent arteriovenous malformation (AVM) of the right foot, undergoing arteriography and magnetic resonance imaging (MRI).

DISCUSSION

History/Indications for Procedure
A 22-year-old woman has a long-standing AVM on the plantar surface of her right foot. She has undergone two previous surgical resections, with recurrence, and she now presents with pain and discomfort.

Procedure
Direct puncture embolization of arteriovenous malformation of the foot

Pre-procedure Imaging
Right lower-extremity arteriogram shows the AVM to be supplied by multiple feeding vessels, including the dorsalis pedis artery and the medial and lateral plantar arteries (Fig. 1).

Intraprocedural Findings
The malformation was punctured directly with ultrasound guidance (Fig. 1), and contrast injection shows reflux into the feeding arteries. The nidus of the malformation was embolized with n-butyl cyanoacrylate (Fig. 2).

Follow-up and Complications
The patient underwent three embolization sessions for complete AVM treatment (Figs. 3 and 4). The patient's symptoms were controlled for 3 years, at which time she developed recurrent pain; MRI showed persistent enhancing soft tissue along the plantar surface of the foot, but no abnormal vessels could be identified with ultrasound. The patient responded to treatment for plantar fasciitis.

Suggested Readings
Tan KT, Simons ME, Rajan DK, Terbrugge K: Peripheral high-flow arteriovenous vascular malformations: A single-center experience. J Vasc Intervent Radiol 15:1071-1080, 2004.

White RI Jr, Pollak J, Persing J, et al: Long-term outcome of embolotherapy and surgery for high-flow extremity arteriovenous malformations. J Vasc Intervent Radiol 11:1285-1295, 2000.

Yakes WF, Rossi P, Odink H: How I do it. Arteriovenous malformation management. Cardiovasc Intervent Radiol 19:65-71, 1996.

Case 120   241

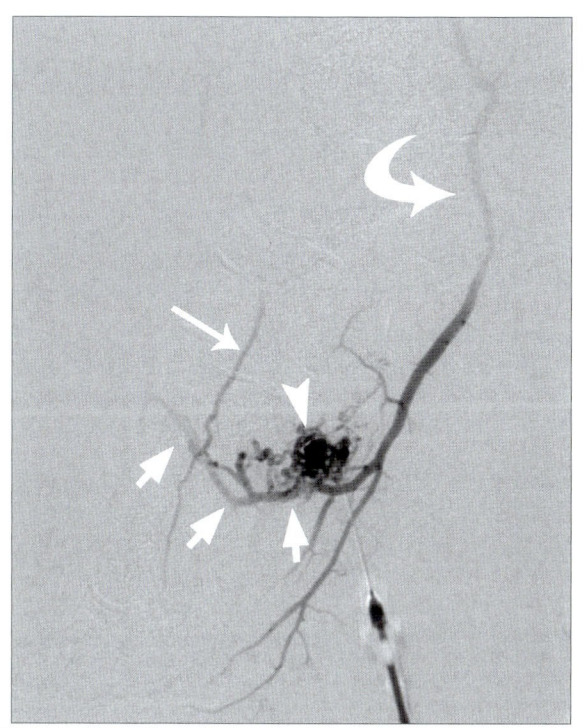

Figure 1. The nidus of the AVM *(arrowhead)* was punctured directly with ultrasound guidance. Contrast is refluxed into the feeding arteries with visualization of the distal posterior tibial artery *(curved arrow)* and plantar arch *(short arrows)*. There is communication with the dorsalis pedis artery *(long arrow)*.

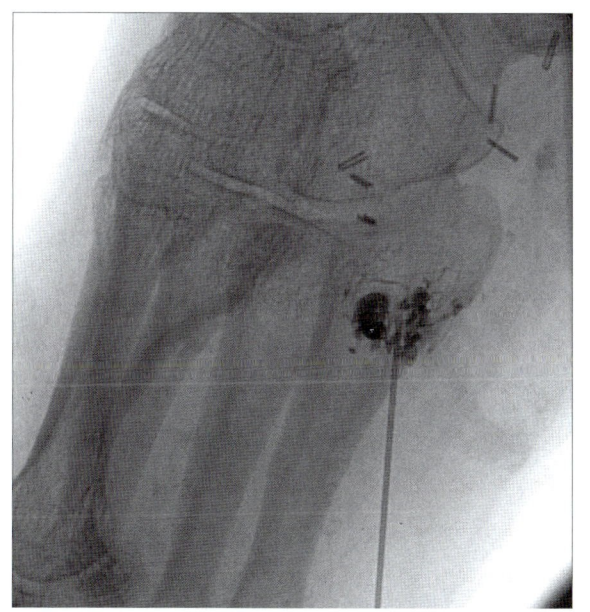

Figure 2. A portion of the nidus is filled with *n*-butyl cyanoacrylate.

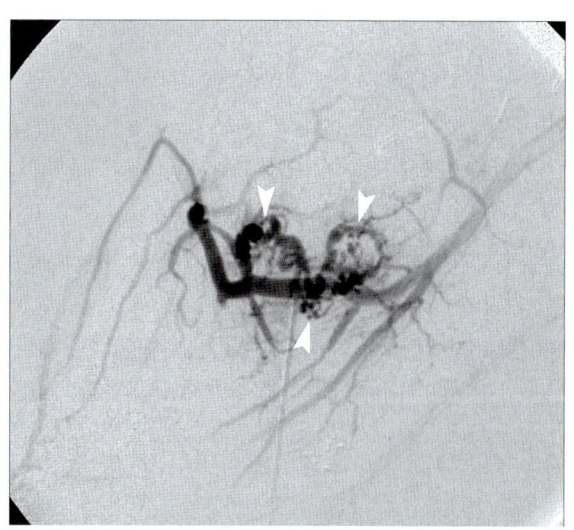

Figure 3. The embolization was staged. The nidus *(arrowheads)* was again punctured directly with ultrasound guidance. Contrast injection shows reflux into the plantar arch and other adjacent arteries.

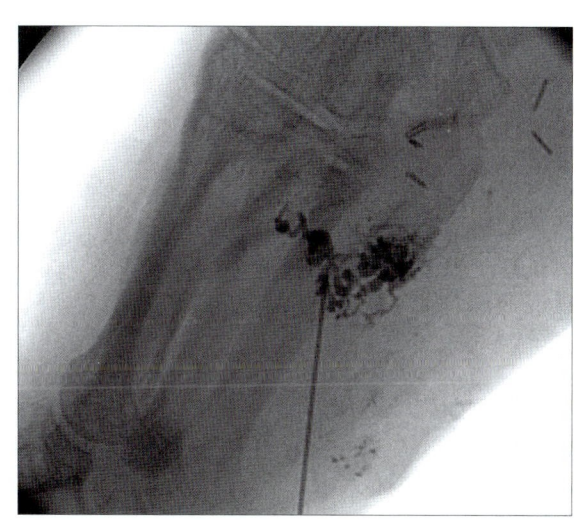

Figure 4. Spot fluoroscopic image after injection of *n*-butyl cyanoacrylate shows that the glue forms a case within the vessels in the nidus of the malformation.

Case 121

DEMOGRAPHICS/CLINICAL HISTORY

A 74-year-old woman with hereditary hemorrhagic telangiectasia and left renal arteriovenous fistula, undergoing computed tomography (CT) and arteriography.

DISCUSSION

History/Indications for Procedure
A 74-year-old woman has hereditary hemorrhagic telangiectasia and a 3-year history of congestive heart failure. She has undergone many prior embolizations for hepatic hemangiomas; she has had chronic gastrointestinal hemorrhage from small-bowel arteriovenous malformations (AVMs) and epistaxis from nasopharyngeal telangiectasias.

Procedure
Endovascular management of renal arteriovenous fistula

Pre-procedure Imaging
Contrast-enhanced CT shows enlarged vessels in the left renal hilum that are consistent with an arteriovenous fistula (Fig. 1).

Intraprocedural Findings
There is a large arteriovenous fistula in the hilum of the left kidney (Figs. 2 and 3). The fistula was embolized with multiple platinum coils (Fig. 4).

Follow-up and Complications
The patient was discharged the day after the embolization. She was able to ambulate without oxygen and continued medical treatment for congestive heart failure.

Suggested Readings
Giavroglou CE, Farmakis TM, Kiskinis D: Idiopathic renal arteriovenous fistula treated by transcatheter embolization. Acta Radiol 46:368-370, 2005.

Guttmacher AE, Marchuk DA, White RI Jr: Hereditary hemorrhagic telangiectasia. N Engl J Med 333:918-924, 1995.

Mori T, Sugimoto K, Taniguchi T, et al: Renal arteriovenous fistula with rapid blood flow successfully treated by transcatheter arterial embolization: Application of interlocking detachable coil as coil anchor. Cardiovasc Intervent Radiol 27:374-376, 2004.

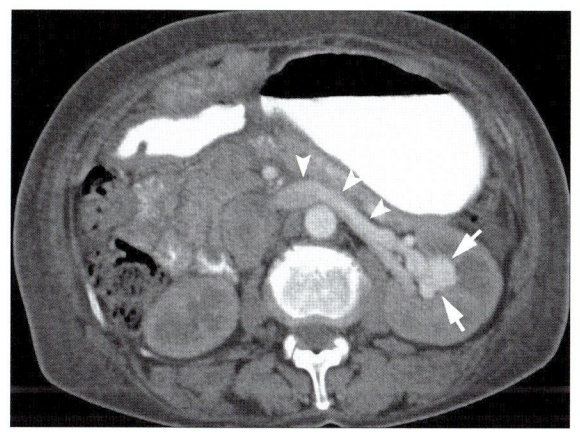

Figure 1. Contrast-enhanced CT scan through the left kidney shows several enlarged vessels in the left renal hilum *(arrows)* with early filling of the left renal vein *(arrowheads)*.

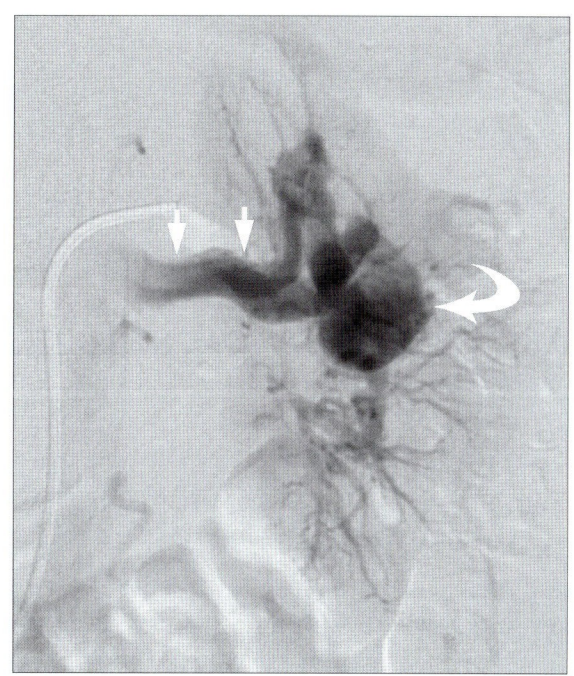

Figure 3. Late arterial phase of a left renal arteriogram shows filling of the venous aneurysm *(curved arrow)* and opacification of the left renal vein *(arrowheads)*.

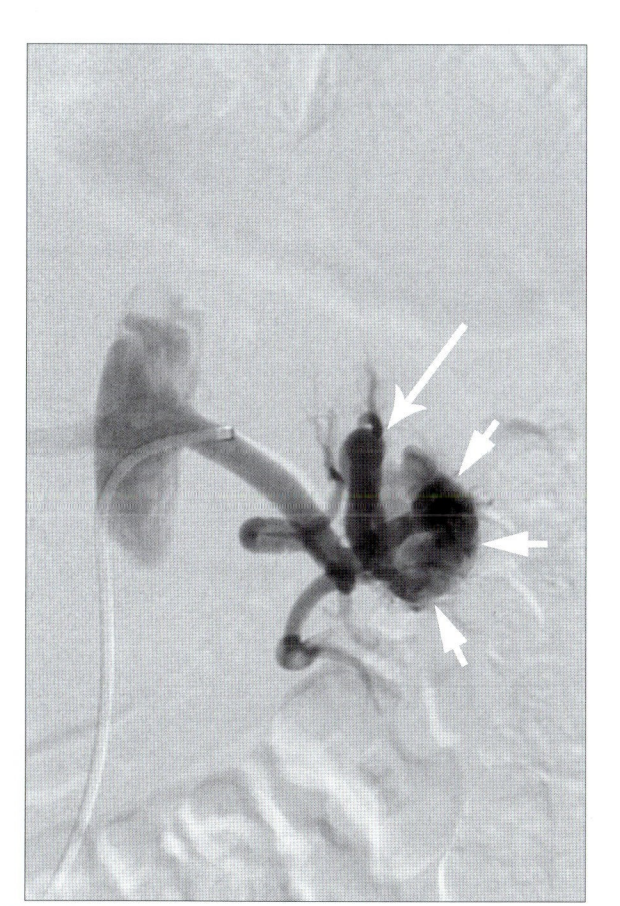

Figure 2. Early arterial phase of a left renal arteriogram shows filling of the arteriovenous fistula *(short arrows)* and early opacification of a renal vein *(long arrow)*.

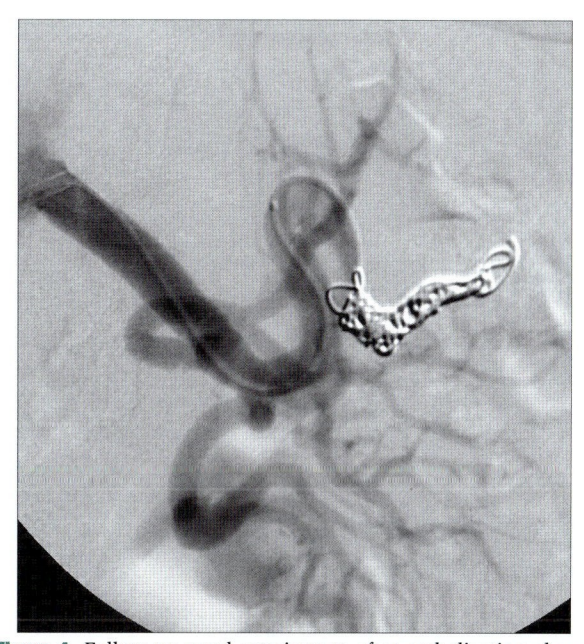

Figure 4. Follow-up renal arteriogram after embolization shows complete occlusion of the feeding artery with coils. There is no further evidence of venous shunting through the arteriovenous fistula.

Case 122

DEMOGRAPHICS/CLINICAL HISTORY

A 66-year-old woman with history of four-vessel coronary bypass and distant ventricular tachycardia for which intravascular defibrillator was placed.

DISCUSSION

History/Indications for Procedure

A 66-year-old woman with history of four-vessel coronary bypass and distant ventricular tachycardia for which intravascular defibrillator was placed. The patient had the defibrillator electively replaced, and 2 weeks later presented with worsening shortness of breath.

Procedure

Endovascular management of iatrogenic injury to LIMA graft

Pre-procedure Imaging

Dobutamine stress test shows decreased function in the anterior septal segment, suggesting ischemia. Cardiac catheterization shows an arteriovenous fistula between the left internal mammary artery (LIMA) bypass graft to the left subclavian vein, with no filling of the distal LIMA graft.

Intraprocedural Findings

There is an AICD lead traversing the LIMA graft, with a resultant pseudoaneurysm and arteriovenous fistula (Fig. 1), and no filling of the distal graft. The site of injury was crossed, and contrast injection shows the distal graft to be patent (Fig. 2); a 4-mm × 19-mm covered stent (Jomed International AB, Helsingborg, Sweden) was placed across the site of injury with restoration of flow to the distal bypass graft (Figs. 3 and 4).

Follow-up and Complications

The patient's shortness of breath symptoms resolved after stent placement. The stent has remained patent over the past 4 years, and the patient has required no further interventions of the LIMA graft.

Suggested Readings

Angle JF, Matsumoto AH, McGraw JK, et al: Percutaneous angioplasty and stenting of left subclavian artery stenosis in patients with left internal mammary-coronary bypass grafts: Clinical experience and long-term follow-up. Vasc Endovasc Surg 37:89-97, 2003.

Barkhordarian S: Stent graft repair of traumatic vertebral pseudoaneurysm with arteriovenous fistula. Vasc Endovasc Surg 41:153-157, 2007.

Sheiban I, Moretti C, Colangelo S: Iatrogenic left internal mammary artery-coronary vein anastomosis treated with covered stent deployment via retrograde percutaneous coronary sinus approach. Catheter Cardiovasc Intervent 68:704-707, 2006.

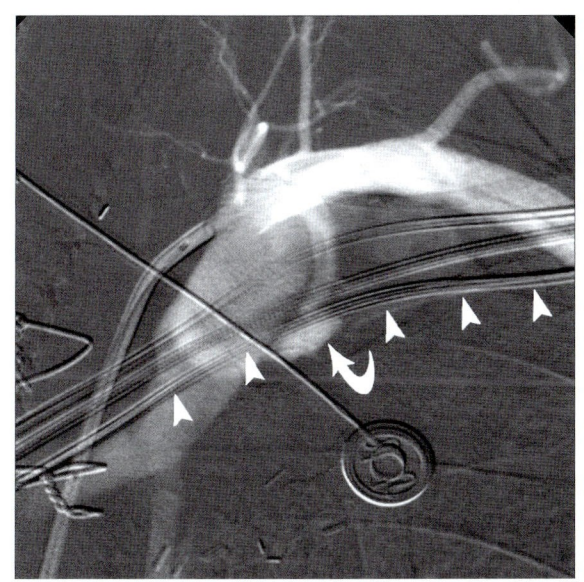

Figure 1. Left subclavian arteriogram shows a pseudoaneurysm and arteriovenous fistula of the proximal left internal mammary artery bypass graft *(curved arrow)*. Note the AICD lead crossing the graft at the site of injury *(arrowheads)*.

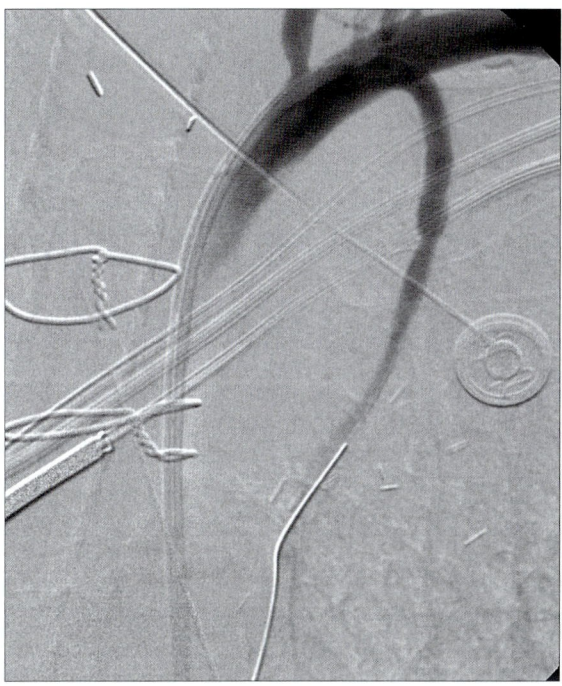

Figure 3. Follow-up arteriogram after stent-graft placement shows exclusion of the pseudoaneurysm and arteriovenous fistula.

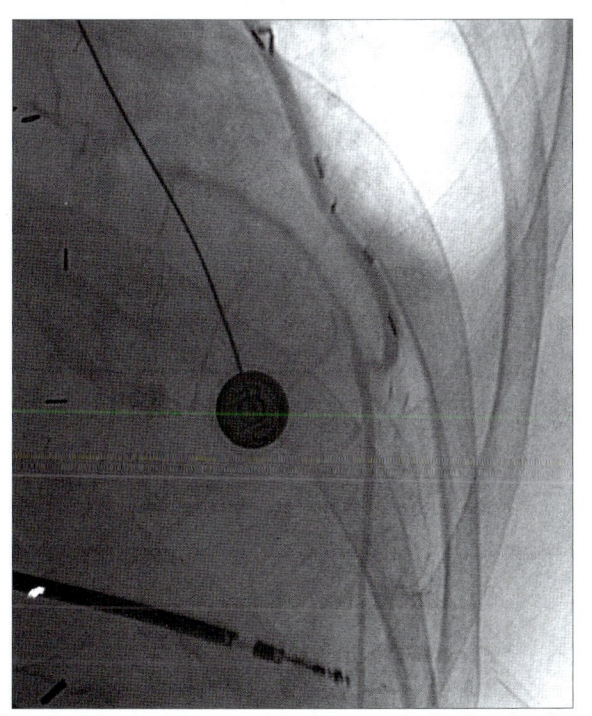

Figure 2. Selective injection of the LIMA graft, distal to the site of injury, shows the distal graft and distal anastamosis to be patent.

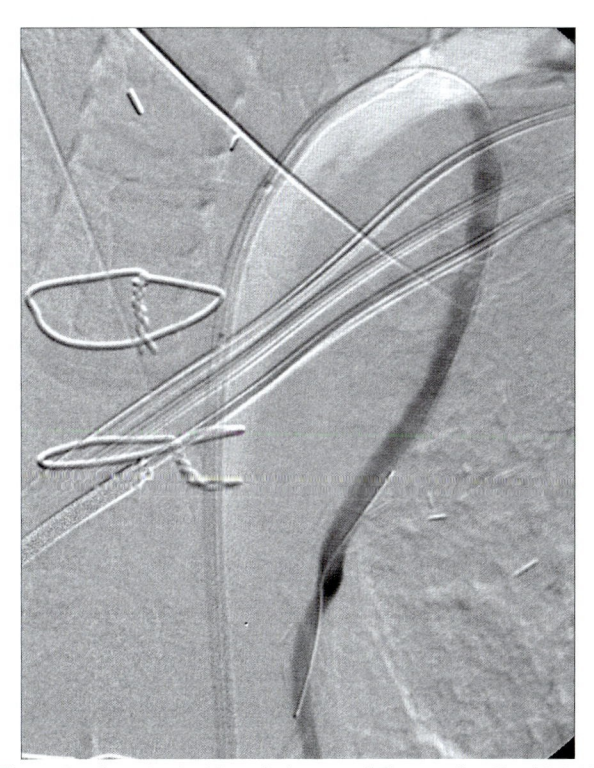

Figure 4. There is significantly improved flow to the distal LIMA graft.

Case 123

DEMOGRAPHICS/CLINICAL HISTORY

A 36-year-old man with hereditary hemorrhagic telangiectasia and increasing shortness of breath with exertion.

DISCUSSION

History/Indications for Procedure
A 36-year-old man with hereditary hemorrhagic telangiectasia and increasing shortness of breath with exertion.

Procedure
Endovascular management of thoracic arteriovenous fistula

Pre-procedure Imaging
Pulmonary arteriogram at an outside hospital was normal. Contrast-enhanced CT of the chest shows abnormal vasculature along the anterior right hemidiaphragm; the abnormal vessels are predominantly supplied by an enlarged right internal mammary artery and inferior phrenic artery.

Intraprocedural Findings
There is a vascular arteriovenous fistula (AVF) between the right inferior phrenic artery and anterior basal branch of the right pulmonary artery (Fig. 1) and between the right internal mammary artery and right inferior pulmonary vein (Fig. 2). The AVFs were occluded with the placement of numerous coils (Figs. 3 and 4).

Follow-up and Complications
Following the embolization, the patient experienced mild right-sided chest pain that was managed using oral pain medications. The patient has not required further embolization in the 2 years since his procedure.

Suggested Readings
Cottin V, Dupuis-Girod S, Lesca G, et al: Pulmonary vascular manifestations of hereditary hemorrhagic telangiectasia (Rendu-Osler disease). Respiration 74:361-78, 2007.

Pollak JS, Saluja S, Thabet A, et al: Clinical and anatomic outcomes after embolotherapy of pulmonary arteriovenous malformations. J Vasc Intervent Radiol 17:35-44, 2006.

White RI Jr, Pollak JS, Wirth JA: Pulmonary arteriovenous malformations: Diagnosis and transcatheter embolotherapy. J Vasc Intervent Radiol 7:787-804, 1996.

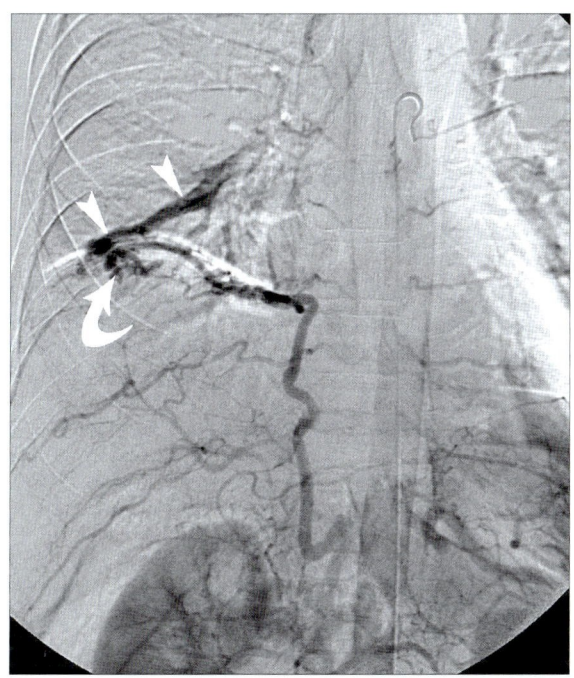

Figure 1. Delayed image from thoracic aortogram shows an enlarged right inferior phrenic artery supplying a small tangle of vessels adjacent to the right hemidiaphragm *(curved arrow)*. There is opacification of the anterior basal branch of the right pulmonary artery *(arrowheads)*.

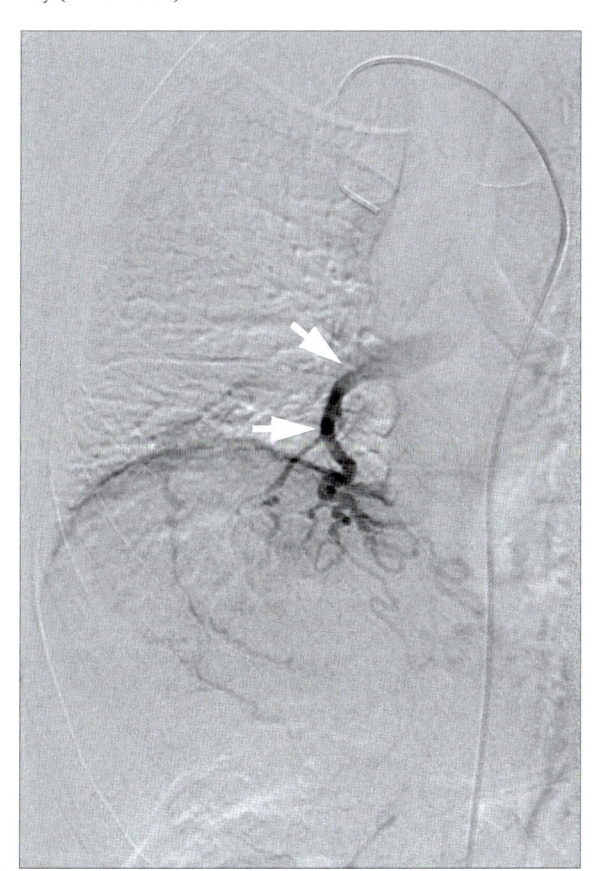

Figure 2. Delayed image from right internal mammary artery injection shows opacification of an abnormal tangle of vessels along the medial right hemidiaphragm and opacification of the right inferior pulmonary vein *(arrows)*.

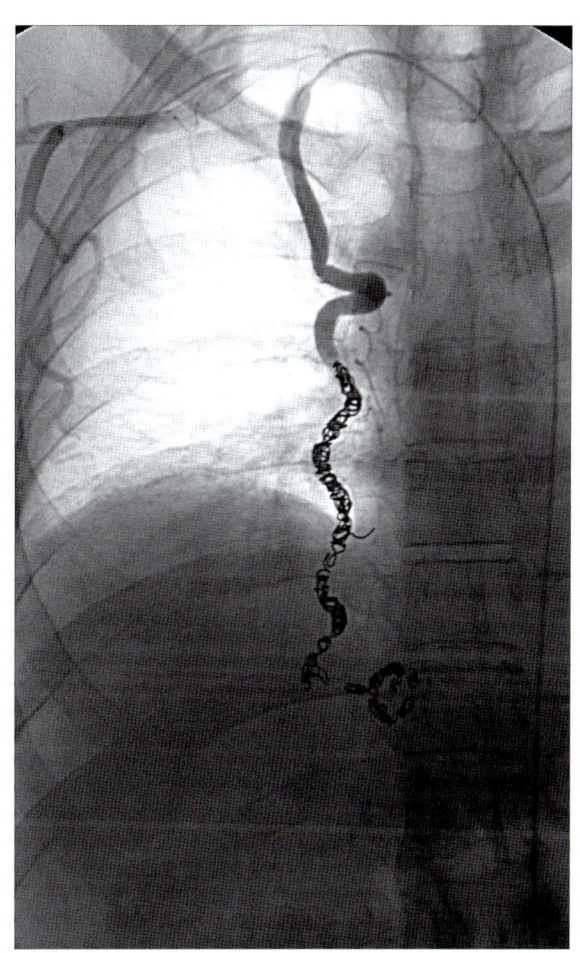

Figure 3. Follow-up arteriogram after embolization. Coils were placed from the inferior epigastric artery into the internal mammary artery. With injection in the right internal mammary artery, there is no further filling of the arteriovenous fistula.

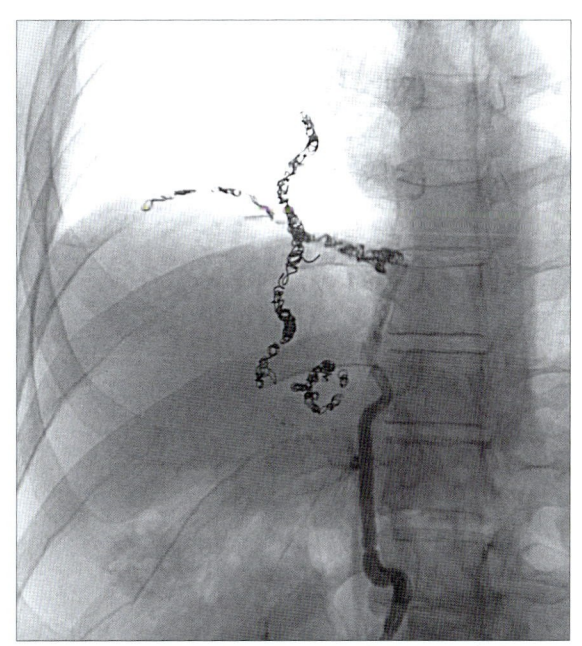

Figure 4. Follow-up arteriogram after embolization. Multiple coils have been placed in the distal inferior phrenic artery occluding the fistula. No further opacification of the pulmonary vein is seen.

Case 124

DEMOGRAPHICS/CLINICAL HISTORY

A 59-year-old man with massive left lower extremity swelling.

DISCUSSION

History/Indications for Procedure
A 59-year-old man presents with massive left lower extremity edema. His symptoms have been present for 1 year; he does have a prior history of gunshot wound to the left lower extremity.

Procedure
Endovascular treatment of pelvic arteriovenous fistula

Pre-procedure Imaging
Contrast-enhanced CT shows early opacification of the left lower extremity venous system and IVC, suggesting the presence of an arteriovenous fistula (Fig. 1). There is marked dilatation of the iliac veins, suggesting this is a chronic condition.

Intraprocedural Findings
There is a large arteriovenous fistula between the left common iliac artery and the common iliac vein (Fig. 2). The fistula was treated by the placement of a stent-graft extending from the common iliac artery into the external iliac artery (Figs. 3 and 4).

Follow-up and Complications
Following stent-graft placement, the patient had gradual improvement in left lower extremity swelling. Follow-up CT shows successful occlusion of the fistula.

Suggested Readings
Criado E, Marston WA, Ligush J, et al: Endovascular repair of peripheral aneurysms, pseudoaneurysms, and arteriovenous fistulas. Ann Vasc Surg 11:256-263, 1997.

Onal B, Ilgit ET, Kosar S, et al: Endovascular treatment of peripheral vascular lesions with stent-grafts. Diagn Intervent Radiol 11:170-174, 2005.

Parodi JC, Schonholz C, Ferreira LM, Bergan J: Endovascular stent-graft treatment of traumatic arterial lesions. Ann Vasc Surg 13:121-129, 1999.

Case 124   249

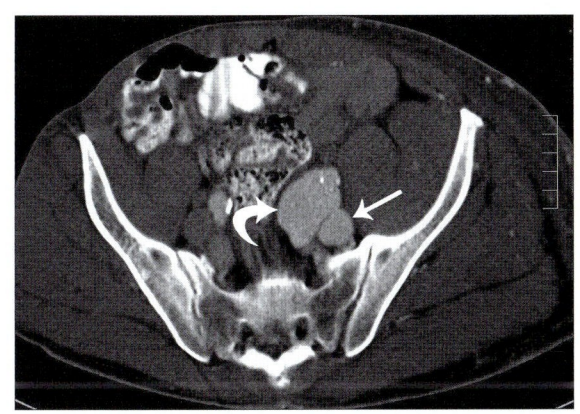

Figure 1. Single image from contrast-enhanced CT shows enlargement and early opacification of the left common iliac vein (*arrow*—common iliac artery; *curved arrow*—common iliac vein).

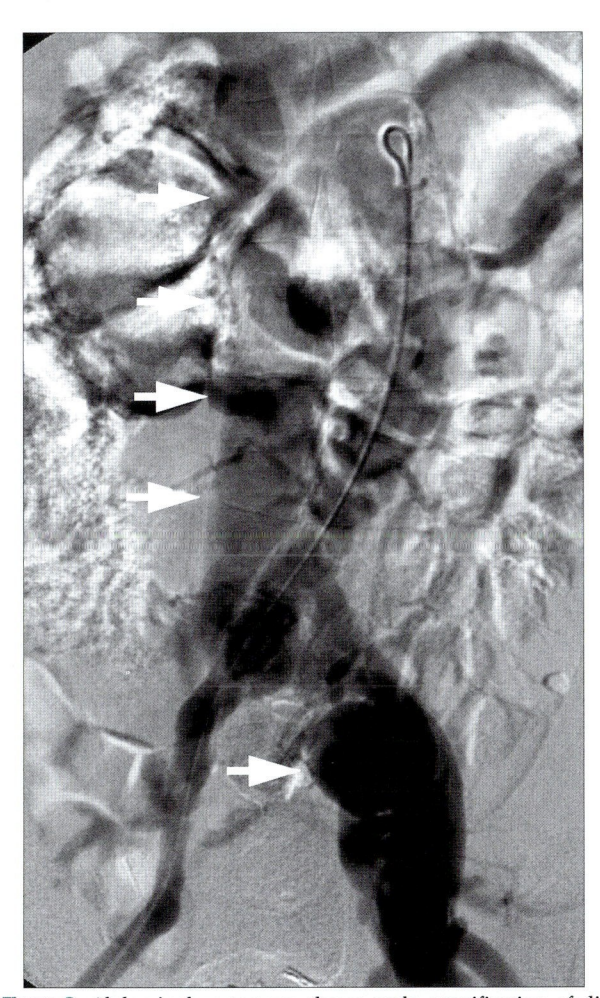

Figure 2. Abdominal aortogram shows early opacification of dilated external and common iliac veins and IVC.

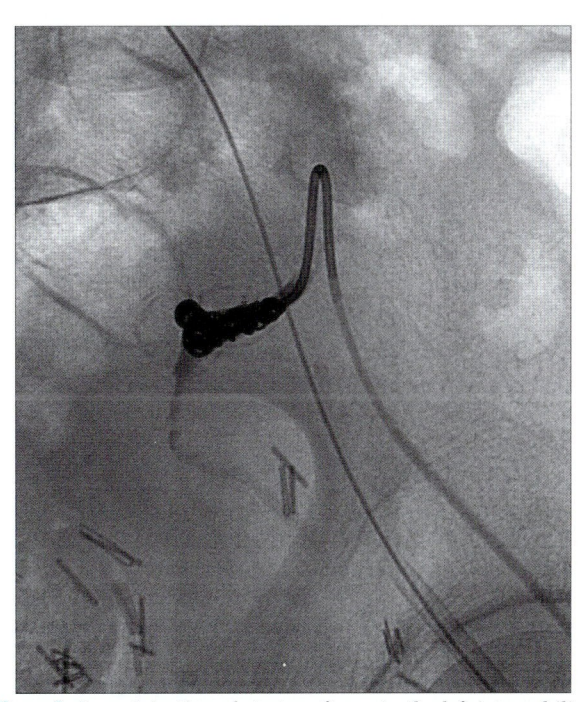

Figure 3. In anticipation of stent-graft repair, the left internal iliac artery was embolized with coils.

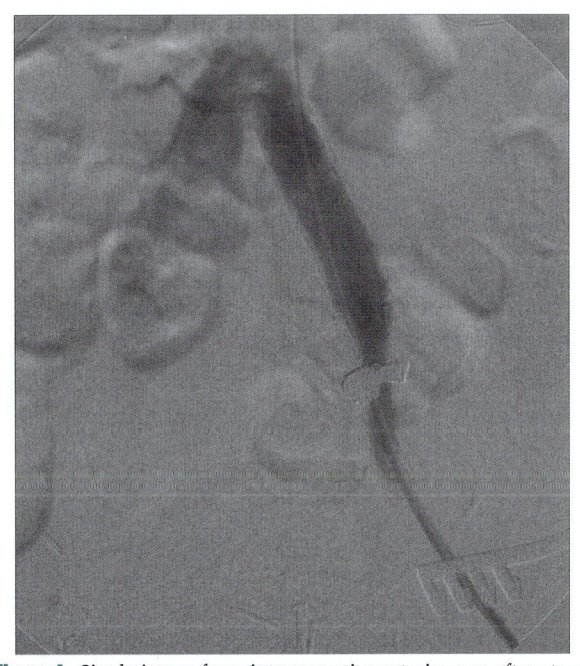

Figure 4. Single image from intraoperative arteriogram after stent-graft placement. The arteriovenous fistula has been successfully occluded.

Case 125

DEMOGRAPHICS/CLINICAL HISTORY

A 22-year-old man with left calf pain, undergoing ultrasound for sclerotherapy.

DISCUSSION

History/Indications for Procedure
A 22-year-old man has left calf pain, which occurs with vigorous exercise and has been increasing in severity over the past 18 months.

Procedure
Endovascular treatment of venous malformation

Pre-procedure Imaging
Magnetic resonance imaging of the left lower extremity showed increased signal intensity within the proximal gastrocnemius muscle.

Intraprocedural Findings
The venous malformation was punctured directly with a 21-gauge needle under ultrasound guidance, and contrast injection showed communication with the deep venous system (Fig. 1). Using direct compression of the popliteal vein, the malformation was sclerosed with alcohol (Fig. 2).

Follow-up and Complications
No further flow was seen by ultrasound after alcohol sclerotherapy. The patient's symptoms significantly improved after a single treatment.

Suggested Readings

Burrows PE, Mason KP: Percutaneous treatment of low-flow vascular malformations. J Vasc Intervent Radiol 15:431-434, 2004.

Lee BB, Do YS, Byun HS, et al: Advanced management of venous malformation with ethanol sclerotherapy: Mid-term results. J Vasc Surg 37:533-538, 2003.

Rautio R, Saarinen J, Laranne J, et al: Endovascular treatment of venous malformation in extremities: Results of sclerotherapy and the quality of life after treatment. Acta Radiol 45:397-403, 2004.

Rimon U, Garniek A, Galili Y, et al: Ethanol sclerotherapy of peripheral venous malformations. Eur J Radiol 52:283-287, 2004.

Case 125   251

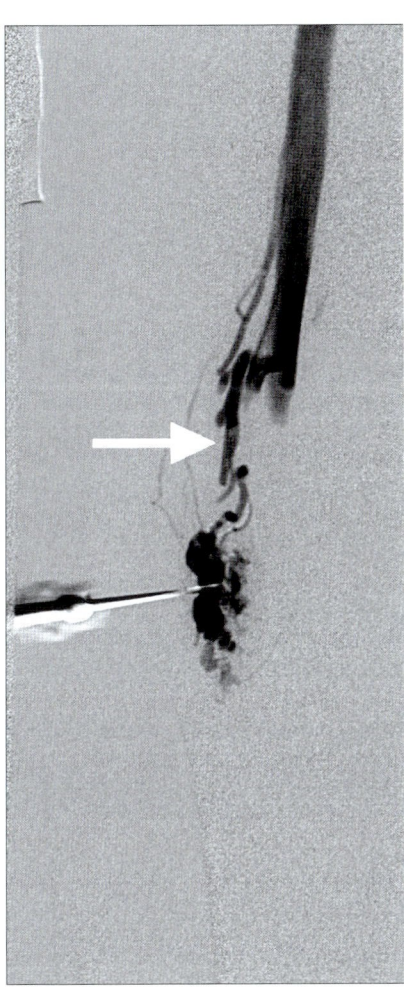

Figure 1. The venous malformation was accessed directly with a 21-gauge needle under ultrasound guidance. Contrast injection shows communication with a small vein that drains directly into the popliteal vein *(arrow)*.

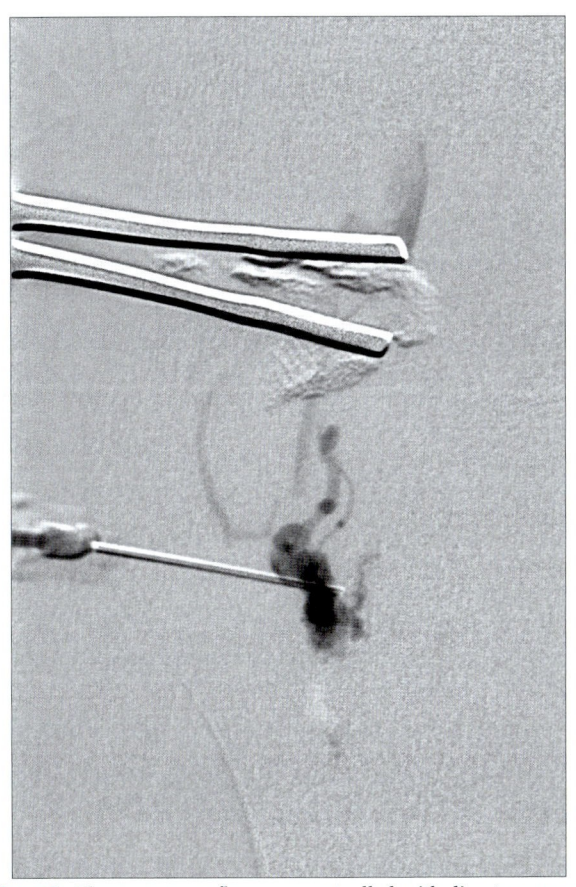

Figure 2. The venous outflow was controlled with direct compression over the site of communication with the deep venous system. This was confirmed with a test injection that was also used to determine the correct volume of alcohol to inject.

Case 126

DEMOGRAPHICS/CLINICAL HISTORY

A 25-year-old woman with a symptomatic venous malformation of the left ankle.

DISCUSSION

History/Indications for Procedure
A 25-year-old woman with a 10-year history of a focal, painful area of the posterior left ankle. The pain has recently been progressive and is exacerbated by standing for long periods and walking long distances.

Procedure
Percutaneous sclerotherapy for lower-extremity venous malformation

Pre-procedure Imaging
Radiograph of the left ankle shows focal soft-tissue swelling in the pre-Achilles fat pad with a single phlebolith (Fig. 1). MRI shows a soft-tissue mass involving the posterior-medial left ankle and extending along the posterior tibial neurovascular bundle into the deep medial mid-foot; the mass is high in T2 signal and shows diffuse contrast enhancement (Fig. 2).

Intraprocedural Findings
The nidus of the malformation was accessed with multiple 20-gauge angiocath needles, and a venogram was performed (Fig. 3). The outflow for the malformation was identified and occluded with tourniquets placed around the lower leg; the malformation was sclerosed with 3% sodium tetradecyl sulfate (STS) mixed with a small volume of Ethiodol (Fig. 4).

Follow-up and Complications
The patient experienced pain and swelling after the sclerotherapy, which was successfully controlled with oral steroids.

Suggested Readings
Burrows PE, Mason KP: Percutaneous treatment of low-flow vascular malformations. J Vasc Intervent Radiol 15:431-434, 2004.

Lee BB, Laredo J, Kim YW, et al: Congenital vascular malformations: General treatment principles. Phlebology 22:258-263, 2007.

Legiehn GM, Heran MK: Venous malformations: Classification, development, diagnosis, and interventional radiologic management. Radiol Clin North Am 46:545-597, 2008.

Rautio R, et al: Endovascular treatment of venous malformation in extremities: Results of sclerotherapy and the quality of life after treatment. Acta Radiol 45:397-403, 2004.

Case 126   253

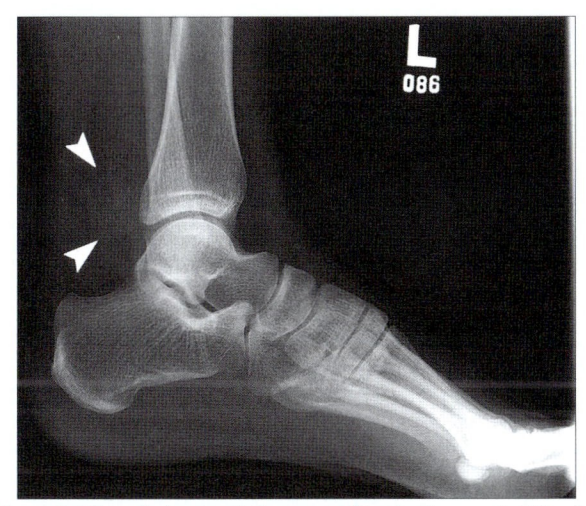

Figure 1. There is focal soft-tissue swelling in the pre-Achilles fat pad (*arrowheads*) with a central phlebolith.

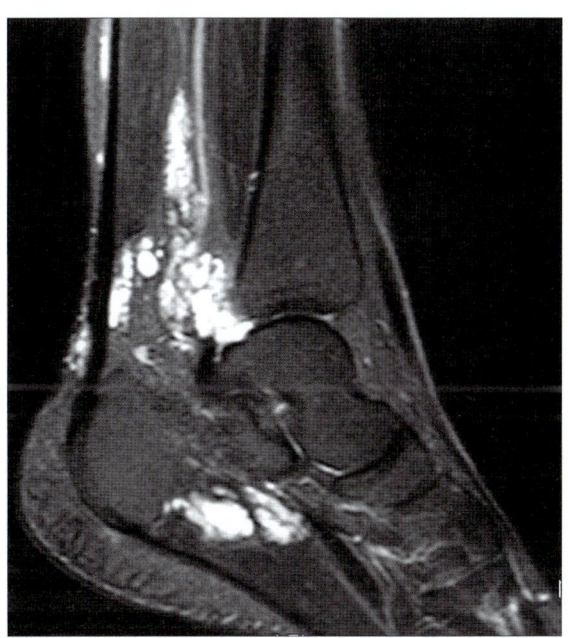

Figure 2. Sagittal image from ankle MRI. The malformation is more extensive than suggested on the radiograph. Cystic spaces of the malformation are seen extending from the lower leg, involving the ankle, and extending to the mid-foot.

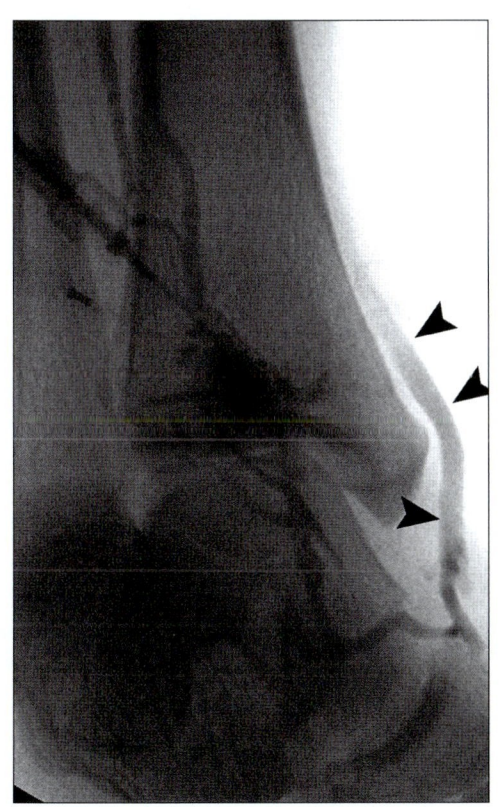

Figure 3. Contrast injection into the nidus of the malformation shows filling of a focal nidus, with outflow into the deep venous system (*arrowheads* indicate anterior tibial vein). The outflow veins were temporarily occluded with the placement of a tourniquet around the lower leg.

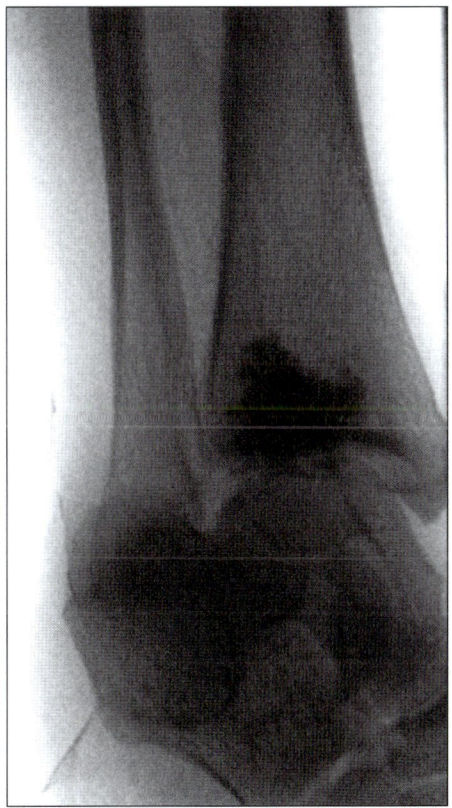

Figure 4. Spot fluorographic image obtained after the sclerotherapy. There is retention of the opacified sclerosant within the nidus of the malformation.

Case 127

DEMOGRAPHICS/CLINICAL HISTORY

A 15-month-old girl with macrocystic lymphatic malformation of the left neck and upper chest, undergoing computed tomography (CT) and magnetic resonance imaging (MRI).

DISCUSSION

History/Indications for Procedure
A 15-month-old girl has a large lymphatic malformation of the left neck and upper chest that was initially diagnosed prenatally (Fig. 1). The malformation has increased in size, and it is causing difficulty feeding.

Procedure
Management of cervical lymphangioma

Pre-procedure Imaging
CT of the neck shows a large, multicystic mass that extends from the angle of the mandible to the sternomanubrial junction (Fig. 2). MRI of the neck confirms the cystic nature of the mass (Fig. 3).

Intraprocedural Findings
Using ultrasound guidance, 18- to 21-gauge needles were placed in each of the largest cysts (Fig. 4). The cysts were aspirated and sclerosed with 3% sodium tetradecyl sulfate.

Follow-up and Complications
The patient was admitted after the procedure for overnight observation and placed on a steroid taper. At the time of discharge, the malformation was palpably smaller, and the child was able to feed without difficulty.

Suggested Readings
Burrows PE, Mason KP: Percutaneous treatment of low-flow vascular malformations. J Vasc Intervent Radiol 15:431-434, 2004.

Molitch HI, Unger ED, Witte CL, vanSonnenberg E: Percutaneous sclerotherapy of lymphangiomas. Radiology 194:343-347, 1995.

Sanlialp I, Karnak I, Tanyel FC, et al: Sclerotherapy for lymphangioma in children. Int J Pediatr Otorhinolaryngol 67:795-800, 2003.

Case 127   255

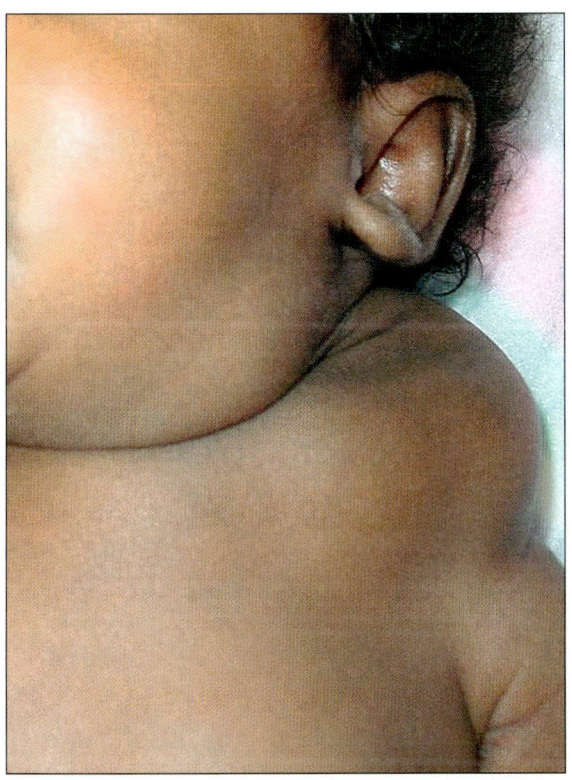

Figure 1. A cystic mass involves the left neck and shoulder.

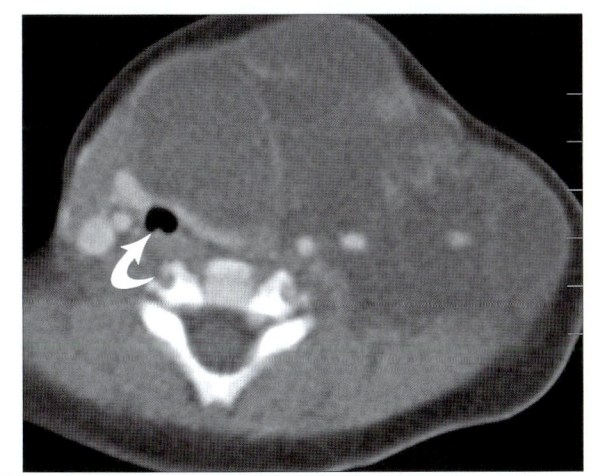

Figure 2. Contrast-enhanced CT through the lower neck shows a large, multicystic mass extending from the neck into the left shoulder. The cysts are large, and they displace the air-filled trachea to the right *(arrow)*.

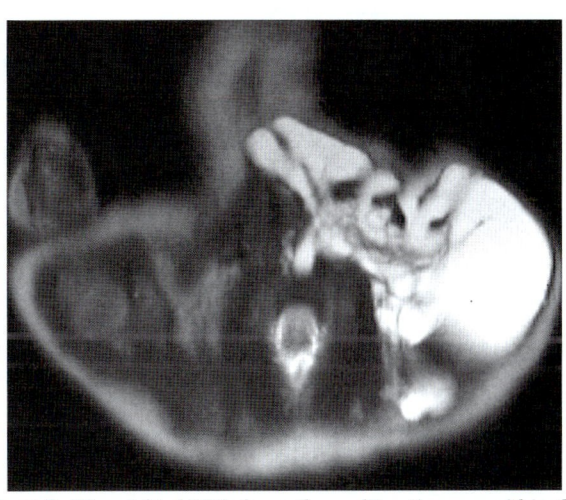

Figure 3. T2-weighted MRI shows the multicystic mass within the lower neck and left chest.

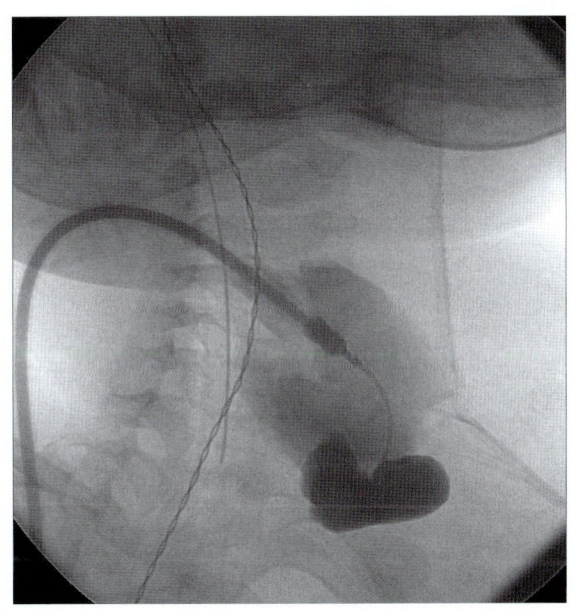

Figure 4. A 22-gauge angiocatheter was placed into the larger cysts with ultrasound guidance. Contrast injection shows filling of one of the larger cysts. The larger cysts were sclerosed after aspiration of their contents.

Case 128

DEMOGRAPHICS/CLINICAL HISTORY

A 5-month-old girl with a 3-month history of right shoulder hemangioma.

DISCUSSION

History/Indications for Procedure
A 5-month-old girl with a right shoulder hemangioma, diagnosed at age 2 months, and associated Kasabach-Merritt syndrome. The patient has had a poor response to systemic steroids and vincristine and remains thrombocytopenic.

Procedure
Percutaneous management of soft-tissue hemangioma

Pre-procedure Imaging
MRI of the right shoulder shows a large, infiltrating mass of the right shoulder and upper chest (Fig. 1). The mass is low T1 signal intensity and heterogeneous T2 signal intensity, with homogeneous contrast enhancement.

Intraprocedural Findings
A large echogenic mass is seen with ultrasound. A total of five 22-gauge angiocatheters were inserted in different locations within the mass (Fig. 2); 3% sodium tetradecyl sulfate mixed with Ethiodol was injected into the mass under fluoroscopy (Fig. 3).

Follow-up and Complications
The platelet count increased from $20 \times 10^9/L$ to $225 \times 10^9/L$. She has since undergone two additional sclerotherapy procedures for recurrent thrombocytopenia (Fig. 4).

Suggested Readings
Burrows PE, Mason KP: Percutaneous treatment of low-flow vascular malformations. J Vasc Intervent Radiol 15:431-434, 2004.

Claudon M, Upton J, Burrows PE: Diffuse venous malformation of the upper limb: Morphologic characterization by MRI and venography. Pediatr Radiol 31:507-514, 2001.

Holt P, Burrows P: Interventional radiology in the treatment of vascular lesions. Facial Plast Surg Clin North Am 9:585-599, 2001.

Case 128   257

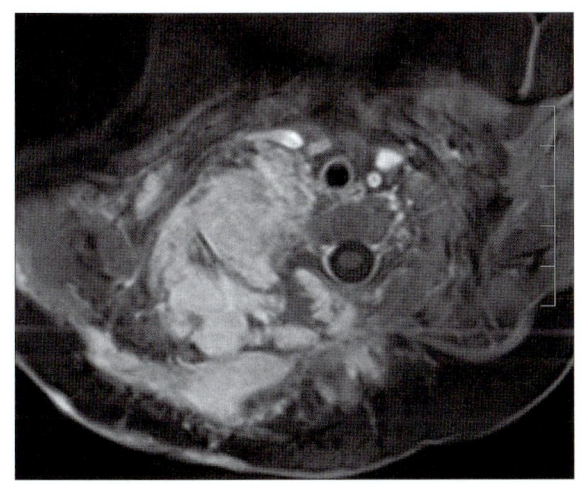

Figure 1. T1, post-contrast, fat-suppressed MR image shows a large, infiltrative mass in the right shoulder and upper chest. The mass enhances homogeneously with contrast.

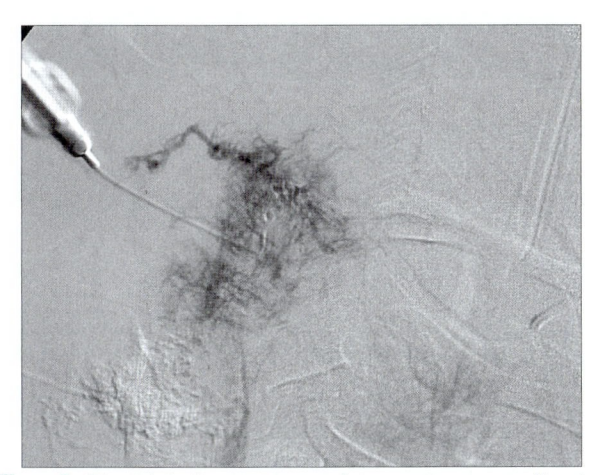

Figure 2. Direct injection venogram shows numerous small, spindly veins within the hemangioma.

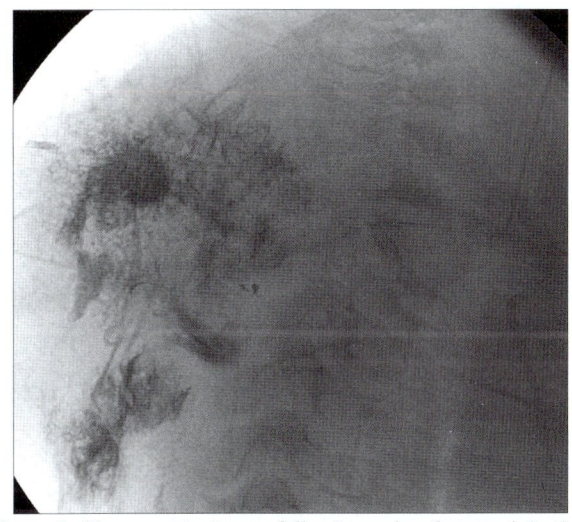

Figure 3. Fluoroscopic image following sclerotherapy injection shows retained Ethiodol throughout the hemangioma. The sodium tetradecyl sulphate was mixed with Ethiodol so that it could be visualized during injection.

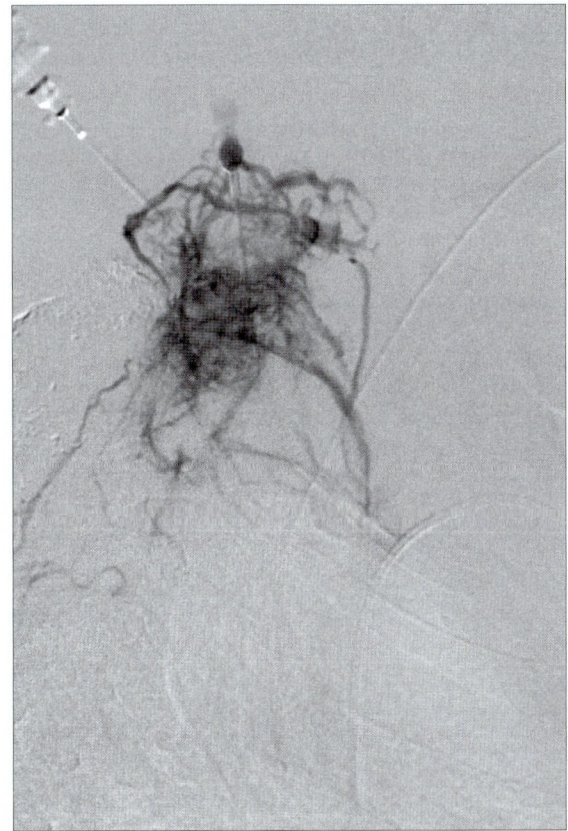

Figure 4. Venogram from later treatment again shows multiple small, spindly veins within the hemangioma. There are several prominent outflow veins. Control of the outflow veins is necessary prior to sclerosant injection.

Case 129

DEMOGRAPHICS/CLINICAL HISTORY

A 6-month-old boy with symptomatic right lower extremity kaposiform hemangioendothelioma undergoing magnetic resonance imaging (MRI).

DISCUSSION

History/Indications for Procedure

A 6-month-old boy with right lower extremity kaposiform hemangioendothelioma that resulted in a consumptive coagulopathy and Kasabach-Merritt syndrome.

Procedure

Percutaneous sclerotherapy for kaposiform hemangioendothelioma of the extremity

Pre-procedure Imaging

Contrast-enhanced MRI of the extremity demonstrated diffuse high signal intensity on T2-weighted sequences throughout the soft tissues of the right lower leg (Fig. 1). The image demonstrates avid enhancement after contrast administration (Fig. 2).

Intraprocedural Findings

Direct-injection venogram demonstrates opacification of numerous, small, delicate, branching venous channels (Fig. 3). Sclerotherapy was performed with a 1.5% solution of sodium tetradecyl sulfate.

Follow-up and Complications

The patient underwent two additional sclerotherapy sessions for this lesion. At this point, the platelet count has stabilized, and the child appears to have less pain associated with the lesion, despite the stable appearance on follow-up imaging (Fig. 4).

Suggested Readings

Burrows PE, Mason KP: Percutaneous treatment of low flow vascular malformations. J Vasc Intervent Radiol 15:431-434, 2004.

Konez O, Burrows PE: Magnetic resonance of vascular anomalies. Magn Reson Imaging Clin N Am 10:363-388, vii, 2002.

Rautio R, Saarinen J, Laranne J, et al: Endovascular treatment of venous malformations in extremities: Results of sclerotherapy and the quality of life after treatment. Acta Radiol 45:397-403, 2004.

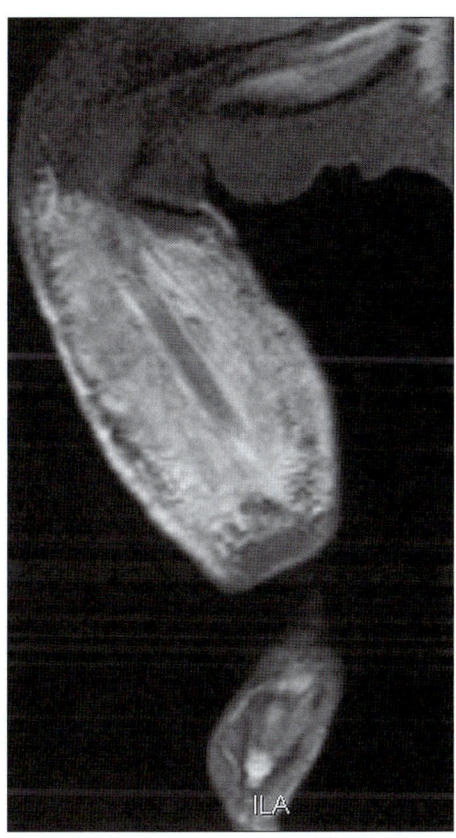

Figure 1. Sagittal T2-weighted MR image of the right lower extremity demonstrates diffuse high signal intensity throughout the soft tissues.

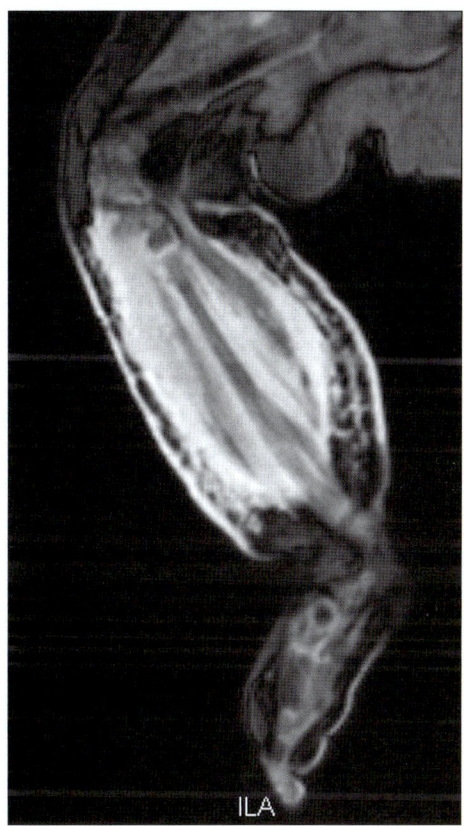

Figure 2. Postcontrast, T1-weighted, fat-saturated image demonstrates avid enhancement of the lesion.

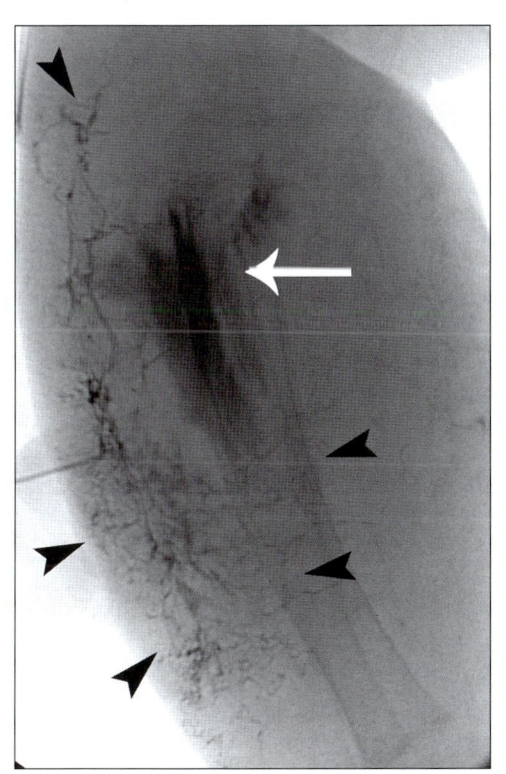

Figure 3. Direct-injection venogram opacifies numerous small, delicate venous channels *(arrowheads)*. There is a small amount of deep muscle contrast extravasation *(arrow)*.

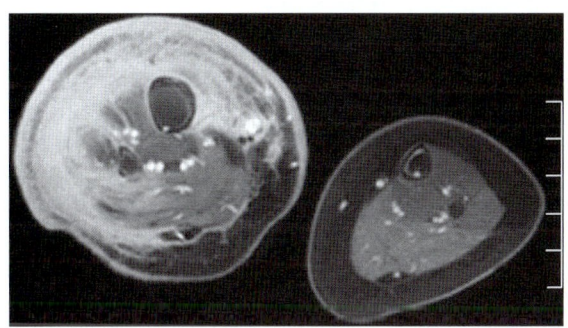

Figure 4. Follow-up MRI was performed 5 months after the initial sclerotherapy session, and a single postcontrast, T1-weighted, fat-saturation sequence demonstrates persistent diffuse enhancement throughout the soft tissues of the right lower extremity that is essentially unchanged. Notice the asymmetry in the size of the lower extremities.

Case 130

DEMOGRAPHICS/CLINICAL HISTORY

A 62-year-old man with alcohol-induced cirrhosis and 5.4-cm hepatocellular carcinoma in segment 8 of the liver, undergoing MRI.

DISCUSSION

History/Indications for Procedure
This patient has an enlarging hepatocellular carcinoma in segment 8 of the liver.

Procedure
Chemoembolization for hepatocellular carcinoma

Pre-procedure Imaging
Contrast-enhanced MRI of the liver shows a 4.4-cm × 5.4-cm mass with peripheral enhancement (Fig. 1). The liver is nodular, and there are secondary signs of portal hypertension.

Intraprocedural Findings
A hypervascular mass is identified near the dome of the liver, supplied by a replaced right hepatic artery (Fig. 2). There is visible accumulation of ethiodized oil (Ethiodol) in the lesion after chemoembolization (Fig. 3).

Follow-up and Complications
Follow-up MRI 3 months after embolization shows the lesion decreased in size and no longer enhancing (Fig. 4). The patient underwent successful liver transplantation 6 months after embolization and is currently disease-free.

Suggested Readings
Liu DM, Salem R, Bui JT, et al: Angiographic considerations in patients undergoing liver-directed therapy. J Vasc Intervent Radiol 16:911-935, 2005.

Llovet JM, Bruix J: A systematic review of randomized trials for unresectable hepatocellular carcinoma chemoembolization improves survival. Hepatology 37:429-442, 2003.

Llovet JM, Fuster J, Bruix J: The Barcelona approach: Diagnosis, staging, and treatment of hepatocellular carcinoma. Liver Transplant 10:115-120, 2004.

Case 130   261

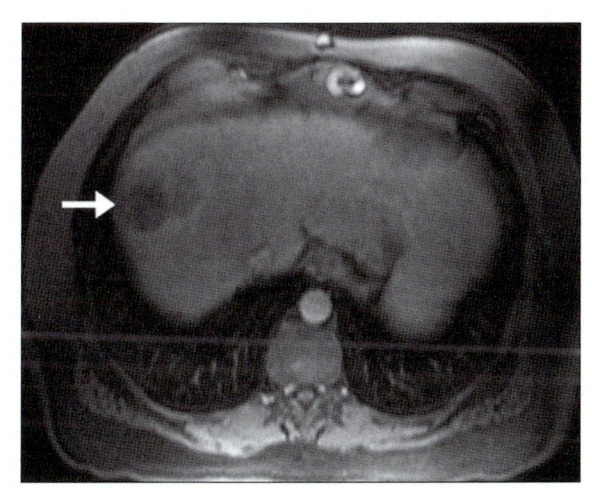

Figure 1. T1-weighted fat-saturated axial image through the liver shows a 5.4-cm mass in segment 8 (arrow).

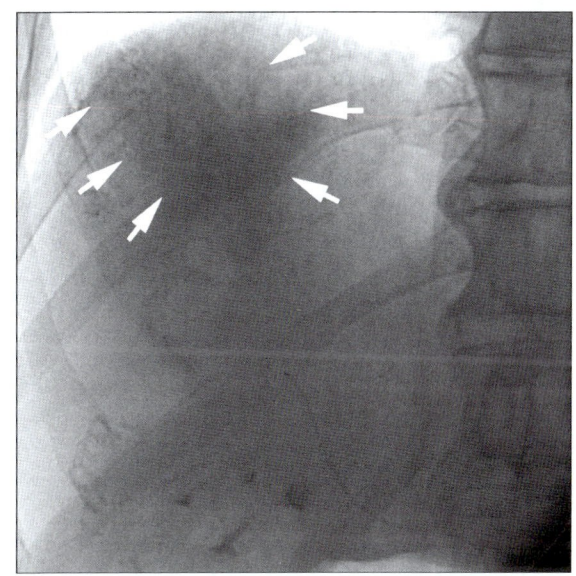

Figure 3. Accumulation of ethiodized oil (Ethiodol) is present within the mass (arrowheads) after chemoembolization.

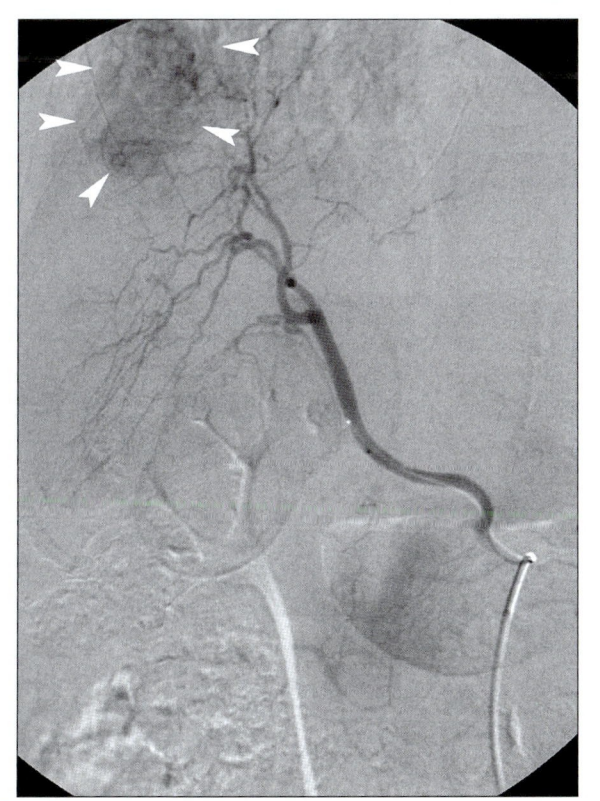

Figure 2. Selective injection of the right hepatic artery shows the lesion to be hypervascular (arrowheads).

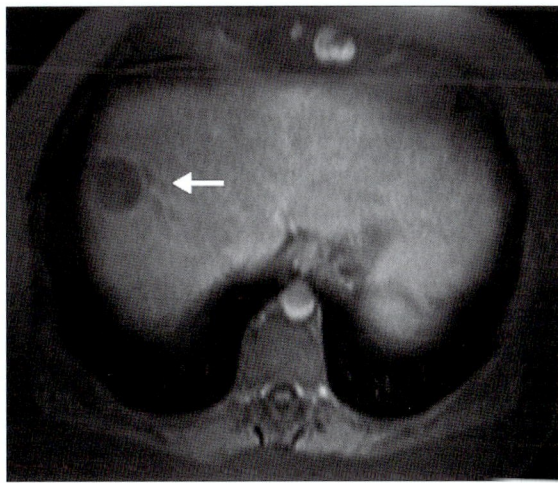

Figure 4. T1-weighted fat-saturated axial image 3 months after embolization shows the lesion to have reduced in size with no appreciable internal enhancement (arrow).

Case 131

DEMOGRAPHICS/CLINICAL HISTORY

A 50-year-old woman with multifocal hepatocellular carcinoma, undergoing magnetic resonance imaging (MRI), arteriography, and transarterial chemoembolization (TACE).

DISCUSSION

History/Indications for Procedure
A 50-year-old woman with no history of liver disease presents with multifocal hepatocellular carcinoma.

Procedure
Transarterial chemoembolization (TACE) for hepatocellular carcinoma

Pre-procedure Imaging
Contrast-enhanced MRI demonstrates many early-enhancing lesions in both lobes of the liver. The largest lesion is located in segment IVb and measures 10 cm × 8 cm (Fig. 1).

Intraprocedural Findings
Celiac arteriogram demonstrates many hypervascular lesions in the liver, with the largest located in segment IVb (Fig. 2). Chemoembolization of the segment IV lesion was performed using a combination of doxorubicin, mitomycin, Ethiodol, and calibrated microspheres (Fig. 3).

Follow-up and Complications
Contrast-enhanced MRI performed 2 months after chemoembolization shows that the mass has decreased in size, now measuring 7 cm × 4 cm (Fig. 4). Enhancement of the mass has been significantly reduced.

Suggested Readings
Llovet JM, Bruix J: A systematic review of randomized trials for unresectable hepatocellular carcinoma chemoembolization improves survival. Hepatology 37:429-442, 2003.
Llovet JM, Burroughs A, Bruix J: Hepatocellular carcinoma. Lancet 362:1907-1917, 2003.
Llovet JM, Fuster J, Bruix J, et al: The Barcelona approach: Diagnosis, staging, and treatment of hepatocellular carcinoma. Liver Transplant 10(Suppl 1):S115-S120, 2004.
LLovet JM, Real MI, Montaña X, et al, for the Barcelona Liver Cancer Group: Arterial embolisation or chemoembolisation versus symptomatic treatment in patients with unresectable hepatocellular carcinoma: A randomized controlled trial. Lancet 359:1734-1739, 2002.
Lo CM, Ngan H, Tso WK, et al: Randomized controlled trial of transarterial lipiodol chemoebolization for unresectable hepatocellular carcinoma. Hepatology 35:1164-1171, 2002.

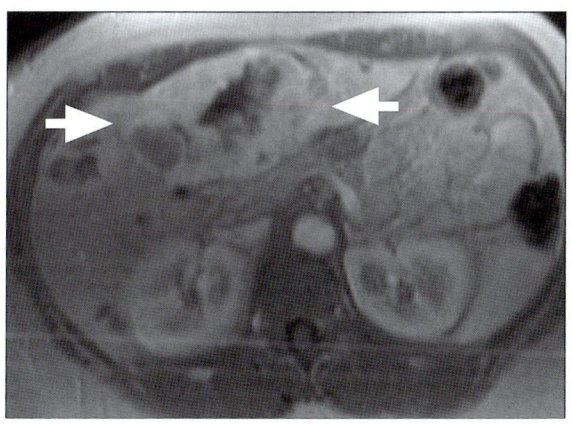

Figure 1. T1-axial image through the abdomen after gadolinium administration demonstrates a large hypervascular mass with central necrosis (arrows).

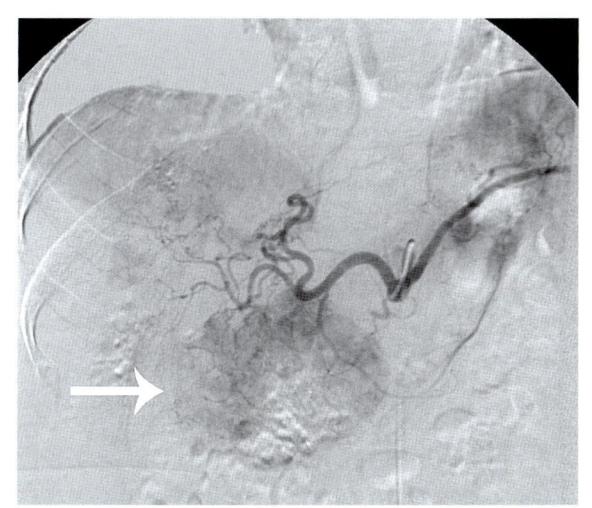

Figure 2. Celiac arteriogram confirms the mass is hypervascular (arrow). Several smaller lesions also were identified.

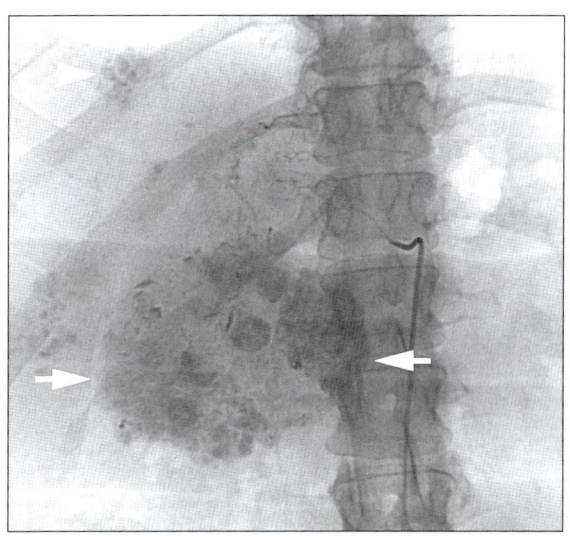

Figure 3. There is retention of Ethiodol throughout the mass after chemoembolization (arrows).

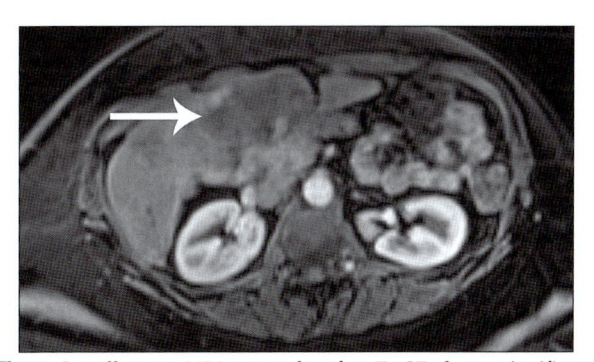

Figure 4. Follow-up MRI 2 months after TACE shows significant reduction in the size and enhancement of the mass (arrow).

Case 132

DEMOGRAPHICS/CLINICAL HISTORY

A 51-year-old man with hepatitis C–related cirrhosis and hepatocellular carcinoma, undergoing computed tomography (CT), arteriography, and fluoroscopy.

DISCUSSION

History/Indications for Procedure
A 51-year-old man has hepatitis C–related cirrhosis. He underwent abdominal CT for acute epigastric pain that revealed a mass in the caudate lobe of the liver.

Procedure
Transarterial chemoembolization of hepatocellular carcinoma

Pre-procedure Imaging
Contrast-enhanced CT shows a 5-cm × 6.2-cm, heterogeneously enhancing mass in the caudate lobe of the liver (Fig. 1). The mass has an adjacent high-attenuation fluid collection that is consistent with recent hemorrhage.

Intraprocedural Findings
Hepatic arteriography showed a hypervascular mass supplied by a branch of the left hepatic artery. A 3-French microcatheter was used for superselective catheterization of the feeding artery (Fig. 2), and chemoembolization was carried out using mitomycin and doxorubicin mixed with Ethiodol, followed by 300-μm to 500-μm calibrated microspheres (Fig. 3).

Follow-up and Complications
The patient was observed overnight in the hospital and treated for postembolization pain and nausea. Contrast-enhanced CT performed 1 year after embolization shows the mass to be stable in size as compared with earlier follow-up scans, with some retained Ethiodol and no visible enhancement (Fig. 4).

Suggested Readings
Lau KY, Wong TP, Wong WW, et al: Emergency embolization of spontaneous ruptured hepatocellular carcinoma: Correlation between survival and Child-Pugh classification. Australas Radiol 47:231-235, 2003.

Llovet JM, Bruix J: A systematic review of randomized trials for unresectable hepatocellular carcinoma chemoembolization improves survival. Hepatology 37:429-442, 2003.

Llovet JM, Burroughs A, Bruix J: Hepatocellular carcinoma. Lancet 362:1907-1917, 2003.

Case 132   265

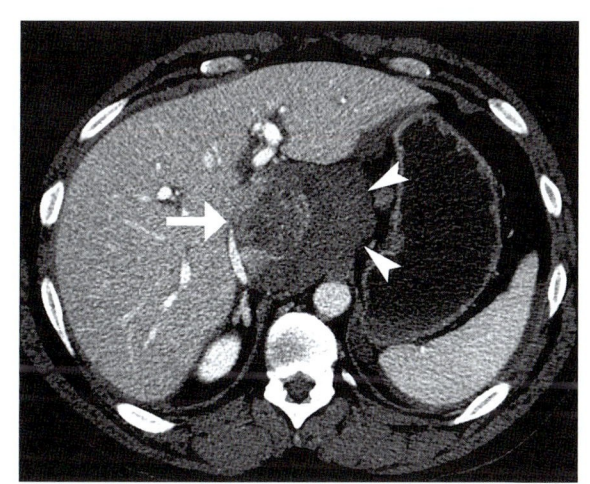

Figure 1. Contrast-enhanced CT through the liver shows a heterogeneously enhancing mass within the caudate lobe *(arrow)* compressing the inferior vena cava. The surrounding fluid *(arrowheads)* is consistent with recent hemorrhage.

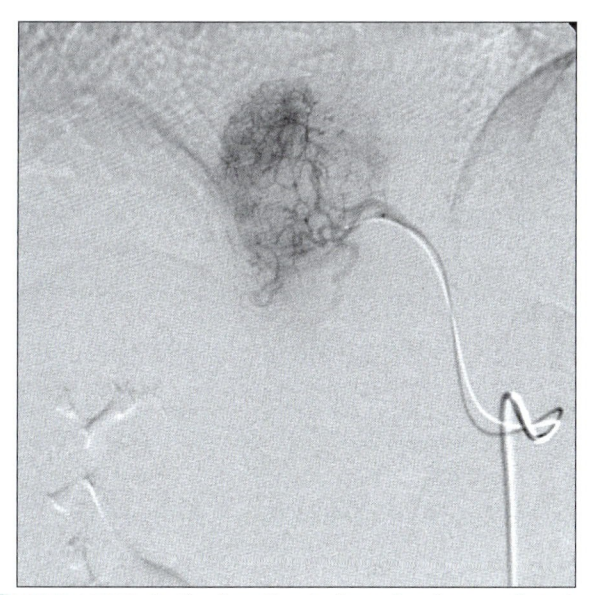

Figure 2. Superselective hepatic arteriography shows catheterization of the artery supplying the tumor. The microcatheter was advanced as close to the tumor as possible.

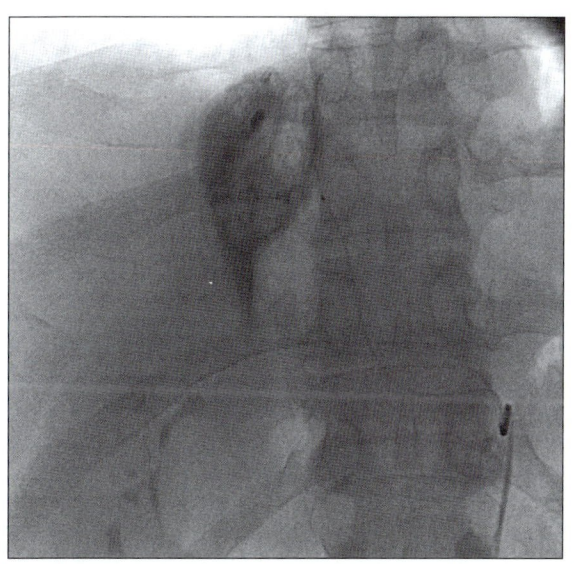

Figure 3. Fluoroscopy after chemoembolization shows retained contrast within the lesion.

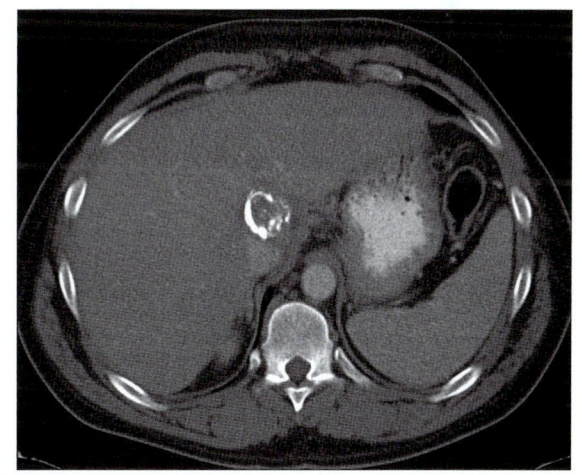

Figure 4. Contrast-enhanced CT performed 1 year after embolization shows that the lesion has decreased in size to 3 cm × 2.8 cm, and has is no visible enhancement. The lesion size had remained stable as compared with earlier postembolization studies.

Case 133

DEMOGRAPHICS/CLINICAL HISTORY
A 63-year-old man with hepatocellular carcinoma.

DISCUSSION

History/Indications for Procedure
A 63-year-old man diagnosed with hepatitis C 18 years prior. Over the past several months, he noted increasing weight loss, decreasing muscle mass, and increasing ascites.

Procedure
Chemoembolization for hepatocellular carcinoma

Pre-procedure Imaging
MRI of the liver shows a 3.9-cm × 2.9-cm enhancing mass within the caudate lobe (Fig. 1). The mass shows early arterial enhancement with rapid washout and late capsular enhancement, compatible with hepatocellular carcinoma.

Intraprocedural Findings
The hypervascular mass is identified on angiography (Fig.2). A 3-French microcatheter was used to selectively catheterize the feeding artery, and chemoembolization was performed with mitomycin and doxorubicin (Fig. 3).

Follow-up and Complications
Contrast-enhanced MRI performed 3 months after chemoembolization shows the mass to be decreased in size, measuring 3.3 cm × 2.7 cm, with no visible enhancement. MRI performed 8 months after chemoembolization shows no evidence of tumor growth of the caudate mass (Fig. 4) but the development of new lesions in segments IV and VII.

Suggested Readings
Brown DB, Geschwind JF, Soullen MC, et al: Society of Interventional Radiology position statement on chemoembolization of hepatic malignancies. J Vasc Interv Radiol 17:217-223, 2006.

Llovet JM, Brux J: A systematic review of randomized trials for unresectable hepatocellular carcinoma chemoembolization improves survival. Hepatology 37:429-442, 2003.

Ramsey DE, Kernagis LY, Soulen MC, et al: Chemoembolization of hepatocellular carcinoma. J Vasc Intervent Radiol 13:S211-S221, 2002.

Vogl TJ, Naguib NN, Nour-Eldin NE, et al: Review on transarterial chemoembolization in hepatocellular carcinoma: Palliative, combined, neoadjuvant, bridging, and symptomatic indications. Eur J Radiol [preprint e-pub], 2008.

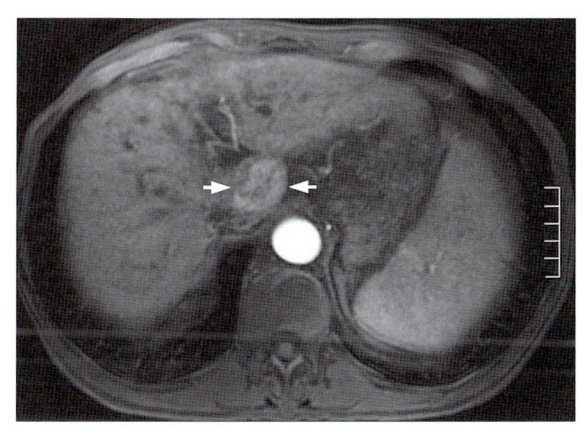

Figure 1. T1, post-contrast MR image with fat saturation shows an enhancing lesion in the caudate lobe *(arrows)*. The lesion shows early arterial enhancement and rapid wash-out. In the setting of underlying cirrhosis, this is compatible with hepatocellular carcinoma.

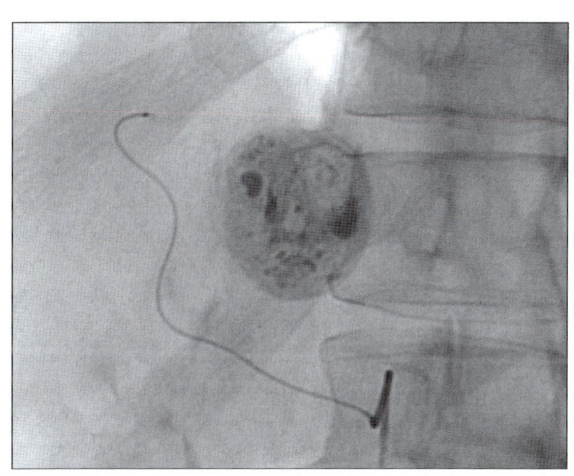

Figure 3. Fluoroscopic image after chemoembolization shows accumulation of the Ethiodol within the mass.

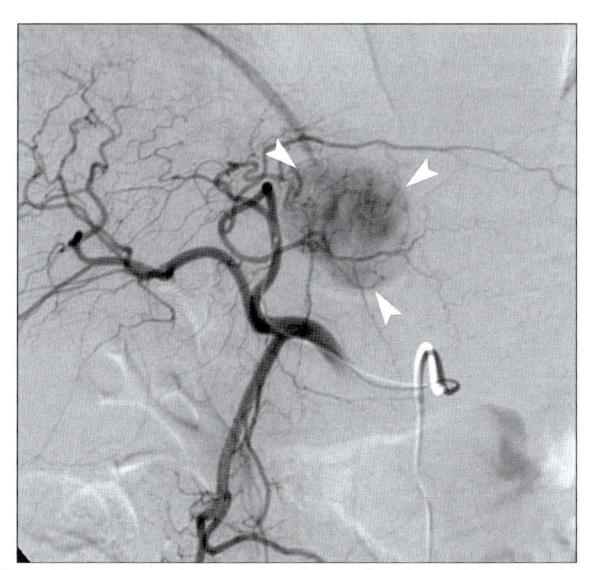

Figure 2. Hepatic arteriogram. A 3-French microcatheter has been used to selectively catheterize the left hepatic artery. The hypervascular mass in the caudate lobe is clearly seen *(arrowheads)*, supplied by branches of the left hepatic artery.

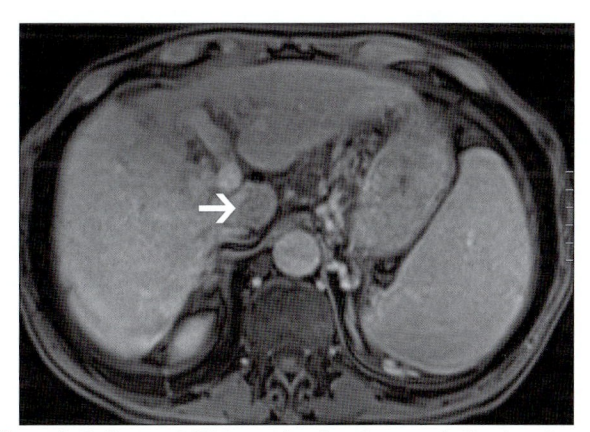

Figure 4. Follow-up MRI 8 months after chemoembolization shows that the mass has decreased in size *(arrow)*. There is minimal enhancement within the lesion.

Case 134

DEMOGRAPHICS/CLINICAL HISTORY

A 58-year-old woman with hepatocellular carcinoma.

DISCUSSION

History/Indications for Procedure
A 58-year-old woman with non-alcoholic steatohepatitis (NASH).

Procedure
Transarterial chemoembolization for hepatocellular carcinoma

Pre-procedure Imaging
Contrast-enhanced CT performed at an outside hospital shows a 4-cm enhancing mass within segment 5 of the liver (Fig. 1). Contrast-enhanced MRI of the liver shows the mass to have early arterial enhancement with central wash-out, compatible with hepatocellular carcinoma.

Intraprocedural Findings
A hyperenhancing mass is identified in segment 5, corresponding to the lesion identified on CT and MRI (Fig. 2). Attempts at superselective catheterization of the segment 5 branch of the right hepatic artery were not successful; a combination of mitomycin and doxorubicin with Ethiodol was injected into the distal right hepatic artery, followed by embolization using 300-µm to 500-µm calibrated microspheres (Fig. 3).

Follow-up and Complications
The patient returned 6 weeks later and underwent CT-guided radiofrequency ablation (RFA) of the tumor (Fig. 4); there was no residual lesion enhancement on follow-up MRI. Three months after the RFA, the patient underwent liver transplantation; there was no viable tumor at pathology, and the patient has had no recurrence on follow-up.

Suggested Readings
Brown DB, Geschwind JF, Soullen MC, et al: Society of Interventional Radiology position statement on chemoembolization of hepatic malignancies. J Vasc Intervent Radiol 17:217-223, 2006.

Higgins MC, Soulen MC: Multimodality approaches for control of hepatocellular carcinoma. Tech Vasc Intervent Radiol 10:64-66, 2007.

Llovet JM, Brux J: A systematic review of randomized trials for unresectable hepatocellular carcinoma chemoembolization improves survival. Hepatology 37:429-442, 2003.

Llovet JM, Fuster J, Bruix J: The Barcelona approach: Diagnosis, staging, and treatment of hepatocellular carcinoma. Liver Transplant 10:S115-S120, 2004.

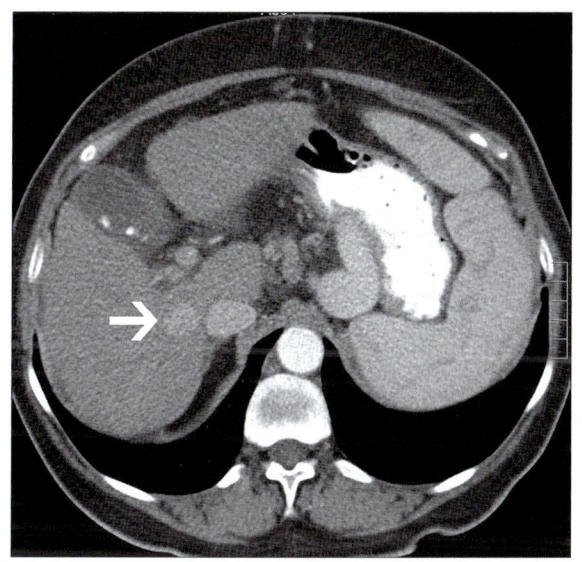

Figure 1. Contrast-enhanced CT of the abdomen shows a homogeneously enhancing mass (arrow) in segment 5 of the liver, compatible with hepatocellular carcinoma.

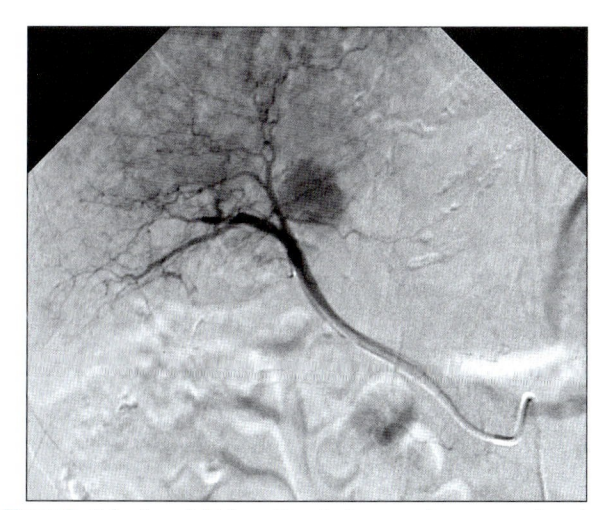

Figure 2. Selective right hepatic arteriogram shows an enhancing mass within the right hepatic lobe.

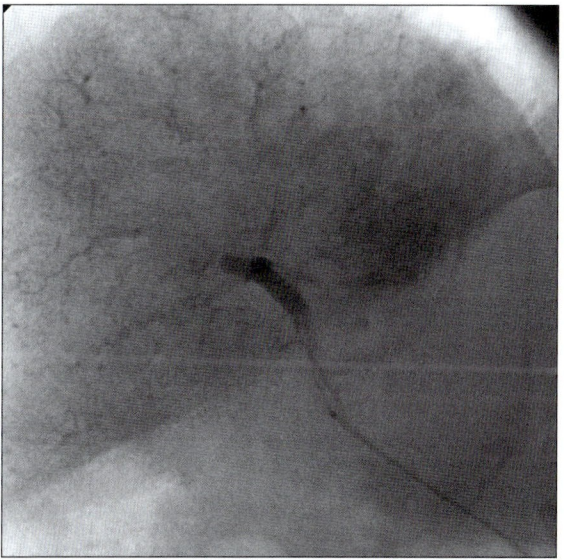

Figure 3. Spot fluoroscopic image after chemoembolization. Because of the small size of the segment 5 branch, superselective catheterization was not possible. Chemoembolization was performed through a 3-French microcatheter positioned in the distal right hepatic artery. After chemoembolization, Ethiodol is seen throughout the right hepatic lobe, with stasis of contrast in the distal right hepatic artery.

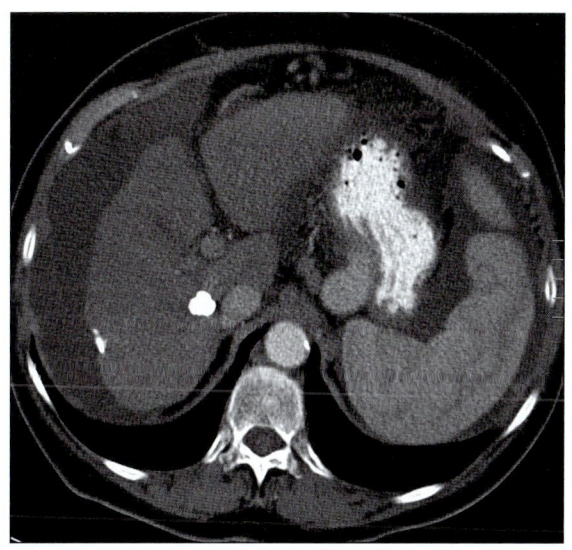

Figure 4. Contrast-enhanced CT performed at the time of RFA, 6 weeks after chemoembolization. The lesion is clearly visible because of the retained Ethiodol.

Case 135

DEMOGRAPHICS/CLINICAL HISTORY

A 48-year-old man with metastatic melanoma to the liver.

DISCUSSION

History/Indications for Procedure
A 48-year-old man with metastatic melanoma to the liver. The liver lesions have not responded to systemic chemotherapy.

Procedure
Hepatic chemoembolization for metastatic melanoma

Pre-procedure Imaging
Contrast-enhanced CT of the abdomen shows near complete replacement of the left hepatic lobe by a heterogeneously enhancing mass (Fig.1). The mass extends into the right lobe and numerous right lobe lesions are also present.

Intraprocedural Findings
There is a large hypervascular mass within the left hepatic lobe and multiple hyperenhancing masses throughout the right hepatic lobe (Figs. 2 and 3). A dose of 100 mg of carmustine (BCNU) mixed with 10 ml of Ethiodol was injected into the left hepatic artery, followed by embolization with 300-μm to 500-μm calibrated microspheres (Embospheres, Biosphere Medical, Rockland, Mass).

Follow-up and Complications
Contrast-enhanced CT performed 2 months after treatment shows reduction in tumor size of the left hepatic lobe lesions with retained Ethiodol throughout much of the tumor (Fig. 4). Multiple untreated lesions are present in the right hepatic lobe.

Suggested Readings
Patel K, Sullivan K, Berd D, et al: Chemoembolization of the hepatic artery with BCNU for metastatic uveal melanoma: Results of a phase II study. Melanoma Res 15:297-304, 2005.

Sharma KV, Gould JE, Harbour JW, et al: Hepatic arterial chemoembolization for management of metastatic melanoma. AJR Am J Roentgenol 190:99-104, 2008.

Vogl T, Eichler K, Zangos S, et al: Preliminary experience with transarterial chemoembolization (TACE) in liver metastases of uveal malignant melanoma: Local tumor control and survival. J Cancer Res Clin Oncol 133:177-184, 2007.

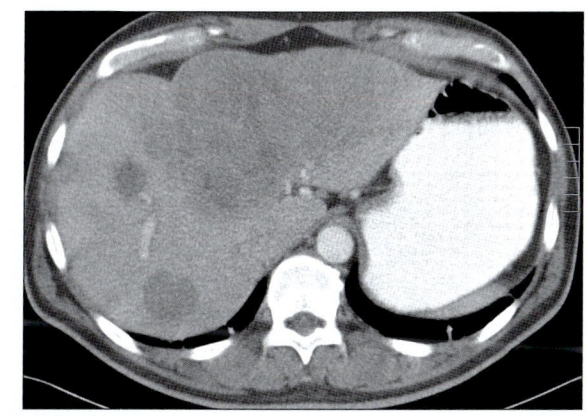

Figure 1. Single axial image from contrast-enhanced CT of the abdomen demonstrates multiple hypodense masses throughout the left and right hepatic lobes. There is nearly complete replacement of the left hepatic lobe by tumor.

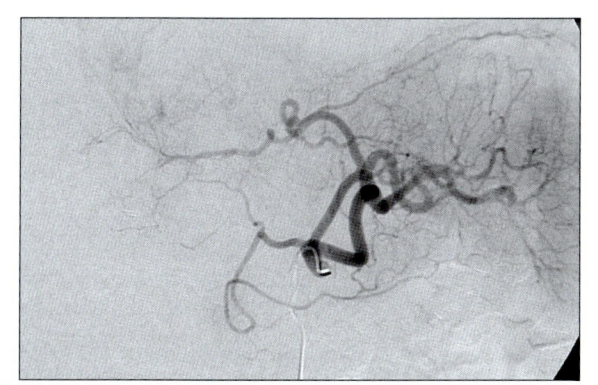

Figure 2. Celiac angiogram shows the left hepatic artery to arise from the left gastric artery. Subtle tumor vascularity is evident in the left hepatic lobe.

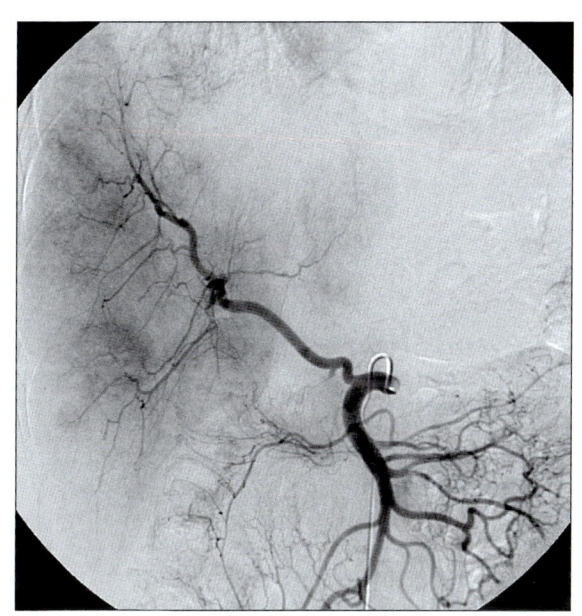

Figure 3. Selective angiogram with the catheter in the superior mesenteric artery shows a replaced right hepatic artery. Multiple hypervascular masses are present throughout the right hepatic lobe, supplied by the right hepatic artery.

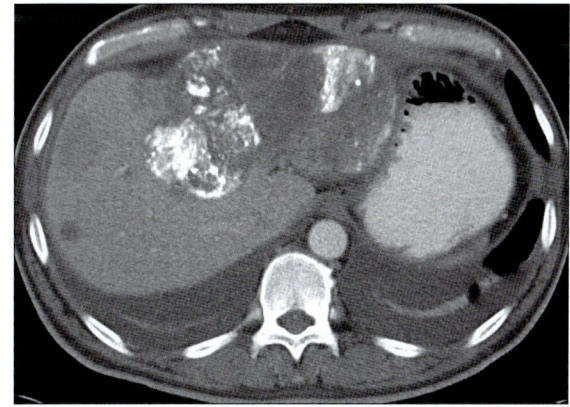

Figure 4. Single image from contrast-enhanced CT performed 2 months after TACE shows retained Ethiodol throughout much of the tumor in the left hepatic lobe. The tumor has slightly decreased in size when compared with the pre-treatment scan.

Case 136

DEMOGRAPHICS/CLINICAL HISTORY

Bland embolization for a 59-year-old woman with small bowel carcinoid tumor metastatic to the liver, undergoing magnetic resonance imaging (MRI), arteriography, and embolization.

DISCUSSION

History/Indications for Procedure
A 59-year-old woman has small bowel carcinoid tumor metastatic to the liver. The patient has right upper quadrant discomfort and mild diarrhea.

Procedure
Bland embolization for metastatic carcinoid tumor

Pre-procedure Imaging
Contrast-enhanced MRI shows several enhancing lesions in the liver that were consistent with metastatic neuroendocrine tumor. Most lesions are located in the right lobe.

Intraprocedural Findings
Hepatic arteriogram reveals several small areas of abnormal enhancement that are consistent with the patient's known metastatic disease (Fig. 1). The right hepatic artery was embolized with 100-μm to 300-μm and 300-μm to 500-μm calibrated microspheres (Fig. 2).

Follow-up and Complications
The patient's symptoms resolved after embolization, and MRI demonstrated a satisfactory response to embolization (Fig. 3). One year later, the symptoms returned, and the patient underwent repeat hepatic embolization.

Suggested Readings
Brown KT, Nevins AB, Getrajdman GI, et al: Particle embolization of hepatic neuroendocrine metastases for control of pain and hormonal symptoms. J Vasc Intervent Radiol 10:397-403, 1999.

Gupta S, Johnson MM, Murthy R, et al: Hepatic arterial embolization and chemoembolization for the treatment of patients with metastatic neuroendocrine tumors: Variables affecting response rates and survival. Cancer 104:1590-1602, 2005.

Madoff DC, Gupta S, Ahrar K, et al: Update on the management of neuroendocrine hepatic metastases. J Vasc Intervent Radiol 17:1235-1250, 2006.

Case 136   273

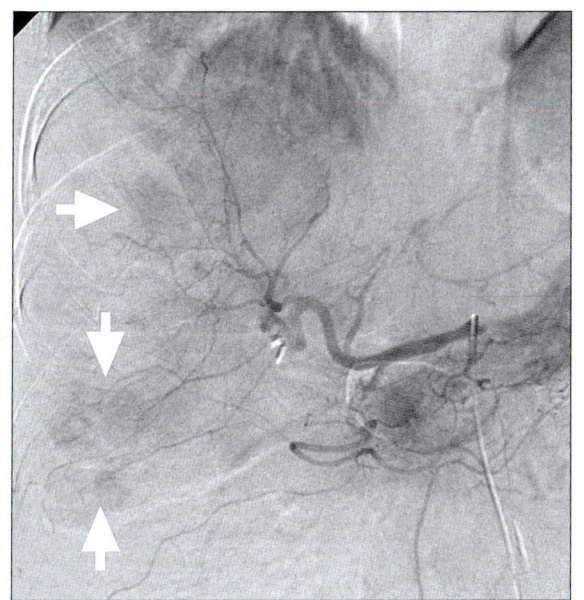

Figure 1. Hepatic arteriogram demonstrates many faintly hypervascular lesions throughout the right hepatic lobe (*arrows*). They correspond to the lesions seen on MRI.

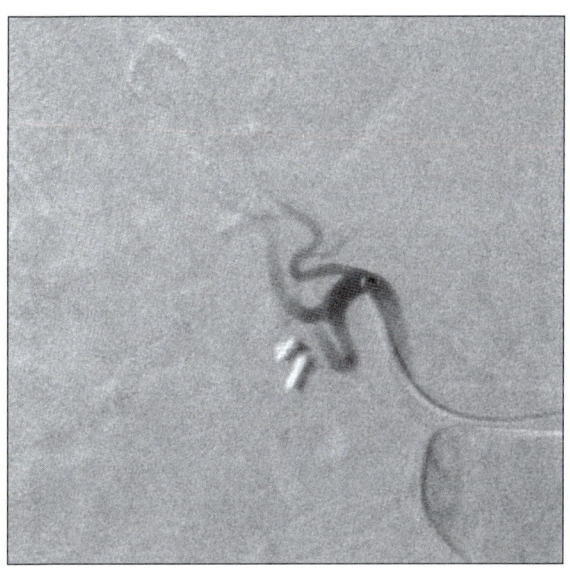

Figure 2. The right hepatic artery was embolized to stasis with 100-μm to 300-μm and 300-μm to 500-μm calibrated microspheres.

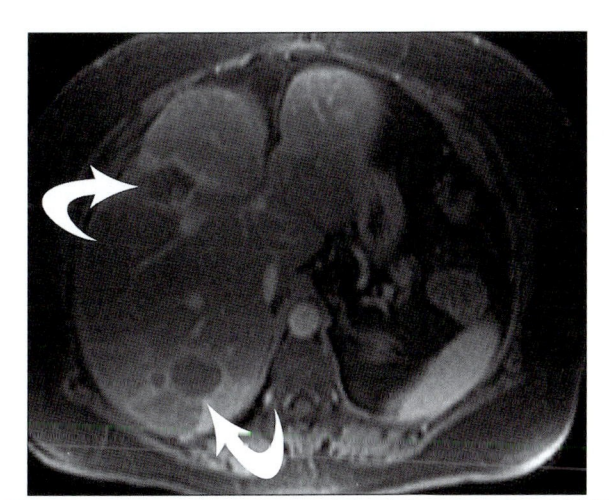

Figure 3. Contrast-enhanced, T1-weighted, fat-saturated, axial MR image demonstrates many hypoenhancing lesions in the right hepatic lobe that are consistent with treated metastases (*arrows*).

Case 137

DEMOGRAPHICS/CLINICAL HISTORY

A 47-year-old man with hepatitis C, undergoing surveillance MRI.

DISCUSSION

History/Indications for Procedure
This patient has a history of hepatitis C and exophytic hepatocellular carcinoma arising from segment 6. The lesion has enlarged on surveillance MRI.

Procedure
Bland embolization of hepatocellular carcinoma

Pre-procedure Imaging
Contrast-enhanced MRI shows a heterogeneous 5.5-cm exophytic mass arising from the right hepatic lobe (Fig. 1).

Intraprocedural Findings
The hypervascular mass was identified on angiography (Fig. 2). Superselective catheterization was performed, and the mass was embolized with 300-μm to 500-μm Embospheres.

Follow-up and Complications
Three months after embolization, the mass measured 2.6 cm with only minimal peripheral enhancement (Fig. 3). The mass has remained stable in size at 1-year follow-up (Fig. 4).

Suggested Readings
Brown KT, Nevins AB, Getrajdman GI, et al: Particle embolization of hepatocellular carcinoma. J Vasc Intervent Radiol 9:822-828, 1998.

Llovet JM, Real MI, Montana X, et al; Barcelona Clinic Liver Cancer Group: Arterial embolisation or chemoembolisation versus symptomatic treatment in patients with unresectable hepatocellular carcinoma: A randomized controlled trial. Lancet 359:1734-1739, 2002.

Maluccio M, Covey AM, Gandhi R, et al: Comparison of survival rates after bland embolization and ablation versus surgical resection for treating patients with solitary hepatocellular carcinoma up to 7 cm. J Vasc Intervent Radiol 16:955-961, 2005.

Case 137   275

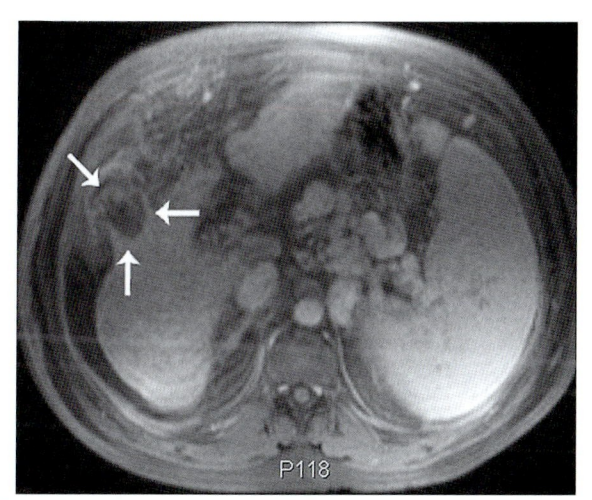

Figure 1. Contrast-enhanced MRI shows an exophytic mass *(arrows)* arising from segment 6 of the liver.

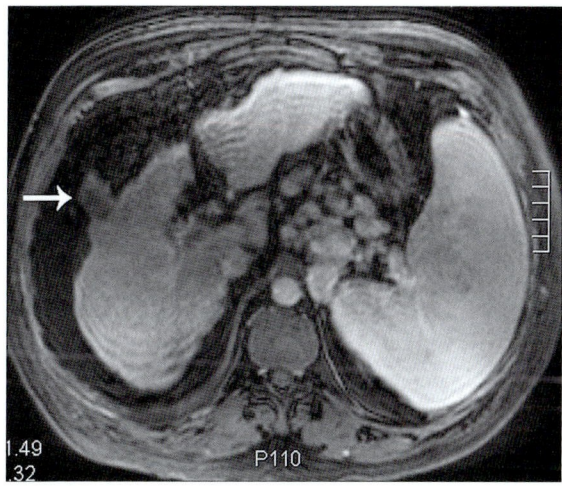

Figure 3. Single image from contrast-enhanced MRI performed 3 months after embolization shows the lesion has decreased in size *(arrow)*.

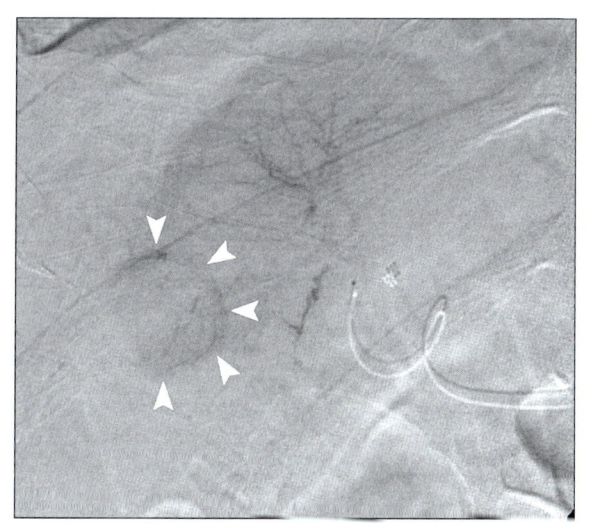

Figure 2. Hepatic angiogram, capillary phase, shows the hypervascular rim around the mass *(arrowheads)*.

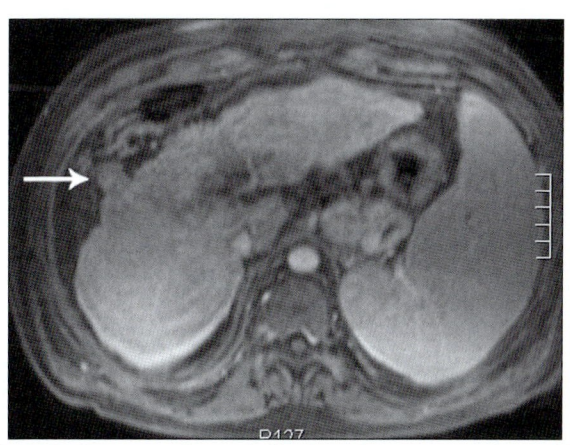

Figure 4. One year after embolization, the mass remains stable *(arrow)* on MRI without any further treatment.

Case 138

DEMOGRAPHICS/CLINICAL HISTORY

An 18-year-old man with a large hepatic adenoma, undergoing magnetic resonance imaging (MRI), angiography, and computed tomography (CT).

DISCUSSION

History/Indications for Procedure
An 18-year-old man with a large hepatic adenoma.

Procedure
Hepatic adenoma embolization

Pre-procedure Imaging
Contrast-enhanced MRI shows multiple liver masses; the largest was 6 cm × 5.4 cm and was located in the right hepatic lobe (Fig. 1). The masses show heterogeneous arterial enhancement with delayed wash-out. Percutaneous biopsy confirmed the diagnosis of hepatic adenoma.

Intraprocedural Findings
After injection, angiography shows a large, hypervascular mass in the right hepatic lobe (Fig. 2). The vessels supplying the mass were selectively catheterized and embolized with 100-μm to 300-μm calibrated microspheres and Ethiodol.

Follow-up and Complications
The patient returned to the emergency department with right upper quadrant pain 1 week after the embolization, and CT performed at the time showed postembolization changes (Fig. 3). Follow-up MRI 3 months after embolization showed complete infarction of the mass (Fig. 4).

Suggested Readings

Ault GT, Wren SM, Ralls PW, et al: Selective management of hepatic adenomas. Am Surg 10:825-829, 1996.

Erdogan D, van Delden OM, Busch OR, et al: Selective transcatheter arterial embolization for treatment of bleeding complications or reduction of tumor mass of hepatocellular adenomas. Cardiovasc Intervent Radiol 30:1252-1258, 2007.

Kim YI, Chung JW, Park JH: Feasibility of transcatheter arterial chemoembolization for hepatic adenoma. J Vasc Intervent Radiol 18:862-867, 2007.

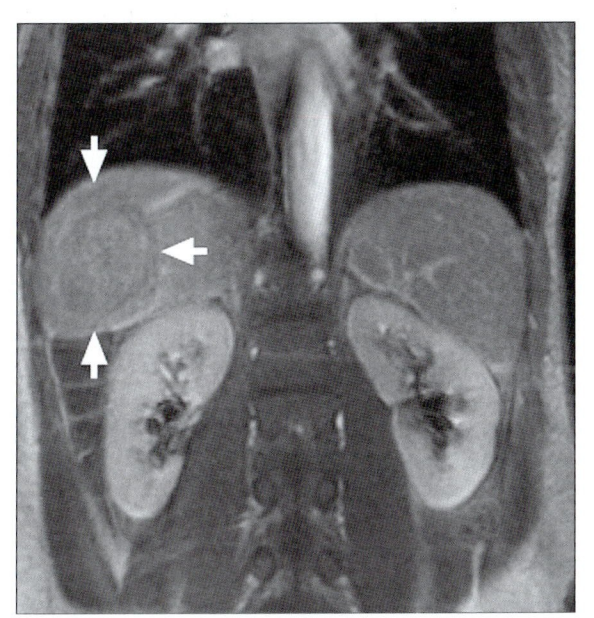

Figure 1. Coronal MRI after gadolinium administration shows a heterogeneously enhancing mass in the right hepatic lobe (*arrows*).

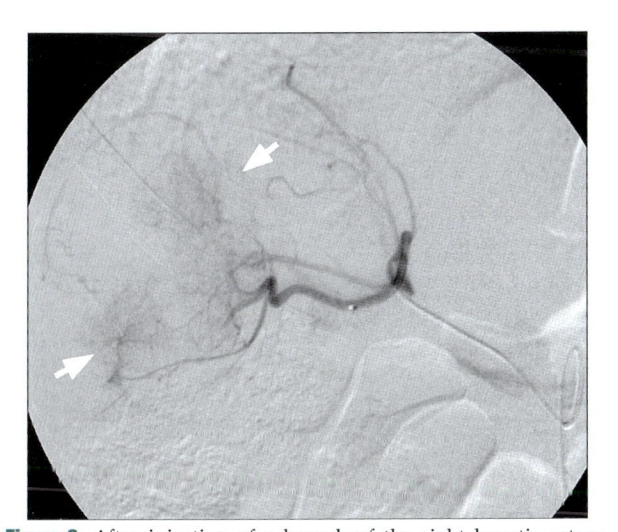

Figure 2. After injection of a branch of the right hepatic artery, angiography shows abnormal vascularity (*arrows*) in the right hepatic lobe within the large adenoma.

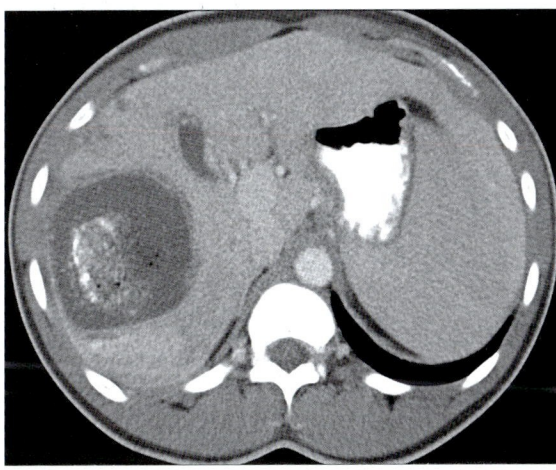

Figure 3. Contrast-enhanced CT performed 1 week after the embolization shows fluid density in the mass. There is some retained Ethiodol and gas bubbles in the mass, characteristic of postembolization changes. The patient responded to conservative management.

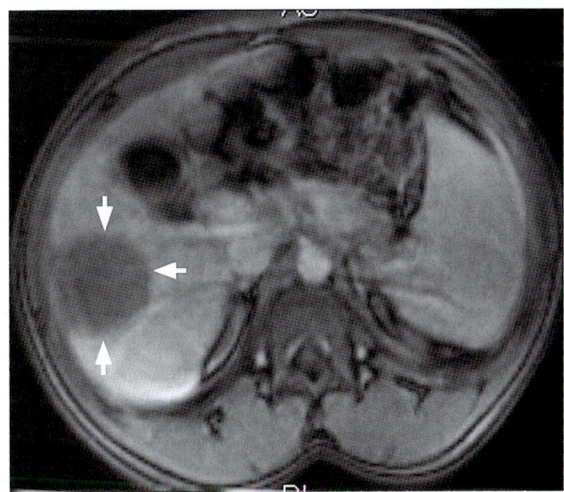

Figure 4. T1-weighted, post-contrast MRI 3 months after embolization shows no enhancement within the mass (*arrows*).

Case 139

DEMOGRAPHICS/CLINICAL HISTORY

A 5-year-old girl with hepatic hemangioendothelioma, undergoing angiography.

DISCUSSION

History/Indications for Procedure
This patient presented with spontaneous hemorrhage secondary to a large hepatic hemangioendothelioma.

Procedure
Embolization of hepatic hemangioendothelioma

Pre-procedure Imaging
CT scan of the abdomen shows a large vascular mass within the left lobe of the liver (Fig. 1). Dense ascites is present, consistent with the patient's history of spontaneous intraperitoneal hemorrhage.

Intraprocedural Findings
A diagnostic arteriogram performed through the superior mesenteric artery shows filling of multiple vascular channels in the left hepatic lobe (Figs. 2 and 3). The mass was embolized with small calibrated microspheres.

Follow-up and Complications
The patient showed no further evidence of bleeding after the embolization and went on to liver transplantation. The patient died 4 days after liver transplant.

Suggested Readings

Burke DR, Verstandig A, Edwards O, et al: Infantile hemangioendothelioma: Angiographic features and factors determining efficacy of hepatic artery embolization. Cardiovasc Intervent Radiol 9:154-157, 1986.

Kullendorff CM, et al: Embolization of hepatic hemangiomas in infants. Eur J Pediatr Surg 12:348-352, 2002.

Stanley P, Grinnell VS, Stanton RE, et al: Therapeutic embolization of infantile hepatic hemangiomas with polyvinyl alcohol. AJR Am J Roentgenol 41:1047, 1983.

Case 139   279

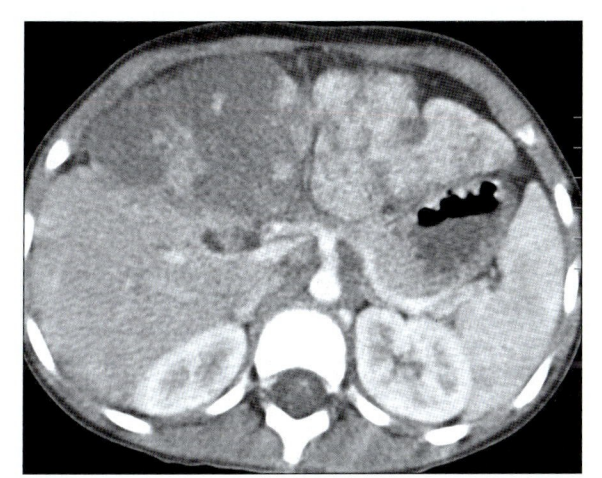

Figure 1. Single image from contrast-enhanced abdominal CT shows a large mass replacing most of the left hepatic lobe parenchyma.

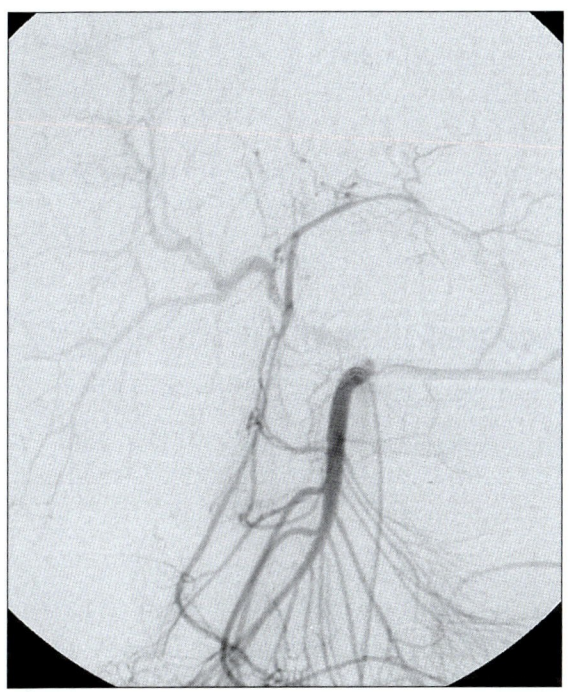

Figure 2. Superior mesenteric angiogram fills the hepatic artery through hypertrophied pancreaticoduodenal arteries.

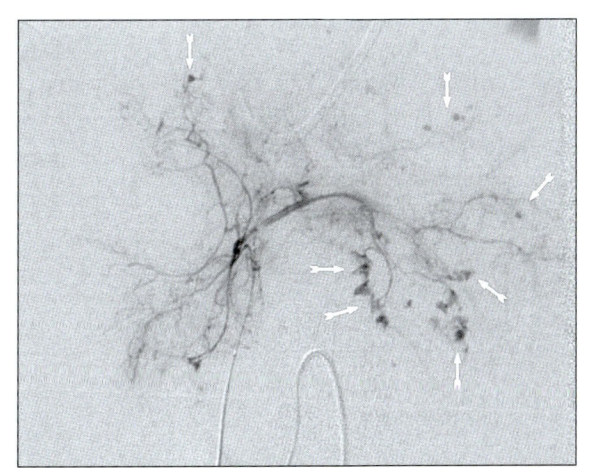

Figure 3. Selective injection of the left hepatic artery in the capillary phase shows filling of numerous abnormal vascular spaces *(arrows)* consistent with a hemangioendothelioma.

Case 140

DEMOGRAPHICS/CLINICAL HISTORY

A 76-year-old woman with hepatitis C, hepatic cirrhosis, and a new 1.3-cm mass in the right hepatic lobe, undergoing magnetic resonance imaging (MRI), computed tomography (CT), arteriography, radiofrequency ablation (RFA), and embolization.

DISCUSSION

History/Indications for Procedure
A 76-year-old woman has hepatitis C and hepatic cirrhosis. A new, 1.3-cm, enhancing mass was identified in the right hepatic lobe on screening MRI.

Procedure
Bland embolization for hepatic malignancies

Pre-procedure Imaging
Contrast-enhanced MRI demonstrates an early enhancing lesion in the right hepatic lobe that also exhibits early wash-out. The lesion is not visible on noncontrast CT, although it is visible after the intravenous administration of contrast.

Intraprocedural Findings
Right hepatic arteriogram demonstrates an enhancing mass in the right hepatic lobe (Fig. 1). Using a 3-French microcatheter, the supplying vessels were selectively catheterized and embolized using a combination of 300-μm to 500-μm calibrated microspheres and Ethiodol (Fig. 2).

Follow-up and Complications
The patient returned 1 month after the embolization and underwent CT-guided RFA of the mass (Fig. 3). Contrast-enhanced MRI performed 4 months after the embolization showed no evidence of viable tumor (Fig. 4).

Suggested Readings
Brown KT, Nevins AB, Getrajdman GI, et al: Particle embolization of hepatocellular carcinoma. J Vasc Intervent Radiol 9:822-828, 1998.

Llovet JM, Real MI, Montaña X, et al, for the Barcelona Clinic Liver Cancer Group: Arterial embolisation or chemoembolisation versus symptomatic treatment in patients with unresectable hepatocellular carcinoma: A randomized controlled trial. Lancet 359:1734-1739, 2002.

Lo CM, Ngan H, Tso WK, et al: Randomized controlled trial of transarterial lipiodol chemoembolization for unresectable hepatocellular carcinoma. Hepatology 35:1164-1171, 2002.

Maluccio M, Covey AM, Gandhi R, et al: Comparison of survival rates after bland embolization and ablation versus surgical resection for treating patients with solitary hepatocellular carcinoma up to 7 cm. J Vasc Intervent Radiol 16:955-961, 2005.

Case 140   281

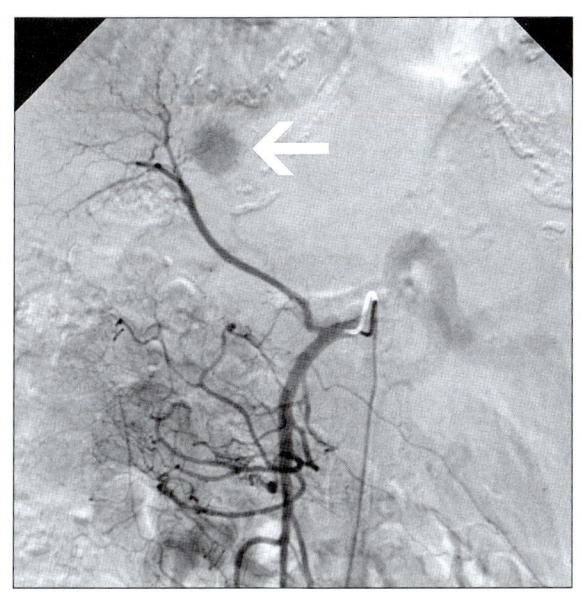

Figure 1. Selective injection of the superior mesenteric artery demonstrates a replaced right hepatic artery. There is a small round, enhancing mass in the right hepatic lobe *(arrow)*.

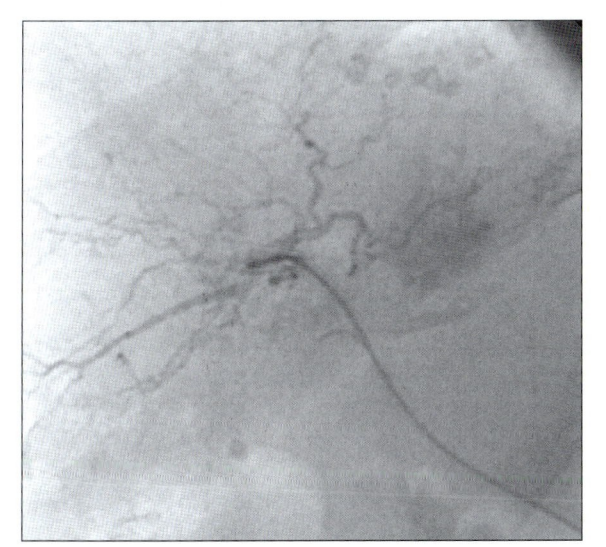

Figure 2. The feeding vessels were superselectively catheterized with a microcatheter, and the mass was embolized with a combination of Ethiodol and calibrated microspheres.

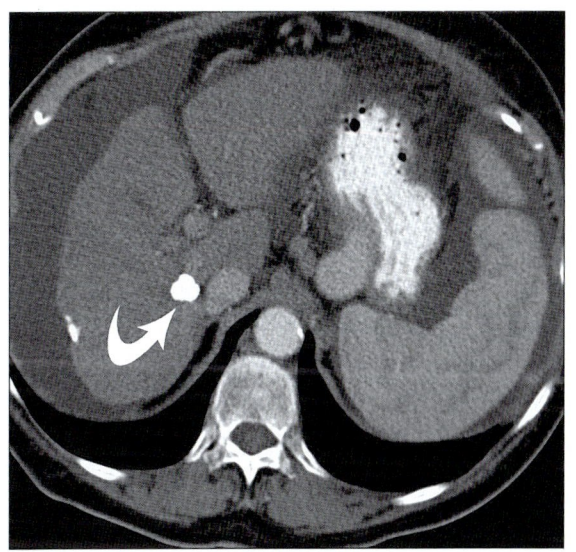

Figure 3. Unenhanced CT performed 1 month later shows retention of the Ethiodol within the lesion *(arrow)*. The lesion was ablated with radiofrequency energy at this time.

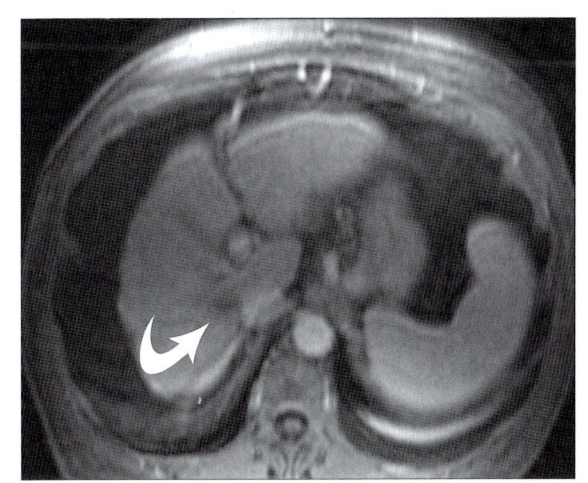

Figure 4. Contrast-enhanced MRI performed 4 months after the embolization shows decreased signal intensity in the region of the lesion *(arrow)*. No enhancement is seen.

Case 141

DEMOGRAPHICS/CLINICAL HISTORY

A 72-year-old man with a 15-cm hepatocellular carcinoma, undergoing magnetic resonance imaging (MRI), arteriography, and embolization.

DISCUSSION

History/Indications for Procedure

A 72-year-old man has a 15-cm hepatocellular carcinoma. He had undergone right portal vein embolization in anticipation of hepatic resection, but there was insufficient hypertrophy of the left hepatic lobe, and the plan for resection was aborted.

Procedure

Radioembolization for hepatocellular carcinoma

Pre-procedure Imaging

Contrast-enhanced MRI demonstrates a hypervascular mass in the right hepatic lobe measuring 15 cm × 10 cm (Fig. 1), and the right portal vein is thrombosed from prior portal vein embolization. The shunt study before using TheraSpheres revealed a 3.5% lung shunt.

Intraprocedural Findings

Selective injection of the right hepatic artery demonstrates a large, hypervascular mass in the right lobe of the liver (Figs. 2 and 3). An amount of approximately 3 GBq of TheraSpheres was administered to the tumor.

Follow-up and Complications

The patient showed an acceptable response to the initial radioembolization procedure (Fig. 4) and was treated a second time. Follow-up MRI after the second treatment demonstrated that the mass was slightly smaller in size, with a significant reduction in vascular enhancement.

Suggested Readings

Geschwind JF, Salem R, Carr BI, et al: Yttrium-90 microspheres for the treatment of hepatocellular carcinoma. Gastroenterology 127(Suppl 1):S194-S205, 2004.

Goin JE, Salem R, Carr BI, et al: Treatment of unresectable hepatocellular carcinoma with intrahepatic yttrium 90 microspheres: Factors associated with liver toxicities. J Vasc Intervent Radiol 16:205-213, 2005.

Salem R, Lewandowski R, Atassi B, et al: Treatment of unresectable hepatocellular carcinoma with use of ^{90}Y microspheres (TheraSphere): Safety, tumor response, and survival. J Vasc Intervent Radiol 16:1627-1639, 2005.

Salem R, Lewandowski R, Roberts C, et al: Use of yttrium-90 glass microspheres (TheraSphere) for the treatment of unresectable hepatocellular carcinoma in patients with portal vein thrombosis. J Vasc Intervent Radiol 15:335-345, 2004.

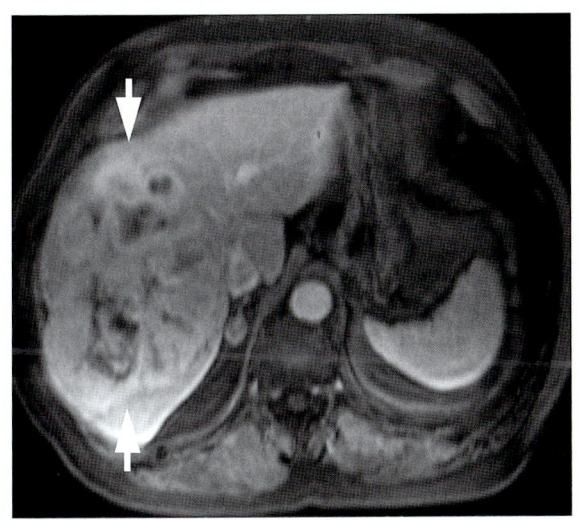

Figure 1. Pretreatment, contrast-enhanced, T1-weighted, post-gadolinium, fat-saturated, axial MR image shows a very large hypervascular mass within the right hepatic lobe *(arrows)*.

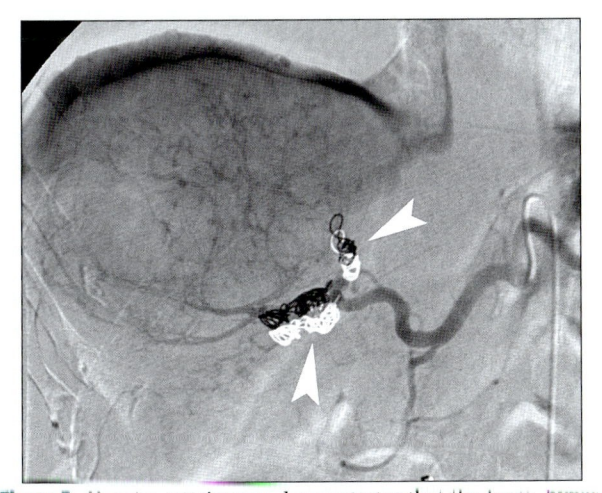

Figure 2. Hepatic arteriogram demonstrates that the large, hypervascular mass is supplied almost entirely by the right hepatic artery *(arrows)*. Metallic coils are present from a previous portal vein embolization.

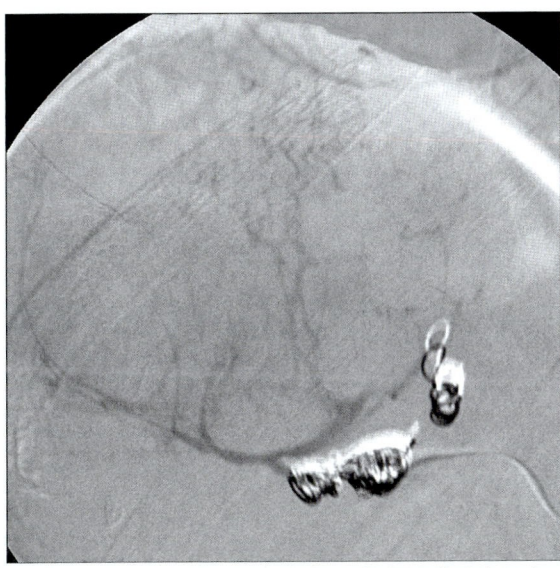

Figure 3. Contrast injection occurred just before administration of the radioactive microspheres. A microcatheter has been advanced into the distal right hepatic artery, where the ^{90}Y particles were administered.

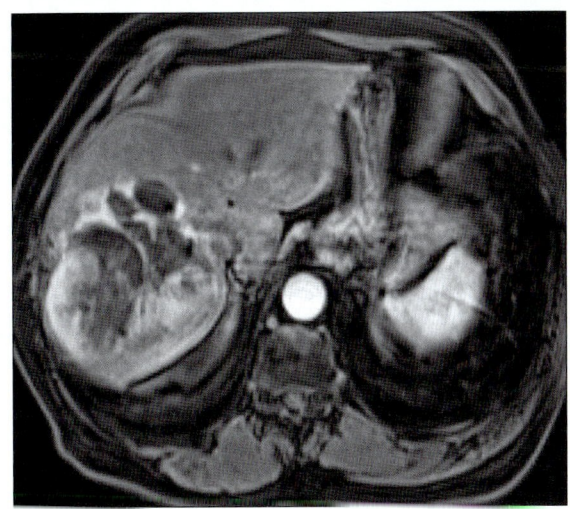

Figure 4. Follow-up MRI was performed after two treatments. The T1-weighted, post-gadolinium, fat-saturated, axial MR image demonstrates that the mass has slightly decreased in size, and there is significant reduction in tumor vascularity.

Case 142

DEMOGRAPHICS/CLINICAL HISTORY

A 77-year-old man with hepatocellular carcinoma and right upper quadrant pain.

DISCUSSION

History/Indications for Procedure
A 77-year-old man with biopsy-proven, well-differentiated hepatocellular carcinoma. The mass was discovered during a workup of unexplained right upper quadrant pain.

Procedure
Intra-arterial radioembolization for hepatocellular carcinoma

Pre-procedure Imaging
Unenhanced CT of the abdomen shows a large mass in the right hepatic lobe measuring 13 cm at greatest diameter (Fig. 1). Pre-treatment hepatic arteriogram shows the mass to be supplied by the right hepatic artery.

Intraprocedural Findings
A 3-French microcatheter was used to selectively catheterize the distal right hepatic artery, and selective arteriogram confirms the presence of the large hypervascular mass (Fig. 2). With the catheter in this location, the ^{90}Y beads (Theraspheres, MDS Nordian, Ottawa, Canada) were safely injected.

Follow-up and Complications
The patient experienced anorexia and malaise for 1 to 2 weeks after the procedure. His right upper quadrant pain improved after the treatment, and subsequent CT scans have shown progressive reduction in tumor size (Figs. 3 and 4).

Suggested Readings

Ibrahim SM, Lewandowski RJ, Sato KT, et al: Radioembolization for the treatment of unresectable hepatocellular carcinoma: A clinical review. World J Gastroenterol 21:1664-1669, 2008.

Kulik LM, Carr BI, Mulcahy MF, et al: Safety and efficacy of ^{90}Y radiotherapy for hepatocellular carcinoma with and without portal vein thrombosis. Hepatology 47:71-81, 2008.

Lewandowski RJ, Sato KT, Atassi B, et al: Radioembolization with ^{90}Y microspheres: Angiographic and technical considerations. Cardiovasc Intervent Radiol 30:571-592, 2007.

Salem R, Lewandowski RJ, Sato KT, et al: Technical aspects of radioembolization with ^{90}Y microspheres. Tech Vasc Intervent Radiol 10:12-29, 2007.

Case 142   285

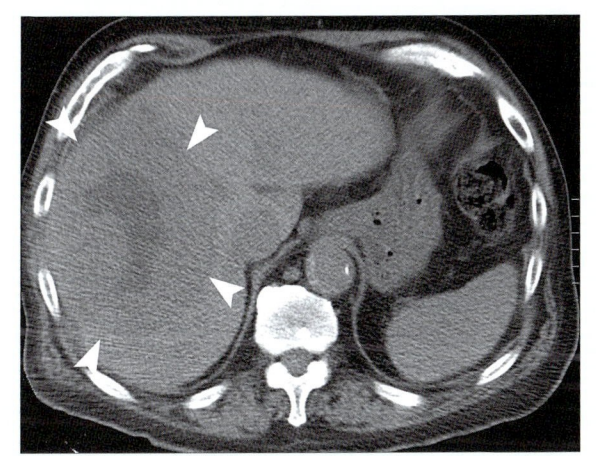

Figure 1. Unenhanced CT through the liver shows a large mass occupying much of the right hepatic lobe *(arrowheads)*. The mass exhibits central low attenuation, suggesting central necrosis.

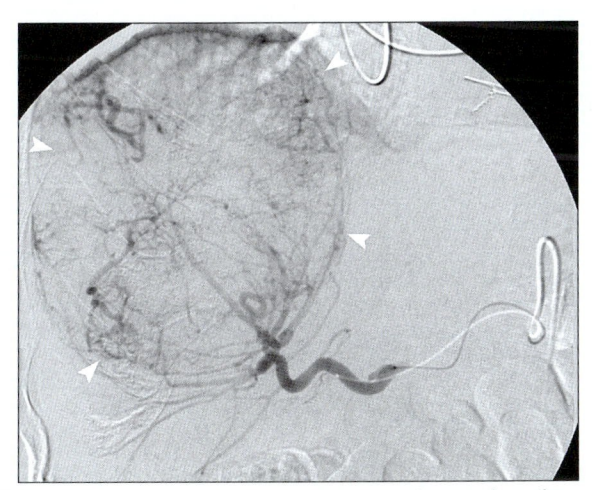

Figure 2. Selective right hepatic arteriogram shows a large hypervascular mass in the right hepatic lobe *(arrowheads)*.

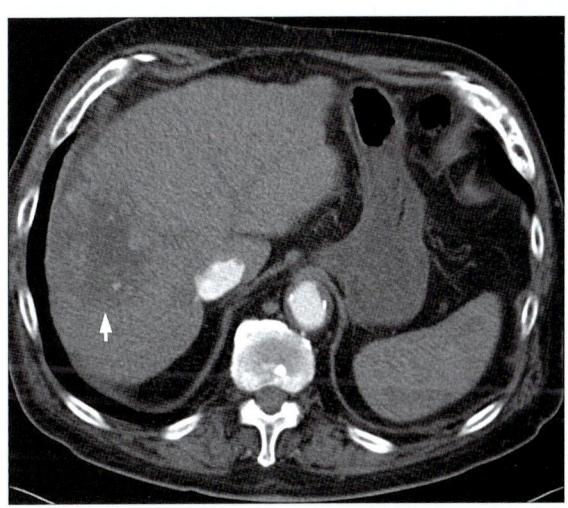

Figure 3. Follow-up contrast-enhanced CT performed 8 months after radioembolization shows the mass to be smaller in size *(arrow)*. The mass now measures 8.4 cm at greatest diameter.

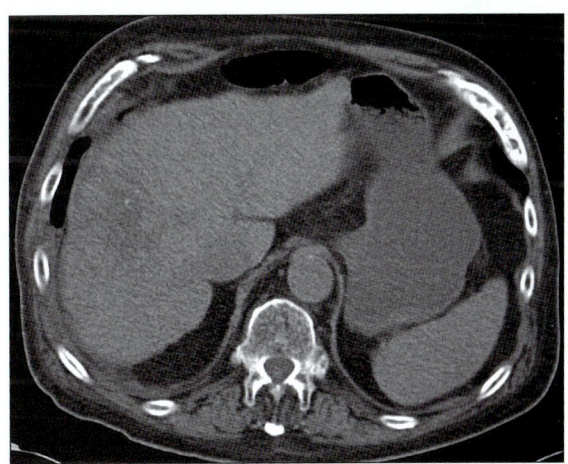

Figure 4. Unenhanced CT performed 13 months after radioembolization shows further reduction in size of the mass, which now measures 7.9 cm at greatest diameter.

Case 143

DEMOGRAPHICS/CLINICAL HISTORY

A 50-year-old man with advanced metastatic gastrinoma, undergoing magnetic resonance imaging (MRI) and arteriography.

DISCUSSION

History/Indications for Procedure

A 50-year-old man has advanced metastatic gastrinoma and a history of many hospital admissions for bleeding duodenal ulcers resulting from Zollinger-Ellison syndrome.

Procedure

Radioembolization for metastatic liver gastrinoma

Pre-procedure Imaging

Contrast-enhanced MRI of the abdomen shows numerous, hypervascular, metastatic lesions in bilateral lobes of the liver. The dominant lesion is located in the posterior right hepatic lobe and is 10 cm in diameter (Fig. 1).

Intraprocedural Findings

Visceral arteriogram shows conventional hepatic arterial anatomy with hepatomegaly with numerous, hypervascular masses (Fig. 2). TheraSpheres (MDS Nordion, Ottawa, ON, Canada), which are yttrium 90–labeled beads, were administered into the right hepatic artery.

Follow-up and Complications

Follow-up MRI shows a cystic change of the dominant lesion in the right hepatic lobe, with a slight overall decrease in enhancement of the remaining right hepatic lobe lesions (Fig. 3); there was progression of disease in the left hepatic lobe, and the patient underwent radioembolization of the left hepatic lobe approximately 6 months later. The dominant right lobe lesion remained stable until 1 year after the initial treatment, when MRI showed the lesion beginning to increase in size.

Suggested Readings

Atassi B, Bangash AK, Bahrani A, et al: Multimodality imaging following ^{90}Y radioembolization: A comprehensive review and pictorial essay. Radiographics 28:81-99, 2008.

Salem R, Thurston KG: Radioembolization with ^{90}yttrium microspheres—a state of the art brachytherapy treatment for primary and secondary liver malignancies. Part 1. Technical and methodological considerations. J Vasc Intervent Radiol 17:1251-1278, 2006.

Sato KT, Lewandowski RJ, Mulcahy MF, et al: Unresectable chemorefractory liver metastases: Radioembolization with ^{90}Y microspheres—safety, efficacy, and survival. Radiology 247:507-515, 2008.

Case 143   287

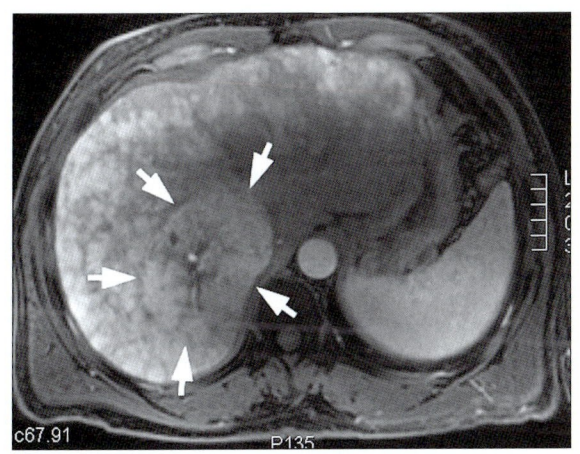

Figure 1. T1-weighted, fat-saturated, post-contrast MRI shows numerous, hyperenhancing hepatic lesions in both lobes of the liver. There is a dominant mass in segment VI *(arrows)*.

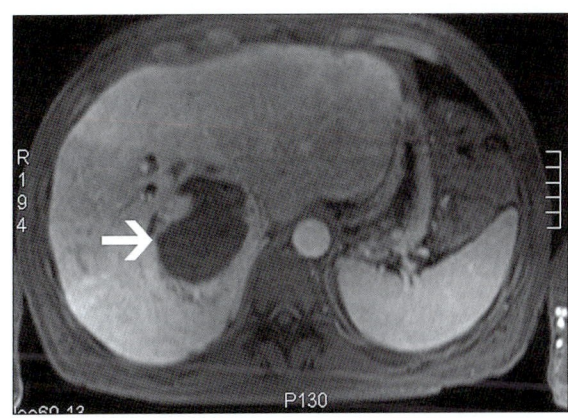

Figure 3. Follow-up MRI performed 3 months after radioembolization shows an interval cystic change of the dominant lesion in the right hepatic lobe *(arrow)*. The remaining right lobe lesions do show reduced enhancement relative to the pretreatment study levels.

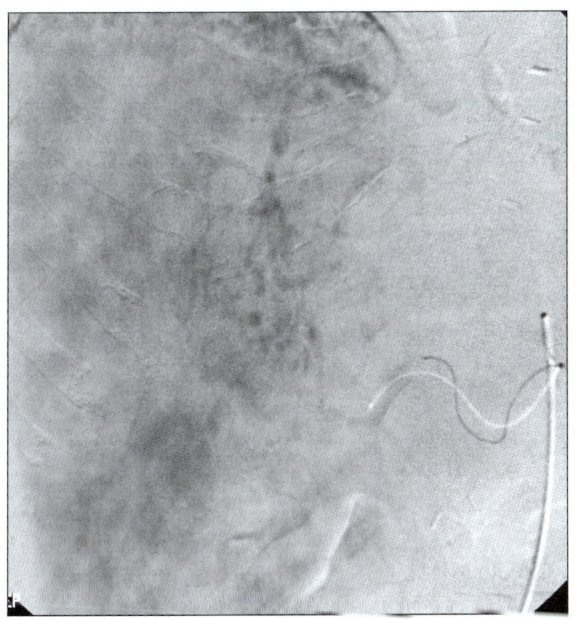

Figure 2. Delayed image of a selective right hepatic arteriogram shows hepatomegaly with numerous hypervascular masses.

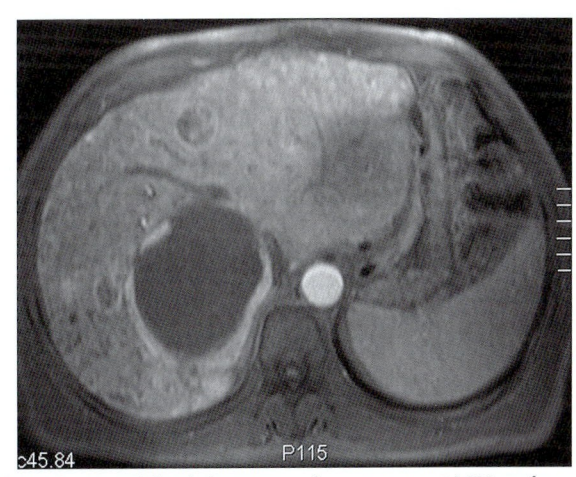

Figure 4. T1-weighted, fat-saturated, post-contrast MRI performed 1 year after the initial treatment shows continued cystic change of the dominant mass. The mass has started to increase in size, indicating viable tumor.

Case 144

DEMOGRAPHICS/CLINICAL HISTORY

A 71-year-old woman with carcinoid tumor metastatic to the liver, undergoing magnetic resonance imaging (MRI) and arteriography.

DISCUSSION

History/Indications for Procedure

A 71-year-old woman has small bowel carcinoid metastatic to the liver. Progression of the disease in the right hepatic lobe has been confirmed on surveillance imaging.

Procedure

Radioembolization for metastatic carcinoid

Pre-procedure Imaging

Contrast-enhanced MRI of the abdomen shows multiple, enhancing lesions in the right hepatic lobe (Fig. 1). The largest is 3.2 cm × 2.6 cm.

Intraprocedural Findings

A 3-French microcatheter was used to selectively catheterize the distal right hepatic artery (Fig. 2). The ^{90}Y beads were administered from this location.

Follow-up and Complications

Contrast-enhanced MRI performed 1 month after radioembolization shows a reduction in the size and enhancement of the right hepatic lesions (Fig. 3). MRI performed approximately 1 year later shows fibrosis of the right hepatic lobe in the region of the previously treated lesions, and several new, enhancing metastases have developed (Fig. 4).

Suggested Readings

Kennedy AS, Dezarn WA, McNeillie P, et al: Radioembolization for unresectable neuroendocrine hepatic metastases using resin ^{90}Y-microspheres: Early results in 148 patients. Am J Clin Oncol 31: 271-279, 2008.

King J, Quinn R, Glenn DM, et al: Radioembolization with selective internal radiation microspheres for neuroendocrine liver metastases. Cancer 113:921-929, 2008.

Murthy R, Kamat P, Nunez R, et al: Yttrium-90 microsphere radioembolotherapy of hepatic metastatic neuroendocrine carcinomas after hepatic arterial embolization. J Vasc Intervent Radiol 19:145-151, 2008.

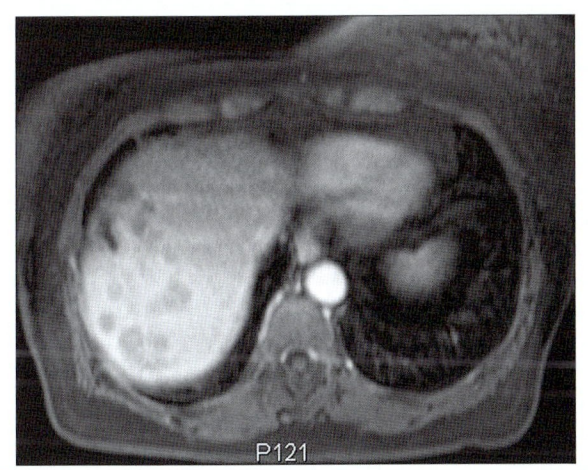

Figure 1. Contrast-enhanced MRI of the liver shows multiple lesions in the right hepatic lobe.

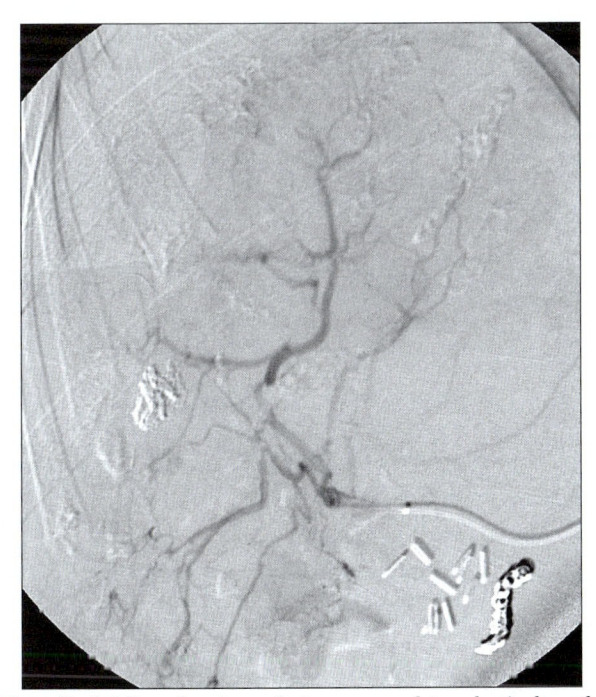

Figure 2. A 3-French microcatheter was used to selectively catheterize the right hepatic artery. The hepatic arteriogram shows some irregularity of the distal hepatic artery branches, likely from prior embolizations. The ^{90}Y beads were administered from this catheter location.

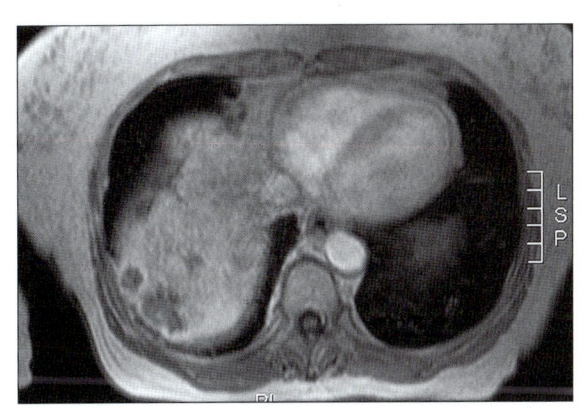

Figure 3. MRI 1 month after radioembolization shows that the lesions in the right hepatic lobe are smaller in size and have reduced enhancement, consistent with the effect of treatment.

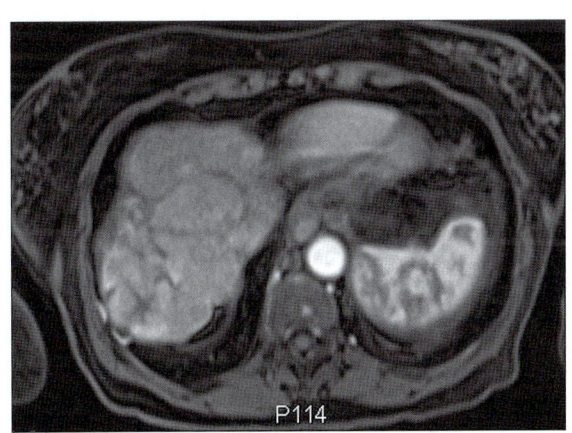

Figure 4. MRI 14 months after radioembolization shows fibrosis and scarring of the right hepatic lobe. The previous lesions are no longer seen, but several new hypervascular lesions have developed.

Case 145

DEMOGRAPHICS/CLINICAL HISTORY

A 62-year-old man with adenocarcinoma of the rectum metastatic to the liver, undergoing ultrasound.

DISCUSSION

History/Indications for Procedure
A 62-year-old man with adenocarcinoma of the rectum metastatic to the liver is preparing to undergo extended right hepatectomy.

Procedure
Portal vein embolization

Pre-procedure Imaging
A contrast-enhanced CT scan of the abdomen shows an 8.8-cm × 4.4-cm mass within the right lobe of the liver.

Intraprocedural Findings
The right portal vein was accessed with ultrasound using an ipsilateral approach (Fig. 1). The right portal vein was embolized using 100-μm to 300-μm microspheres followed by platinum coils (Figs. 2 and 3).

Follow-up and Complications
The volume of the future liver remnant increased from 21% to 38% after the portal vein embolization. The patient subsequently underwent a successful extended right hepatectomy.

Suggested Readings
Abulkhir A, Limongelli P, Healey AJ, et al: Preoperative portal vein embolization for major liver resection: A meta-analysis. Ann Surg 247:49, 2008.

Madoff DC, Abdalla EK, Gupta S, et al: Transhepatic ipsilateral right portal vein embolization extended to segment IV: Improving hypertrophy and resection outcomes with spherical particles and coils. J Vasc Intervent Radiol 16:215, 2005.

Madoff DC, Hicks ME, Abdalla EK, et al: Portal vein embolization with polyvinyl alcohol particles and coils in preparation for major liver resection for hepatobiliary malignancy: Safety and effectiveness—study in 26 patients. Radiology 227:251, 2003.

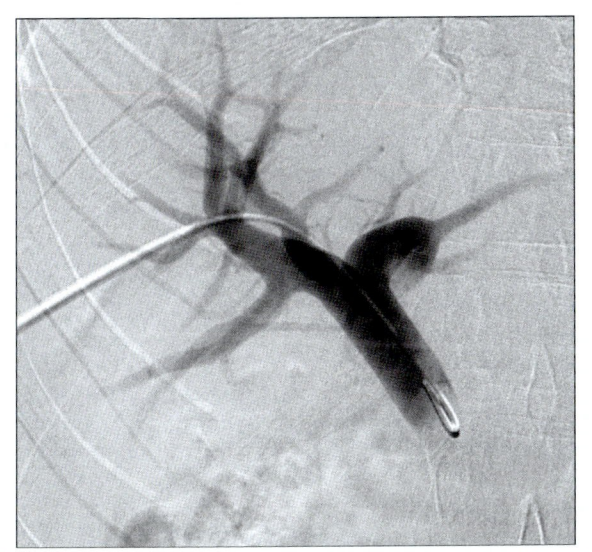

Figure 1. Portal venogram before embolization. Peripheral branch of right portal vein has been accessed using ultrasound guidance.

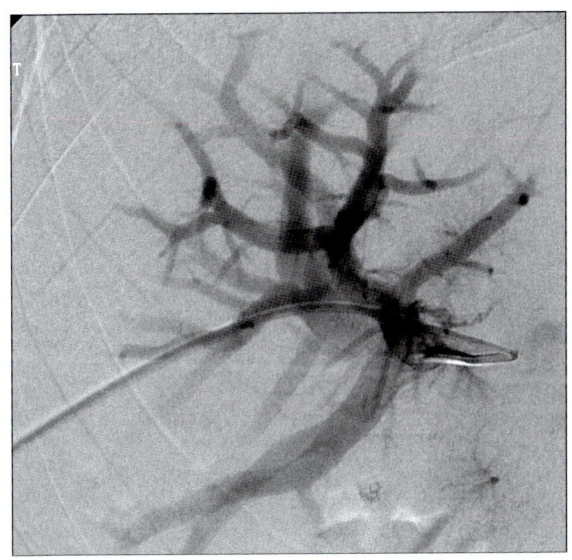

Figure 2. Portal venogram after particulate embolization. There is distal occlusion of right portal vein branches and sluggish flow within right portal vein.

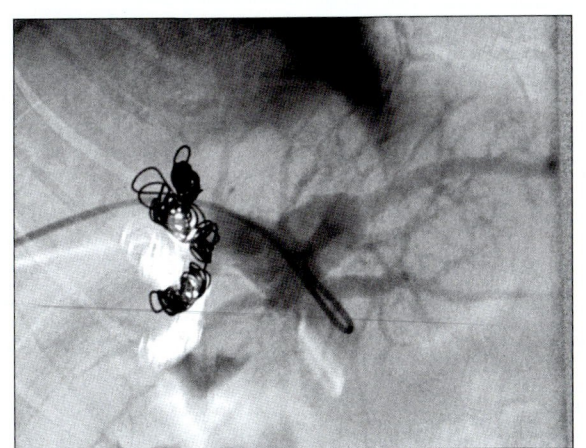

Figure 3. Postembolization portal venogram shows occlusion of right portal vein and preferential flow to segment-II and III branches of left portal vein

Case 146

DEMOGRAPHICS/CLINICAL HISTORY

An 87-year-old man who developed acalculous cholecystitis after a severe burn, undergoing ultrasound, arteriography, cholecystostomy catheter placement, and open cholecystectomy.

DISCUSSION

History/Indications for Procedure
An 87-year-old man suffered a severe burn as a result of a kerosene heater explosion. After a protracted stay in the intensive care unit, the patient developed abnormal liver function test results and findings consistent with acalculous cholecystitis.

Procedure
Hemorrhage after cholecystostomy catheter placement

Pre-procedure Imaging
Right upper quadrant ultrasound demonstrates a thickened, edematous gallbladder containing debris (Fig. 1).

Intraprocedural Findings
A cholecystostomy catheter was placed at the bedside with ultrasound guidance. The patient had significant hemorrhage from the cholecystostomy catheter, and extravasation from a branch of the cystic artery was identified on arteriography (Figs. 2 and 3).

Follow-up and Complications
Because the cystic artery could not be catheterized, coils were placed across the origin of the cystic artery (Fig. 4). The patient continued to have hemorrhagic output from the catheter, necessitating an open cholecystectomy.

Suggested Readings
Akhan O, Akinci D, Oxmen MN: Percutaneous cholecystostomy. Eur J Radiol 43:229-236, 2002.

Boland GW, Lee MJ, Leung J, Mueller PR: Percutaneous cholecystostomy in critically ill patients: Early response and final outcome in 82 patients. AJR Am J Roentgenol 163:339-342, 1994.

van Sonnenberg E, D'Agostino HB, Goodacre BW, et al: Percutaneous gallbladder puncture and cholecystostomy: Results, complications, and caveats for safety. Radiology 183:167-170, 1992.

van Sonnenberg E, Wittich GR, Casola G, et al: Diagnostic and therapeutic percutaneous gallbladder procedures. Radiology 160:23-26, 1986.

Yusoff IF, Barkun JS, Barkun AN: Diagnosis and management of cholecystitis and cholangitis. Gastroenterol Clin North Am 32:1145-1168, 2003.

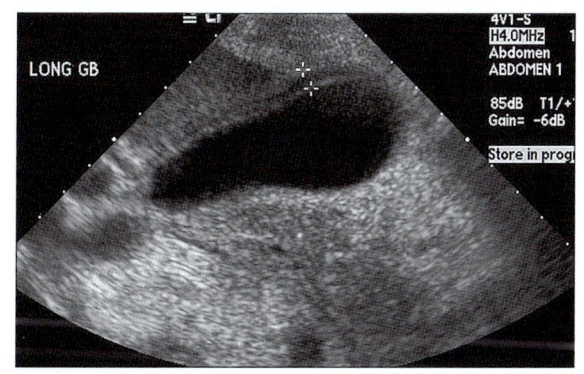

Figure 1. Right upper quadrant ultrasound demonstrates a thickened, edematous gallbladder.

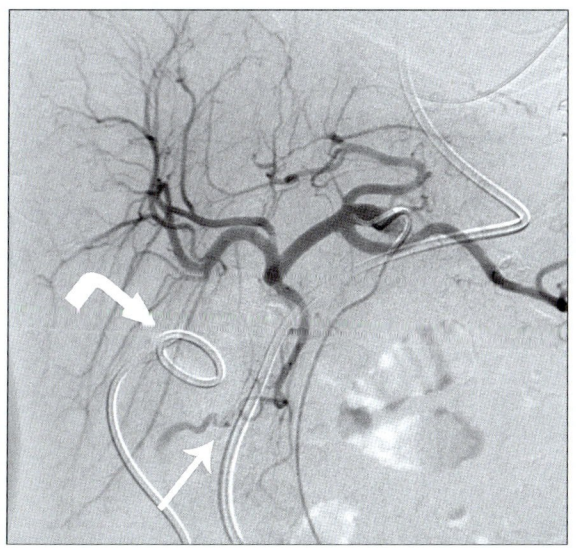

Figure 2. Celiac arteriogram 1 day after cholecystostomy catheter *(curved arrow)* placement demonstrates contrast extravasation into the gallbladder *(arrow)*.

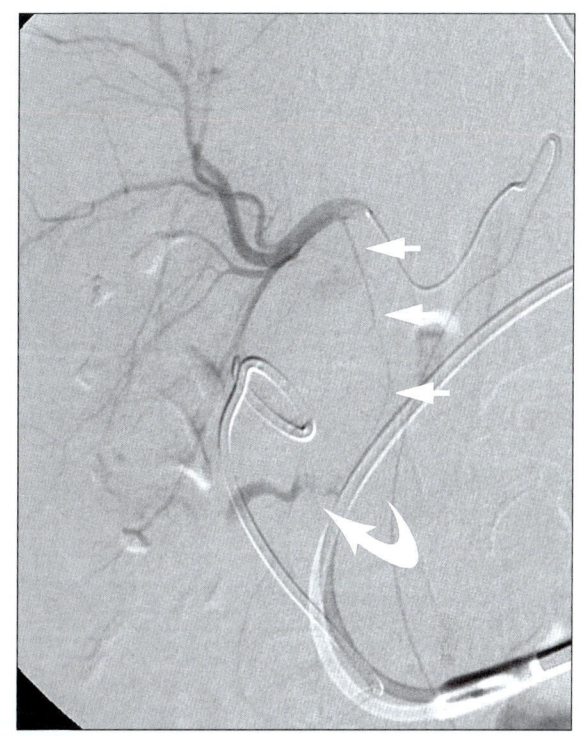

Figure 3. Selective injection of the right hepatic artery confirms the extravasation *(curved arrow)* from the cystic artery. Attempts to catheterize the cystic artery were unsuccessful *(arrows)*.

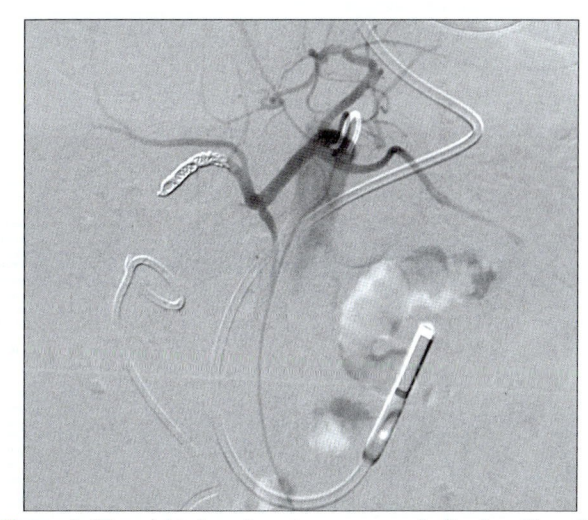

Figure 4. The right hepatic artery was embolized with coils deployed across the origin of the cystic artery. No further extravasation was seen after embolization.

Case 147

DEMOGRAPHICS/CLINICAL HISTORY

A 61-year-old man involved in a motor vehicle accident, undergoing CT.

DISCUSSION

History/Indications for Procedure
This patient has a severe liver laceration with active contrast extravasation on CT.

Procedure
Endovascular management for traumatic liver laceration

Pre-procedure Imaging
Contrast-enhanced CT shows a large, complex liver laceration with active contrast extravasation (Fig. 1).

Intraprocedural Findings
Hepatic angiography shows multiple areas of contrast extravasation throughout the right hepatic lobe (Fig. 2). The right hepatic artery was embolized with Gelfoam slurry (Fig. 3).

Follow-up and Complications
The patient stabilized after the embolization and was transferred to the intensive care unit. The patient had a complicated hospital course and died approximately 1 month after the embolization from multiorgan failure secondary to sepsis.

Suggested Readings
Ciraulo DL, Luk S, Palter M, et al: Selective hepatic arterial embolization of grade IV and V blunt hepatic injuries: An extension of resuscitation in the nonoperative management of traumatic hepatic injuries. J Trauma 45:353-358, 1998.

Hagiwara A, Yukioka T, Ohta S, et al: Nonsurgical management of patients with blunt hepatic injury: Efficacy of transcatheter arterial embolization. AJR Am J Roentgenol 169:1151-1156, 1997.

Hashimoto S, Hiramatsu K, Ido K, et al: Expanding role of emergency embolization in the management of severe blunt hepatic trauma. Cardiovasc Intervent Radiol 13:193-197, 1990.

Schwartz RA, Teitelbaum GP, Katz MD, et al: Effectiveness of transcatheter embolization in the control of hepatic vascular injuries. J Vasc Intervent Radiol 4:359-365, 1993.

Case 147   295

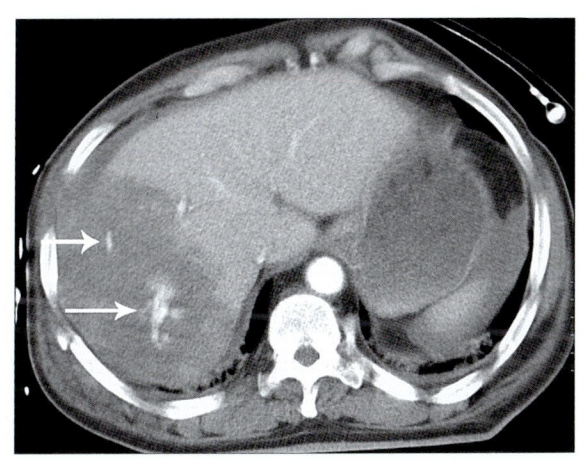

Figure 1. Contrast-enhanced CT scan shows a large laceration involving the right hepatic lobe with multiple areas of active contrast extravasation *(arrows)*.

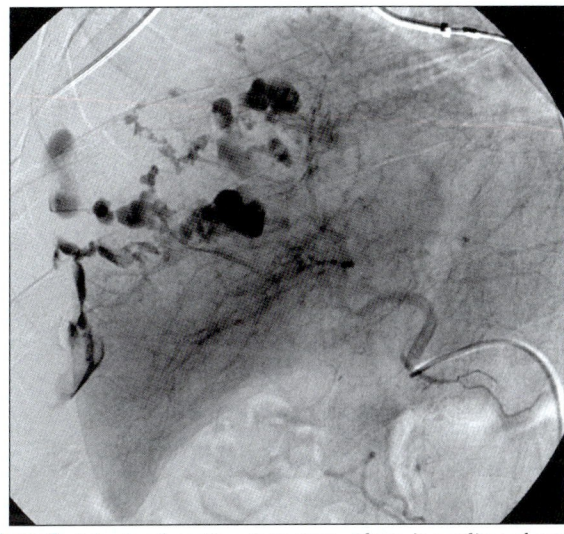

Figure 2. Selective hepatic arteriogram. There is pooling of extravascular contrast material throughout the large laceration.

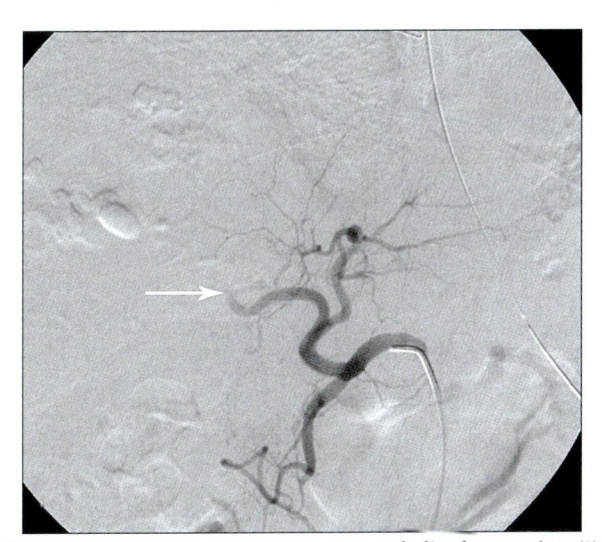

Figure 3. The right hepatic artery was embolized to stasis with Gelfoam slurry *(arrow)*.

Case 148

DEMOGRAPHICS/CLINICAL HISTORY

A 40-year-old woman involved in a motor vehicle collision, undergoing CT and arteriography.

DISCUSSION

History/Indications for Procedure
A 40-year-old woman was involved in a motor vehicle collision. On arrival to the emergency department, she had abdominal distention and tachycardia, and remained hypotensive despite aggressive fluid resuscitation and blood transfusions.

Procedure
Hepatic artery embolization for traumatic liver laceration

Pre-procedure Imaging
A contrast-enhanced CT scan shows a large, complex (grade IV) liver laceration with hemoperitoneum (Fig. 1).

Intraprocedural Findings
There is brisk contrast extravasation from the anterior branch of the right hepatic artery (Fig. 2). The anterior branch of the right hepatic artery was embolized with a combination of Gelfoam and coils (Fig. 3).

Follow-up and Complications
The patient's blood pressure stabilized after the procedure. A follow-up CT scan of the abdomen performed 2 weeks after the accident shows resolving intrahepatic hematoma (Fig. 4).

Suggested Readings
Fang JF, Wong YC, Lin BC, et al: The CT risk factors for the need of operative treatment in initially hemodynamically stable patients after blunt hepatic trauma. J Trauma 61:547, 2006.

Hashimoto S, Ido K, Hiramatsu K, et al: Expanding role of emergency embolization in the management of severe blunt hepatic trauma. Cardiovasc Intervent Radiol 13:193, 1990.

Schwartz RA, Teitelbaum GP, Katz MD, et al: Effectiveness of transcatheter embolization in the control of hepatic vascular injuries. J Vasc Intervent Radiol 4:359, 1993.

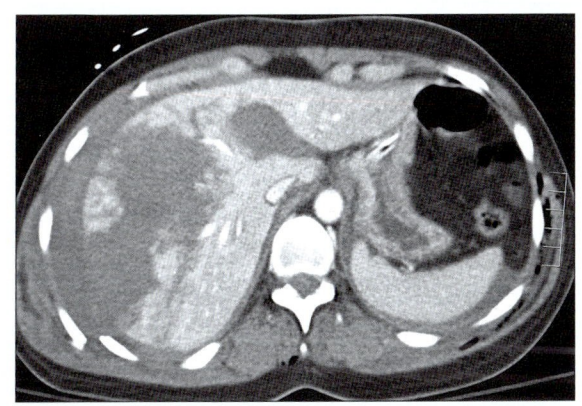

Figure 1. Contrast-enhanced CT scan through liver shows complex liver laceration in right hepatic lobe with adjacent perihepatic hematoma.

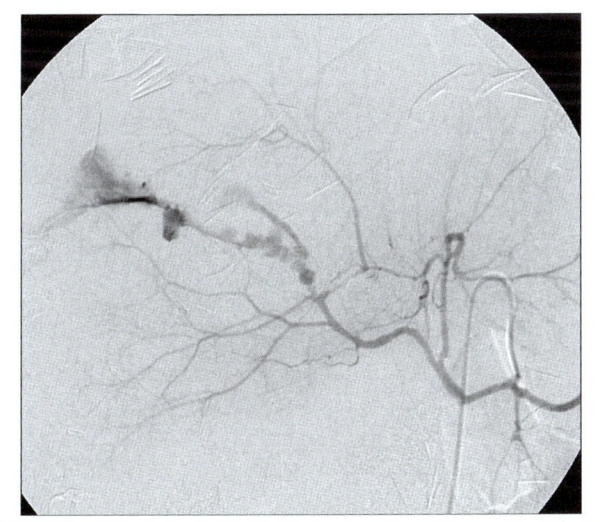

Figure 2. Celiac arteriogram shows massive extravasation from anterior branch of right hepatic artery.

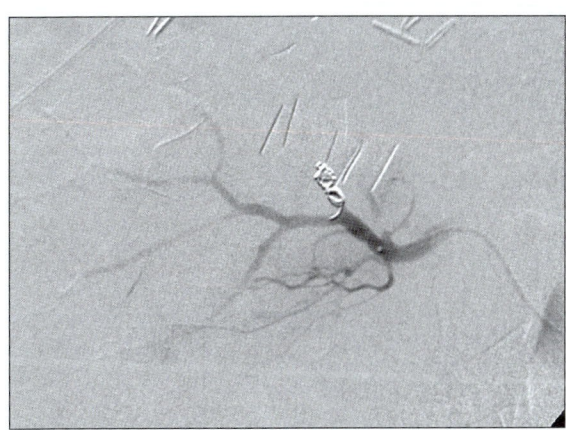

Figure 3. Anterior branch of right hepatic artery was embolized with combination of Gelfoam and coils.

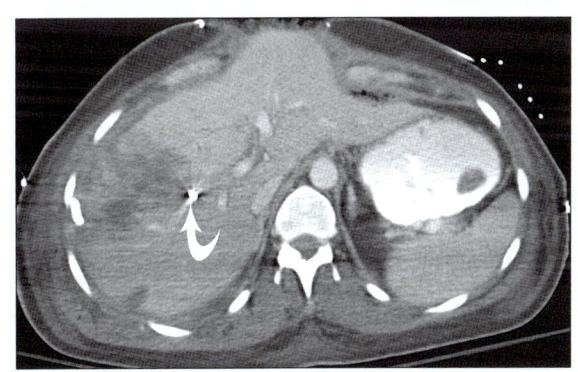

Figure 4. Follow-up CT scan performed 2 weeks after accident shows coils at edge of liver laceration (*arrow*). There is evidence for interval healing of the large laceration.

Case 149

DEMOGRAPHICS/CLINICAL HISTORY

A 24-year-old man with liver laceration after a fall, undergoing computed tomography (CT), arteriography, and embolization.

DISCUSSION

History/Indications for Procedure
A 24-year-old man fell 15 feet from a tree. The patient was hemodynamically unstable on presentation to the emergency department.

Procedure
Embolization for hepatic artery trauma

Pre-procedure Imaging
Contrast-enhanced CT of the abdomen demonstrates a complex laceration of the right hepatic lobe with active contrast extravasation (Fig. 1). There were several small splenic lacerations, with hemoperitoneum around the liver and spleen (Figs. 1 and 2).

Intraprocedural Findings
Hepatic arteriogram demonstrates active contrast extravasation from a branch of the right hepatic artery in the posterior right hepatic lobe (Fig. 3). The right hepatic artery was embolized with Gelfoam (Fig. 4).

Follow-up and Complications
The patient's vital signs stabilized after embolization, and he was observed in the hospital and discharged home with no further evidence of hemorrhage. The patient has remained asymptomatic on follow-up.

Suggested Readings

Hagiwara A, Yukioka T, Ohta S, et al: Nonsurgical management of patients with blunt hepatic injury: Efficacy of transcatheter arterial embolization. AJR Am J Roentgenol 169:1151-1156, 1997.

Hagiwara A, Yukioka T, Shimazaki S, et al: Delayed hemorrhage following catheter arterial embolization for blunt hepatic injury. Cardiovasc Intervent Radiol 16:380-383, 1993.

Schwartz RA, Teitelbaum GP, Katz MD, Pentecost MJ: Effectiveness of transcatheter embolization in the control of hepatic vascular injuries. J Vasc Intervent Radiol 4:359-365, 1993.

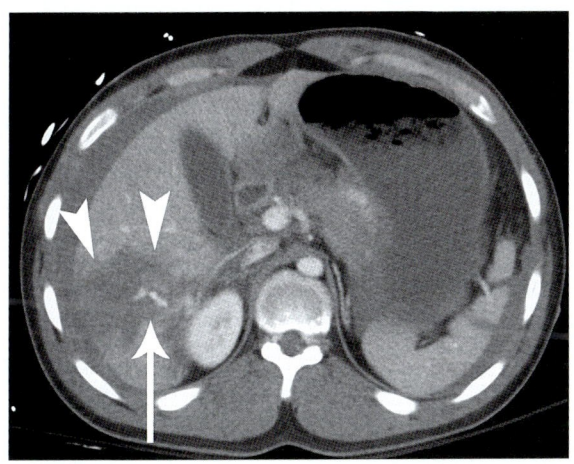

Figure 1. Contrast-enhanced, axial CT image of the abdomen demonstrates a complex laceration of the posterior right hepatic lobe *(arrowheads)*. There is active contrast extravasation within the laceration *(arrow)*.

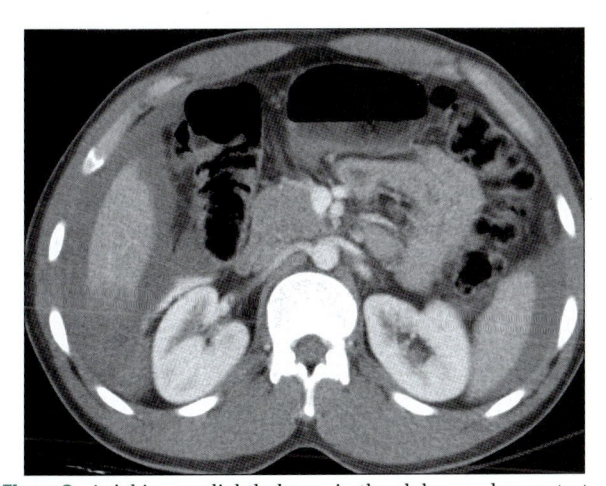

Figure 2. Axial image slightly lower in the abdomen demonstrates a moderate amount of high-density fluid around the liver and spleen, which is consistent with hemoperitoneum.

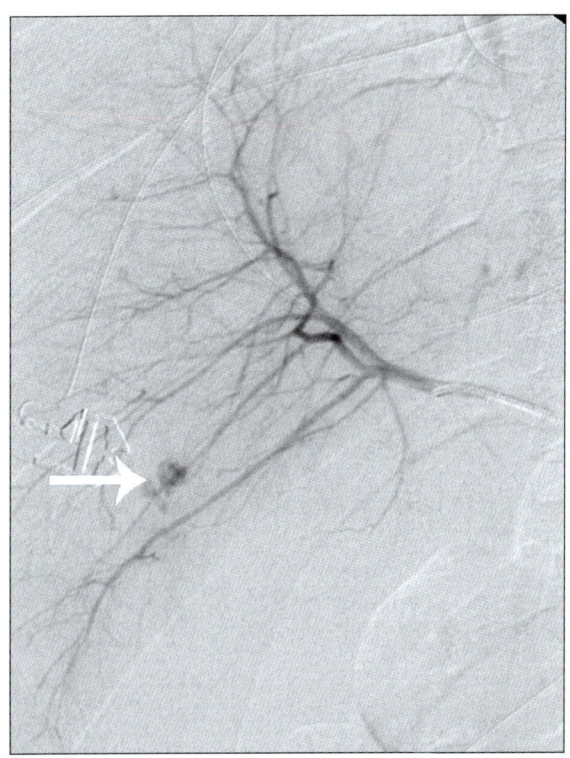

Figure 3. Selective right hepatic arteriogram demonstrates extravasation *(arrow)* from a branch within the posterior right hepatic lobe.

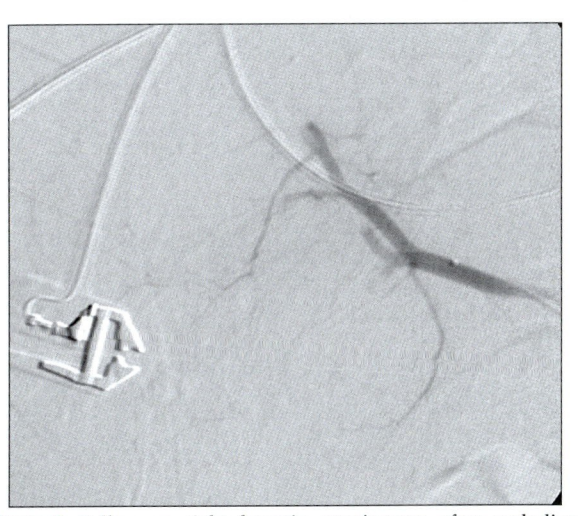

Figure 4. Follow-up right hepatic arteriogram after embolization shows truncation of the branches of the right hepatic artery. No further extravasation was seen, and the patient's vital signs stabilized.

Case 150

DEMOGRAPHICS/CLINICAL HISTORY

A 47-year-old woman with severe liver injury after a motor vehicle accident, undergoing computed tomography (CT), arteriography, and embolization.

History/Indications for Procedure
A 47-year-old woman was involved in a head-on motor vehicle accident. On presentation to the emergency department, she is stable, with a blood pressure responsive to fluid and blood replacement.

Procedure
Liver trauma

Pre-procedure Imaging
Contrast-enhanced CT scan shows a grade V liver laceration with active contrast extravasation (Fig. 1). There is a large amount of free fluid or blood seen throughout the abdomen and pelvis.

Intraprocedural Findings
Selective right arteriogram demonstrates active contrast extravasation (Fig. 2). The right hepatic artery was embolized with a Gelfoam slurry (Fig. 3).

Follow-up and Complications
The patient was observed, and serial hematocrit levels were stable. She developed recurrent abdominal pain 6 weeks after the trauma, and a CT scan performed at that time showed a healing liver laceration with near-complete resolution of a perihepatic hematoma (Fig. 4).

Suggested Readings
Hagiwara A, Yukioka T, Ohta S, et al: Nonsurgical management of patients with blunt hepatic injury: Efficacy of transcatheter arterial embolization. AJR Am J Roentgenol 169:1151-1156, 1997.

Schwartz RA, Teitelbaum GP, Katz MD, Pentecost MJ: Effectiveness of transcatheter embolization in the control of hepatic vascular injuries. J Vasc Intervent Radiol 4:359-365, 1993.

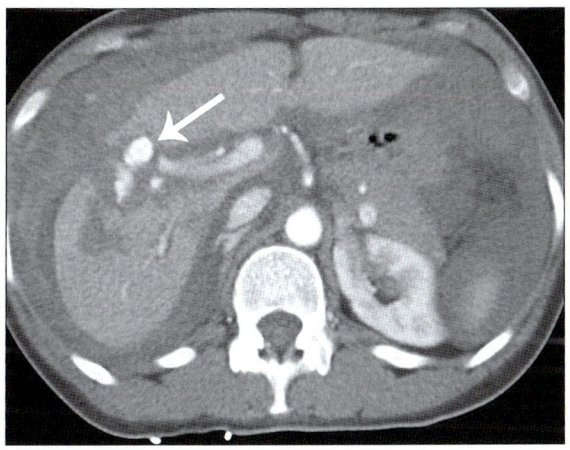

Figure 1. Contrast-enhanced CT demonstrates a complex laceration through the right hepatic lobe with a large area of active contrast extravasation *(arrow)*.

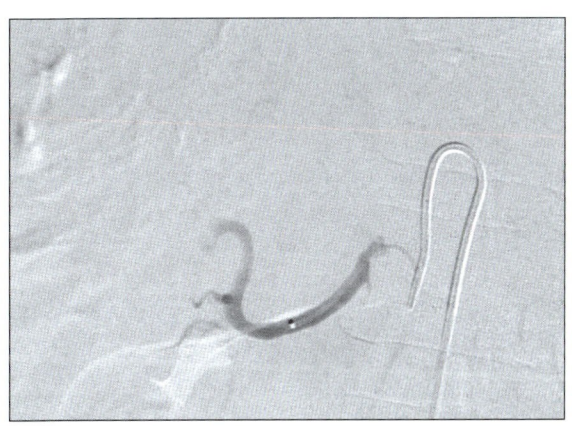

Figure 3. The right hepatic artery was embolized to stasis with a Gelfoam slurry.

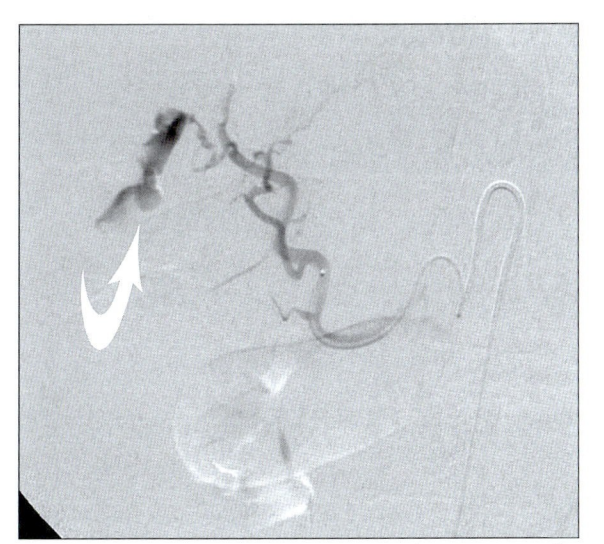

Figure 2. Selective right hepatic arteriogram demonstrates a large amount of active extravasation.

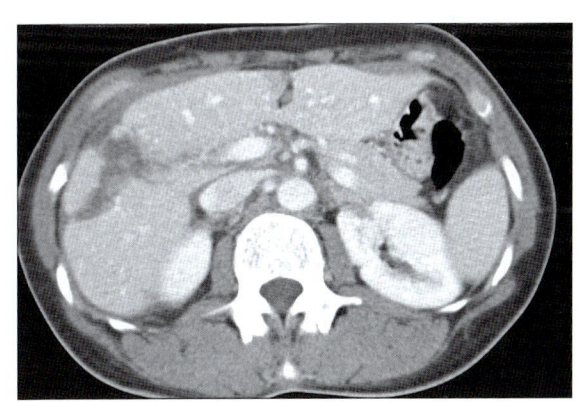

Figure 4. Follow-up contrast-enhanced CT demonstrates healing of the liver laceration with nearly complete resolution of perihepatic hematoma.

Case 151

DEMOGRAPHICS/CLINICAL HISTORY

An 80-year-old man with abdominal pain and hypotension after a fall.

DISCUSSION

History/Indications for Procedure
An 80-year-old man with left-sided abdominal pain after a fall. The patient is hypotensive on presentation to the emergency department.

Procedure
Management of post-traumatic splenic pseudoaneurysm and arteriovenous fistula

Pre-procedure Imaging
Contrast-enhanced CT of the abdomen demonstrates a splenic laceration with pooling of contrast and early opacification of the splenic vein (Fig. 1). There is high-density fluid throughout the abdomen consistent with hemoperitoneum.

Intraprocedural Findings
There is focal pseudoaneurysm in the mid-spleen with an associated arteriovenous fistula (Figs. 2 and 3). The feeding artery was selectively catheterized and embolized with coils (Fig. 4).

Follow-up and Complications
The patient was observed following the procedure, and the blood pressure and hematocrit levels remained stable. The patient's recovery was prolonged by the development of a hospital-acquired pneumonia but was otherwise uneventful.

Suggested Readings
Davis KA, Fabian TC, Croce MA, et al: Improved success in nonoperative management of blunt splenic injuries: Embolization of splenic artery pseudoaneurysms. J Trauma 44:1008-1013, 1998.

Marmery H, Shanmuganathan K, Alexander MT, et al: Optimization of selection for nonoperative management of blunt splenic injury: Comparison of MDCT grading systems. AJR Am J Roentgenol 189:1421-1427, 2007.

Sclafani SJ, Shaftan GW, Scalea TM, et al: Nonoperative salvage of computed tomography-diagnosed splenic injuries: Utilization of angiography for triage and embolization for hemostasis. J Trauma 39:818-825, 1995.

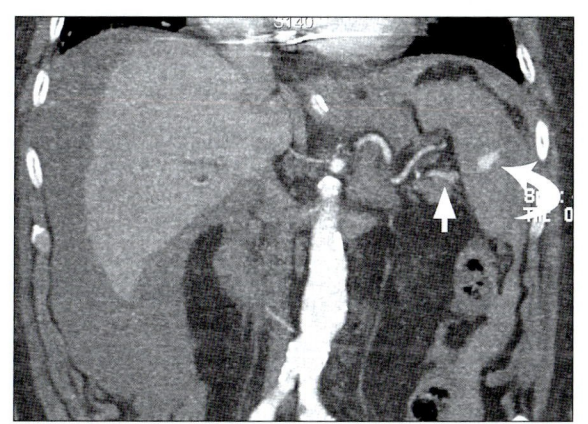

Figure 1. Coronal reconstruction from CT angiogram of the abdomen shows a focal collection of contrast within the splenic parenchyma *(curved arrow)*. There is also early opacification of the splenic vein *(arrow)*, indicating an arteriovenous fistula.

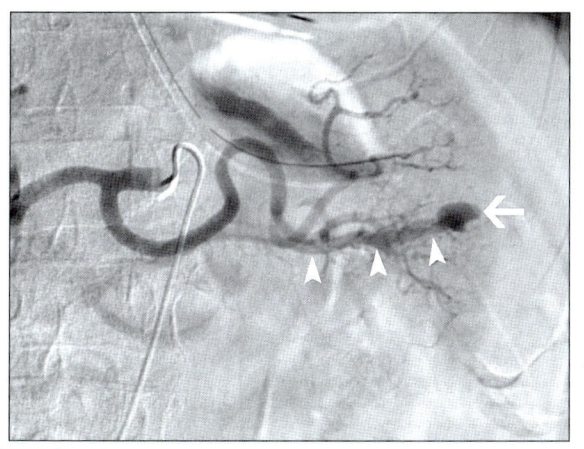

Figure 2. Celiac arteriogram shows a pseudoaneurysm in the splenic parenchyma *(arrow)*. There is an associated arteriovenous fistula with early opacification of the splenic vein *(arrowheads)*.

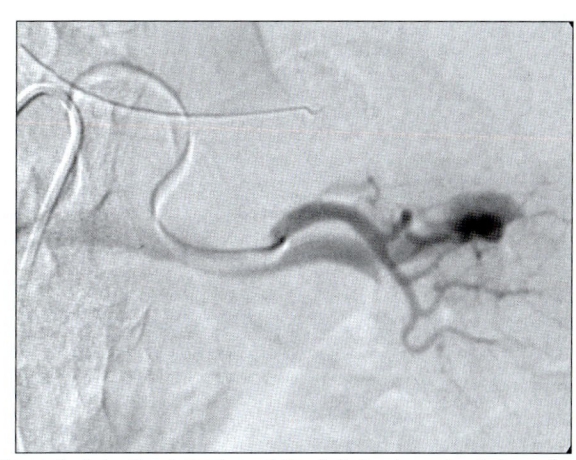

Figure 3. Selective injection of the inferior branch of the splenic artery shows opacification of the pseudoaneurysm and arteriovenous fistula.

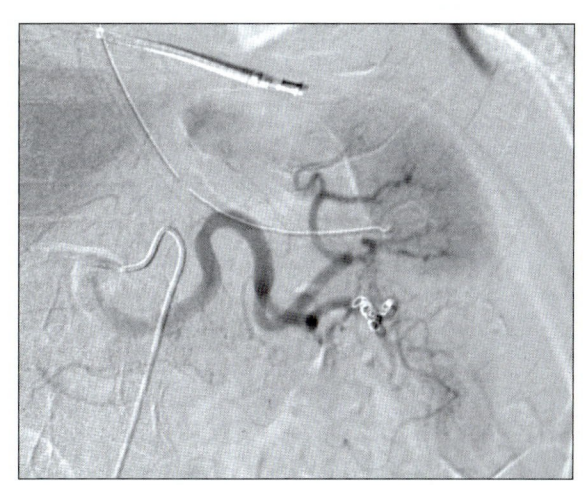

Figure 4. Follow-up celiac arteriogram after embolization shows successful exclusion of the pseudoaneurysm with preservation of much of the splenic parenchyma. There is no longer filling of the arteriovenous fistula.

Case 152

DEMOGRAPHICS/CLINICAL HISTORY

A 20-year-old man with history of blunt splenic trauma and left upper quadrant pain, undergoing computed tomography (CT), arteriography, and embolization.

DISCUSSION

History/Indications for Procedure
A 20-year-old man has a history of many episodes of blunt splenic trauma. The patient has new-onset left upper quadrant pain.

Procedure
Endovascular management of splenic traumas

Pre-procedure Imaging
Contrast-enhanced CT through the abdomen demonstrates a large, splenic subcapsular hematoma (Fig. 1). Within the subcapsular hematoma are several areas of increased attenuation that are consistent with active contrast extravasation (Fig. 2).

Intraprocedural Findings
Splenic arteriogram reveals the mass effect from the subcapsular hematoma and numerous, small, punctate areas of extravasation within the splenic parenchyma (Fig. 3). The main splenic artery was embolized with coils (Fig. 4).

Follow-up and Complications
The patient's hemoglobin levels remained stable after the embolization. He underwent an elective splenectomy 2 days later.

Suggested Readings

Bessoud B, Denys A, Calmes JM, et al: Nonoperative management of traumatic splenic injuries: Is there a role for proximal splenic artery embolization? AJR Am J Roentgenol 186:779-785, 2006.

Hagiwara A, Fukushima H, Murata A, et al: Blunt splenic injury: Usefulness of transcatheter arterial embolization in patients with a transient response to fluid resuscitation. Radiology 235:57-64, 2005.

Hagiwara A, Yukioka T, Ohta S, et al: Nonsurgical management of patients with blunt splenic injury: Efficacy of transcatheter arterial embolization. AJR Am J Roentgenol 167:159-166, 1996.

Sclafani SJ, Weisberg A, Scalea TM, et al: Blunt splenic injuries: Nonsurgical treatment with CT, arteriography and transcatheter arterial embolization of the splenic artery. Radiology 181:189-196, 1991.

Case 152   305

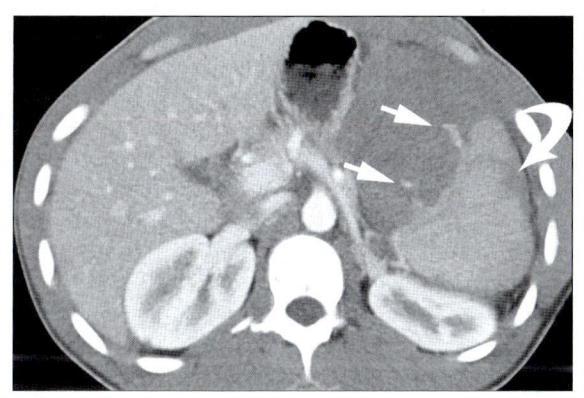

Figure 1. Contrast-enhanced CT through the upper abdomen demonstrates a large, perisplenic hematoma containing active contrast extravasation *(arrows)*.

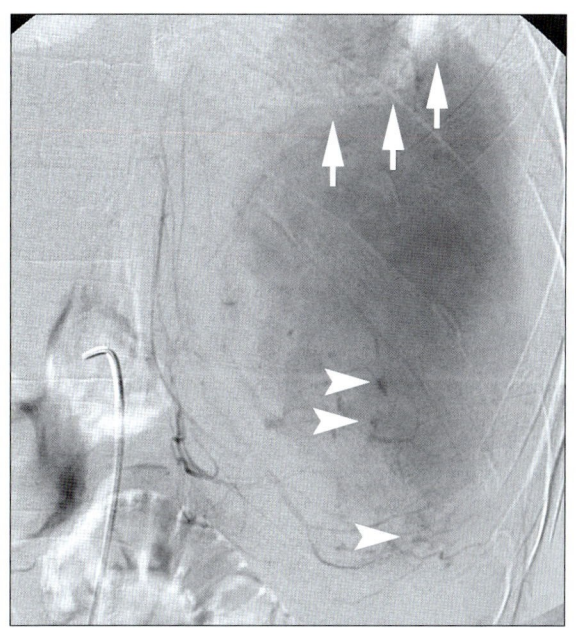

Figure 3. The capillary phase of a splenic arteriogram shows filling-in of punctate intraparenchymal hemorrhages *(arrowheads)*. The linear hypovascular region corresponds to a large splenic laceration *(arrows)*.

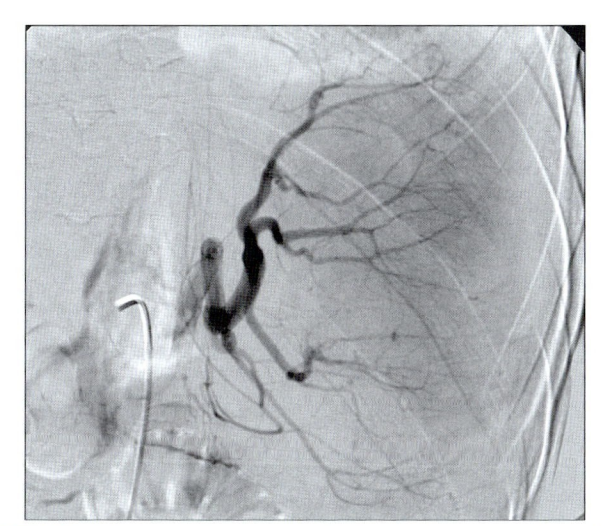

Figure 2. Splenic arteriogram, arterial phase, shows several small, punctate areas of contrast extravasation.

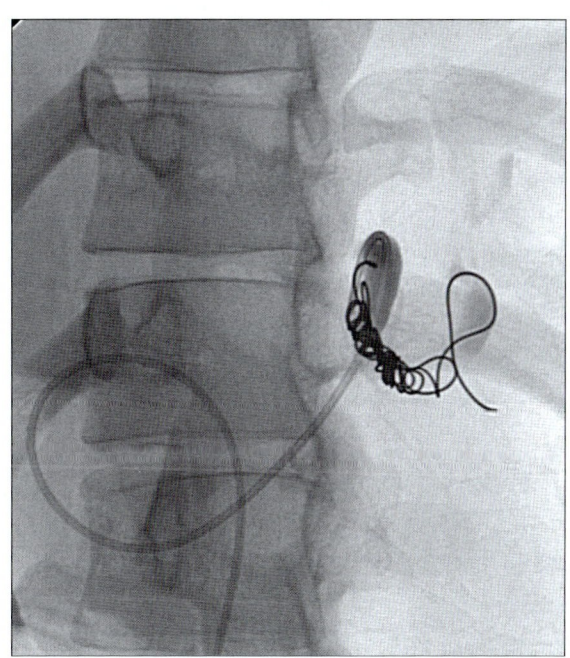

Figure 4. The main splenic artery was embolized with platinum coils.

Case 153

DEMOGRAPHICS/CLINICAL HISTORY

A 30-year-old man involved in an ATV roll-over accident, undergoing CT and angiography.

DISCUSSION

History/Indications for Procedure
This patient initially was managed nonoperatively. He presented 3 weeks later with abdominal pain.

Procedure
Splenic artery embolization

Pre-procedure Imaging
Contrast-enhanced CT scan showed an 8-cm × 7-cm pseudoaneurysm within the spleen (Fig. 1).

Intraprocedural Findings
A celiac angiogram confirmed the large pseudoaneurysm within the mid-spleen (Fig. 2). The feeding arteries were selectively embolized with platinum coils (Fig. 3).

Follow-up and Complications
CT scan performed the day after embolization showed thrombosis of the pseudoaneurysm (Fig. 4). The patient was asymptomatic at last follow-up, 1 month after the embolization.

Suggested Readings
Davis KA, Fabian TC, Croce MA, et al: Improved success in nonoperative management of blunt splenic injuries: Embolization of splenic artery pseudoaneurysms. J Trauma 44:1008-1013, 1998.

Dent D, Alsabrook G, Erickson BA, et al: Blunt splenic injuries: High nonoperative management rate can be achieved with selective embolization. J Trauma 56:1063-1067, 2004.

Marmery H, Shanmuganathan K, Alexander MT, et al: Optimization of selection for nonoperative management of blunt splenic injury: Comparison of MDCT grading systems. AJR Am J Roentgenol 189:1421-1427, 2007.

Sclafani SJ, Weisberg A, Scalea TM, et al: Blunt splenic injuries: Nonsurgical treatment with CT, arteriography and transcatheter arterial embolization of the splenic artery. Radiology 181:189-196, 1991.

Wu SC, Chow KC, Lee KH, et al: Early selective angioembolization improves success of nonoperative management of blunt splenic injury. Am Surg 73:897-902, 2007.

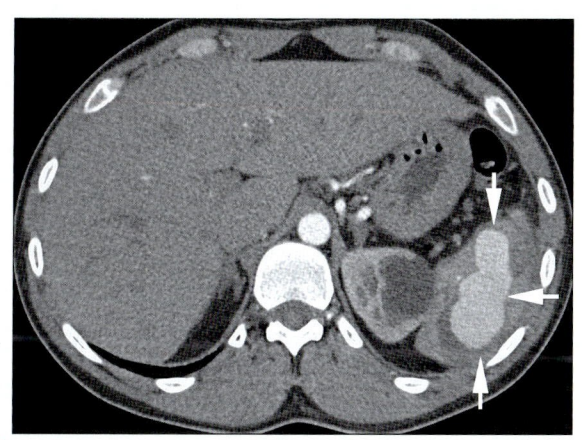

Figure 1. Contrast-enhanced CT scan shows a large pseudoaneurysm within the spleen *(arrows)*.

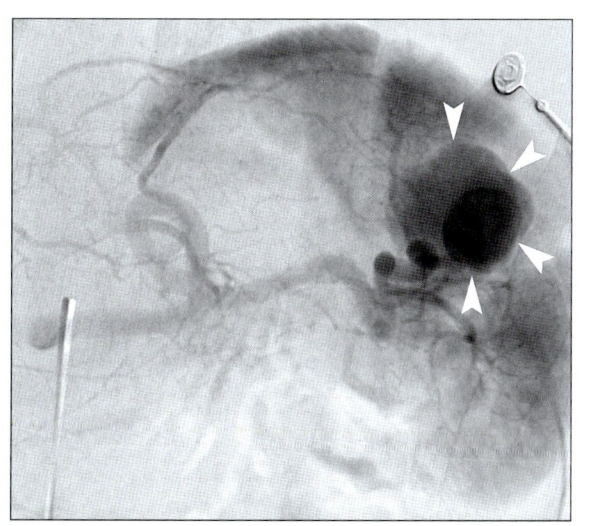

Figure 2. Celiac angiogram confirms the presence of the large pseudoaneurysm *(arrowheads)*.

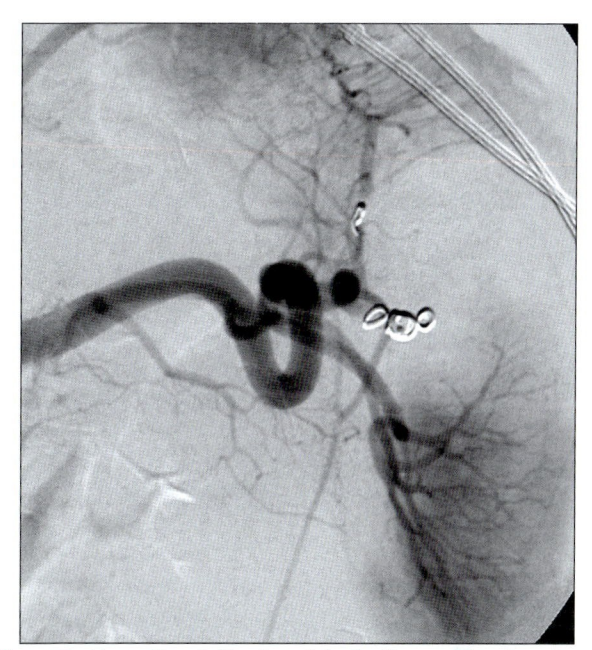

Figure 3. After coil embolization of the feeding arteries, there is no filling of the pseudoaneurysm.

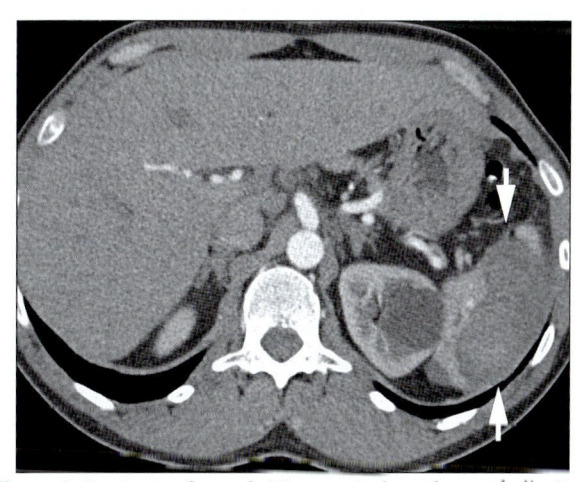

Figure 4. Contrast-enhanced CT scan 1 day after embolization shows a large hematoma within the splenic parenchyma *(arrows)*. No enhancement of the pseudoaneurysm was present.

Case 154

DEMOGRAPHICS/CLINICAL HISTORY

A 27-year-old man with splenomegaly, bleeding gastric varices, and thrombocytopenia.

DISCUSSION

History/Indications for Procedure
A 27-year-old man with portal vein thrombosis since childhood. The patient now presents with bleeding gastric varices and a platelet count of 61×10^9/L (normal 150 to 440×10^9/L).

Procedure
Embolization, splenic, for thrombocytopenia

Pre-procedure Imaging
Contrast-enhanced MRI of the abdomen shows cavernous transformation of the portal vein. The spleen is massively enlarged, measuring 24 cm in length.

Intraprocedural Findings
Splenic arteriogram was performed showing massive splenomegaly (Fig. 1). The upper pole branch and a lower pole branch were each selectively catheterized and embolized with Gelfoam slurry (Figs. 2 and 3), embolizing approximately 75% of the splenic parenchyma.

Follow-up and Complications
The patient's platelet count normalized after the procedure, and he has had no further episodes of gastrointestinal bleeding. A contrast-enhanced CT was performed 2 weeks after the embolization that showed infarction of the majority of the splenic parenchyma (Fig. 4).

Suggested Readings
Koconis KG, Singh H, Soares G: Partial splenic embolization in the treatment of patients with portal hypertension: A review of the English language literature. J Vasc Intervent Radiol 18:463-481, 2007.

Madoff DC, Denys A, Wallace MJ, et al: Splenic arterial interventions: Anatomy, indications, technical considerations, and potential complications. Radiographics 25:S191-S211, 2005.

Romano M, Giojelli A, Capuano G, et al: Partial splenic embolization in patients with idiopathic portal hypertension. Eur J Radiol 49:268-273, 2004.

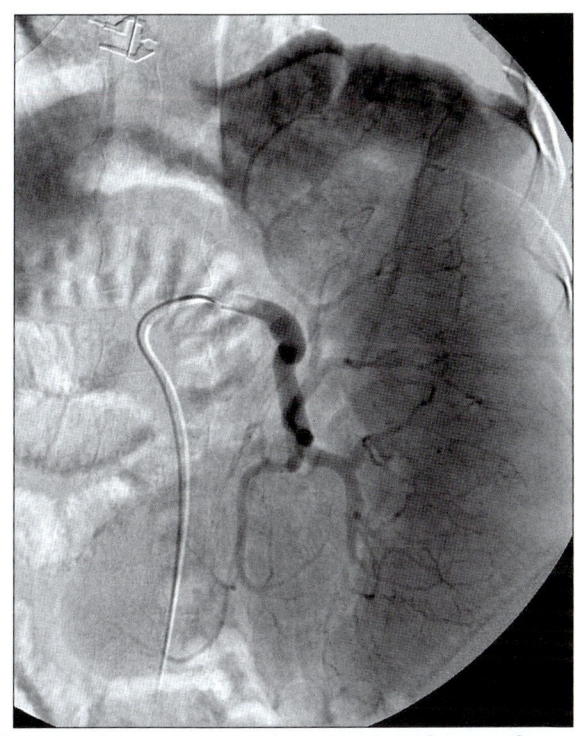

Figure 1. Splenic arteriogram shows massive splenomegaly.

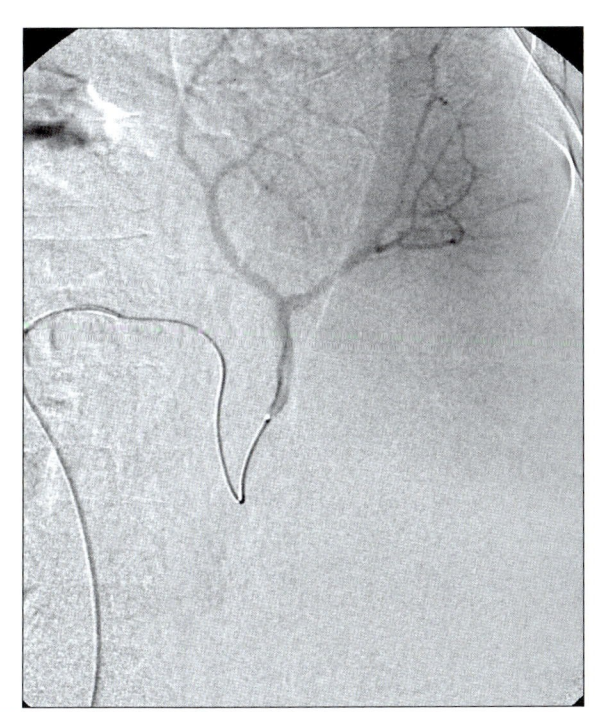

Figure 2. A 3-French microcatheter was used to selectively catheterize the upper pole branch of the splenic artery. This branch was embolized with Gelfoam slurry.

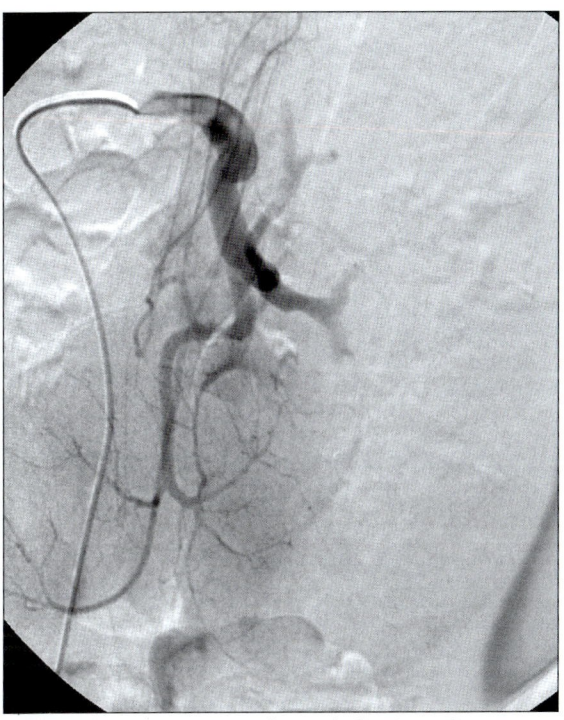

Figure 3. Splenic arteriogram after embolization. The upper pole and a portion of the lower pole of the spleen have been completely embolized. A small amount of residual splenic parenchyma remains in the medial lower pole.

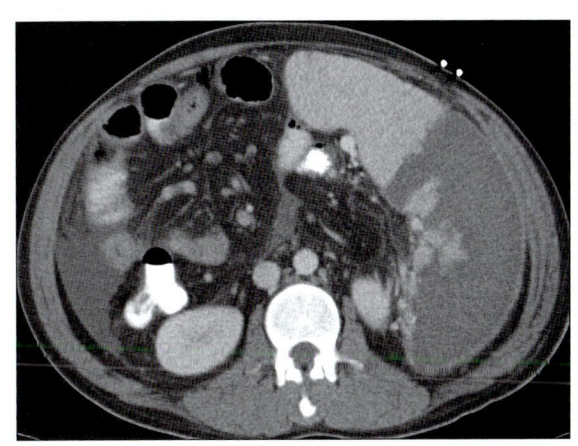

Figure 4. Follow-up contrast-enhanced CT 2 weeks after embolization shows infarction of a large volume of splenic parenchyma.

Case 155

DEMOGRAPHICS/CLINICAL HISTORY

A 31-year-old man with a history of spontaneous gastrointestinal bleeding from gastric varices.

DISCUSSION

History/Indications for Procedure
A 31-year-old man with chronic superior mesenteric and portal vein thrombosis. The patient has a history of gastrointestinal bleeding from grade III gastric varices.

Procedure
Splenic artery embolization for management of gastric varices

Pre-procedure Imaging
CT of the abdomen shows massive splenomegaly (Fig. 1). There is cavernous transformation of the portal vein, and gastrohepatic and parasplenic varices are present.

Intraprocedural Findings
Splenic arteriogram shows massive splenomegaly (Fig. 2). Embolization of the upper pole branch and a prominent lower pole branch was performed using a combination of calibrated microspheres and coils (Fig. 3); a small branch perfusing a portion of the lower pole of the spleen was left untreated.

Follow-up and Complications
The patient had significant left upper quadrant pain after embolization, and follow-up CT shows infarction of a majority of the splenic parenchyma (Fig. 4). The patient's gastric varices completely resolved on follow-up endoscopy, and the patient has had no further episodes of upper GI hemorrhage.

Suggested Readings
Koconis KG, Singh H, Soares G: Partial splenic embolization in the treatment of patients with portal hypertension: A review of the English language literature. J Vasc Intervent Radiol 18:463-481, 2007.

Romano M, Giojelli A, Capuano G, et al: Partial splenic embolization in patients with idiopathic portal hypertension. Eur J Radiol 49: 268-273, 2004.

Yoshida H, Mamada Y, Taniai N, et al: New methods for the management of gastric varices. World J Gastroenterol 12:5926-5931, 2006.

Case 155   311

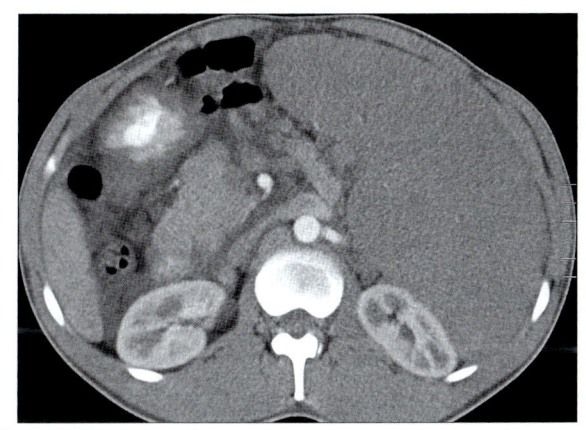

Figure 1. CT of the abdomen shows massive splenomegaly.

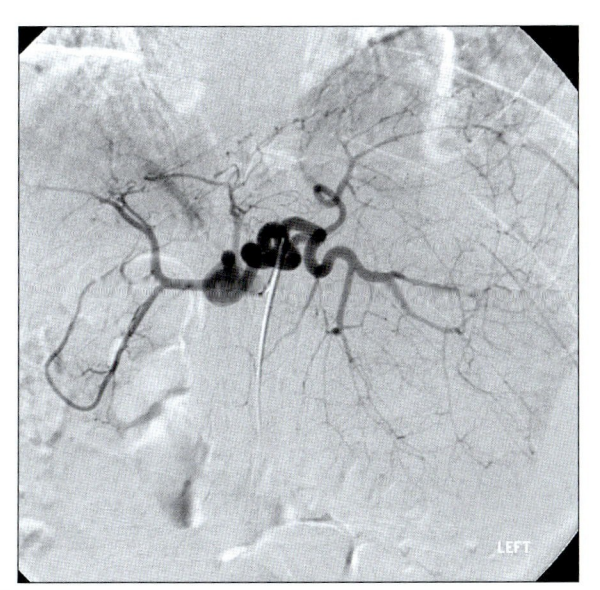

Figure 2. Celiac arteriogram shows a very tortuous splenic artery and a massively enlarged spleen.

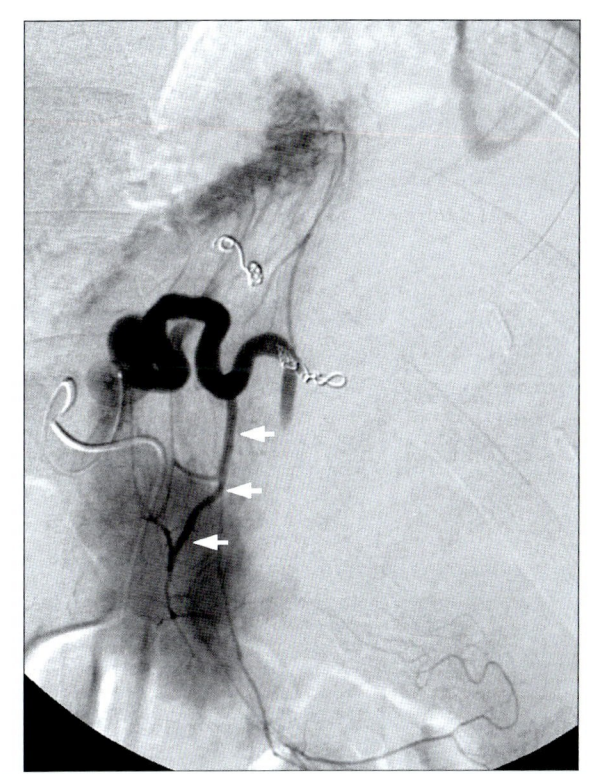

Figure 3. The upper pole and a majority of the lower pole of the spleen were embolized using a combination of calibrated microspheres and coils. A small branch supplying the medial tip of the lower pole of the spleen remains patent *(arrows)*.

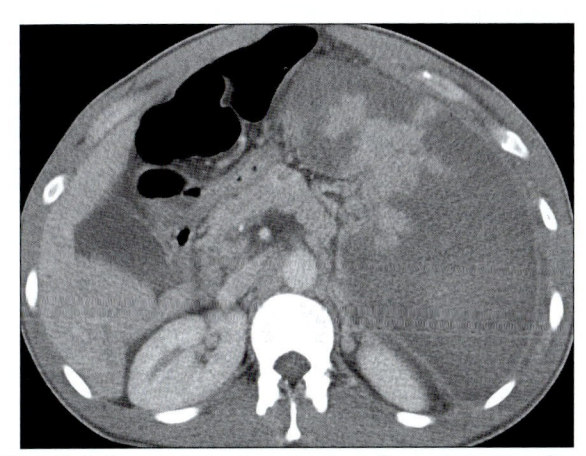

Figure 4. Follow-up CT performed 2 days after embolization shows infarction of the majority of the splenic parenchyma. There is a small volume of viable tissue near the splenic hilum.

Case 156

DEMOGRAPHICS/CLINICAL HISTORY

A 44-year-old woman with menorrhagia, undergoing MRI and arteriography.

DISCUSSION

History/Indications for Procedure
A 44-year-old woman with menorrhagia.

Procedure
Uterine fibroid embolization

Pre-procedure Imaging
Contrast-enhanced MRI shows multiple enhancing, intramural uterine leiomyomas (Figs. 1 and 2).

Intraprocedural Findings
Bilateral selective uterine arteriograms were performed, confirming the presence of multiple hypervascular leiomyomas (Fig. 3). Both uterine arteries were embolized with 700-µm to 900-µm calibrated microspheres.

Follow-up and Complications
The patient experienced significant improvement in symptoms 3 months after the procedure (Fig. 4). The symptomatic improvement persisted at 1-year follow-up.

Suggested Readings
Pron G, Bennett J, Common A, et al: The Ontario Uterine Fibroid Embolization Collaboration Group: The Ontario Uterine Fibroid Embolization Trial, Part 2: Uterine fibroid reduction and symptom relief after uterine artery embolization for fibroids. Fertil Steril 79:120-127, 2003.

Spies JB, Bruno J, Czeyda-Pommersheim F, et al: Long-term outcome of uterine artery embolization of leiomyomas. Obstet Gynecol 106:933-939, 2005.

Spies JB, Myers ER, Worthington-Kirsch R, et al: FIBROID Registry Investigators: The FIBROID Registry: Symptom and quality-of-life status 1 year after therapy. Obstet Gynecol 106:1309-1318, 2005.

Worthington-Kirsch R, Spies J, Myers ER, et al: FIBROID Investigators: The Fibroid Registry for outcomes data (FIBROID) for uterine artery embolization: Short term outcomes. Obstet Gynecol 106:52-59, 2005.

Case 156 313

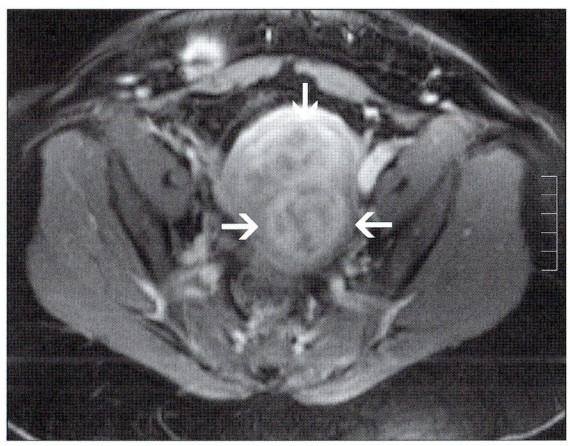

Figure 1. Axial contrast-enhanced MR image of the pelvis shows multiple enhancing leiomyomas within the uterus (arrows).

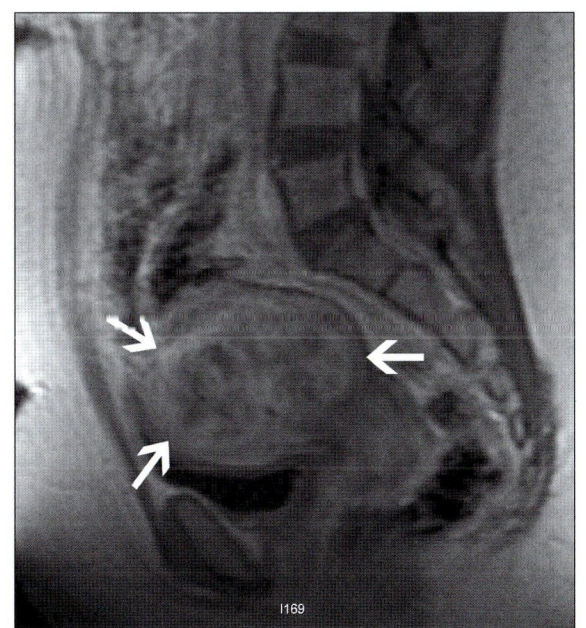

Figure 2. Sagittal contrast-enhanced MR image of the pelvis also shows multiple enhancing leiomyomas within the uterus (arrows).

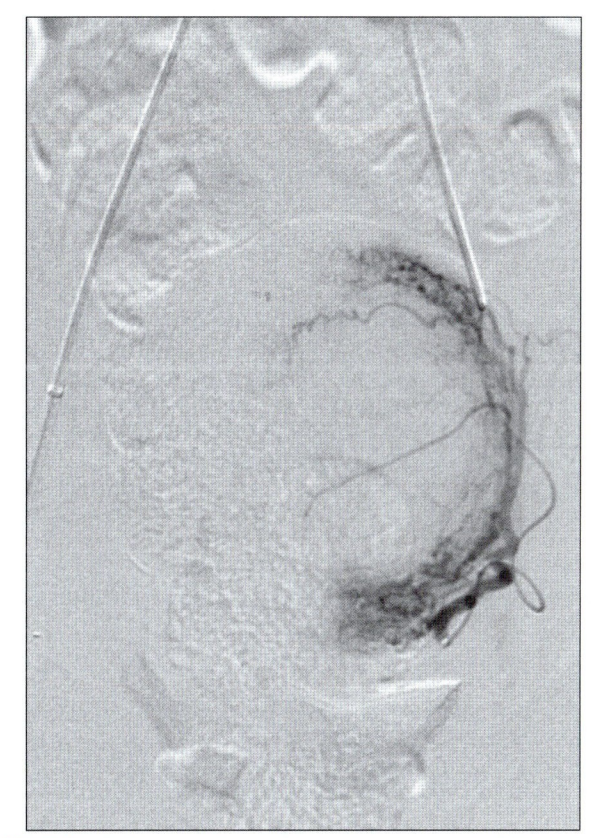

Figure 3. Single image from selective injection of the left uterine artery. The left uterine artery is enlarged and supplying a large uterine leiomyoma.

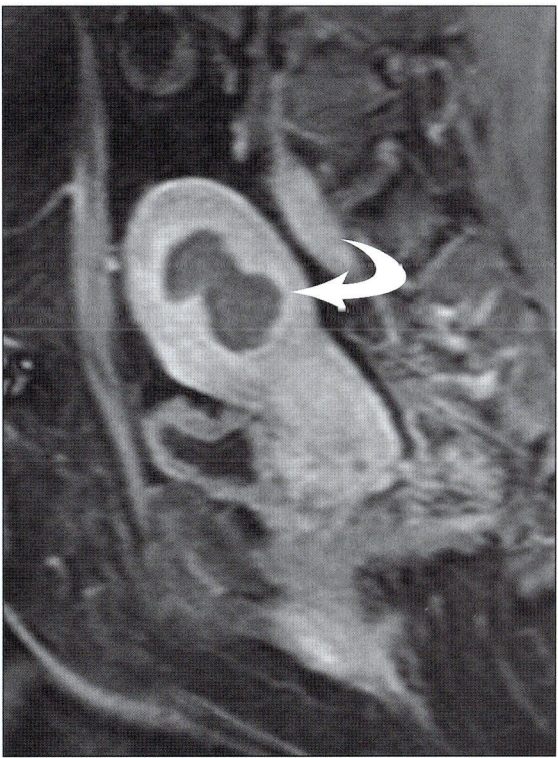

Figure 4. Sagittal contrast-enhanced MR image performed 3 months after uterine fibroid embolization. The image shows a devascularized leiomyoma within the uterine fundus.

Case 157

DEMOGRAPHICS/CLINICAL HISTORY

A 48-year-old woman with menorrhagia, undergoing uterine fibroid embolization.

DISCUSSION

History/Indications for Procedure
A 48-year-old woman has menorrhagia that has been increasing over the past several years.

Procedure
Uterine fibroid embolization

Pre-procedure Imaging
Pelvic MRI shows a dominant, heterogeneously enhancing, intramural and submucosal fibroid (Fig. 1). The fibroid is 11 cm in diameter.

Intraprocedural Findings
The large fibroid was supplied predominantly by the right uterine artery (Fig. 2). Bilateral uterine arteries were embolized with 500-μm to 700-μm Embospheres (Biosphere Medical, Rockland, MA).

Follow-up and Complications
The fibroid showed continued enhancement on follow-up MRI (Fig. 3), and the patient therefore underwent repeat embolization. MRI performed 7 months after the second procedure shows complete infarction of the fibroid (Fig. 4); the patient's symptoms significantly improved after the second embolization.

Suggested Readings
Spies J, Myers ER, Worthington-Kitsch R, et al: The FIBROID Registry: Symptom and quality-of-life status 1 year after therapy. Obstet Gynecol 106:1309-1318, 2005.

Spies JB, Patel AA, Epstein NB, White AM: Recent advances in uterine fibroid embolization. Curr Opin Obstet Gynecol 17:562-567, 2005.

Worthington-Kirsch R, Spies JB, Myers ER, et al: The Fibroid Registry for Outcomes Data (FIBROID) for uterine artery embolization: Short term outcomes. Obstet Gynecol 106:52-59, 2005.

Case 157 315

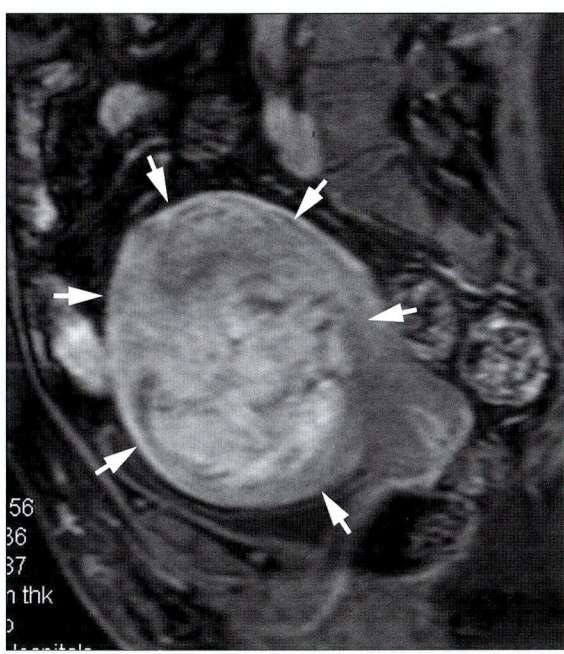

Figure 1. Sagittal, T1-weighted, postgadolinium MRI of the pelvis shows a large, heterogeneously enhancing, intramural and submucosal fibroid *(arrows)*.

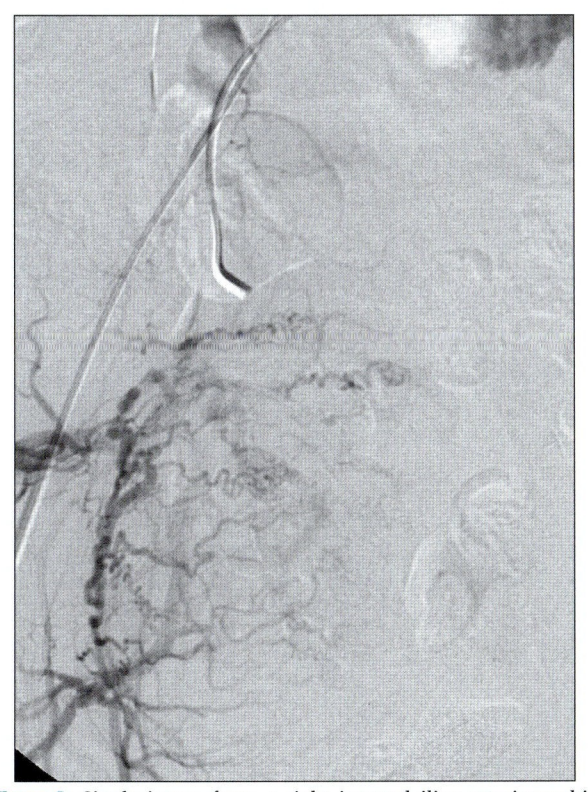

Figure 2. Single image from a right internal iliac arteriographic study shows the large, hypervascular fibroid supplied predominantly by the right uterine artery.

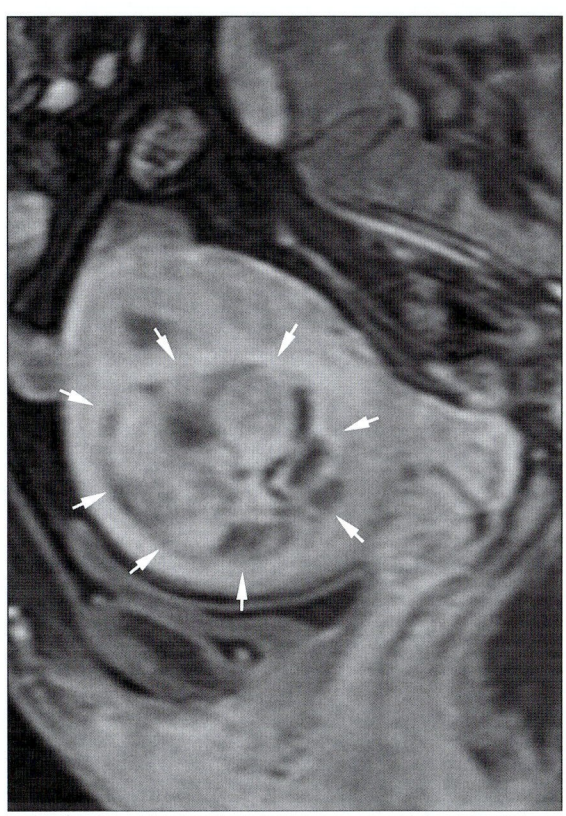

Figure 3. Follow-up MRI performed 3 months after the initial embolization shows significant residual enhancement within the fibroid *(arrows)*.

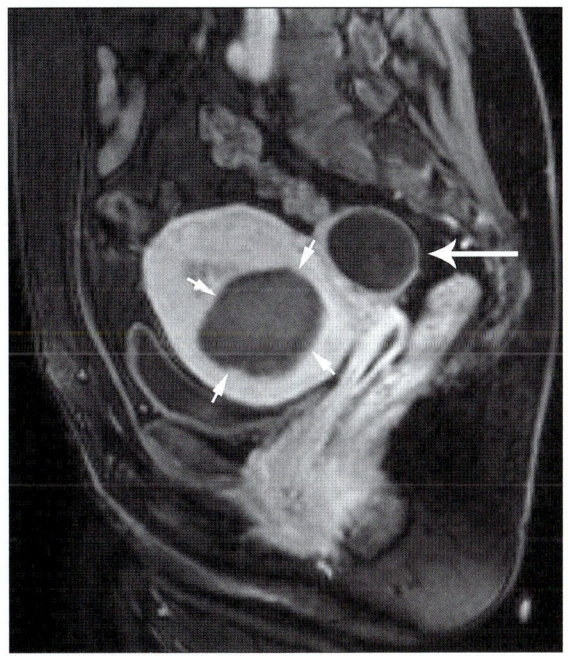

Figure 4. Sagittal, T1-weighted, contrast-enhanced MRI through the uterus shows volume loss by the fibroid *(short arrows)* and no further enhancement. A new right adnexal cyst *(long arrow)* was incidentally identified.

Case 158

DEMOGRAPHICS/CLINICAL HISTORY

A 33-year-old woman with menorrhagia, undergoing magnetic resonance imaging (MRI) and arteriography.

DISCUSSION

History/Indications for Procedure
On physical examination, a 33-year-old woman with menorrhagia was found to have a 5-cm to 6-cm, prolapsing fibroid.

Procedure
Uterine artery embolization for cervical leiomyomas

Pre-procedure Imaging
MRI of the pelvis shows three cervical fibroids; the largest is 6.1-cm × 5.7-cm × 6.2-cm (Fig. 1). All three fibroids show homogenous enhancement.

Intraprocedural Findings
Pelvic arteriography shows that the hypervascular masses are supplied by branches of the uterine arteries (Figs. 2 and 3). Bilateral uterine arteries were embolized with 500-μm to 700-μm calibrated microspheres (Embospheres, BioSphere Medical, Inc., Rockland, MA).

Follow-up and Complications
The patient had some sloughing of the fibroid after the embolization, but overall, she was faring well at follow-up. Follow-up MRI shows a marked decrease in size of the cervical fibroids (Fig. 4).

Suggested Readings

Bruno J, Allison S, McCullough M, et al: Recovery after uterine artery embolization for leiomyomas: A detailed analysis of its duration and severity. J Vasc Intervent Radiol 15:801-807, 2004.

Jha R, Ascher S, Imaoka I, Spies J: Symptomatic fibroleiomyomata: MR imaging of the uterus before and after uterine arterial embolization. Radiology 217:228-235, 2000.

Pelage J, Guaou N, Jha R, et al: Long term imaging outcome after embolization for uterine fibroid tumors. Radiology 230:803-809, 2004.

Spies JB, Patel AA, Epstein NB, White AM: Recent advances in uterine fibroid embolization. Curr Opin Obstet Gynecol 17:562-567, 2005.

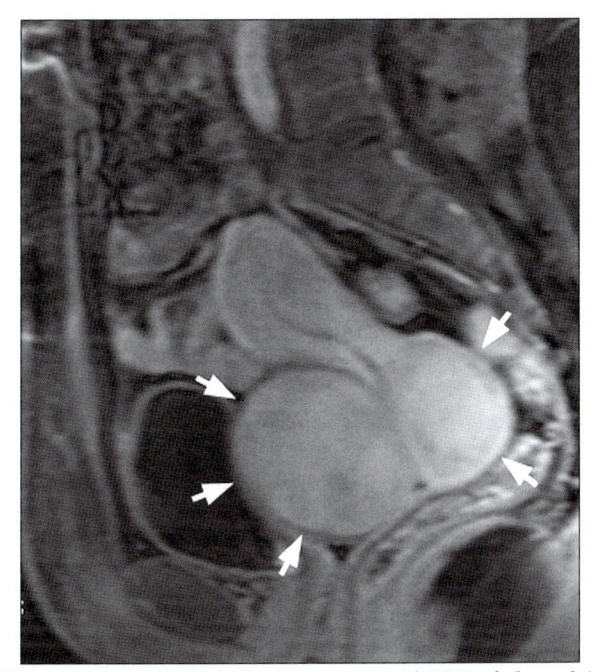

Figure 1. T1-weighted, post-contrast, sagittal MRI of the pelvis shows two, large, homogeneously enhancing masses *(arrows)* arising from the cervix, which are consistent with cervical fibroids.

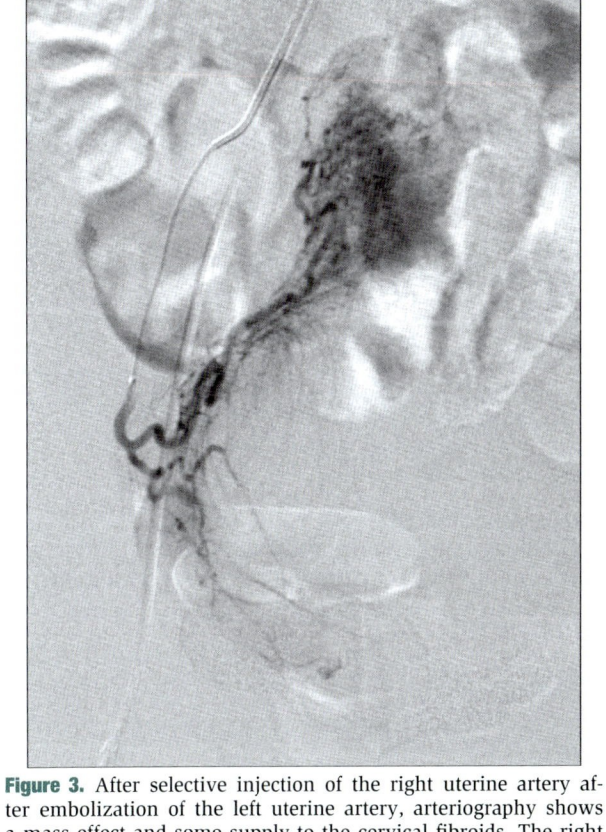

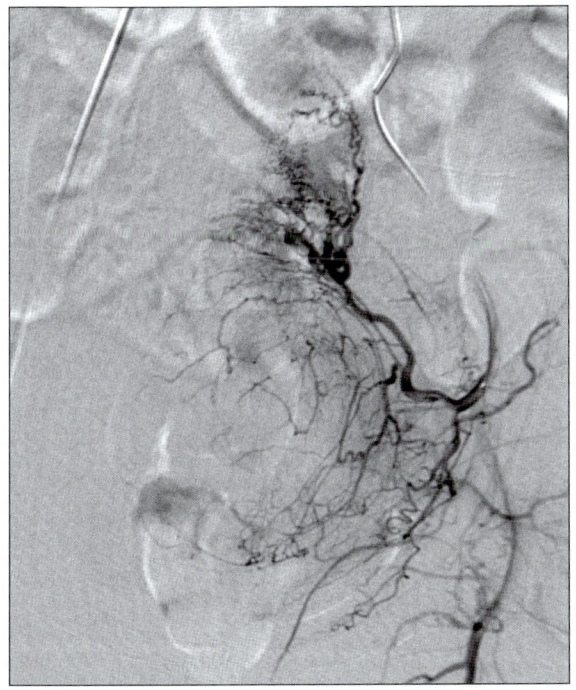

Figure 2. After selective injection of the left uterine artery before embolization, arteriography shows a large, hypervascular fibroid. The left uterine artery was embolized to near stasis with microspheres.

Figure 3. After selective injection of the right uterine artery after embolization of the left uterine artery, arteriography shows a mass effect and some supply to the cervical fibroids. The right uterine artery was also embolized with microspheres.

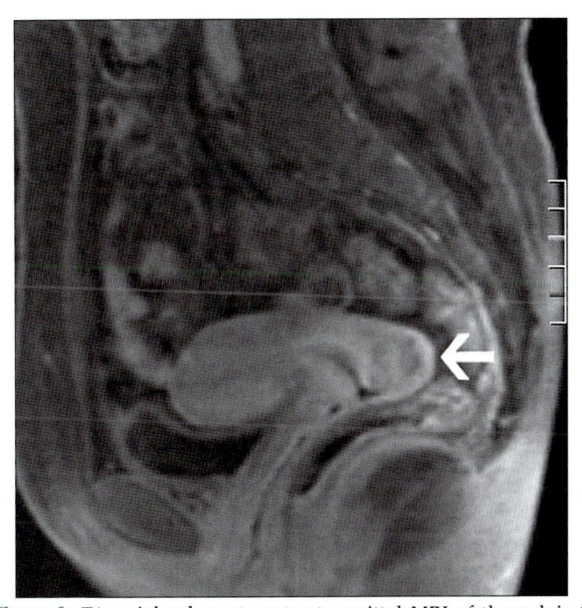

Figure 4. T1-weighted, post-contrast, sagittal MRI of the pelvis 3 months after embolization shows nearly complete resolution of the large cervical fibroids. A small, necrotic fibroid remains within the posterior cervix *(arrow)*.

Case 159

DEMOGRAPHICS/CLINICAL HISTORY

A 27-year-old woman with uncontrollable uterine hemorrhage, undergoing angiography.

DISCUSSION

History/Indications for Procedure
This patient underwent dilatation and curettage for retained fetal products after intrauterine fetal demise in a 14-week pregnancy. Significant uterine bleeding developed during the procedure.

Procedure
Pelvic embolization for postpartum hemorrhage

Intraprocedural Findings
A pelvic angiogram shows active extravasation in the left pelvis (Figs. 1 and 2). Bilateral internal iliac arteries were embolized with a Gelfoam slurry (Fig. 3).

Follow-up and Complications
The patient had no further evidence of bleeding during her hospital stay.

Suggested Readings
Greenwood LH, Glickman MG, Schwartz PE, et al: Obstetric and non-malignant gynecologic bleeding: Treatment with angiographic embolization. Radiology 164:155-159, 1987.

Pelage JP, Le Dref O, Mateo J, et al: Life-threatening primary postpartum hemorrhage: Treatment with emergency selective arterial embolization. Radiology 208:359-362, 1998.

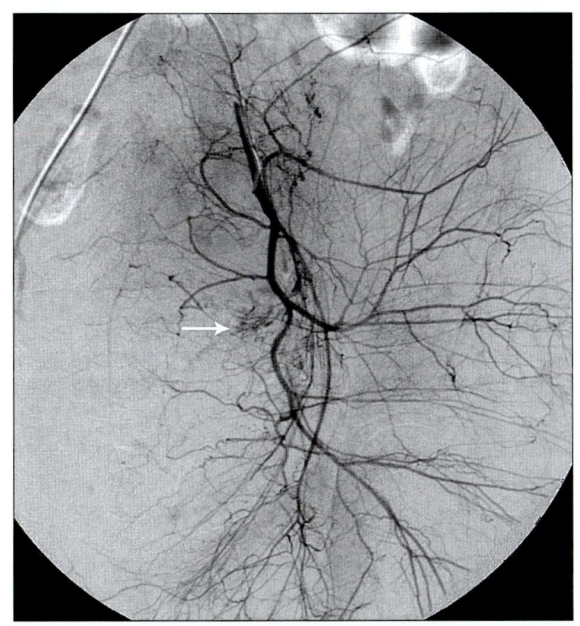

Figure 1. Selective left internal iliac angiogram in the arterial phase shows an abnormal area of hypervascularity in the left pelvis *(arrow)*.

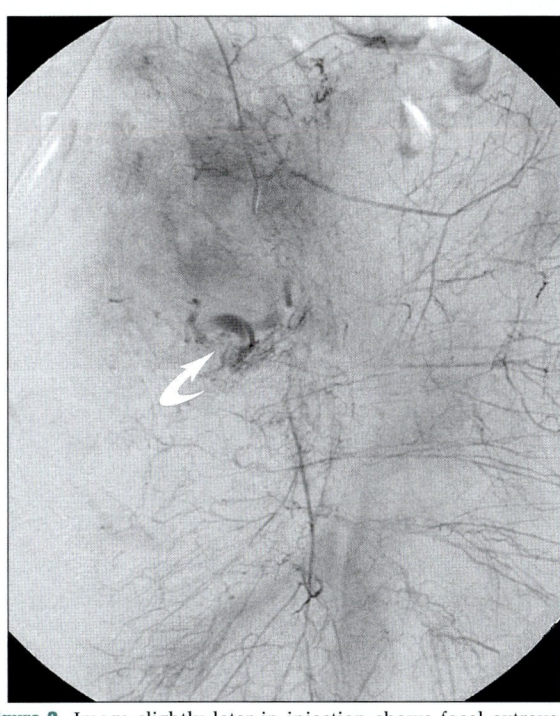

Figure 2. Image slightly later in injection shows focal extravasation *(curved arrow)* in the area of abnormality.

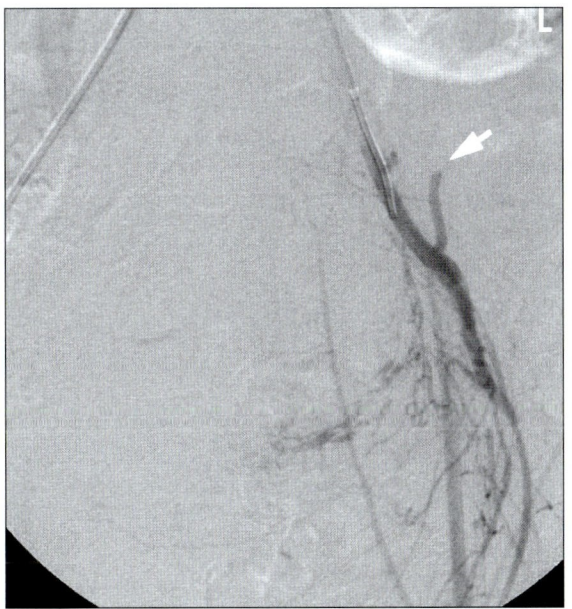

Figure 3. Image from follow-up injection after embolization with Gelfoam slurry shows no further extravasation. Note the truncation of the superior gluteal artery *(arrow)* from nontarget embolization.

Case 160

DEMOGRAPHICS/CLINICAL HISTORY

A 27-year-old woman, 31 weeks pregnant, with placenta percreta, undergoing cesarean section.

DISCUSSION

History/Indications for Procedure
A 27-year-old woman, 31 weeks pregnant, with placenta percreta, undergoing cesarean section. Because of the risk of severe hemorrhage from possible invasion of adjacent structures, the placenta was left in situ, to be removed at a later date.

Procedure
Uterine artery embolization for management of placenta percreta

Pre-procedure Imaging
Unenhanced MRI of the pelvis performed at 15 weeks' pregnancy shows the placenta invading the uterine myometrium of the lower uterine segment (Fig. 1). There is poor delineation between the anterior uterine wall and bladder wall, suggesting possible invasion.

Intraprocedural Findings
Occlusion balloons were placed into the internal iliac arteries bilaterally in the event of uncontrollable hemorrhage during the cesarean section (Fig. 2). After the cesarean section, the patient returned to the angiographic suite, and pelvic arteriogram shows massive hypervascularity to the placenta (Fig. 3); bilateral uterine arteries were embolized with 700-μm to 900-μm and 900-μm to 1200-μm calibrated microspheres (Fig. 4).

Follow-up and Complications
The patient was started on methotrexate after the cesarean section. Postoperatively, she had no pelvic hemorrhage; 6 weeks later, she underwent an uncomplicated hysterectomy.

Suggested Readings
Sumigama S, Itakura A, Ota T, et al: Placenta previa increta/percreta in Japan: A retrospective study of ultrasound findings, management and clinical course. J Obstet Gynaecol Res 33:606-611, 2007.

Tan CH, Tay KH, Sheah K, et al: Perioperative endovascular internal iliac artery occlusion balloon placement in management of placenta accreta. AJR Am J Roentgenol 189:1158-1163, 2007.

Case 160   321

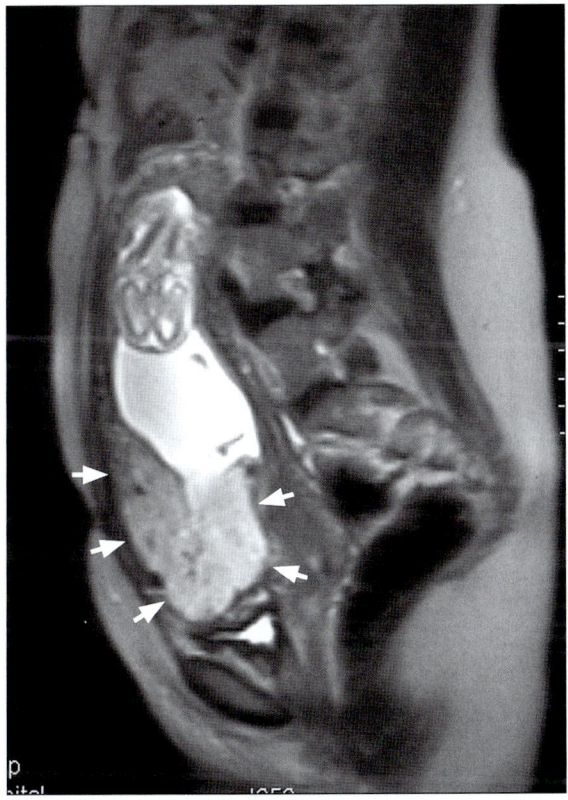

Figure 1. Sagittal T2-weighted MRI of the pelvis shows a prominent placenta *(arrows)* that is invading the myometrium of the lower uterine segment.

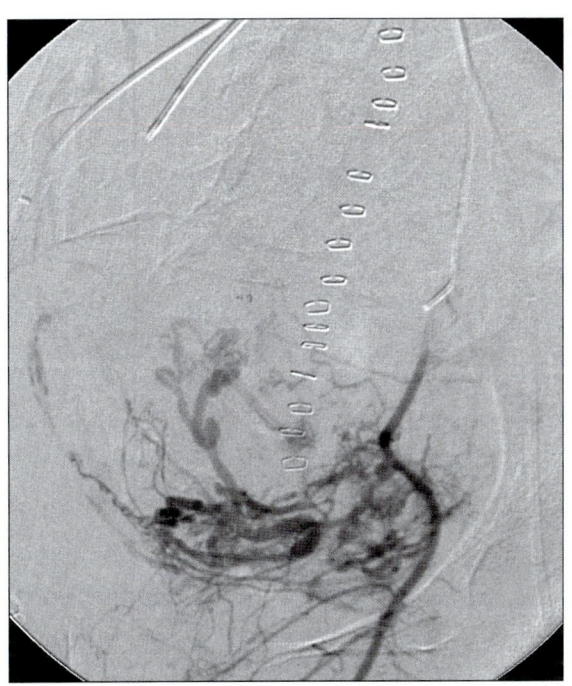

Figure 3. Selective injection of the anterior division of the left internal iliac artery after cesarean section. There is marked pelvic hypervascuarity from the retained placenta.

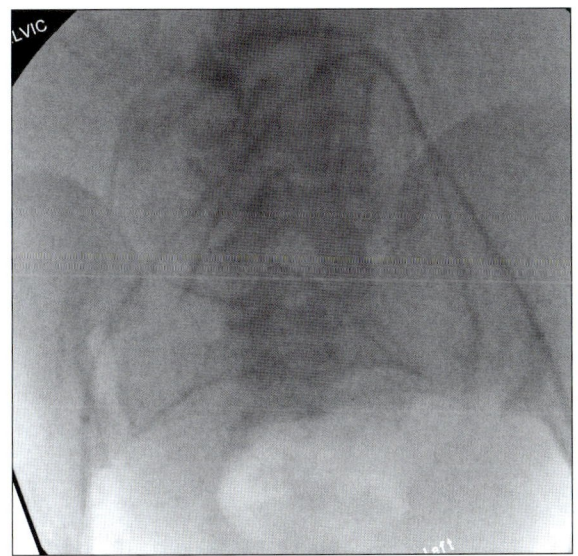

Figure 2. Immediately prior to cesarean section, occlusion balloons were placed in the internal iliac arteries.

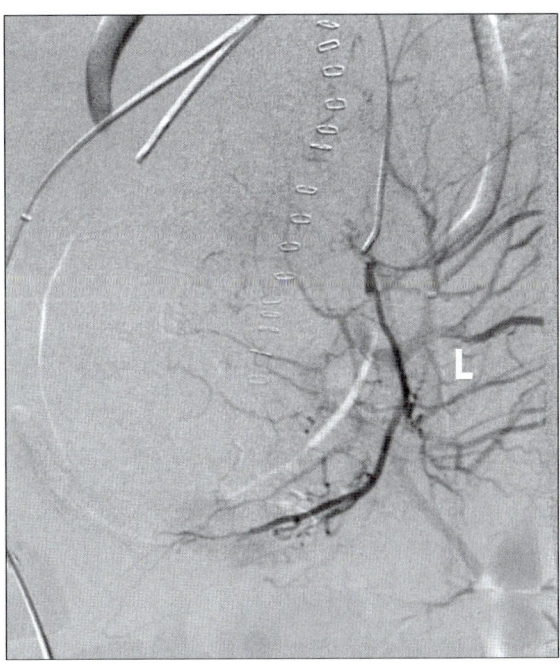

Figure 4. Follow-up arteriogram following embolization. There is no longer filling of large pelvic vessels supplying the uterus and placenta.

Case 161

DEMOGRAPHICS/CLINICAL HISTORY

A 49-year-old man with hepatic artery stenosis 6 months after liver transplantation undergoing angioplasty.

DISCUSSION

History/Indications for Procedure

A 49-year-old man underwent liver transplantation for hepatitis C cirrhosis 6 months earlier. He is asymptomatic and has a mildly elevated gamma-glutamyl transferase (GGT) level.

Procedure

Percutaneous angioplasty for hepatic artery stenosis

Pre-procedure Imaging

Doppler ultrasound of the liver suggests development of hepatic artery stenosis because of the decrease in hepatic artery resistive indices (RIs). The RI of the common hepatic artery is 0.48, which was lower than the value of 0.71 calculated during the prior ultrasound.

Intraprocedural Findings

There is a high-grade stenosis at the hepatic artery anastomosis (Fig. 1). The patient was given intravenous heparin and intra-arterial nitroglycerin; the lesion was crossed with a 0.014-inch guidewire, and angioplasty was performed with a 5-mm balloon (Fig. 2).

Follow-up and Complications

The follow-up angiogram after angioplasty demonstrated significantly improved vessel caliber at the anastomosis (Fig. 3). There was no evidence for recurrent stenosis on Doppler ultrasound performed 6 months after the angioplasty.

Suggested Readings

Abbasoglu O, Levy MF, Vodapally MS, et al: Hepatic artery stenosis after liver transplantation—incidence, presentation, treatment, and long term outcome. Transplantation 63:250-255, 1997.

Mondragon RS, Karani JB, Heaton ND, et al: The use of percutaneous transluminal angioplasty in hepatic artery stenosis after transplantation. Transplantation 57:228-231, 1994.

Saad WE, Davies MG, Sahler L, et al: Hepatic artery stenosis in liver transplant recipients: Primary treatment with percutaneous transluminal angioplasty. J Vasc Intervent Radiol 16:795-805, 2005.

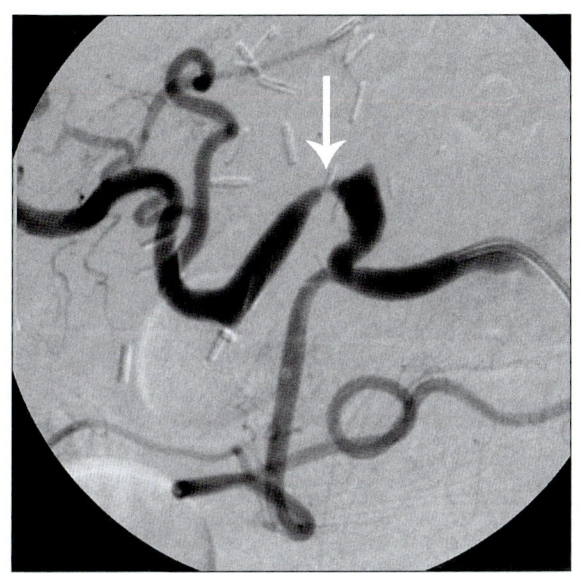

Figure 1. Hepatic arteriogram shows the catheter positioned in the common hepatic artery and demonstrates a high-grade stenosis at the hepatic artery anastomosis *(arrow)*.

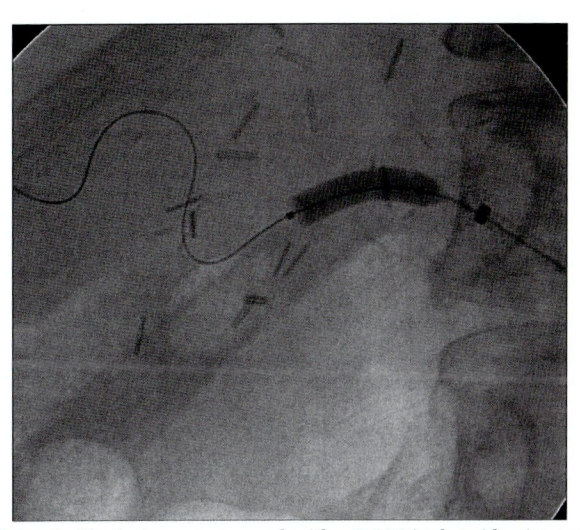

Figure 2. The lesion was crossed with a 0.014-inch guidewire and dilated with a 5-mm balloon.

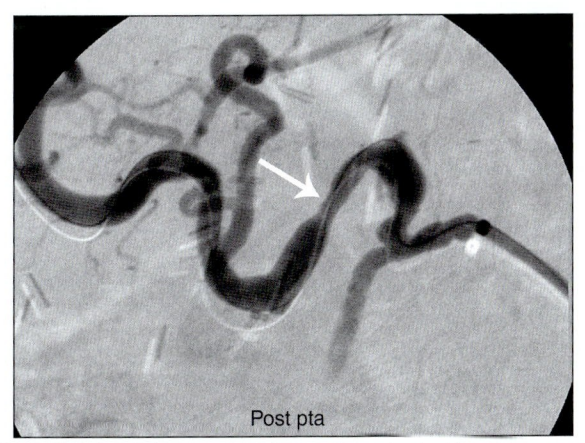

Figure 3. After balloon angioplasty, there is significant improvement in vessel caliber at the arterial anastomosis *(arrow)*.

Case 162

DEMOGRAPHICS/CLINICAL HISTORY

A 49-year-old man who underwent liver transplantation for end-stage liver disease attributed to hepatitis C cirrhosis, undergoing ultrasound.

DISCUSSION

History/Indications for Procedure
A 49-year-old man underwent liver transplantation 3 months before presentation. He has newly elevated levels of liver transaminases.

Procedure
Hepatic artery stenosis management in the liver transplant patient

Pre-procedure Imaging
Doppler ultrasound of the liver demonstrates a parvus tardus waveform in the hepatic artery, and the resistive index in the common hepatic artery is decreased, measuring 0.44.

Intraprocedural Findings
Hepatic arteriogram demonstrates a high-grade stenosis in the hepatic artery transplant (Fig. 1). Angioplasty of the stenosis was performed with a 4-mm balloon (Figs. 2 to 4).

Follow-up and Complications
The patient was observed overnight and discharged the next day. He has done well and has not required further arterial intervention in the 5 years since the angioplasty was performed.

Suggested Readings
Abbasoglu O, Levy MF, Vodapally MS, et al: Hepatic artery stenosis after liver transplantation—incidence, presentation, treatment, and long term outcome. Transplantation 63:250-255, 1997.

Mondragon RS, Karani JB, Heaton ND, et al: The use of percutaneous transluminal angioplasty in hepatic artery stenosis after transplantation. Transplantation 57:228-231, 1994.

Saad WE, Davies MG, Sahler L, et al: Hepatic artery stenosis in liver transplant recipients: Primary treatment with percutaneous transluminal angioplasty. J Vasc Intervent Radiol 16:795-805, 2005.

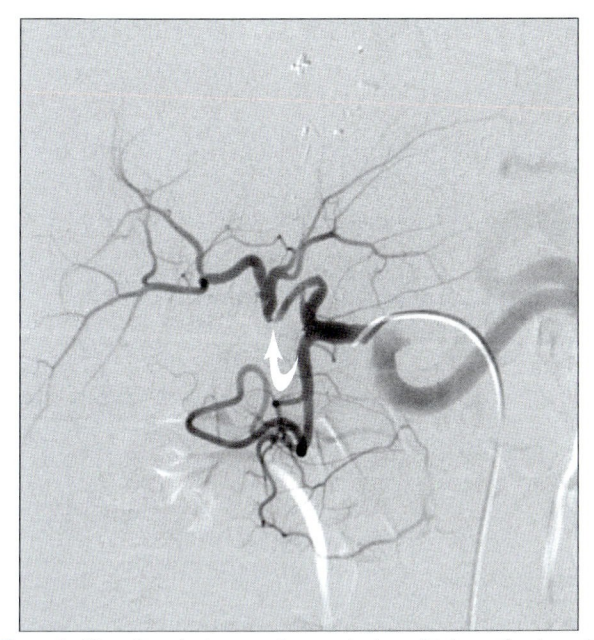

Figure 1. Hepatic arteriogram demonstrates a high-grade stenosis within the hepatic artery transplant *(arrow)*.

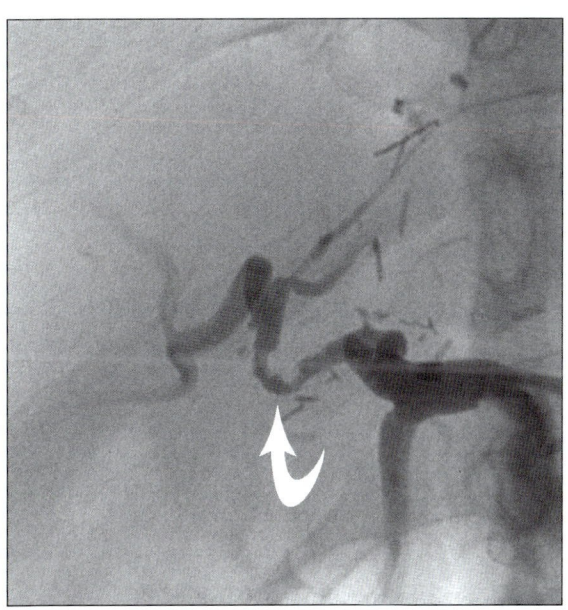

Figure 3. Follow-up arteriogram after balloon dilatation demonstrates the improved caliber of the stenotic portion of the vessel. The vessel is irregular in appearance *(arrow)*, possibly because of the presence of the guidewire straightening the vessel.

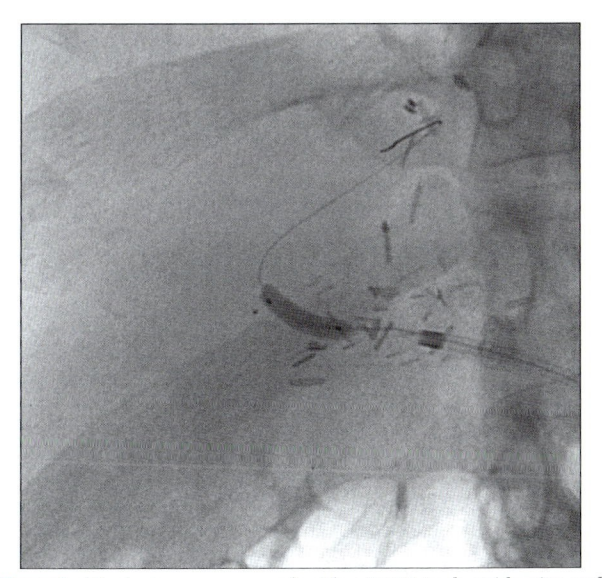

Figure 2. The lesion was crossed with a 0.014-inch guidewire and dilated with a 4-mm monorail balloon.

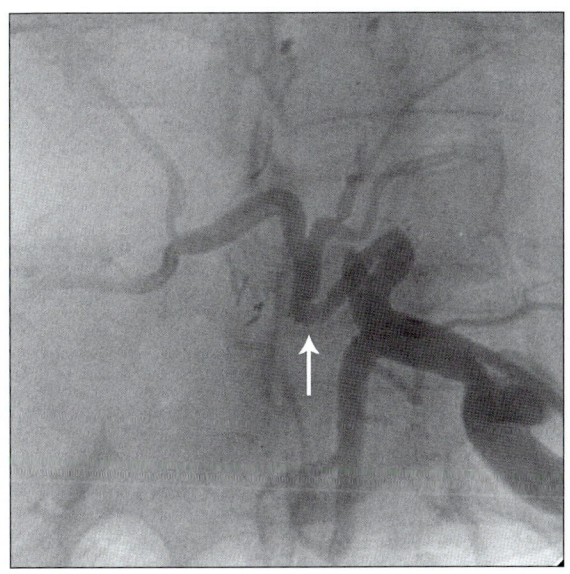

Figure 4. Repeat hepatic arteriogram after removing the guidewire shows that the irregularity of the hepatic artery no longer is present and there is only mild residual narrowing at the site of the original stenosis *(arrow)*.

Case 163

DEMOGRAPHICS/CLINICAL HISTORY

A 17-year-old girl after liver transplantation with a hepatic artery stenosis discovered on ultrasound, undergoing arteriography.

DISCUSSION

History/Indications for Procedure
A 17-year-old girl 1 month after liver transplantation has elevated liver function test results.

Procedure
Hepatic artery stenosis after liver transplantation

Pre-procedure Imaging
Doppler ultrasound of the liver showed a decrease in the resistive indices of the hepatic arteries (0.17 to 0.38), suggesting a hepatic artery stenosis.

Intraprocedural Findings
Hepatic angiography confirms a focal, high-grade stenosis of the hepatic artery (Fig. 1). Because the lesion showed significant elastic recoil after balloon angioplasty, a 5-mm, balloon-expandable stent was deployed across the lesion (Figs. 2 and 3).

Follow-up and Complications
The patient did well for 3 years (Fig. 4), at which time the hepatic arterial resistive indices again began to fall.

Suggested Readings
Cotroneo AR, Di Stasi C, Cina A, et al: Stent placement in four patients with hepatic artery stenosis or thrombosis after liver transplantation. J Vasc Intervent Radiol 13:619-623, 2002.

Denys A, Chevallier P, Doenz F, et al: Interventional radiology in the management of complications after liver transplantation. Eur Radiol 14:431-439, 2004.

Karani JB, Yu DF, Kane PA: Interventional radiology in liver transplantation. Cardiovasc Intervent Radiol 28:271-283, 2005.

Saad WE, Davies MG, Sahler L, et al: Hepatic artery stenosis in liver transplant recipients: Primary treatment with percutaneous transluminal angioplasty. J Vasc Intervent Radiol 16:795-805, 2005.

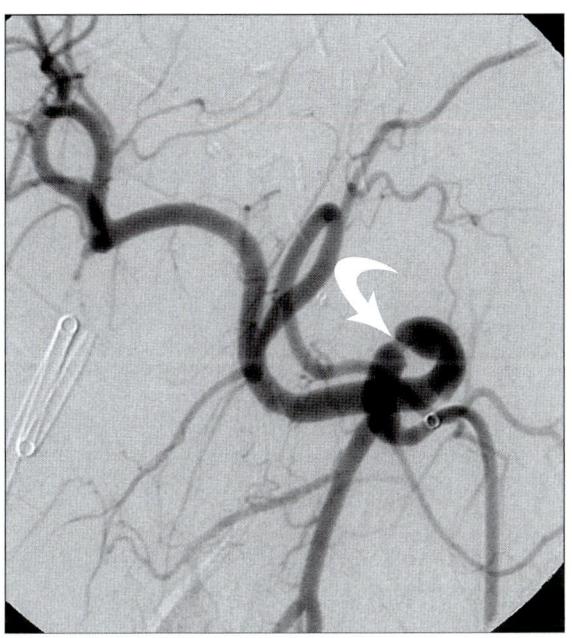

Figure 1. Selective hepatic arteriogram shows a focal stenosis in the region of the hepatic artery anastomosis *(arrow)*.

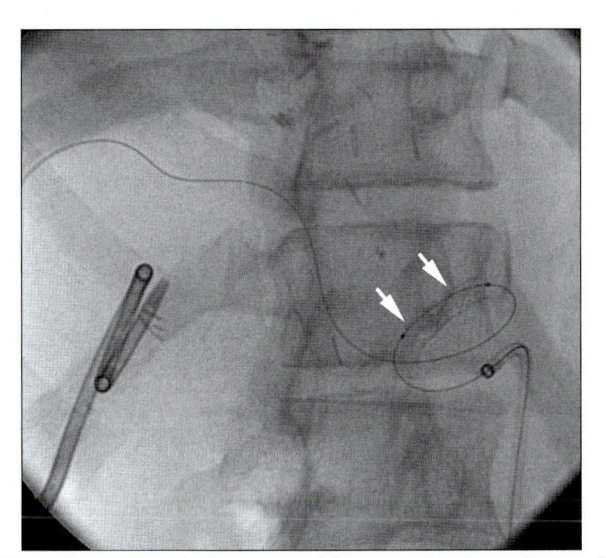

Figure 2. A 5-mm, balloon-expandable stent has been deployed across the stenosis *(arrows)*.

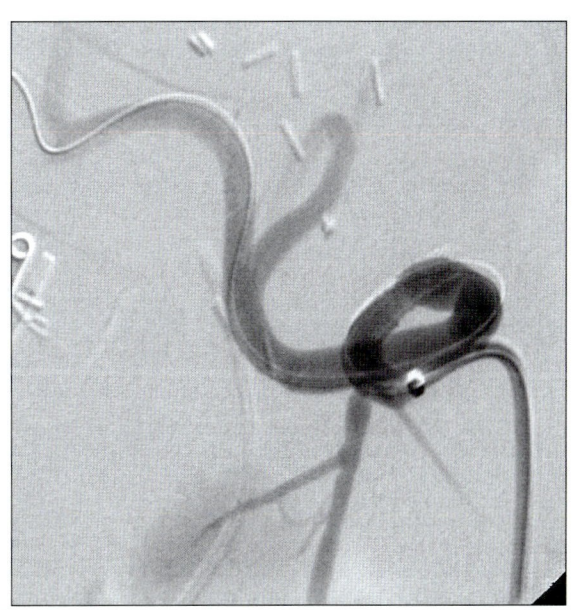

Figure 3. Follow-up arteriogram after stent placement shows no residual stenosis, and no complications were seen.

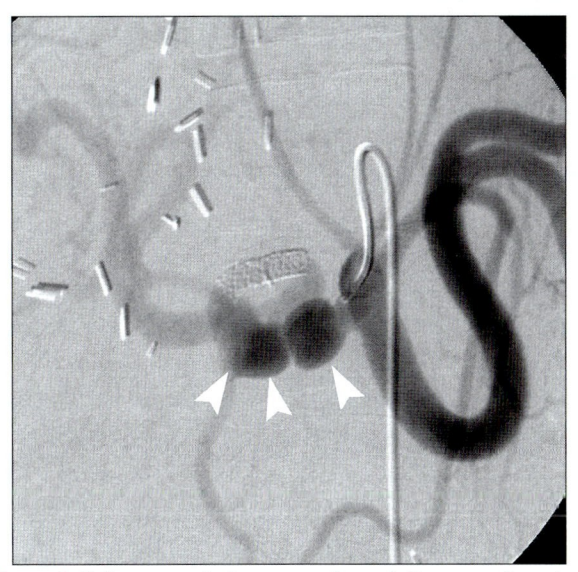

Figure 4. Follow-up arteriogram performed 3 years after stent placement shows the stent remains widely patent. There is new aneurysmal dilatation of the patient's native common hepatic artery proximal to the stent *(arrowheads)*.

Case 164

DEMOGRAPHICS/CLINICAL HISTORY

A 56-year-old man who underwent liver transplant 1 year earlier now presenting with hepatic artery stenosis, undergoing ultrasound and arteriography.

DISCUSSION

History/Indications for Procedure
A 56-year-old man who underwent liver transplant 1 year earlier now presents with hepatic artery stenosis.

Procedure
Percutaneous angioplasty for hepatic artery stenosis in a liver transplant patient

Pre-procedure Imaging
Doppler ultrasound of the liver shows tardus parvus waveforms of the intrahepatic arteries consistent with a stenosis at the hepatic artery anastomosis (Fig. 1).

Intraprocedural Findings
Hepatic arteriogram shows a focal, high-grade stenosis at the hepatic arterial anastomosis (Fig. 2). A 6 French guiding catheter was used for selective catheterization of the common hepatic artery. Angioplasty of the hepatic artery stenosis was performed with a 6-mm balloon (Fig. 3).

Follow-up and Complications
A small, non–flow-limiting dissection was identified after angioplasty. Follow-up ultrasound showed normalization of velocities and waveforms of the intrahepatic arteries (Fig. 4).

Suggested Readings
Saad WE: Management of hepatic artery steno-occlusive complications after liver transplantation. Tech Vasc Intervent Radiol 10:207, 2007.

Saad WE, Davies MG, Sahler L, et al: Hepatic artery stenosis in liver transplant recipients: Primary treatment with percutaneous transluminal angioplasty. J Vasc Intervent Radiol 16:795, 2005.

Zhou J, Lu SC, Yan LN, et al: Incidence and treatment of hepatic artery complications after orthotopic liver transplantation. World J Gastroenterol 9:2853, 2003.

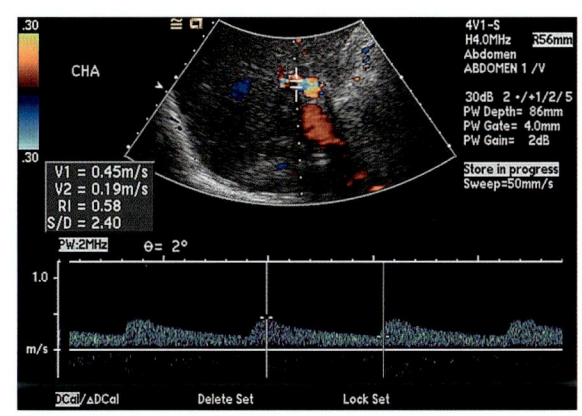

Figure 1. Doppler ultrasound of common hepatic artery shows reduced velocity and tardus parvus waveform suggesting more proximal stenosis.

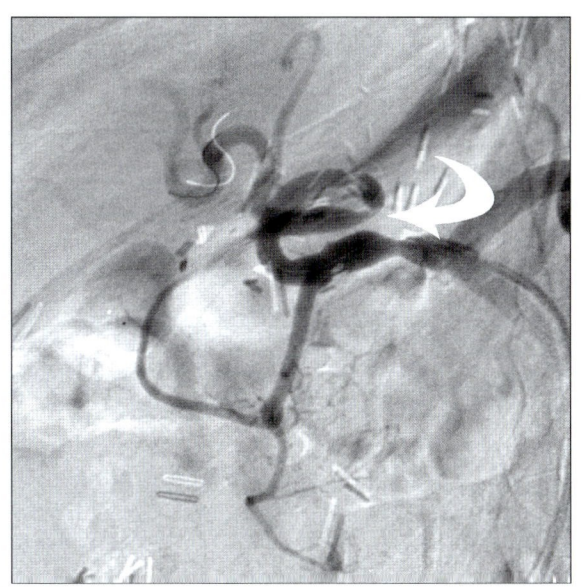

Figure 2. Hepatic arteriogram shows high-grade stenosis at anastomosis (*curved arrow*).

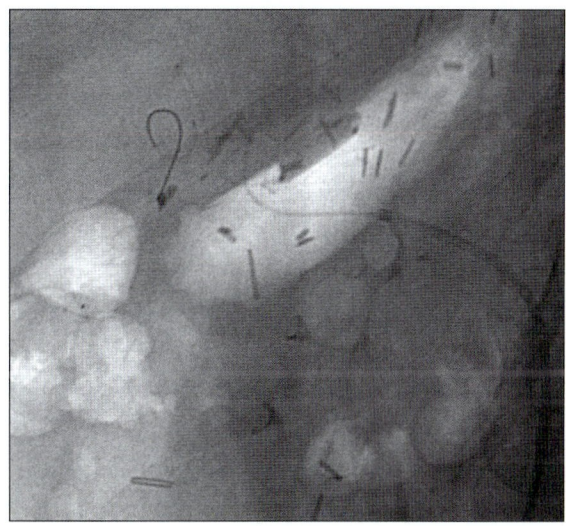

Figure 3. A 6 French guiding catheter has been advanced into common hepatic artery, and lesion has been crossed with 0.014-inch guidewire. A 6-mm balloon is inflated across stenosis.

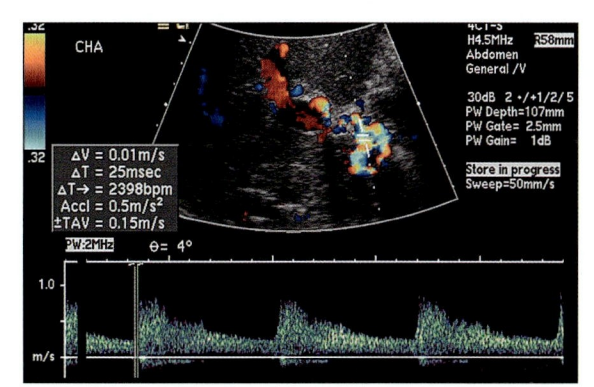

Figure 4. Follow-up Doppler ultrasound of common hepatic artery shows interval increase in hepatic artery velocity and normalization of arterial waveform.

Case 165

DEMOGRAPHICS/CLINICAL HISTORY

A 66-year-old man with abnormal surveillance ultrasound after liver transplant.

DISCUSSION

History/Indications for Procedure
A 66-year-old man who underwent liver transplantation 6 weeks prior presents with an abnormal surveillance ultrasound.

Procedure
Celiac artery stent placement for arterial steal syndrome in a liver transplant patient

Pre-procedure Imaging
Doppler ultrasound of the liver shows a slight tardus parvus waveform of the hepatic artery suggesting hepatic artery stenosis. CT angiogram shows a web-like stenosis of the proximal celiac trunk (Fig. 1); the hepatic artery anastamosis is widely patent.

Intraprocedural Findings
Visceral arteriogram shows a focal, high-grade stenosis of the celiac trunk with filling of the hepatic artery to pancreaticoduodenal arterial collaterals (Fig. 2). Because of the downward angulation of the origin of the celiac trunk, a left brachial arterial approach was used; the lesion was crossed with a 0.014-in guidewire and predilated to 4-mm (Fig. 3), and a 7-mm × 15-mm balloon-expandable stent was deployed (Fig. 4).

Follow-up and Complications
Follow-up Doppler ultrasound showed improvement in hepatic arterial waveform.

Suggested Readings
Kirbas I, Ulu EM, Ozturk A, et al: Multidetector computed tomographic angiography findings of splenic artery steal syndrome in liver transplantation. Transplant Proc 39:1178-1180, 2007.

Sevmis S, Boyvat F, Aytekin C, et al: Arterial steal syndrome after orthotopic liver transplantation. Transplant Proc 38:3651-3655, 2006.

Yilmaz S, Ceken K, Gurkan A, et al: Endovascular treatment of a recipient celiac trunk stenosis after orthotopic liver transplantation. J Endovasc Ther 10:376-380, 2003.

Case 165   331

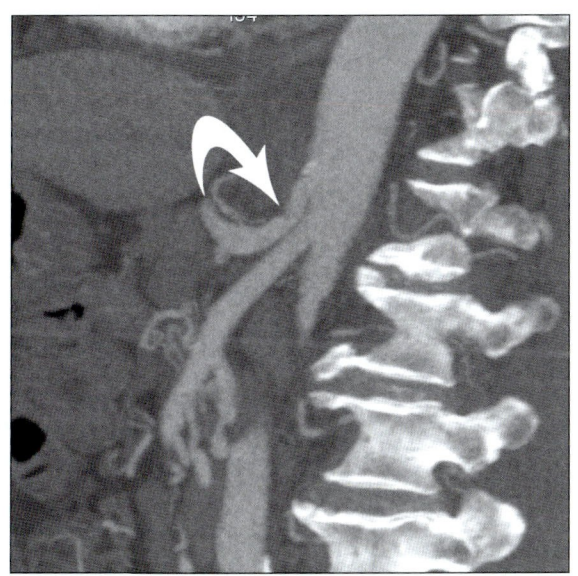

Figure 1. Sagittal reconstruction from CT angiogram of the abdomen shows a web-like stenosis of the proximal celiac trunk *(arrow)*.

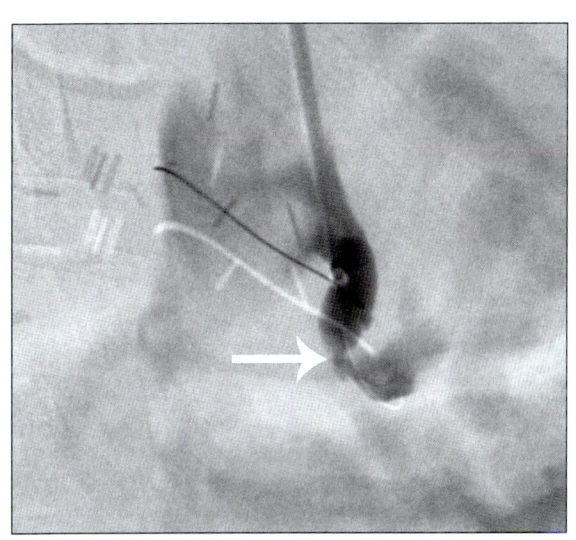

Figure 3. A 5-French sheath has been advanced into the proximal celiac trunk from a left brachial approach. Angiogram after predilatation of the stenosis shows the high-grade celiac artery stenosis *(arrow)*.

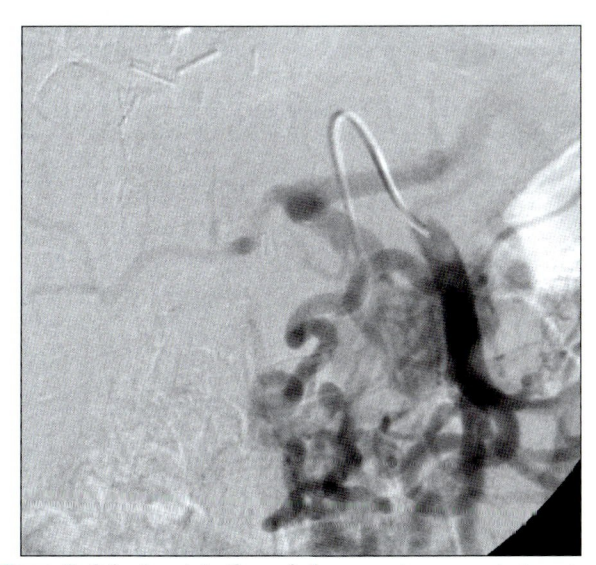

Figure 2. Selective injection of the superior mesenteric artery shows massively hypertrophied pancreaticoduodenal arteries and retrograde filling of the gastroduodenal and hepatic arteries.

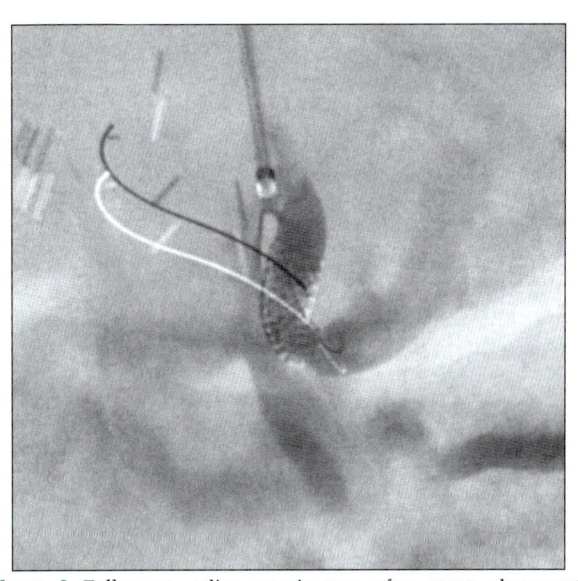

Figure 4. Follow-up celiac arteriogram after stent placement. A balloon-expandable stent has been placed across the lesion with no residual narrowing.

Case 166

DEMOGRAPHICS/CLINICAL HISTORY

A 66-year-old woman with new portal vein stenosis after liver transplantation, undergoing ultrasound and portal venography.

DISCUSSION

History/Indications for Procedure
A 66-year-old woman has new right upper quadrant abdominal pain after undergoing liver transplantation for biliary adenomatosis 6 years earlier.

Procedure
Portal vein stenosis after liver transplantation

Pre-procedure Imaging
Doppler ultrasound of the liver demonstrated a fivefold increase in velocity across the portal vein anastomosis.

Intraprocedural Findings
The portal vein was accessed with a transhepatic approach (Fig. 1). Portal venogram demonstrates a focal, high-grade stenosis at the portal vein anastomosis that is associated with a pressure gradient of 6 mm Hg.

Follow-up and Complications
The portal vein stenosis was successfully treated with angioplasty using a 9-mm balloon (Fig. 2), reducing the pressure gradient to 1 mm Hg. After the procedure, the patient's abdominal pain persisted, but ultrasound demonstrated that the portal vein velocities returned to baseline (Fig. 3), and the patient required no further portal vein interventions.

Suggested Readings

Buell JF, Funaki B, Cronin DC, et al: Long-term venous complications after full-size and segmental pediatric liver transplantation. Ann Surg 236:658-666, 2002.

Denys A, Chavallier P, Doenz F, et al: Interventional radiology in the management of complications after liver transplantation. Eur Radiol 14:431-439, 2004.

Funaki B, Rosenblum JD, Leef JA, et al: Percutaneous treatment of portal venous stenosis in children and adolescents with segmental hepatic transplants: Long-term results. Radiology 215:147-151, 2000.

Karani JB, Yu DF, Kane PA: Interventional radiology in liver transplantation. Cardiovasc Intervent Radiol 28:271-283, 2005.

Zajko AB, Bron KM, Orons PD: Vascular complications in liver transplant recipients: Angiographic diagnosis and treatment. Semin Intervent Radiol 9:270-281, 1992.

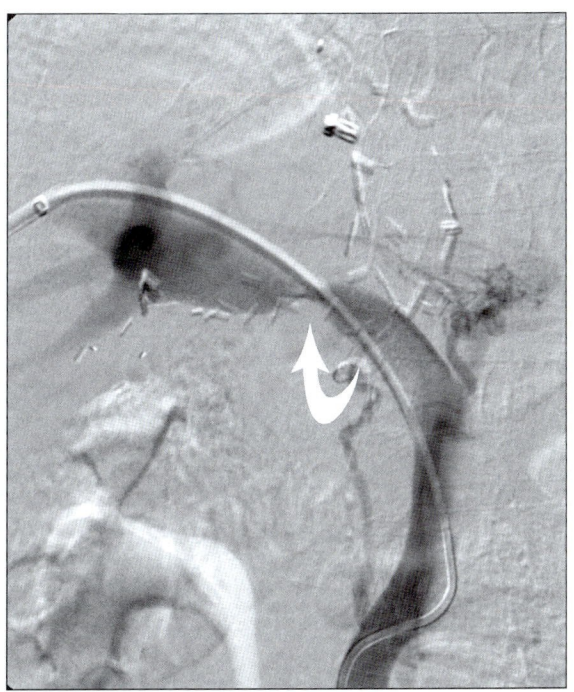

Figure 1. Transhepatic portogram demonstrates a focal portal vein stenosis at the anastomosis *(arrow)*. This stenosis was associated with a pressure gradient of 6 mm Hg.

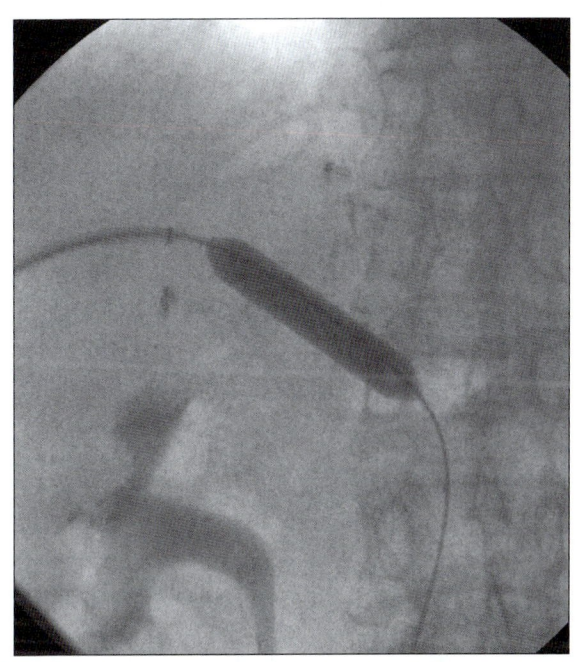

Figure 2. The stenosis was treated with angioplasty using a 9-mm balloon.

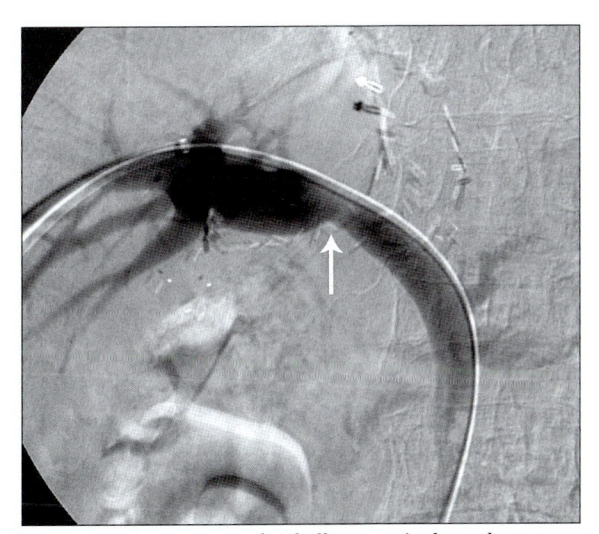

Figure 3. Portal venogram after balloon angioplasty demonstrates only mild residual narrowing at the portal vein anastomosis *(arrow)*. The pressure gradient at this point was only 1 mm Hg.

Case 167

DEMOGRAPHICS/CLINICAL HISTORY

A 44-year-old man who underwent liver transplantation 1 year earlier for hepatitis C.

DISCUSSION

History/Indications for Procedure
A 44-year-old man who underwent liver transplantation 1 year earlier for hepatitis C. The patient is currently asymptomatic, but he has had a recent elevation in liver enzymes.

Procedure
Management of portal vein stenosis in a liver transplant patient

Pre-procedure Imaging
Doppler ultrasound of the liver shows a stenosis at the site of the portal vein anastomosis with an elevation in blood flow velocity at this location (Fig. 1).

Intraprocedural Findings
There is a focal, high-grade stenosis of the portal vein at the level of the anastomosis; this stenosis is associated with a 4 mm Hg pressure gradient and there is competing flow out the enlarged coronary vein (Fig. 2). The stenosis was angioplastied to 14 mm Hg (Fig. 3) with only mild portal vein narrowing following the angioplasty and no residual pressure gradient across the anastomosis (Fig. 4).

Suggested Readings
Shibata T, Itoh K, Kubo T, et al.: Percutaneous transhepatic balloon dilation of portal venous stenosis in patient with living donor liver transplantation. Radiology 235:1078-1083, 2005.

Woo DH, Laberge JM, Gordon RL, et al.: Management of portal venous complications after liver transplantation. Tech Vasc Intervent Radiol 10:233-239, 2007.

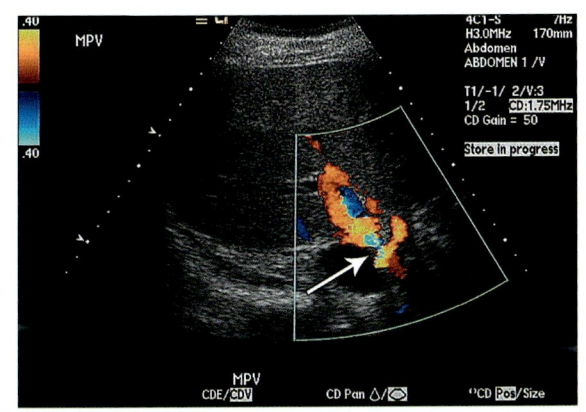

Figure 1. Color Doppler ultrasound shows narrowing of the main portal vein (arrow) with associated elevated blood flow velocities.

Figure 3. The portal vein stenosis was angioplastied to 14 mm.

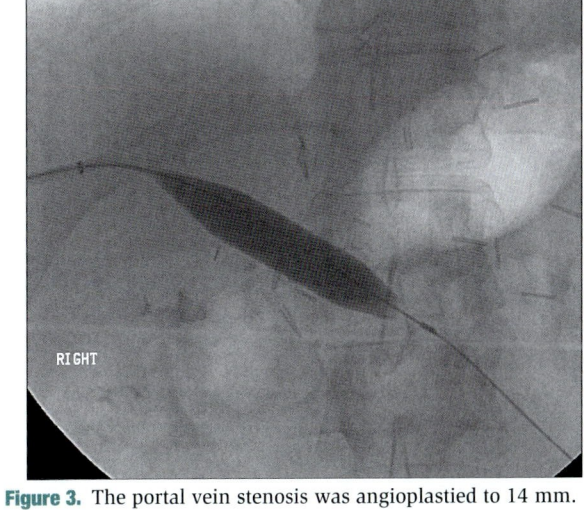

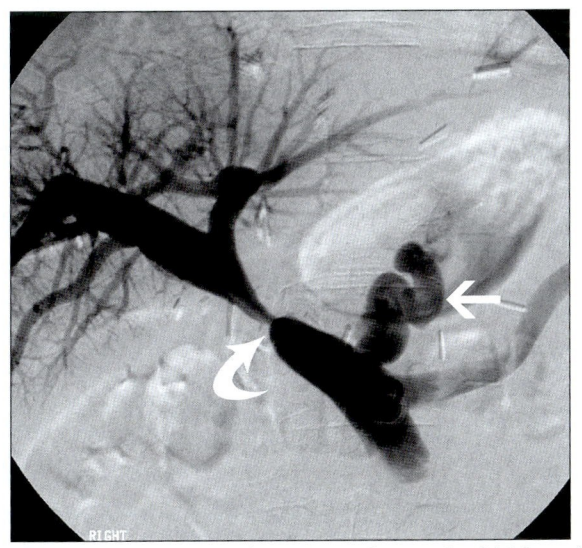

Figure 2. Transhepatic portal venogram shows a focal high-grade stenosis of the main portal vein (curved arrow) with filling of a large coronary vein (arrow).

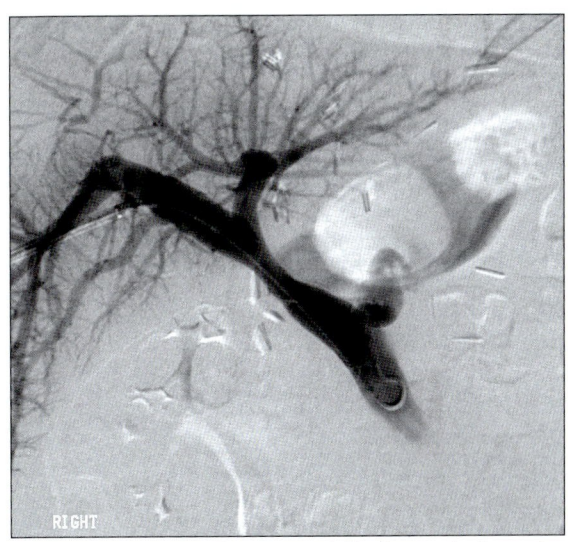

Figure 4. Follow-up portal venogram following angioplasty shows markedly improved caliber of the main portal vein. Despite the mild residual narrowing, there was no associated pressure gradient

Case 168

DEMOGRAPHICS/CLINICAL HISTORY

A 51-year-old woman after liver transplantation for hepatitis C–induced cirrhosis, undergoing ultrasonography and portography.

DISCUSSION

History/Indications for Procedure
A 51-year-old woman who underwent liver transplantation for hepatitis C–induced cirrhosis presents with worsening ascites.

Procedure
Portal vein thrombosis in a liver transplant recipient

Pre-procedure Imaging
Doppler ultrasound of the liver shows a large thrombus in the main portal vein (Fig. 1).

Intraprocedural Findings
Transhepatic portography shows a large thrombus in the main portal vein (Fig. 2). The thrombus was macerated with a 20-mm Dormia basket, and the remaining thrombus was treated with an overnight infusion of urokinase.

Follow-up and Complications
The thrombus in the portal vein had largely resolved after 24 hours of catheter-directed thrombolysis (Fig. 3). The portal vein remained patent at the time of the last follow-up, 4 years after the thrombolysis procedure.

Suggested Readings

Bhattacharjya T, Olliff SP, Bhattacharjya S, et al: Percutaneous portal vein thrombolysis and endovascular stent for management of posttransplant portal venous conduit thrombosis. Transplantation 69:2195-2198, 2000.

Cherukuri R, Haskal ZJ, Naji A, Shaked A: Percutaneous thrombolysis and stent placement for the treatment of portal vein thrombosis after liver transplantation: Long-term follow-up. Transplantation 65:1124-1126, 1998.

Durham JD, LaBerge JM, Altman S, et al: Portal vein thrombolysis and closure of competitive shunts following liver transplantation. J Vasc Intervent Radiol 5:611-615, 1994.

Karani JB, Yu DF, Kane PA: Interventional radiology in liver transplantation. Cardiovasc Intervent Radiol 28:271-283, 2005.

Case 168   337

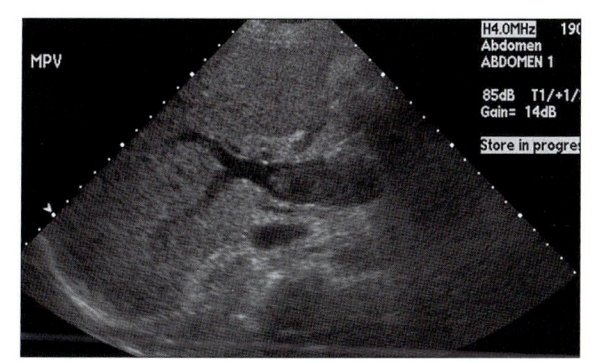

Figure 1. Ultrasound image shows a large thrombus in the main portal vein *(arrow)*. The intrahepatic portal vein branches are patent.

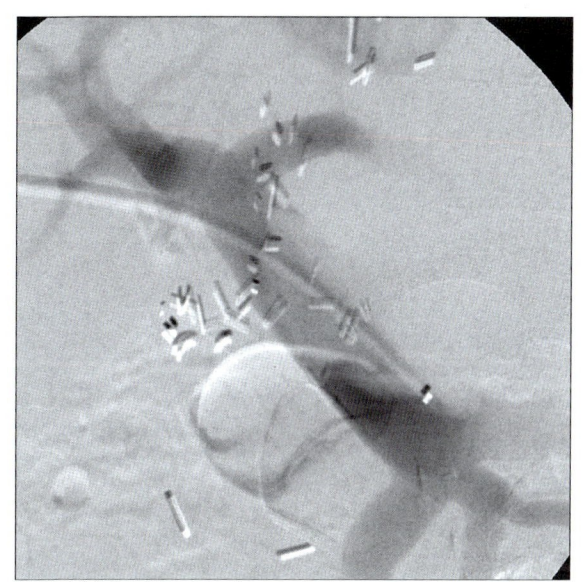

Figure 2. Transhepatic portogram shows a large filling defect in the main portal vein that is consistent with thrombus.

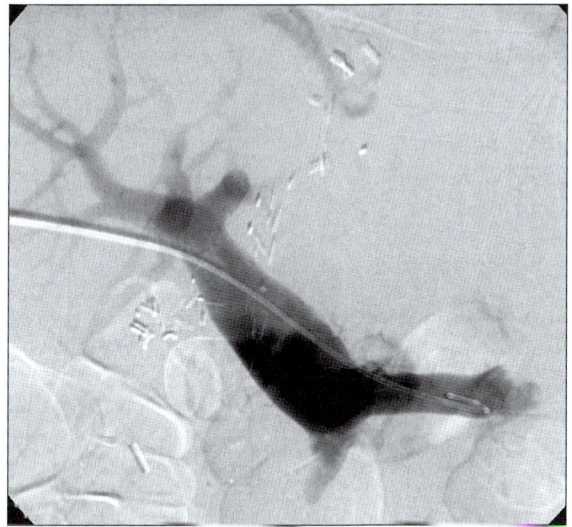

Figure 3. Follow-up portogram after thrombolysis shows nearly complete resolution of the portal vein clot.

Case 169

DEMOGRAPHICS/CLINICAL HISTORY

A 39-year-old woman, status post–liver transplantation with poor liver function, undergoing inferior venacavography.

DISCUSSION

History/Indications for Procedure
At 8 days status post–liver transplantation, this patient presented with worsening ascites and liver function.

Procedure
Inferior vena cava (IVC) stenting in a liver transplant patient

Pre-procedure Imaging
Doppler ultrasound of the liver reveals increasing size of the liver and slight decrease in hepatic vein phasicity.

Intraprocedural Findings
A focal stenosis is identified in the suprahepatic inferior vena cava (IVC) with a pressure gradient of 20 mm Hg (Fig. 1). This lesion was stented with a 20-mm Gianturco stent; the hepatic venous outflow also was treated with the placement of a Wallstent from the right hepatic vein into the IVC (Figs. 2 and 3).

Follow-up and Complications
Follow-up Doppler ultrasound of the liver showed reduction in size of the liver with restoration of triphasic waveforms within the hepatic veins.

Suggested Readings
Orons PD, Hari AK, Zajko JB, et al: Thrombolysis and endovascular stent placement for inferior vena caval thrombosis in a liver transplant recipient. Transplantation 64:1357-1361, 1997.

Weeks SM, Gerber DA, Jaques PF, et al: Primary Gianturco stent placement for inferior vena cava abnormalities following liver transplantation. J Vasc Intervent Radiol 11(2 Pt 1):177-187, 2000.

Wittich GR, Goodacre BW, Kennedy PT, et al: Anchoring a migrating inferior vena cava stent with use of a T-fastener. J Vasc Intervent Radiol 12:994-996, 2001.

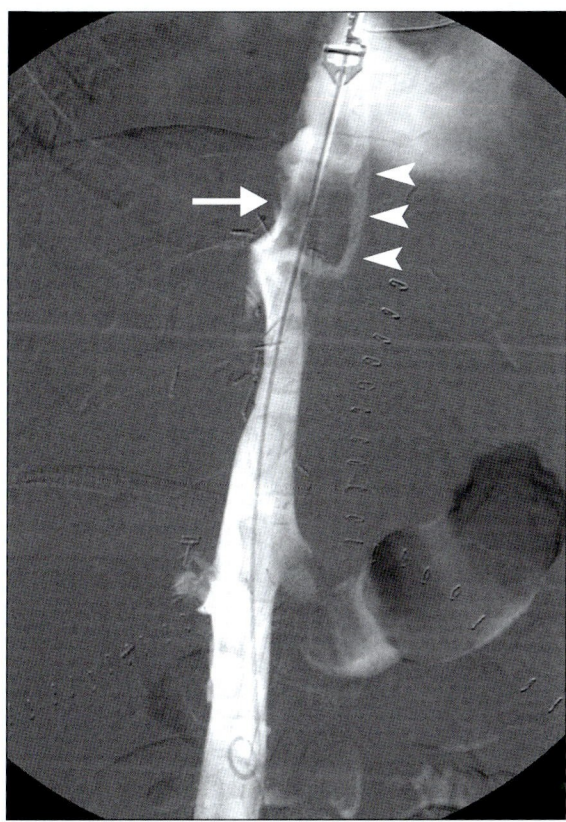

Figure 1. Inferior venacavogram shows stenosis of the suprahepatic IVC *(arrow)*. Note the presence of a prominent collateral vein *(arrowheads)*.

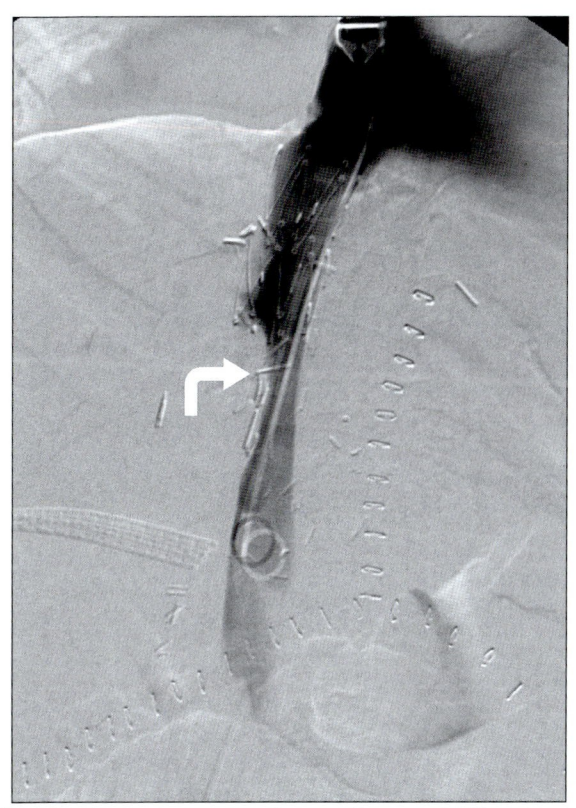

Figure 2. Gianturco stent placed across the stenosis. There is now mild narrowing of the IVC below the stent *(arrow)*, probably the result of twisting of the IVC.

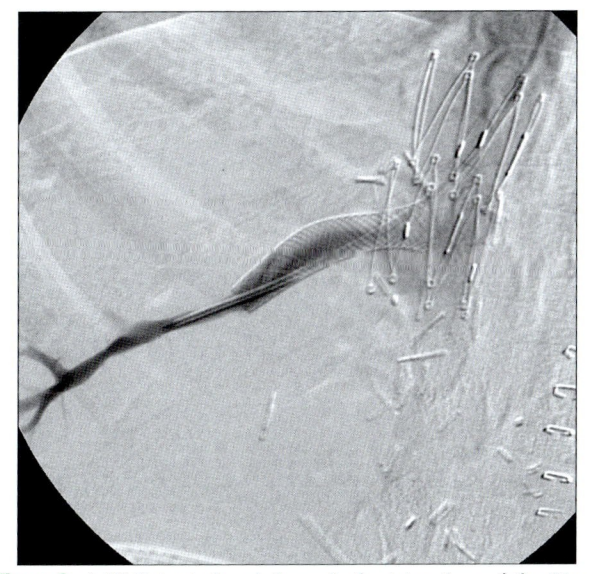

Figure 3. A Wallstent placed through the interstices of the Gianturco stent was used to improve hepatic venous outflow.

Case 170

DEMOGRAPHICS/CLINICAL HISTORY

A 52-year-old man with inferior vena cava (IVC) stenosis 3 weeks after liver transplantation, undergoing ultrasound.

DISCUSSION

History/Indications for Procedure
A 52-year-old man underwent liver transplantation for hepatitis C cirrhosis. Postoperatively, the patient developed severe ascites.

Procedure
Inferior vena cava stenosis in a liver transplant patient

Pre-procedure Imaging
Doppler ultrasound demonstrated narrowing of the IVC just inferior to the caval anastomosis. The Doppler waveforms within the IVC were damped and monophasic.

Intraprocedural Findings
The long-segment stenosis of the intrahepatic IVC (Fig. 1) is associated with a 12-mm Hg pressure gradient. The stenosis was stented with two overlapping, self-expanding Gianturco stents.

Follow-up and Complications
After stent placement, the gradient across the intrahepatic IVC was 1 mm Hg (Figs. 2 and 3). The patient was discharged from the hospital 1 week after stent placement (4 weeks after liver transplantation), and he continues to do well and has had no further IVC interventions in the 2 years since stent placement.

Suggested Readings
Orons PD, Hari AK, Zajko AB, Marsh JW: Thrombolysis and endovascular stent placement for inferior vena caval thrombosis in a liver transplant recipient. Transplantation 64:1357-1361, 1997.

Weeks SM, Gerber DA, Jaques PF, et al: Primary Gianturco stent placement for inferior vena cava abnormalities following liver transplantation. J Vasc Intervent Radiol 11(Pt 1):177-187, 2000.

Wittich GR, Goodacre BW, Kennedy PT, Mathew P: Anchoring a migrating inferior vena cava stent with use of a T-fastener. J Vasc Intervent Radiol 12:994-996, 2001.

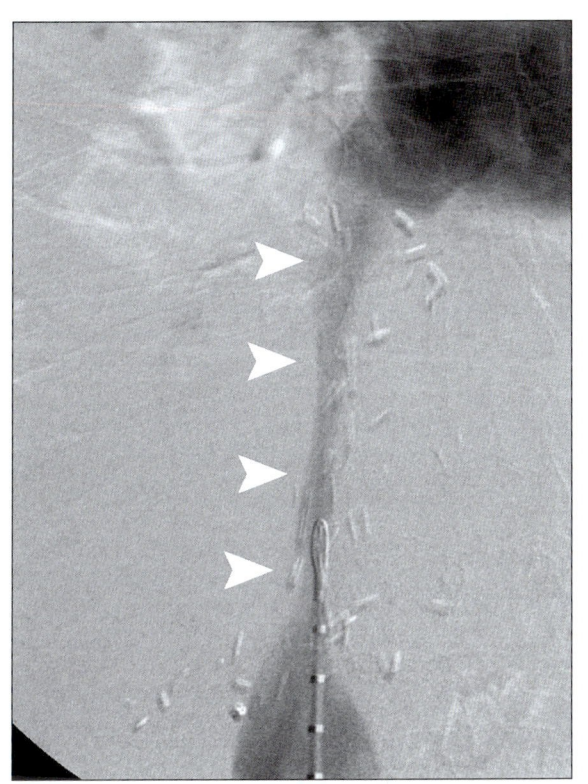

Figure 1. Inferior venacavogram from a femoral approach demonstrates diffuse narrowing of the intrahepatic IVC *(arrowheads)*. This stenosis was associated with a 12-mm Hg pressure gradient.

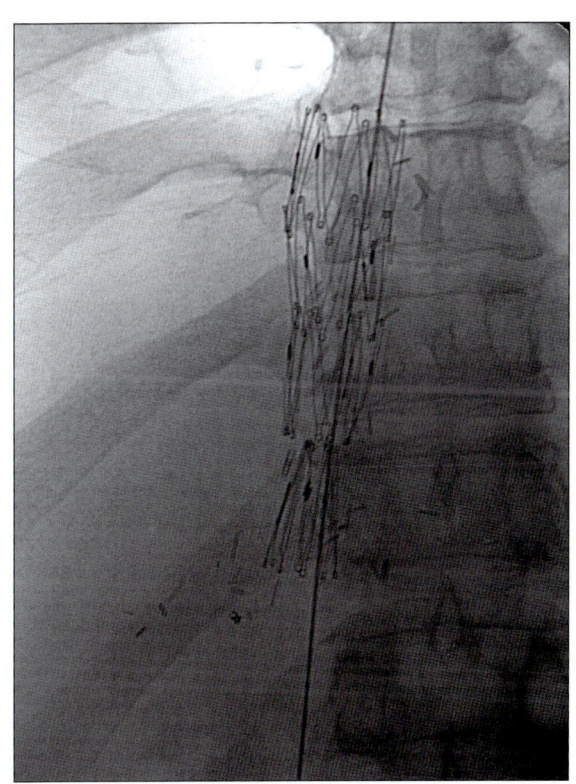

Figure 2. The lesion was treated with the placement of two overlapping, self-expanding Gianturco stents.

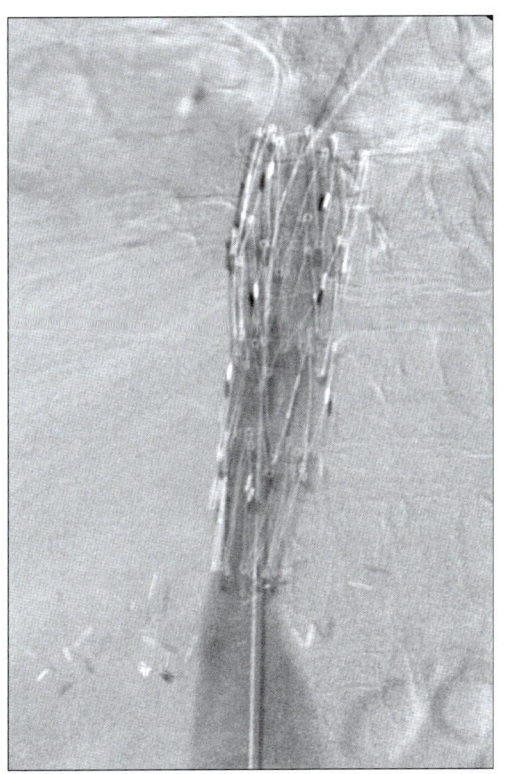

Figure 3. Follow-up cavogram after stent placement demonstrates improved flow through the intrahepatic IVC. The pressure gradient was 1 mm Hg after stent placement.

Case 171

DEMOGRAPHICS/CLINICAL HISTORY

A 9-year-old girl who has undergone liver transplantation with recurrent inferior vena cava (IVC) stenosis, undergoing cavography.

DISCUSSION

History/Indications for Procedure

A 9-year-old girl who underwent a second liver transplantation 2 years earlier presents with recurrent IVC stenosis. The patient has had multiple episodes of hypoalbuminemia over the past year, requiring IVC angioplasty on an increasingly frequent basis.

Procedure

Inferior vena cava stent placement in a liver transplant patient

Pre-procedure Imaging

Cavography shows a recurrent stenosis at the cavoatrial junction (Fig. 1). The infrarenal IVC is occluded, and there is filling of numerous venous collaterals.

Intraprocedural Findings

A 14-mm × 4-cm self-expanding nitinol stent was deployed across the stenosis (Fig. 2). Follow-up cavography shows the stent to be positioned above the hepatic vein anastomosis, extending into the right atrium (Fig. 3).

Follow-up and Complications

Since the stent placement, the patient's albumin levels have remained normal, and she has had no evidence for recurrent stenosis.

Suggested Readings

Carnevale FC, Machado AT, De Gregorio MA, et al: Midterm and long-term results of percutaneous endovascular treatment of venous outflow obstruction after pediatric liver transplantation. J Vasc Intervent Radiol 19:1439, 2008.

Darcy MD: Management of venous outflow complications after liver transplantation. Tech Vasc Intervent Radiol 10:240, 2007.

Lorenz JM, Van Ha T, Funaki B, et al: Percutaneous treatment of venous outflow obstruction in pediatric liver transplants. J Vasc Intervent Radiol 17:1753, 2006.

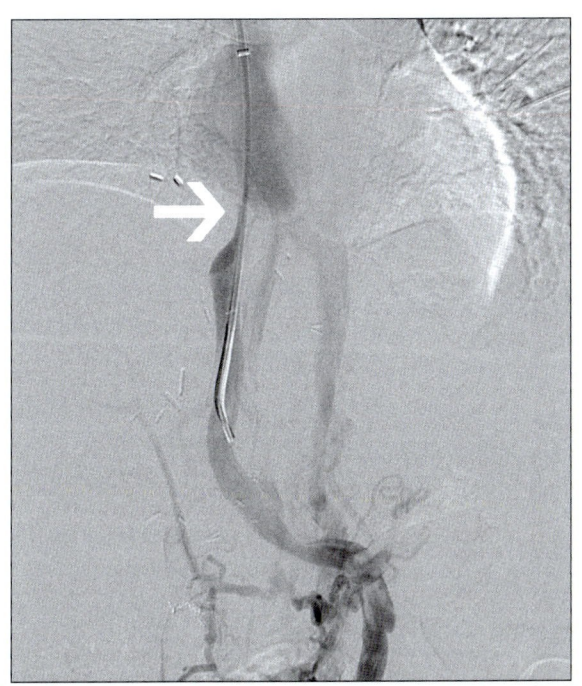

Figure 1. Inferior venacavogram shows chronic occlusion of infrarenal IVC with filling of multiple collateral veins. There is focal, high-grade stenosis of IVC at level of cavoatrial junction (*arrow*).

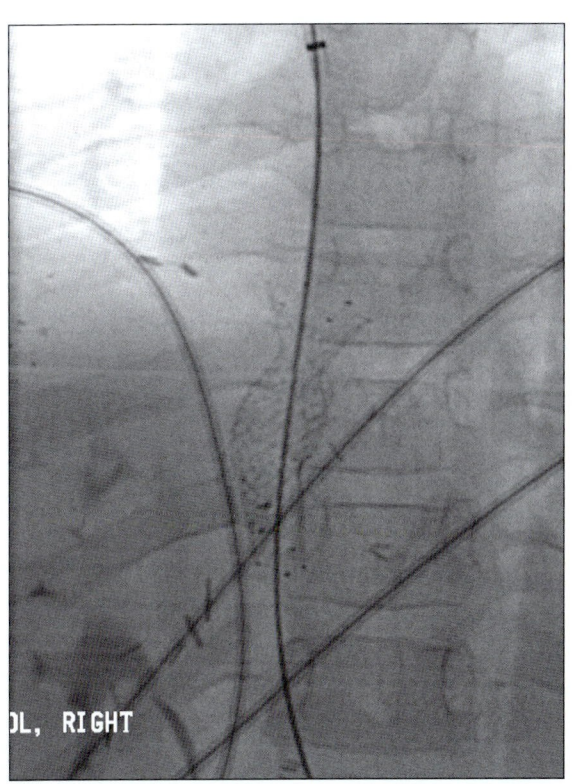

Figure 2. Cavogram shows 14-mm × 4-cm self-expanding nitinol stent has been deployed across stenosis.

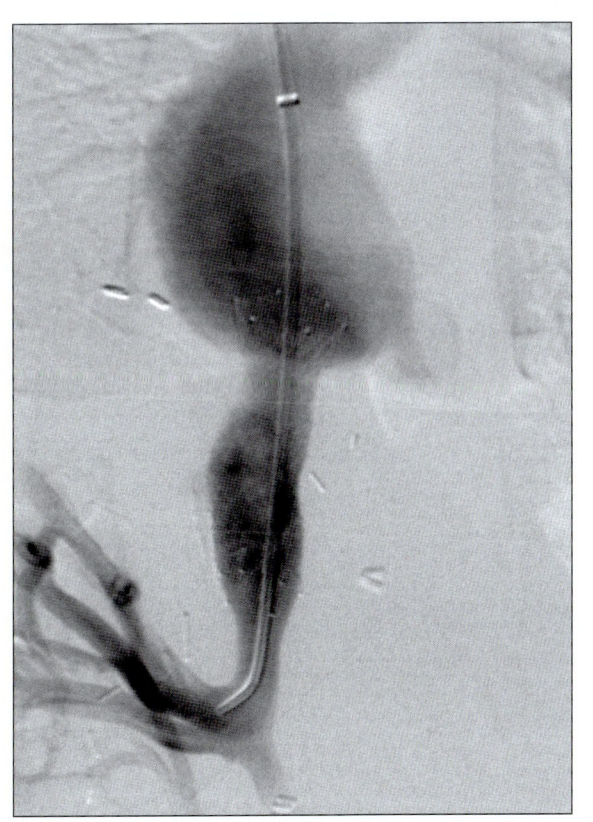

Figure 3. Follow-up cavogram with catheter positioned at level of hepatic veins shows significantly improved venous outflow through stent. There is no longer filling of abdominal venous collaterals.

Case 172

DEMOGRAPHICS/CLINICAL HISTORY

A 49-year-old man with increasing ascites following liver transplantation.

DISCUSSION

History/Indications for Procedure
A 49-year-old man underwent liver transplantation 2 weeks previously with increasing ascites.

Procedure
Hepatic vein stenting following liver transplantation

Pre-procedure Imaging
Doppler ultrasound of the liver demonstrates elevated velocities at the junction of the right hepatic vein and IVC suggesting stenosis at this location (not shown). The intrahepatic IVC is also narrowed.

Intraprocedural Findings
There is narrowing of the intrahepatic IVC with no associated pressure gradient. There is a high-grade stenosis at the junction of the right hepatic vein and IVC associated with a 12-mm Hg pressure gradient; this was treated with the placement of a 20-mm × 5-cm Gianturco stent (Figs. 1 and 2).

Follow-up and Complications
The patient had a follow-up hepatic venogram after an abnormal ultrasound 2 years after stent placement. This follow-up venogram shows the stent to remain patent with no development of a pressure gradient.

Suggested Readings
Darcy MD: Management of venous outflow complications after liver transplantation. Tech Vasc Intervent Radiol 10:240-245, 2007.

Ko GY, Sung KB, Yoon HK, et al: Endovascular treatment of hepatic venous outflow obstruction after living-donor liver transplantation. J Vasc Intervent Radiol 13:591-599, 2002.

Denys A, Chevallier P, Doenz F, et al: Interventional radiology in the management of complications after liver transplantation. Eur Radiol 14:431-439, 2004.

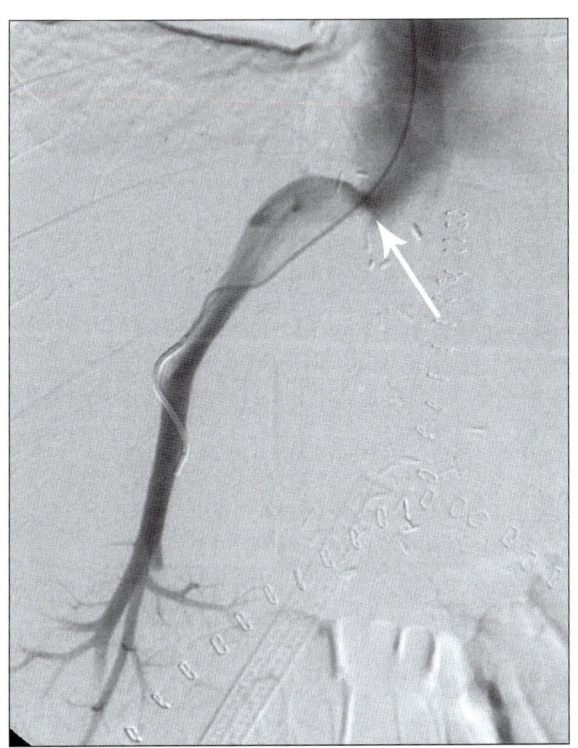

Figure 1. Hepatic venogram shows a focal stenosis at the junction of the hepatic vein and IVC (arrow). This was associated with a 12-mm Hg pressure gradient.

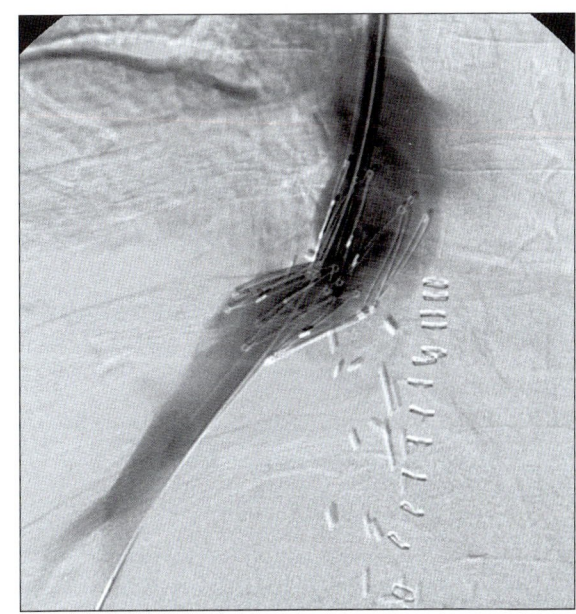

Figure 2. Follow-up venogram following stent placement shows improved venous outflow following Gianturco stent placement.

Case 173

DEMOGRAPHICS/CLINICAL HISTORY

A 61-year-old asymptomatic woman with incidental discovery of pulmonary arteriovenous malformation (AVM), undergoing chest radiography.

DISCUSSION

History/Indications for Procedure
Incidental discovery of a pulmonary AVM measuring > 3 mm in size was made in this patient. The patient also has a history of nosebleeds.

Procedure
Embolization of pulmonary arteriovenous malformation (AVM)

Pre-procedure Imaging
Chest radiograph shows a parenchymal density in the left lower lobe, consistent with the patient's pulmonary AVM (Fig. 1).

Intraprocedural Findings
A pulmonary AVM was identified in the left lung base, supplied by a solitary feeding vessel measuring 5.5 mm in diameter (Figs. 2 and 3). The AVM was embolized with coils (Fig. 4).

Follow-up and Complications
The patient recovered from the embolization uneventfully. She and her family were referred for genetic counseling for hereditary hemorrhagic telangiectasia syndrome.

Suggested Readings
Guttmacher AE, Marchuk DA, White RI Jr: Hereditary hemorrhagic telangiectasia. N Engl J Med 333:918-924, 1995.

Mager JJ, Overtoom TT, Blauw H, et al: Embolotherapy of pulmonary arteriovenous malformations: Long-term results in 112 patients. J Vasc Intervent Radiol 15:451-456, 2004.

Pollak JS, Saluja S, Thabet A, et al: Clinical and anatomic outcomes after embolotherapy of pulmonary arteriovenous malformations. J Vasc Intervent Radiol 17:35-45, 2006.

White RI Jr, Pollak JS, Wirth JA: Pulmonary arteriovenous malformations: Diagnosis and transcatheter embolotherapy. J Vasc Intervent Radiol 7:787-804, 1996.

Case 173   347

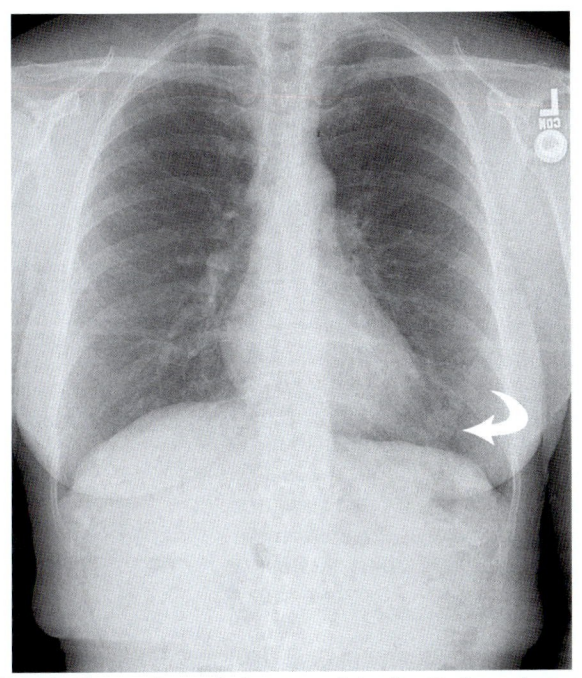

Figure 1. Chest radiograph shows a nodular density *(curved arrow)* in the left lung base.

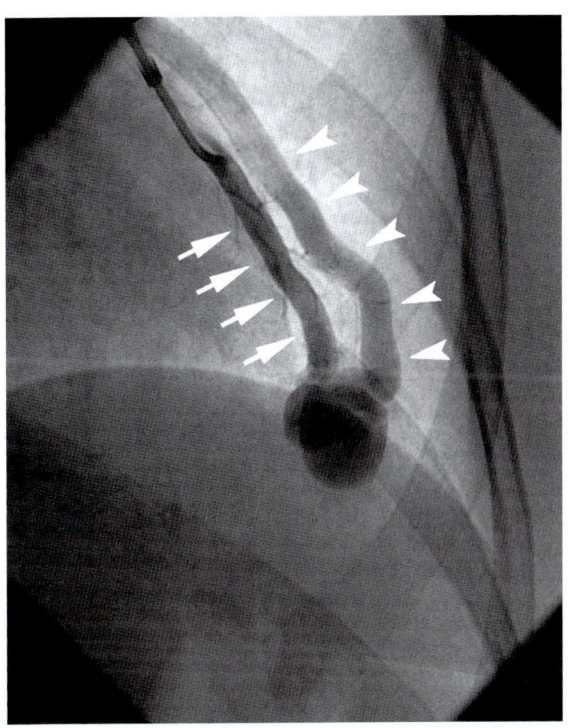

Figure 3. Selective injection confirms only a single feeding artery *(arrows)* and single draining vein *(arrowheads)*.

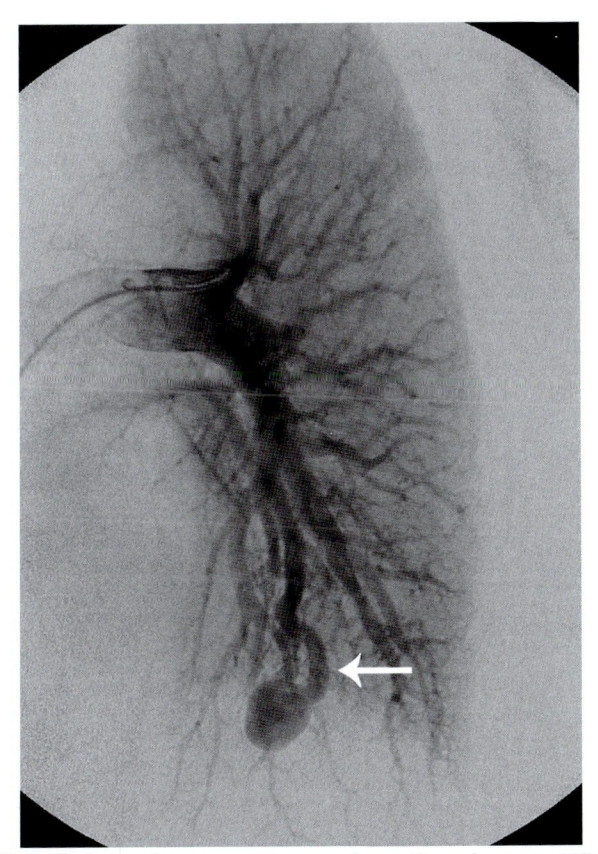

Figure 2. Left pulmonary angiogram shows the pulmonary AVM *(arrow)* in the left lung base.

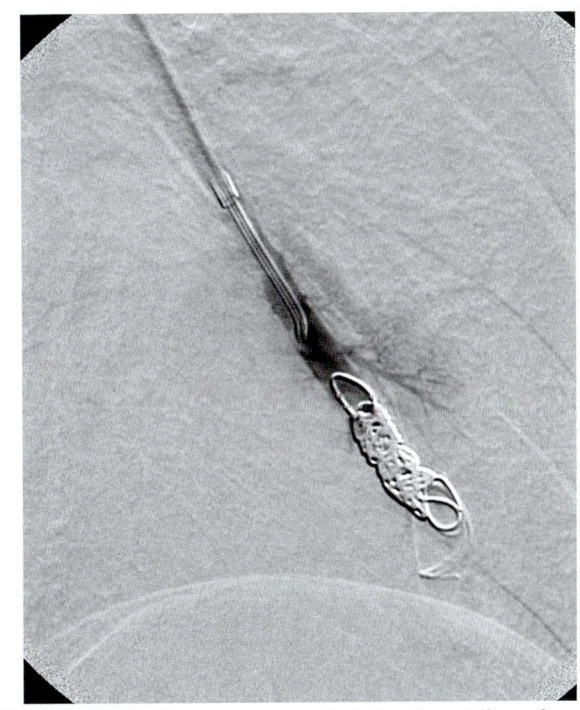

Figure 4. The feeding artery was occluded with metallic coils.

Case 174

DEMOGRAPHICS/CLINICAL HISTORY

A 38-year-old woman with a history of multiple sclerosis and shortness of breath, undergoing CT.

DISCUSSION

History/Indications for Procedure
This patient presented with shortness of breath and was shown to have a pulmonary arteriovenous malformation (AVM).

Procedure
Endovascular management of large pulmonary arteriovenous malformation (AVM).

Pre-procedure Imaging
Contrast-enhanced CT scan of the chest reveals a large pulmonary AVM supplied by a left lower lobe pulmonary artery (Fig. 1). The AVM is associated with a 4.2-cm venous aneurysm (Fig. 2).

Intraprocedural Findings
Pulmonary angiogram shows a large, simple pulmonary AVM with a short feeding artery (Fig. 3). The aneurysm was embolized with a combination of detachable and pushable metallic coils (Fig. 4).

Follow-up and Complications
The patient's oxygen requirement significantly improved after the embolization.

Suggested Readings

Dinkel HP, Triller J: Pulmonary arteriovenous malformations: Embolotherapy with superselective coaxial catheter placement and filling of venous sac with Guglielmi detachable coils. Radiology 223: 709-714, 2002.

White RI Jr, Lynch-Nyhan A, Terry P, et al: Pulmonary arteriovenous malformations: Techniques and long-term outcome of embolotherapy. Radiology 169:663-669, 1988.

White RI Jr, Pollak JS, Wirth JA, et al: Pulmonary arteriovenous malformations: Diagnosis and transcatheter embolotherapy. J Vasc Intervent Radiol 7:787-804, 1996.

White RI Jr, Mitchell SE, Barth KH, et al: Angioarchitecture of pulmonary arteriovenous malformations: An important consideration before embolotherapy. AJR Am J Roentgenol 140:681-686, 1983.

Case 174   349

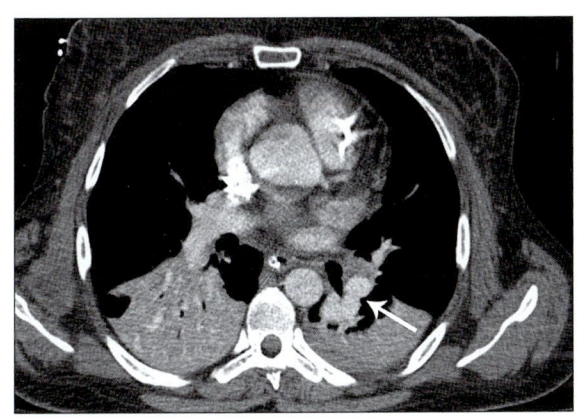

Figure 1. Axial CT scan shows pulmonary AVM *(arrow)* in the left lower lobe. Bilateral lower lobe consolidation also is present.

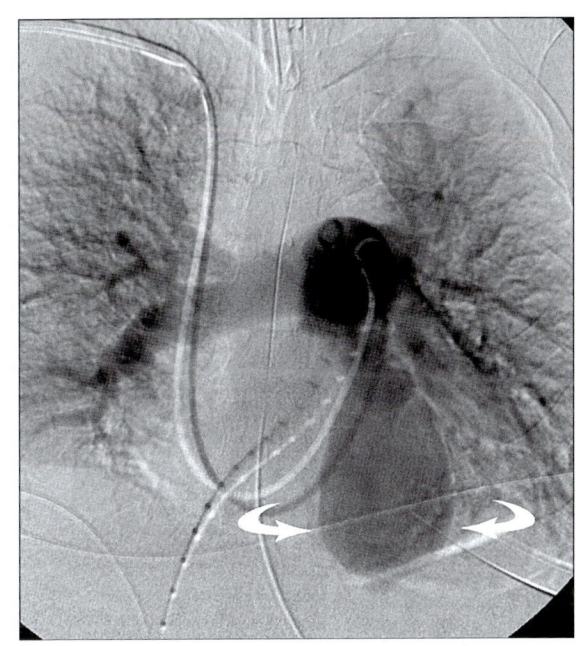

Figure 3. Pulmonary arteriography shows the pulmonary AVM and associated venous aneurysm *(curved arrows)*.

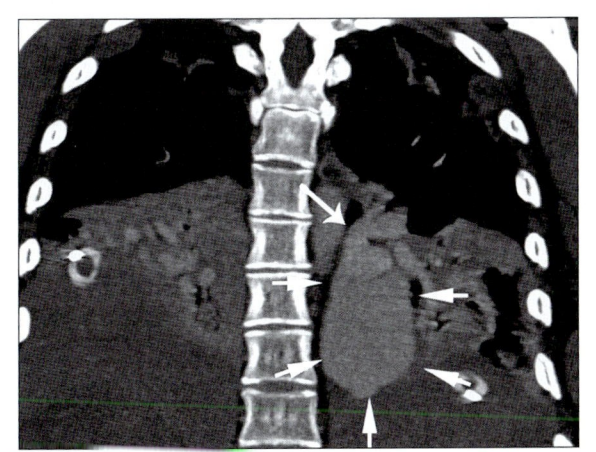

Figure 2. Coronal CT scan shows the pulmonary AVM in the left lower lobe *(arrow)* with an associated 4.2-cm venous aneurysm *(arrowheads)*.

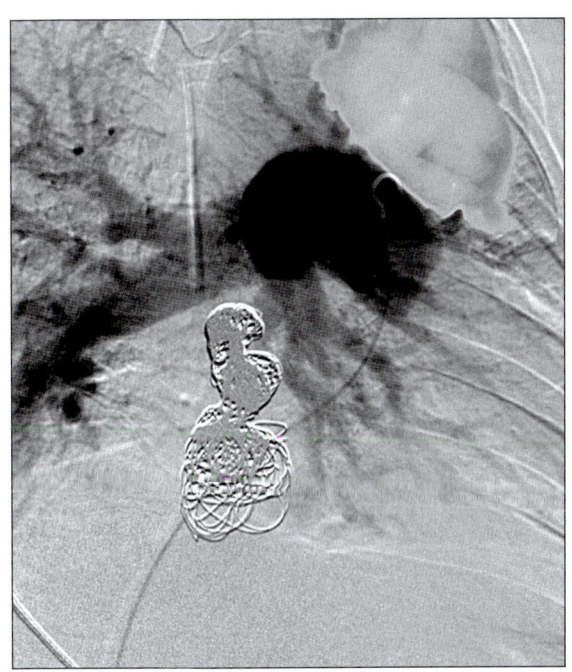

Figure 4. After coil embolization, the AVM has been occluded with no further filling of the venous aneurysm.

Case 175

DEMOGRAPHICS/CLINICAL HISTORY

A 17-year-old boy with polycythemia, mild hypoxia, and finger clubbing, undergoing radiography, arteriography, and computed tomography (CT).

DISCUSSION

History/Indications for Procedure

A 17-year-old boy has polycythemia, mild hypoxia, and finger clubbing. He reports intermittent scleral icterus and headaches.

Procedure

Embolization of pulmonary arteriovenous malformation

Pre-procedure Imaging

Chest radiograph shows an abnormal vessel overlying the right hilum (Fig. 1). Chest CT confirms the presence of a large pulmonary malformation in the superior segment of the right lower lobe (Fig. 2); several smaller pulmonary arteriovenous malformations (AVMs) are present bilaterally.

Intraprocedural Findings

A pulmonary arteriogram performed from a right femoral venous approach confirmed the presence of a large, simple pulmonary AVM (Fig. 3). Because of the high flow through the lesion, embolization was performed using detachable coils (Fig. 4).

Follow-up and Complications

The patient underwent sinonasal endoscopy, during which many telangiectasias were discovered. The patient was referred for genetic counseling for hereditary hemorrhagic telangiectasia.

Suggested Readings

Guttmacher AE, Marchuk DA, White RI Jr: Hereditary hemorrhagic telangiectasia. N Engl J Med 333:918-924, 1995.

Pollak JS, Saluja S, Thabet A, et al: Clinical and anatomic outcomes after embolotherapy of pulmonary arteriovenous malformations. J Vasc Intervent Radiol 17:35-45, 2006.

Shovlin CL, Guttmacher AE, Buscarini E, et al: Diagnostic criteria for hereditary hemorrhagic telangiectasia. Am J Med Genet 91:66-67, 2000.

White RI Jr, Pollak JS, Wirth JA: Pulmonary arteriovenous malformations: Diagnosis and transcatheter embolotherapy. J Vasc Intervent Radiol 7:787-804, 1996.

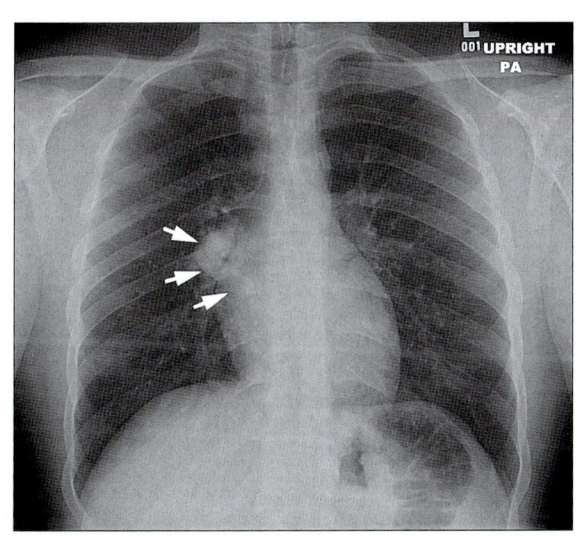

Figure 1. Posteroanterior chest radiograph shows an abnormal tubular density projecting over the right hilum *(arrows)*.

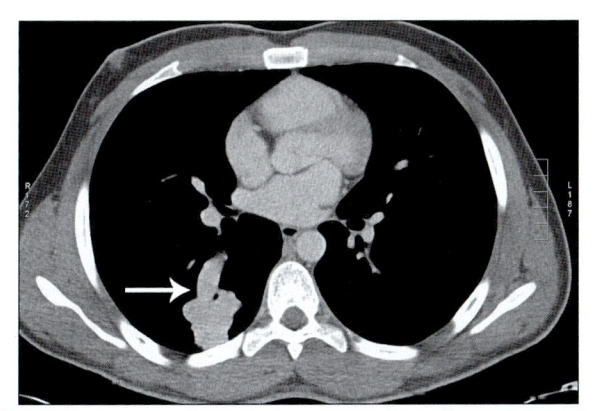

Figure 2. Contrast-enhanced chest CT confirms the presence of a pulmonary AVM in the superior segment of the right lower lobe with a single feeding artery *(arrow)*. Several smaller AVMs were identified bilaterally; each measured less than 3 mm in diameter.

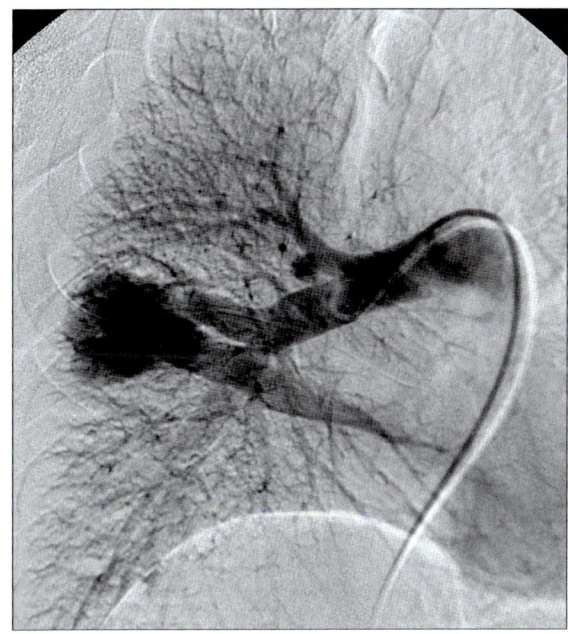

Figure 3. Single image from a right-sided pulmonary arteriographic study shows opacification of the large pulmonary AVM. The AVM had a single feeding artery and a single draining vein.

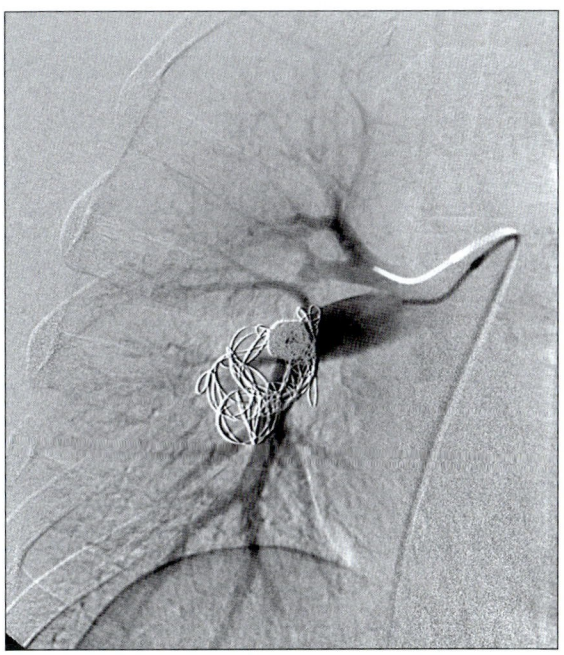

Figure 4. Pulmonary arteriogram after coil embolization shows complete occlusion of the AVM.

Case 176

DEMOGRAPHICS/CLINICAL HISTORY

A 40-year-old man with a 2-week history of shortness of breath, undergoing CT.

DISCUSSION

History/Indications for Procedure
This patient presented with worsening shortness of breath and dyspnea on exertion.

Procedure
Pulmonary artery thrombolysis

Pre-procedure Imaging
Contrast-enhanced CT shows a large saddle embolus with near-complete occlusion of all lobar branches on the right (Fig. 1). Echocardiography also was performed and showed right ventricular dilation with severe right ventricular contractile dysfunction.

Intraprocedural Findings
The pulmonary artery pressure was elevated, measuring 53/7 mm Hg (mean 28 mm Hg). A large right pulmonary embolus was identified on angiography (Fig. 2), and thrombolysis was initiated with tissue plasminogen activator at a rate of 0.5 mg/h.

Follow-up and Complications
The patient underwent 72 hours of thrombolysis with near-complete resolution of the right pulmonary embolus (Figs. 3 and 4). The patient was asymptomatic at the conclusion of the procedure and was placed on long-term anticoagulation.

Suggested Readings
De Gregorio MA, Gimeno MJ, Mainar A, et al: Mechanical and enzymatic thrombolysis for massive pulmonary embolism. J Vasc Intervent Radiol 13:163-169, 2002.

Murphy JM, Mulvihill N, Mulcahy D, et al: Percutaneous catheter and guidewire fragmentation with local administration of recombinant tissue plasminogen activator as a treatment for massive pulmonary embolism. Eur Radiol 9:959-964, 1999.

Stock KW, Jacob AL, Schnabel KJ, et al: Massive pulmonary embolism: Treatment with thrombus fragmentation and local fibrinolysis with recombinant human-tissue plasminogen activator. Cardiovasc Intervent Radiol 20:364-368, 1997.

Uflacker R: Interventional therapy for pulmonary embolism. J Vasc Intervent Radiol 12:147-164, 2001.

Case 176   353

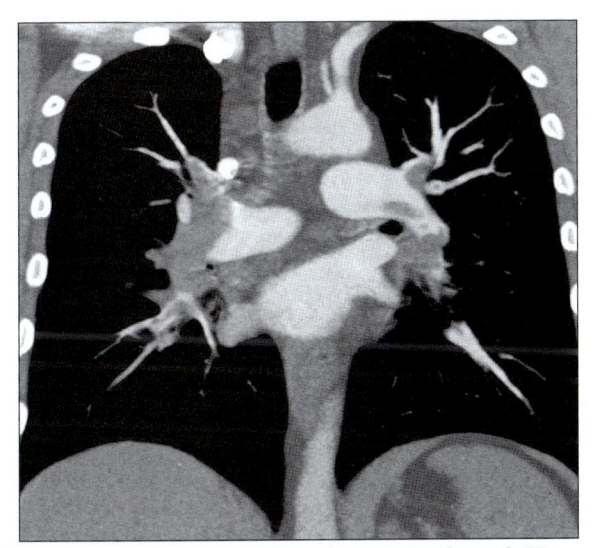

Figure 1. Coronal reconstruction of contrast-enhanced CT scan shows a large saddle pulmonary embolus extending into the lobar branches bilaterally.

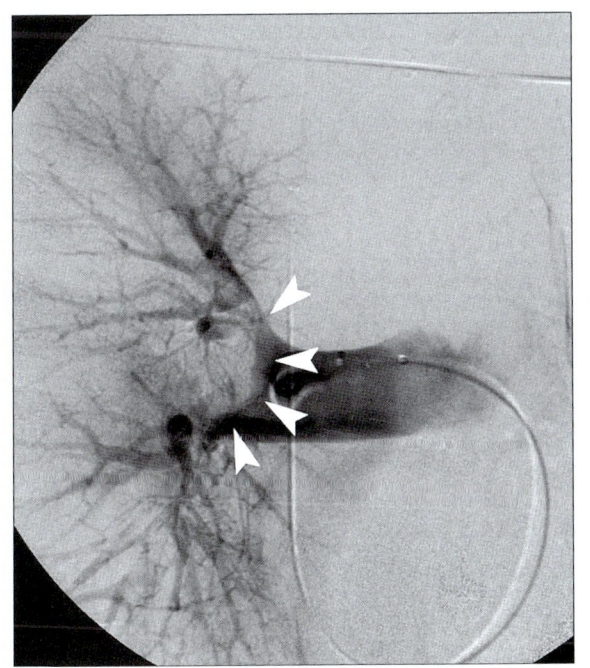

Figure 2. Selective right pulmonary arteriogram confirms the large thrombus in the right pulmonary artery *(arrowheads)*.

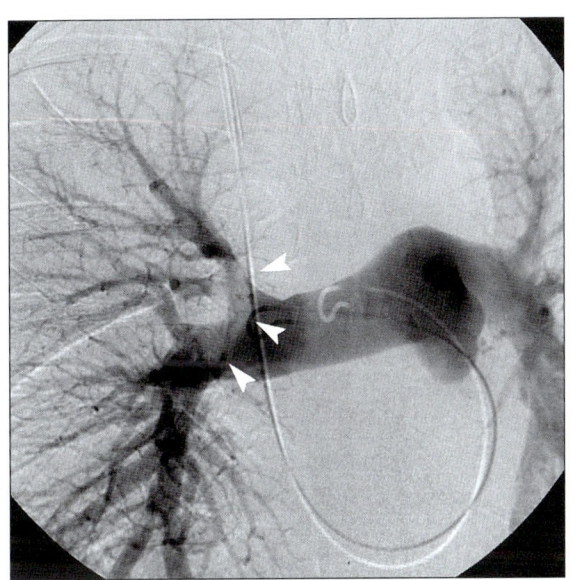

Figure 3. After 24 hours of tissue plasminogen activator thrombolysis, there is a slight reduction in clot *(arrowheads)* with improved perfusion of the right lung.

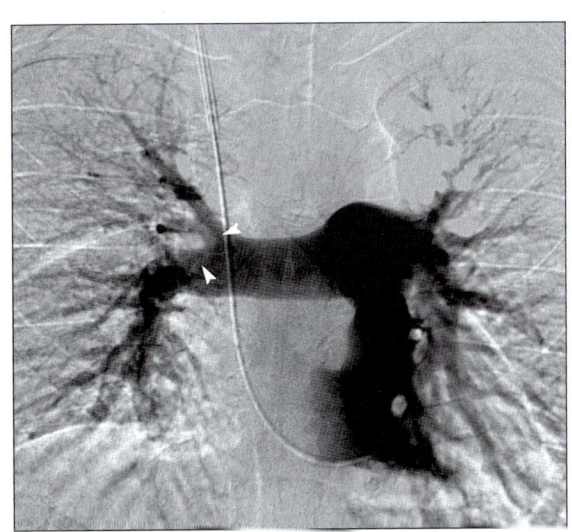

Figure 4. After 72 hours of thrombolysis, there is minimal residual thrombus *(arrowhead)* with significantly improved perfusion of the right lung.

Case 177

DEMOGRAPHICS/CLINICAL HISTORY

A 66-year-old woman with intracranial hemorrhage, upper extremity venous thrombosis, and tenuous respiratory status, undergoing superior venacavogram.

DISCUSSION

History/Indications for Procedure
This patient has intracranial hemorrhage from a ruptured intracranial aneurysm and upper extremity deep vein thrombosis (DVT). She has tenuous respiratory status.

Procedure
Superior vena cava filter placement

Pre-procedure Imaging
A lower extremity venous ultrasound scan was negative for lower extremity DVT. An upper extremity venous ultrasound showed acute thrombus in the right upper extremity brachial and cephalic veins (not shown).

Intraprocedural Findings
The superior vena cava (SVC) was patent with a diameter of 17 mm (Fig. 1). A Günther Tulip filter (Cook, Bloomington, IN) was deployed in the SVC (Fig. 2).

Follow-up and Complications
The patient was discharged to a skilled nursing facility for rehabilitation. She returned 4 months after filter placement for attempted filter removal (Fig. 3); however, the filter could not be freed from the wall of the SVC and was left in place as a permanent device.

Suggested Readings

Ascher E, Hingorani A, Tsemekhin B, Yorkovich W, et al: Lessons learned from a 6-year clinical experience with superior vena cava Greenfield filters. J Vasc Surg 32:881-887, 2000.

Ascer E, Gennaro M, Lorensen E, et al: Superior vena caval Greenfield filters: Indications, techniques, and results. J Vasc Surg 23:498-503, 1996.

Spence LD, Gironta MG, Malde HM, et al: Acute upper extremity deep venous thrombosis: Safety and effectiveness of superior vena caval filters. Radiology 210:53-58, 1999.

Case 177

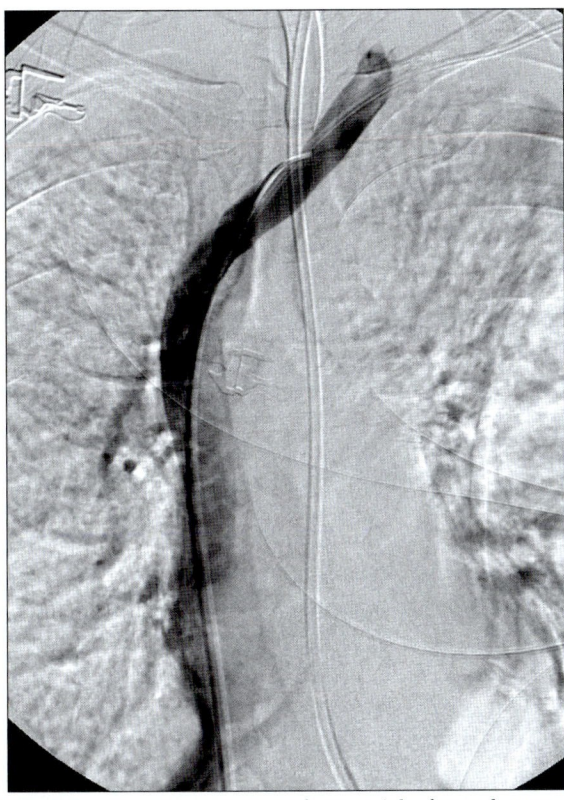

Figure 1. Superior venacavogram from a right femoral approach shows the SVC to be patent. The caval diameter measured 17 mm.

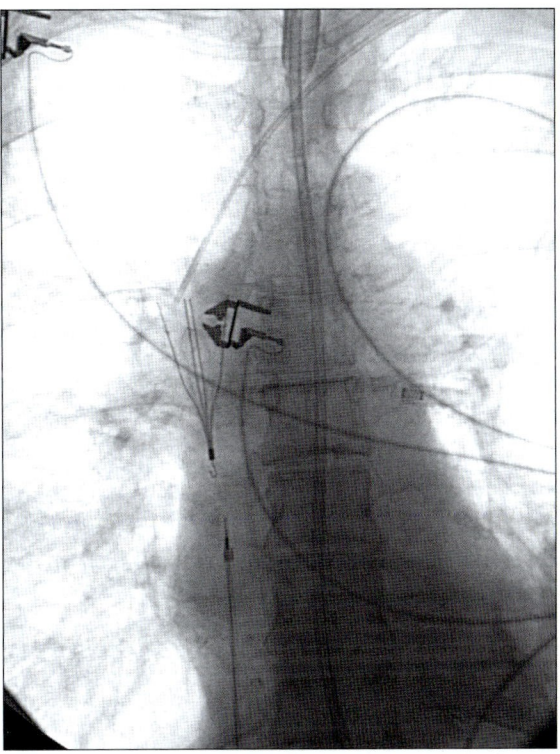

Figure 2. A Günther Tulip filter was deployed just below the confluence of the brachiocephalic veins. The cone is oriented toward the right atrium.

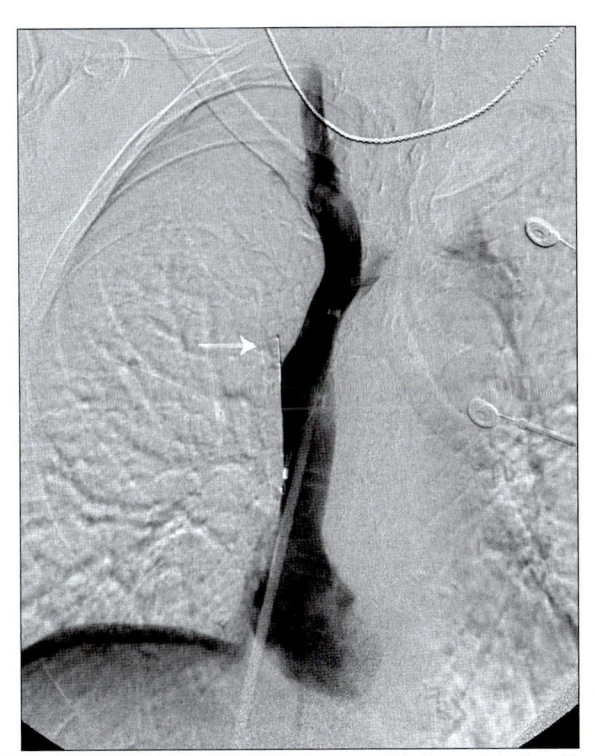

Figure 3. Superior venacavogram performed 4 months after filter placement shows the filter to be tilted within the SVC *(arrow)*. One of the filter legs is protruding outside the flow channel of the SVC. Attempts to retrieve the filter failed because of inability to free the filter legs that were well incorporated into the wall of the SVC.

Case 178

DEMOGRAPHICS/CLINICAL HISTORY

A 55-year-old woman with obesity, undergoing preoperative inferior vena cava (IVC) filter placement with cavography and fluoroscopic guidance.

DISCUSSION

History/Indications for Procedure

A 55-year-old woman with obesity is scheduled to undergo gastric bypass surgery. The patient has an underlying hypercoagulable risk factor with elevated homocystine levels and is referred for preoperative IVC filter placement.

Procedure

Management of inferior vena cava filter migration

Intraprocedural Findings

Anteroposterior cavography showed the IVC diameter measured 22 mm. After filter deployment in the infrarenal IVC (Fig. 1), the filter was observed to migrate to the right atrium, where it was retrieved with a snare (Figs. 2 to 4).

Follow-up and Complications

The patient underwent gastric bypass surgery without a prophylactic IVC filter. She had no periprocedural complications and lost 133 pounds in the first year after the operation.

Suggested Readings

Bochenek KM, Aruny JE, Tal MG, et al: Right atrial migration and percutaneous retrieval of a Gunther Tulip inferior vena cava filter. J Vasc Intervent Radiol 14:1207-1209.

Bui JT, West DL, Pinto C, et al: Right ventricular migration and endovascular removal of an inferior vena cava filter. J Vasc Intervent Radiol 19:141-144, 2008.

Izutani H, Lalude O, Gill IS, Biblo LA: Migration of an inferior vena cava filter to the right ventricle and literature review. Can J Cardiol 20:233-235, 2004.

Kuo WT, Loh CT, Sze DY: Emergency retrieval of a G2 filter after complete migration into the right ventricle. J Vasc Intervent Radiol 18:1177-1182, 2007.

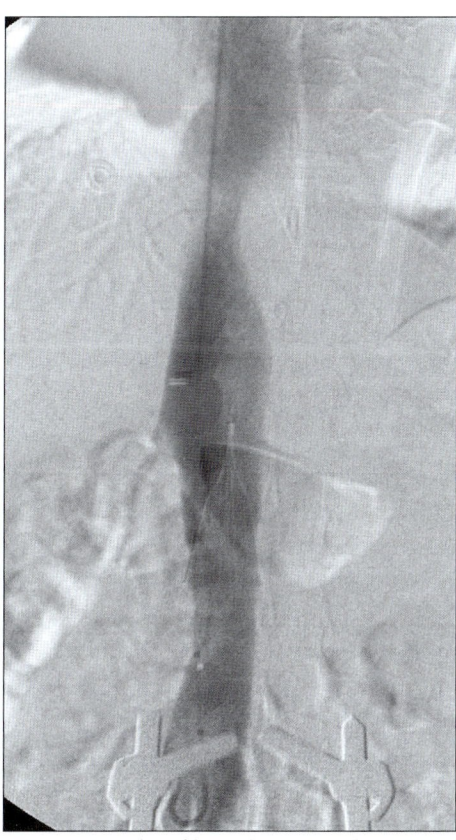

Figure 1. Cavogram after filter placement shows the filter in appropriate position within the infrarenal IVC.

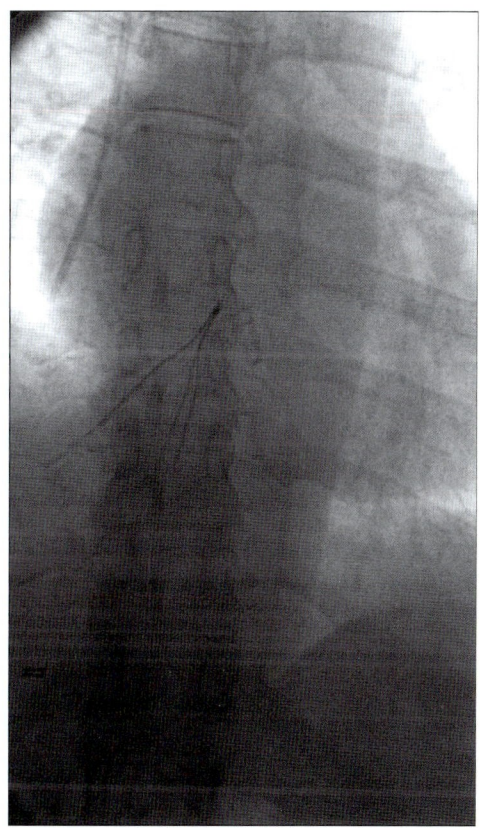

Figure 2. Within minutes of deployment, the filter was observed under fluoroscopy migrating into the right atrium.

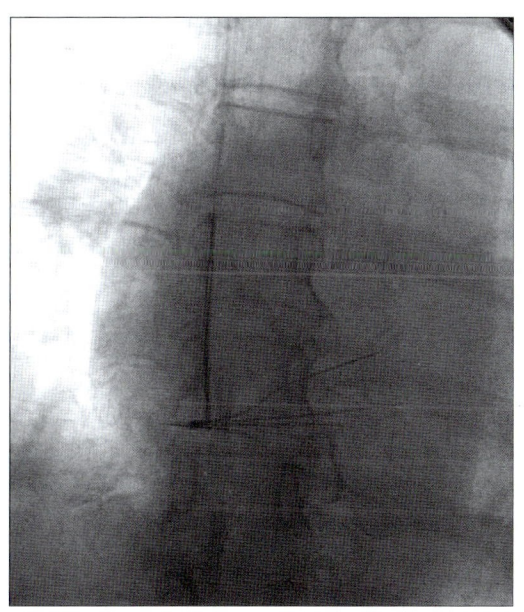

Figure 3. The filter tilted into a horizontal orientation in the right atrium. The top of the filter was captured with a standard gooseneck snare.

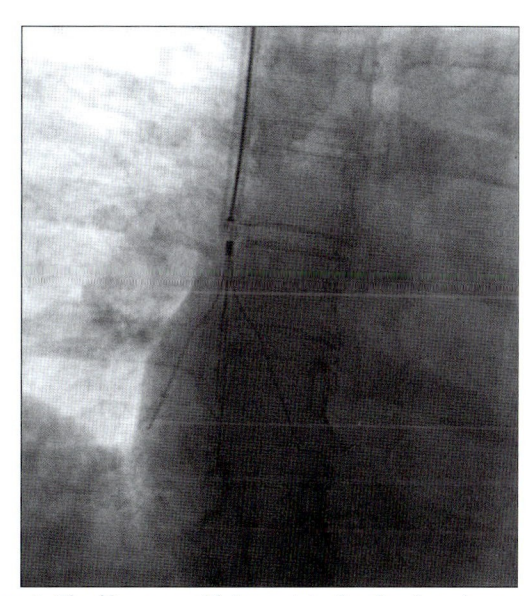

Figure 4. The filter was withdrawn into the sheath and removed.

Case 179

DEMOGRAPHICS/CLINICAL HISTORY

A 42-year-old man presenting for inferior vena cava (IVC) filter removal 3 years after placement following a motor vehicle accident, undergoing CT angiography and cavography.

DISCUSSION

History/Indications for Procedure
A 42-year-old man presents with nonspecific right lower-quadrant pain. The patient had a prophylactic IVC filter placed after a motor vehicle accident 3 years earlier.

Procedure
Removal of chronically embedded inferior vena cava filter

Pre-procedure Imaging
A CT angiogram shows the IVC filter within the IVC, just above the confluence of the right and left common iliac veins (Fig. 1). One of the filter legs is seen protruding through the medial wall of the IVC and overlies the right common iliac artery.

Intraprocedural Findings
Cavography shows the filter hook to be embedded in the wall of the IVC (Fig. 2), and intravascular ultrasound showed the filter leg indenting the wall of the right common iliac artery without any evidence of arterial perforation. The hook of the filter was grasped with bronchoscopic forceps (Fig. 3), and using considerable force, the filter was freed from the wall of the IVC.

Follow-up and Complications
Follow-up cavography after filter removal shows no evidence for caval injury (Fig. 4). The patient's right lower-quadrant pain significantly improved after removal of the filter.

Suggested Readings
Marquess JS, Burke CT, Beecham AH, et al: Factors associated with failed retrieval of the Gunther Tulip inferior vena cava filter. J Vasc Intervent Radiol 19:1321, 2008.

Ray CT Jr, Mitchell E, Zipser S, et al: Outcomes with retrievable inferior vena cava filters: A multicenter study. J Vasc Intervent Radiol 17:1595, 2006.

Stavropoulos SW, Dixon RG, Burke CT, et al: Embedded inferior vena cava filter removal: Use of endobronchial forceps. J Vasc Intervent Radiol 19:1297, 2008.

Stavropoulos SW, Solomon JA, Trerotola SO: Wall-embedded recovery inferior vena cava filters: Imaging features and technique for removal. J Vasc Intervent Radiol 17:379, 2006.

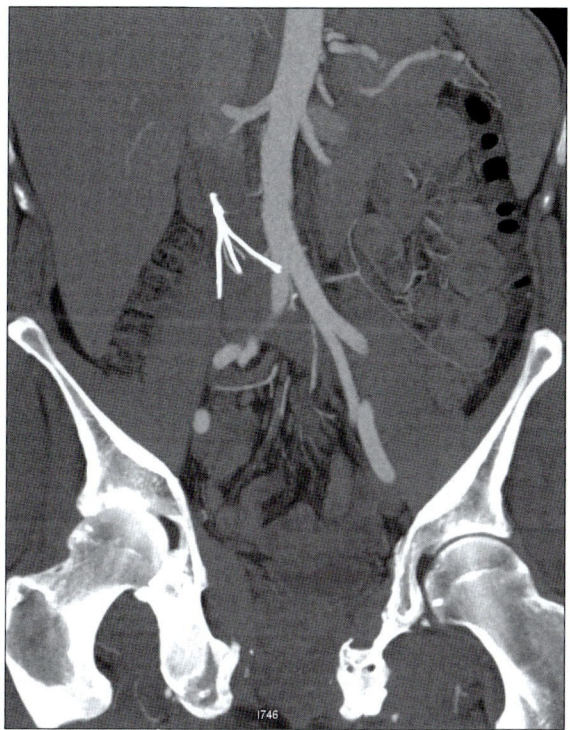

Figure 1. CT angiogram, coronal reconstruction, shows IVC filter slightly tilted within IVC. Filter is located just above confluence of the right and left common iliac veins, and one leg is seen protruding outside the wall of the IVC, overlying right common iliac artery.

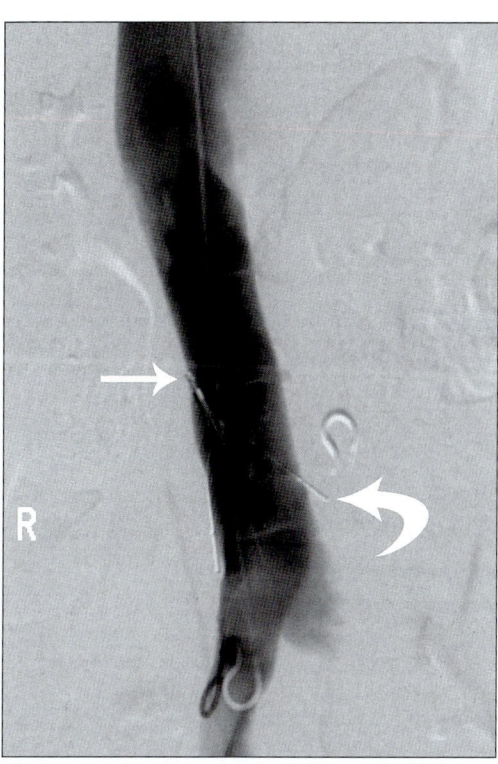

Figure 2. Cavography shows hook of filter embedded in wall of IVC *(straight arrow)*. Filter leg is also seen protruding beyond flow lumen of IVC *(curved arrow)*.

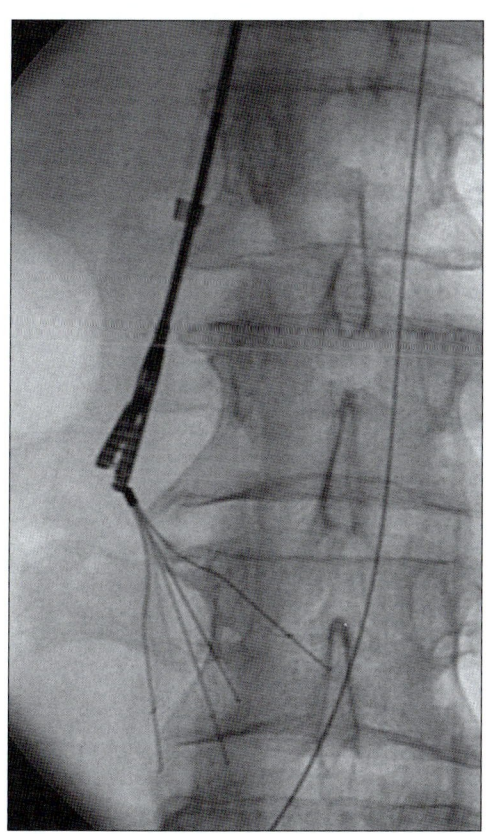

Figure 3. Filter hook was dissected free and grasped using bronchoscopic forceps.

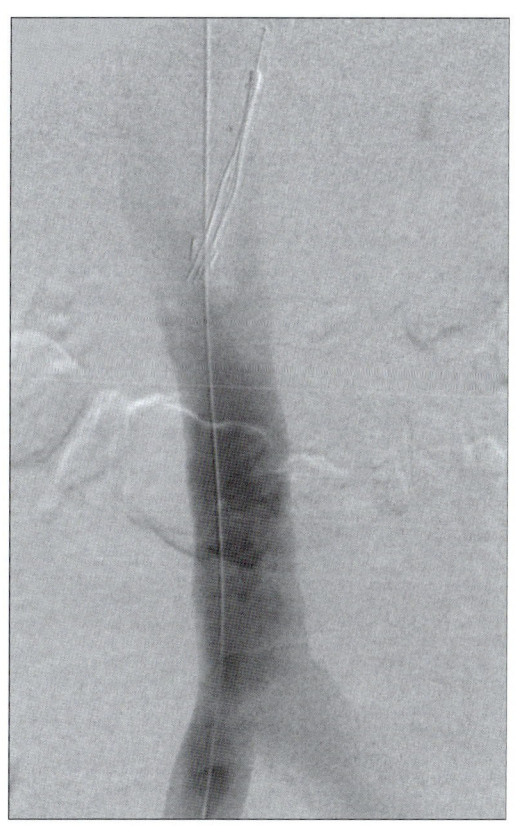

Figure 4. Cavography after filter removal. There is no evidence of injury to IVC after filter removal, despite the considerable force required for filter extraction.

Case 180

DEMOGRAPHICS/CLINICAL HISTORY

A 57-year-old woman with acute onset of left lower extremity swelling and pain.

DISCUSSION

History/Indications for Procedure
A 57-year-old woman with acute onset of left lower extremity swelling and pain. On physical exam, the left leg is erythematous and swollen.

Procedure
Management of acute lower extremity deep venous thrombosis

Pre-procedure Imaging
Doppler ultrasound shows intraluminal obstruction of the deep venous system of the entire left lower extremity.

Intraprocedural Findings
The deep venous system of the left lower extremity was accessed through a popliteal approach, and ascending venogram shows thrombus from the popliteal vein to the external iliac vein (Figs. 1 and 2). The thrombus was treated using the 8-French Trellis device with near-complete removal of thrombus; an overnight infusion of tissue plasminogen activator (tPA) was used to remove the remaining clot.

Follow-up and Complications
Follow-up venogram performed after overnight thrombolytic infusion shows minimal residual thrombus (Figs. 3 and 4). The patient's leg swelling had significantly improved, and she was discharged home on oral anticoagulation.

Suggested Readings
Alesh I, Kayali F, Stein PD: Catheter-directed thrombolysis (intra-thrombus injection) in treatment of deep venous thrombosis: A systematic review. Catheter Cardiovasc Intervent 70:143-148, 2007.

Hilleman DE, Razavi MK: Clinical and economic evaluation of the Trellis-8 infusion catheter for deep vein thrombosis. J Vasc Intervent Radiol 19:377-383, 2008.

O'Sullivan GJ, Lohan DG, Gough N, et al: Pharmacomechanical thrombectomy of acute deep vein thrombosis with the Trellis-8 isolated thrombolysis catheter. J Vasc Intervent Radiol 18:715-724, 2007.

Semba CP, Razavi MK, Kee ST, et al: Thrombolysis for lower extremity deep venous thrombosis. Tech Vasc Intervent Radiol 7:68-78, 2004.

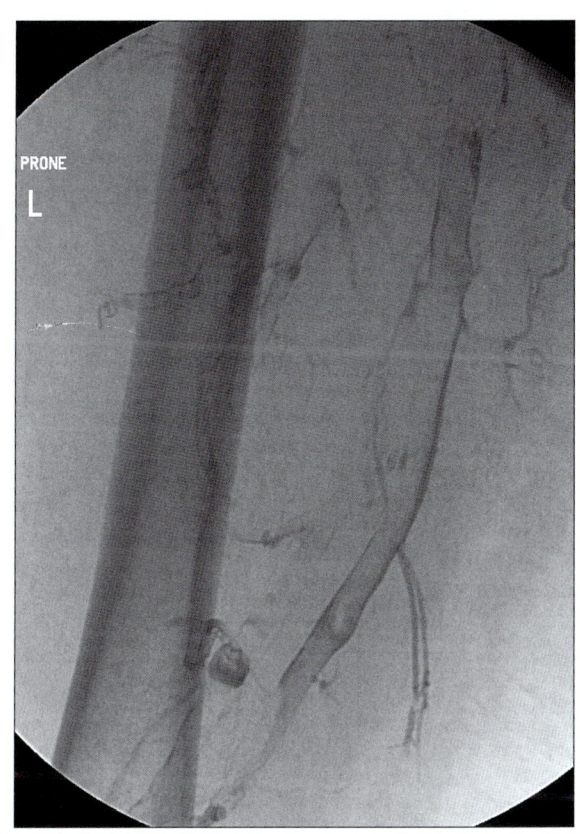

Figure 1. Ascending venogram from a popliteal approach shows a large filling defect throughout the femoral vein consistent with acute thrombus.

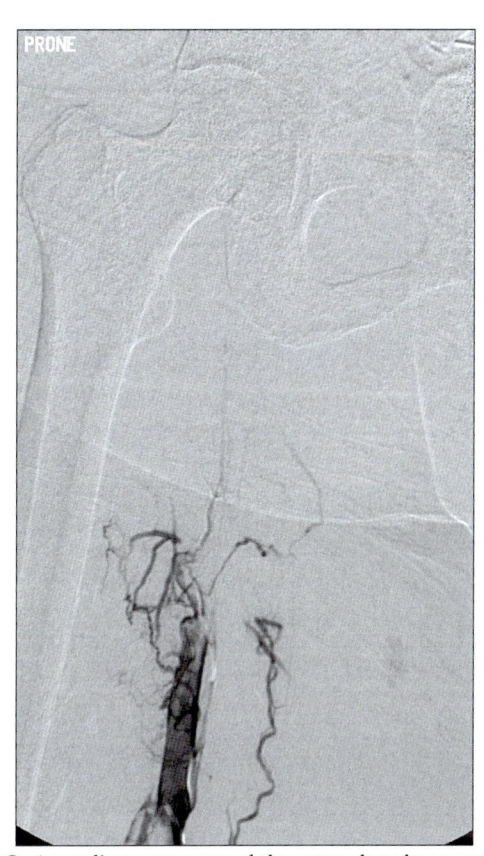

Figure 2. Ascending venogram of the upper leg shows complete occlusion of the femoral vein below the common femoral vein.

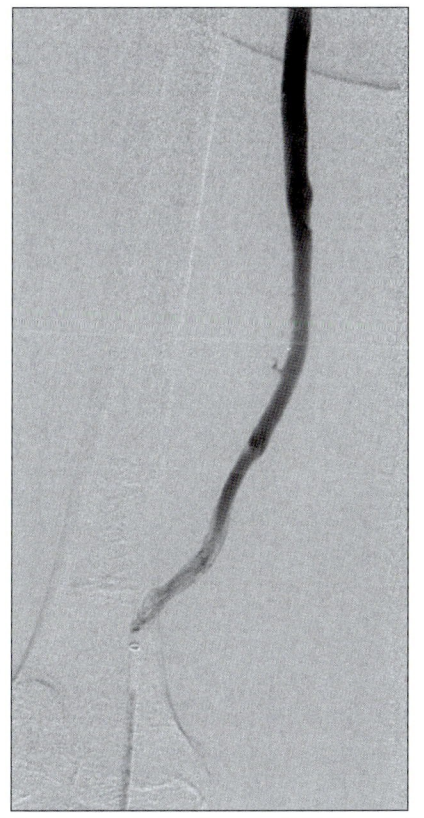

Figure 3. Follow-up venogram after overnight thrombolysis shows no residual thrombus within the femoral vein.

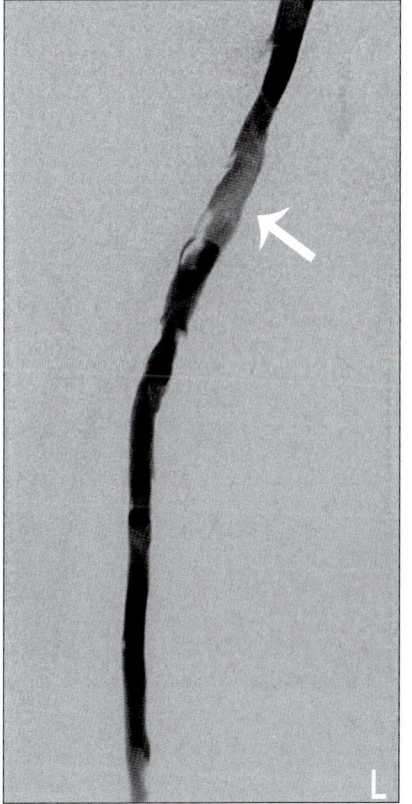

Figure 4. Follow-up venogram shows minimal amount of residual thrombus in the upper portion of the femoral vein *(arrow)*. This did not appear to result in significant flow occlusion.

Case 181

DEMOGRAPHICS/CLINICAL HISTORY

A 64-year-old woman with a 6-month history of increasing left lower extremity swelling, undergoing venography.

DISCUSSION

History/Indications for Procedure
This patient was diagnosed 2 years previously with left lower extremity deep venous thrombosis (DVT), for which she has been receiving anticoagulation.

Procedure
Management of acute lower extremity deep venous thrombosis

Intraprocedural Findings
Acute thrombus was identified in the femoral vein (Fig. 1), and complete occlusion of the iliac veins was identified (Fig. 2). The iliac veins were recanalized and stented (Figs. 3 and 4), and the acute thrombus was treated with a combination of mechanical thrombectomy and thrombolysis.

Follow-up and Complications
The patient's swelling resolved after the procedure. She has had no further episodes of lower extremity swelling for the 3 years since stent placement.

Suggested Readings
Comerota AJ, Throm RC, Mathias SD, et al: Catheter-directed thrombolysis for iliofemoral deep venous thrombosis improves health-related quality of life. J Vasc Surg 32:130-137, 2000.

Grossman C, McPherson S: Safety and efficacy of catheter-directed thrombolysis for iliofemoral venous thrombosis. AJR Am J Roentgenol 172:667-672, 1999.

Murphy KD: Mechanical thrombectomy for DVT. Tech Vasc Intervent Radiol 7:79-85, 2004.

Case 181   363

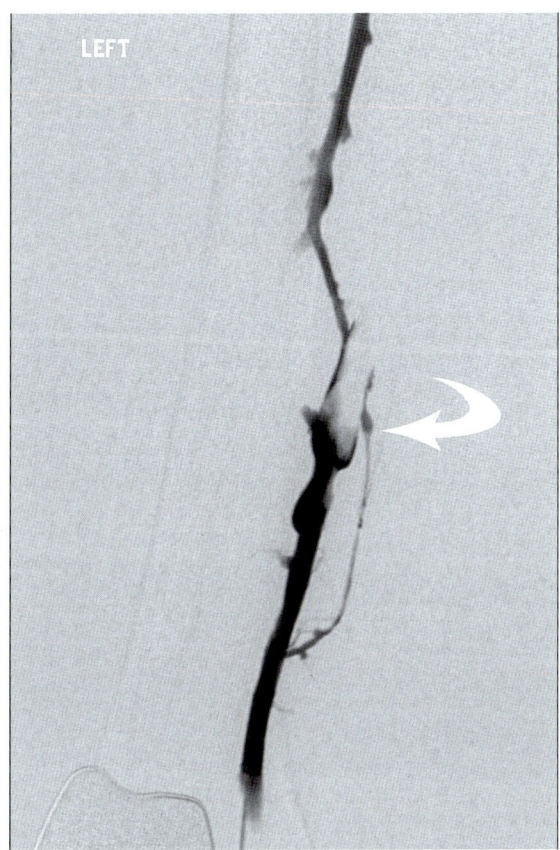

Figure 1. Ascending venogram from a left popliteal vein access shows acute thrombus *(arrow)* and complete occlusion of the femoral vein.

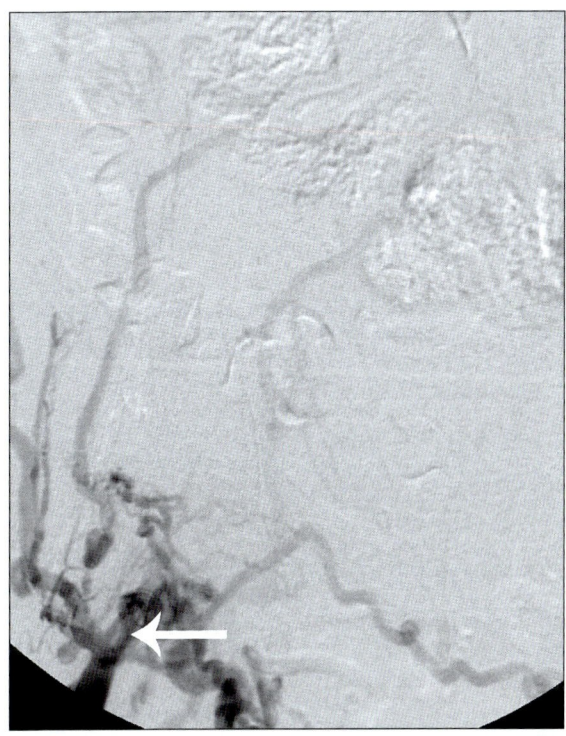

Figure 2. Ascending venogram centered over the pelvis shows complete occlusion of the common femoral and iliac veins. There is filling of numerous collateral veins in the left groin *(arrow)*.

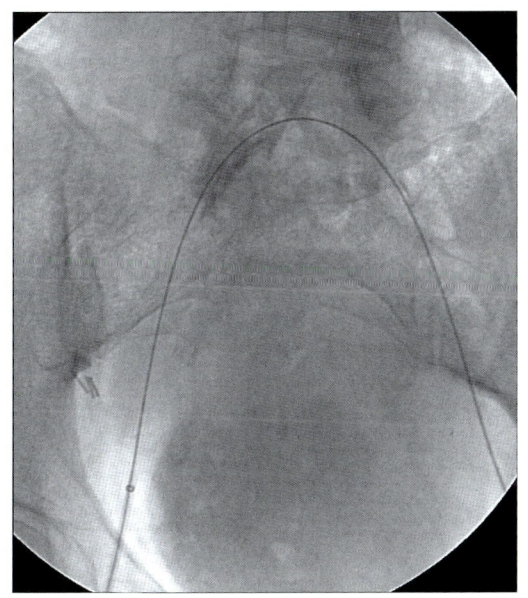

Figure 3. Through-and-through guidewire access was needed to cross the obstruction.

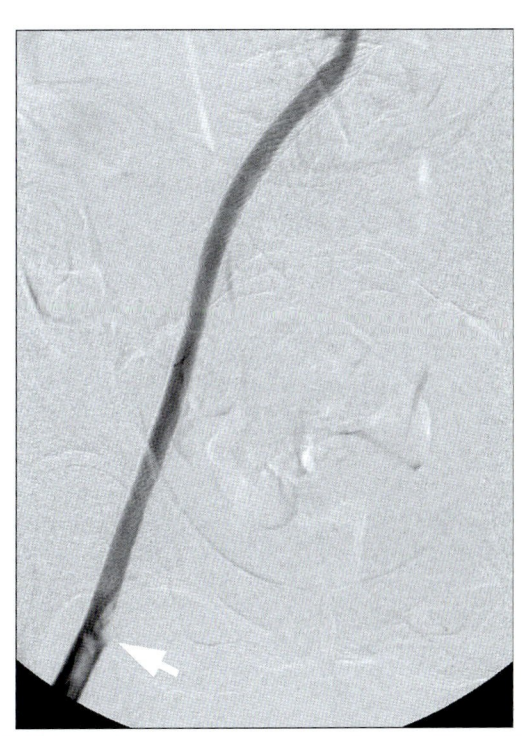

Figure 4. Ascending venogram after stenting shows restoration of antegrade flow within the left iliac system. A small volume of nonocclusive thrombus persists in the lower common femoral vein *(arrow)*.

Case 182

DEMOGRAPHICS/CLINICAL HISTORY

A 36-year-old woman with left lower extremity pain and swelling.

DISCUSSION

History/Indications for Procedure
A 36-year-old woman with acute onset of left lower extremity pain and swelling 3 weeks after undergoing lumbar diskectomy.

Procedure
Thrombolysis for acute lower extremity deep venous thrombosis

Pre-procedure Imaging
Venous ultrasound shows softly echogenic thrombus within the deep veins of the left lower extremity; the veins are distended and non-compressible. CTV shows a low-attenuation filling defect and venous expansion of the deep venous system of the left lower extremity (Fig. 1).

Intraprocedural Findings
The left lower extremity deep venous system was accessed from a popliteal approach, and ascending venography shows acute thrombus in the femoral and iliac veins (Fig. 2). Mechanical thrombolysis was performed using the Angiojet catheter (Possis, Minneapolis, MN), and catheter-directed thrombolysis was initiated.

Follow-up and Complications
On follow-up venogram, a left common iliac vein stenosis was identified and stented with a 14-mm × 6-cm self-expanding stent. The patient underwent a total of 3 days of catheter-directed thrombolysis, with near-complete resolution of intraluminal thrombus (Figs. 3 and 4); the lower extremity swelling was completely resolved at the time of discharge, and she has not been diagnosed in the subsequent 2 years with recurrent DVT.

Suggested Readings
Alesh I, Kayali F, Stein PD: Catheter-directed thrombolysis (intrathrombus injection) in the treatment of deep venous thrombosis: A systemic review. Catheter Cardiovasc Intervent 70:143-48, 2007.

Kim HS, Patra A, Paxton BE, et al: Catheter-directed thrombolysis with percutaneous rheolytic thrombectomy versus thrombolysis alone in upper and lower extremity deep vein thrombosis. Cardiovasc Intervent Radiol 29:1003-07, 2006.

Laiho MK, Oinonen A, Sugano N, et al: Preservation of venous valve function after catheter-directed and systemic thrombolysis for deep venous thrombosis. Eur J Vasc Endovasc Surg 28:391-96, 2004.

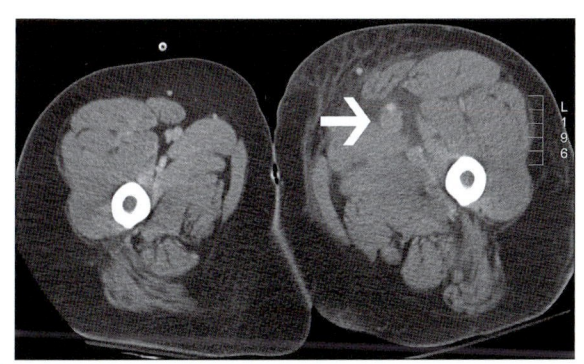

Figure 1. Contrast-enhanced CT of the lower extremities shows acute thrombus in the left femoral vein (arrow). There is perivenous inflammation and left lower extremity edema.

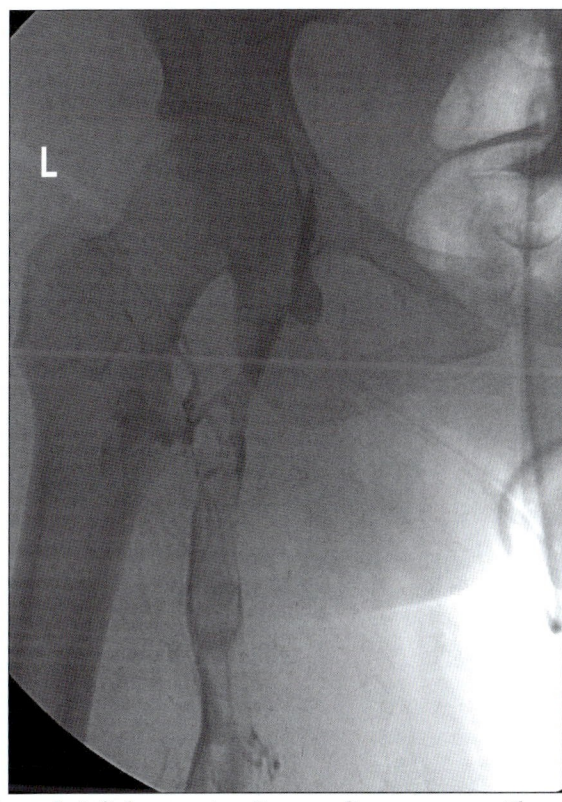

Figure 2. Left lower extremity ascending venogram. There is extensive filling defect within the femoral vein consistent with an acute DVT. There is complete occlusion at the level of the common femoral vein.

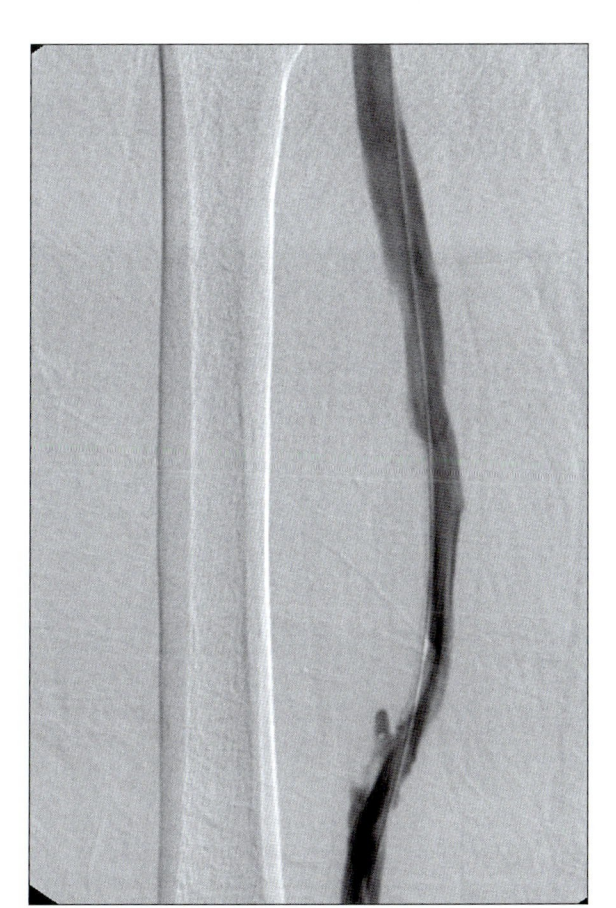

Figure 3. Follow-up venogram after 3 days of catheter-directed thrombolytic therapy shows complete resolution of thrombus within the femoral vein.

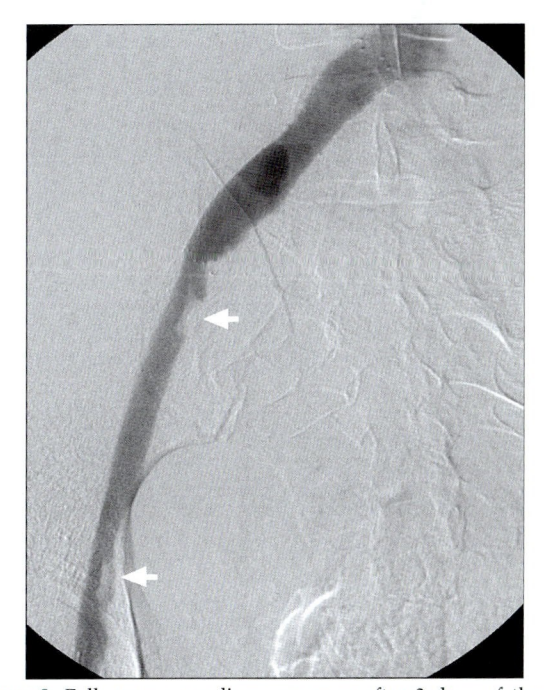

Figure 4. Follow-up ascending venogram after 3 days of thrombolysis shows minimal residual thrombus in the common femoral vein and external iliac vein (arrows). A stent has been placed in the left common iliac vein for a May-Thurner lesion.

Case 183

DEMOGRAPHICS/CLINICAL HISTORY

A 24-year-old woman with a history of prior deep venous thrombosis (DVT) and leg swelling.

DISCUSSION

History/Indications for Procedure
A 24-year-old woman diagnosed with lower extremity DVT and protein S deficiency at age 13. She now presents with chronic bilateral lower extremity swelling.

Procedure
Management of chronic iliac vein and IVC thrombosis

Pre-procedure Imaging
Venous ultrasound shows changes of chronic DVT in the femoral veins bilaterally (not shown). There are abnormal Doppler signals in the common femoral veins, suggesting more central obstruction.

Intraprocedural Findings
Bilateral ascending venograms show changes consistent with chronic DVT in the femoral veins bilaterally; the right common iliac vein is diffusely narrowed, and the left common iliac vein is occluded (Figs. 1–3). The common iliac veins were stented with kissing stents, and the stents were extended to the common femoral veins bilaterally.

Follow-up and Complications
Following stent placement, there was significantly improved flow through the iliac veins (Fig. 4).

Suggested Readings
Hansch E, Razavi M, Semba C, Drake M: Endovascular strategies for inferior vena cava obstruction. Tech Vasc Intervent Radiol 3:40-4, 2000.

O'Sullivan G: Endovascular management of chronic iliac vein occlusion. Tech Vasc Intervent Radiol 3:45-53, 2000.

Sharafuddin M, Sun S, Hoballah J, et al: Endovascular management of venous thrombotic and occlusive diseases of the lower extremities. J Vasc Intervent Radiol 14:405-23, 2003.

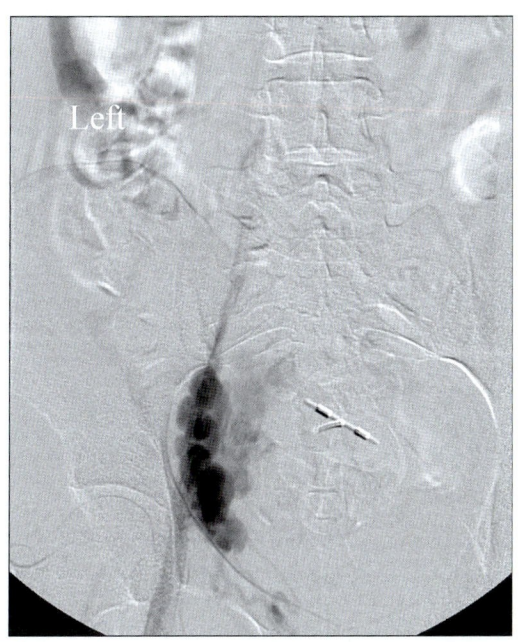

Figure 1. Ascending venogram with the patient prone from a popliteal access. There is complete occlusion of the common iliac vein with filling of large pelvic varicosities.

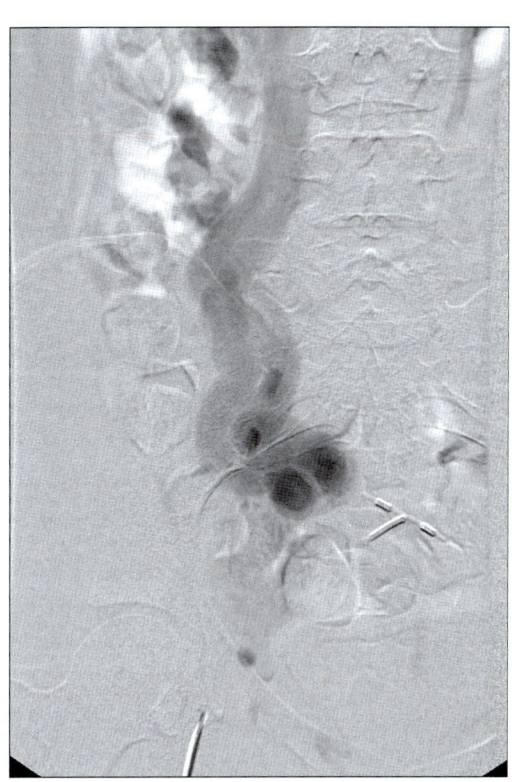

Figure 2. Late image in ascending left lower extremity venogram shows filling of a markedly enlarged left gonadal vein.

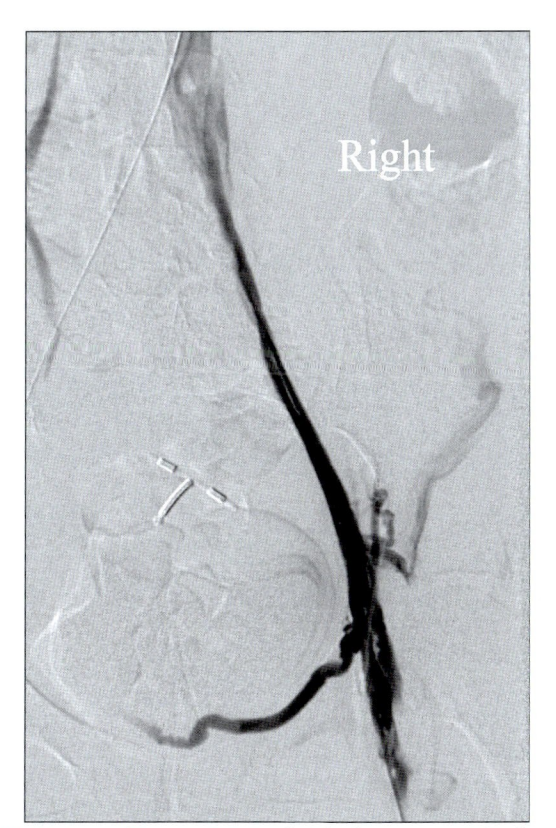

Figure 3. Ascending venogram of right lower extremity from a popliteal approach shows diffuse narrowing of the right common iliac vein.

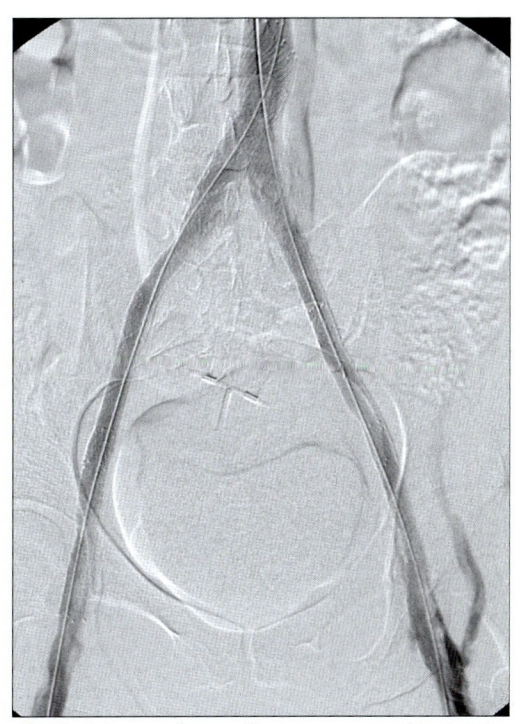

Figure 4. Final image of ascending venogram with simultaneous injection of bilateral popliteal vein sheaths shows markedly improved flow through the iliac veins and lower IVC following stent placement.

Case 184

DEMOGRAPHICS/CLINICAL HISTORY

A 38-year-old woman with chronic left lower extremity swelling, undergoing venography.

DISCUSSION

History/Indications for Procedure
A 38-year-old woman with a history of prior left lower extremity deep venous thrombosis presents with chronic left lower extremity swelling.

Procedure
Endovascular treatment for chronic lower extremity deep venous thrombosis

Pre-procedure Imaging
MR venography shows occlusion of the left common iliac vein and near-complete occlusion of the external iliac vein (not shown). Multiple venous collateral veins are seen in the anterior abdominal wall.

Intraprocedural Findings
The left femoral vein is patent (Fig. 1); there is chronic occlusion of the left iliac veins (Figs. 2 and 3). The occluded segment was successfully crossed and stented with multiple overlapping, self-expanding nitinol stents (Fig. 4).

Follow-up and Complications
The patient's lower extremity swelling nearly completely resolved in the days following the procedure.

Suggested Readings
O'Sullivan G: Endovascular management of chronic iliac vein occlusion. Tech Vasc Intervent Radiol 3:45, 2000.

Raju S, McAllister S, Neglen P: Recanalization of totally occluded iliac and adjacent venous segments. J Vasc Surg 36:903, 2002.

Sharafuddin M, Sun S, Hoballah J, et al: Endovascular management of venous thrombotic and occlusive diseases of the lower extremities. J Vasc Intervent Radiol 14:405, 2003.

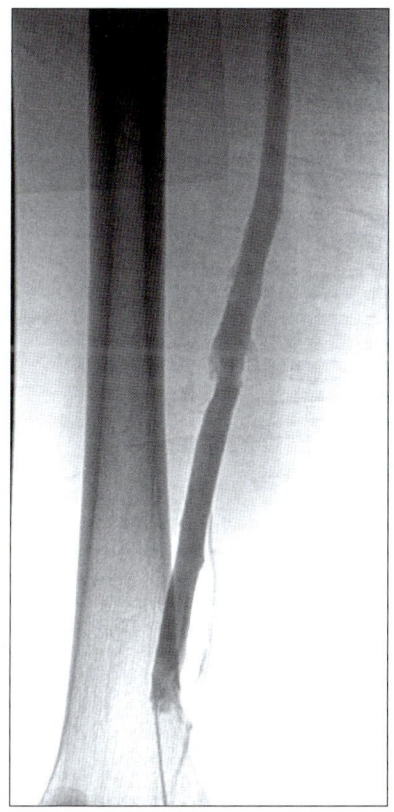

Figure 1. Ascending left lower extremity venogram (with patient prone) from a popliteal approach shows patent femoral vein.

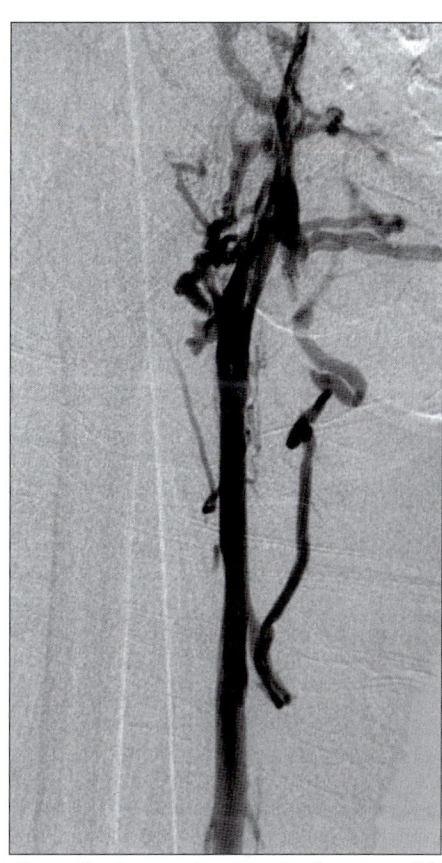

Figure 2. Femoral vein remains open in the upper thigh. Large venous collaterals are seen around left hip.

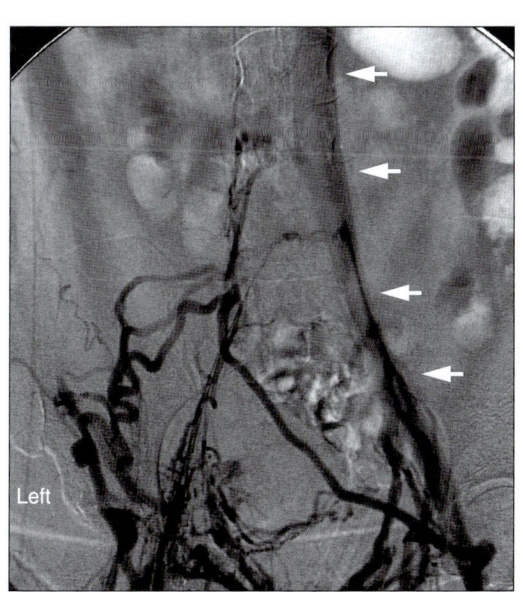

Figure 3. External iliac vein is diminutive, and common iliac vein is occluded. Numerous pelvic collaterals are present with opacification of right iliac venous system and inferior vena cava (*arrows*).

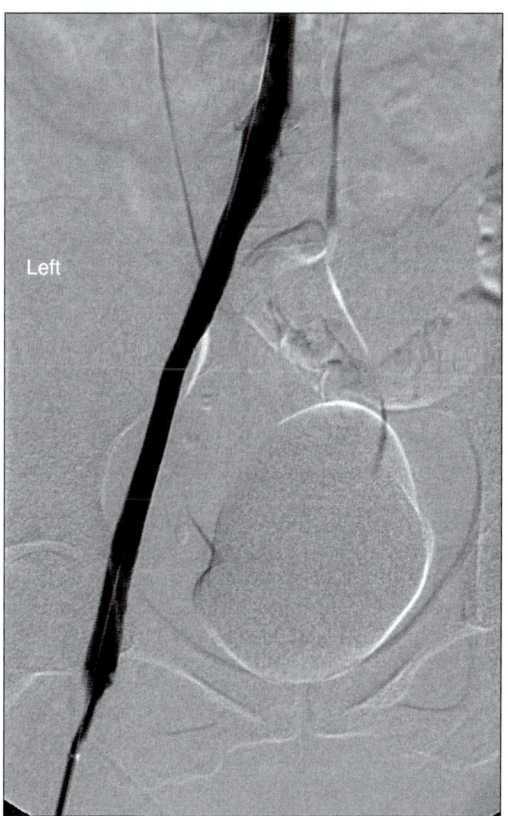

Figure 4. Final venogram after angioplasty and stenting shows marked reduction in venous collaterals with successful recanalization of left iliac system.

Case 185

DEMOGRAPHICS/CLINICAL HISTORY

A 64-year-old man with multiple medical problems, including known mesenteric venous thrombosis and chronic inferior vena cava (IVC) thrombosis, undergoing venography.

DISCUSSION

History/Indications for Procedure
This patient with medical problems including known mesenteric venous thrombosis and chronic IVC thrombosis now has worsening bilateral lower extremity and scrotal edema.

Procedure
Management of chronic inferior vena cava occlusion

Pre-procedure Imaging
Magnetic resonance venography of the abdomen showed patent iliac veins with IVC occlusion.

Intraprocedural Findings
An ascending venogram from a right common femoral vein access showed occlusion of the IVC with venous outflow predominantly through an enlarged ascending lumbar vein that communicated with the azygos and hemiazygos veins (Figs. 1-3). The IVC was recannulated and stented (Fig. 4).

Follow-up and Complications
The patient's edema improved after IVC stenting. Although the hypercoagulability workup failed to identify a hypercoagulable condition, the patient was maintained on life-long anticoagulation.

Suggested Readings
Hansch E, et al: Endovascular strategies for inferior vena cava obstruction. Tech Vasc Intervent Radiol 3:40-44, 2000.
O'Sullivan G: Endovascular management of chronic iliac vein occlusion. Tech Vasc Intervent Radiol 3:45-53, 2000.
Sharafuddin MJ, Sun S, Hoballah JJ, et al: Endovascular management of venous thrombotic and occlusive diseases of the lower extremities. J Vasc Intervent Radiol 14:405-423, 2003.

Case 185   371

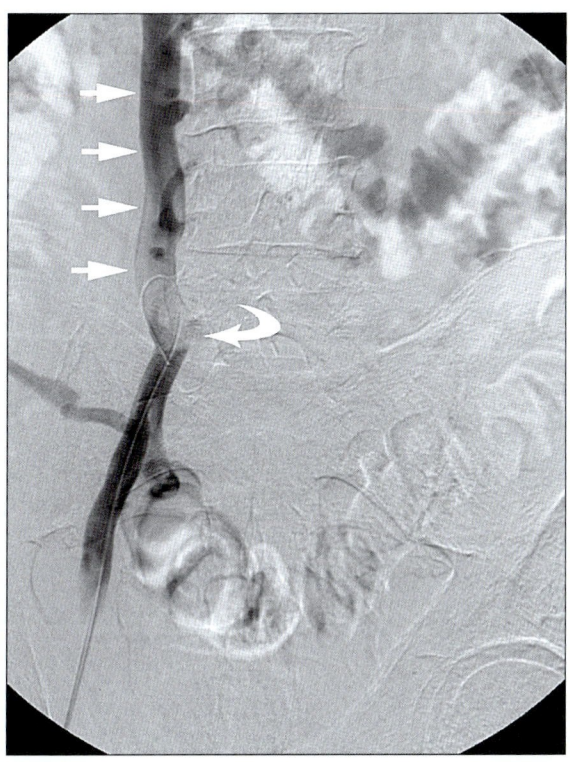

Figure 1. Ascending venogram from right common femoral vein access shows occlusion of the IVC *(curved arrow)*. The lower extremity venous drainage is primarily through an enlarged ascending lumbar vein *(short arrows)*.

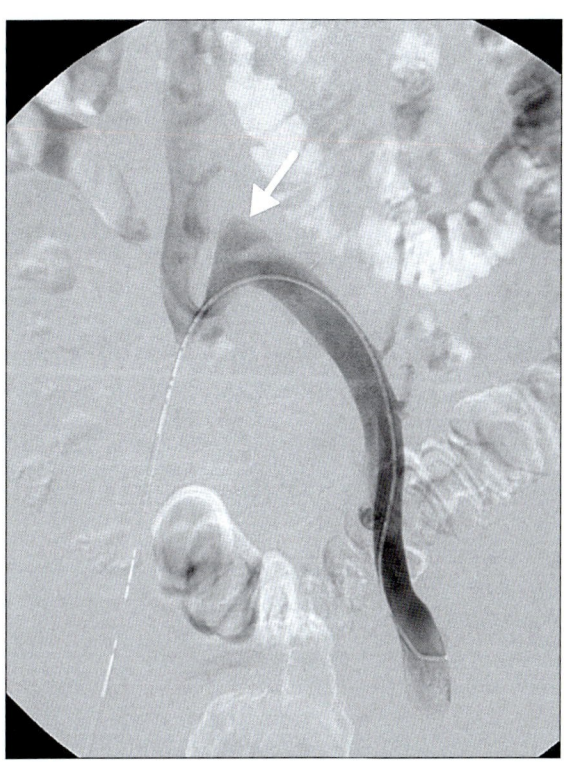

Figure 3. Injection of the left common femoral vein also shows complete IVC occlusion *(arrow)* with venous drainage primarily through the enlarged ascending lumbar vein.

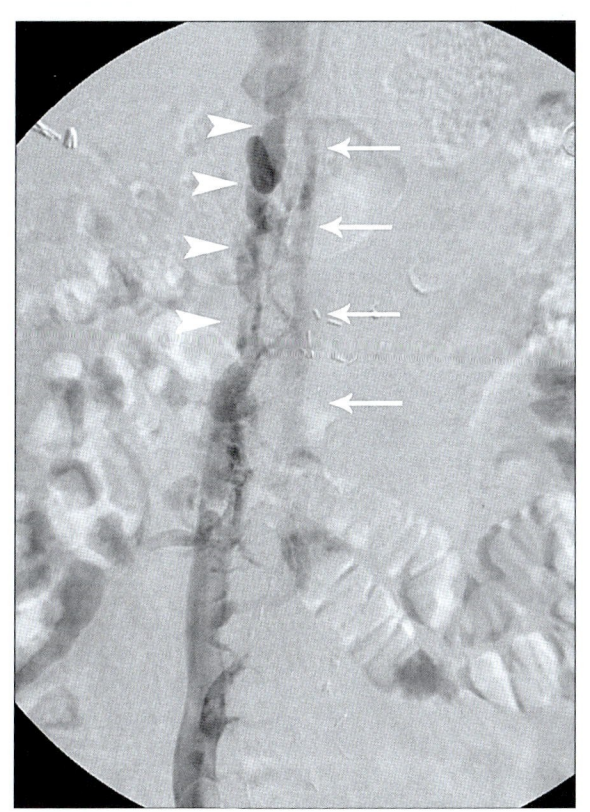

Figure 2. Ascending venogram of the abdomen shows venous drainage primarily through the azygos *(arrowheads)* and hemiazygos *(arrows)* veins.

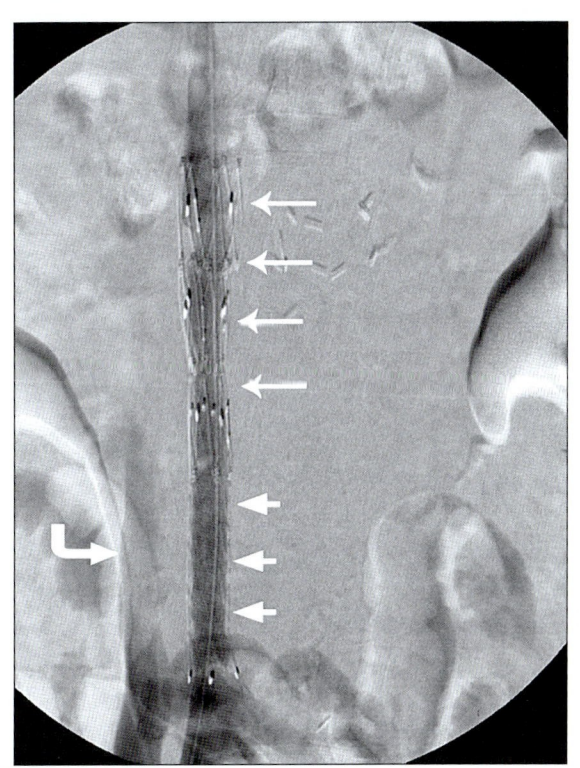

Figure 4. The IVC was reconstructed with a combination of Gianturco *(long arrows)* and self-expanding nitinol stents *(short arrow)*. There is now preferential flow in the native IVC with only faint filling of the ascending lumbar vein *(curved arrow)*.

Case 186

DEMOGRAPHICS/CLINICAL HISTORY

A 37-year-old woman with leg swelling, undergoing Doppler ultrasound, venography, balloon angioplasty, and stenting.

DISCUSSION

History/Indications for Procedure
A 37-year-old woman had a history of spontaneous left lower extremity deep venous thrombosis (DVT) approximately 1 year before the current procedure. She was treated with anticoagulation and compression stockings, but she continued to have intermittent leg pain and swelling.

Procedure
Chronic lower extremity deep venous thrombosis

Pre-procedure Imaging
Doppler ultrasound of the left lower extremity demonstrates reduced phasicity of the common femoral vein, suggesting iliac venous obstruction.

Intraprocedural Findings
Ascending venogram of the left lower extremity from a common femoral vein access demonstrates focal narrowing of the common iliac vein, consistent with a May-Thurner lesion (Fig. 1). The lesion was treated with balloon angioplasty, followed by the placement of a 12-mm × 60-mm Wallstent from the inferior vena cava (IVC) to the external iliac vein (Figs. 2 and 3).

Follow-up and Complications
The patient's symptoms improved after stent placement, but 6 months later, the symptoms recurred, and a repeat venogram demonstrated iliac stent occlusion. The stent was opened with balloon angioplasty, and an additional stent was placed into the external iliac vein.

Suggested Readings
Nazarian GK, Bjarnason H, Dietz CA Jr, et al: Iliofemoral venous stenoses: Effectiveness of treatment with metallic endovascular stents. Radiology 200:193-199, 1996.

O'Sullivan G: Endovascular management of chronic iliac vein occlusion. Tech Vasc Intervent Radiol 3:45-53, 2000.

Sharafuddin M, Sun S, Hoballah JJ, et al: Endovascular management of venous thrombotic and occlusive diseases of the lower extremities. J Vasc Intervent Radiol 14:405-423, 2003.

Case 186   373

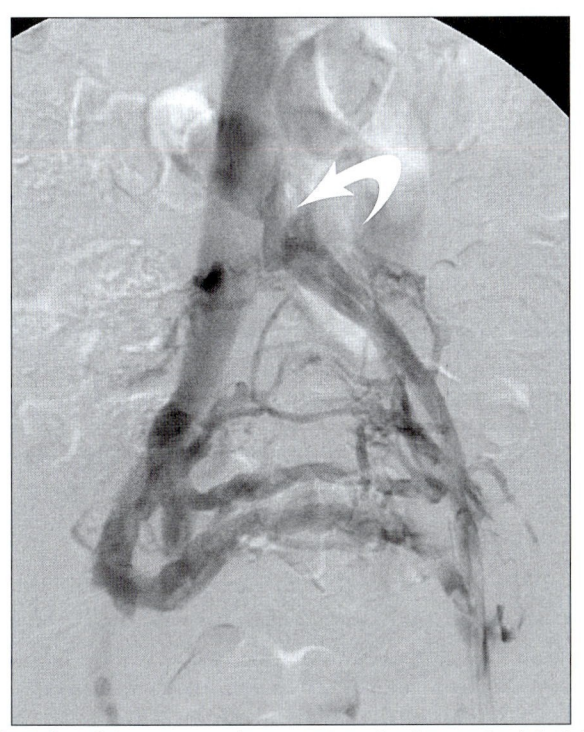

Figure 1. Pelvic venogram demonstrates a focal stenosis of the left common iliac vein *(arrow)* with filling of enlarged lateral sacral veins.

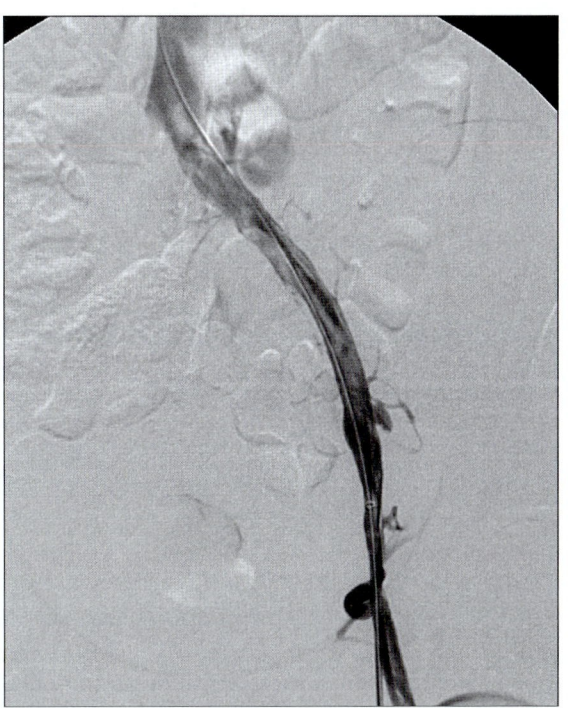

Figure 2. Ascending venogram after balloon angioplasty demonstrates significant improvement in flow through the left iliac veins. There is continued irregularity of the left common and external iliac veins, but the lateral sacral collaterals are no longer filling.

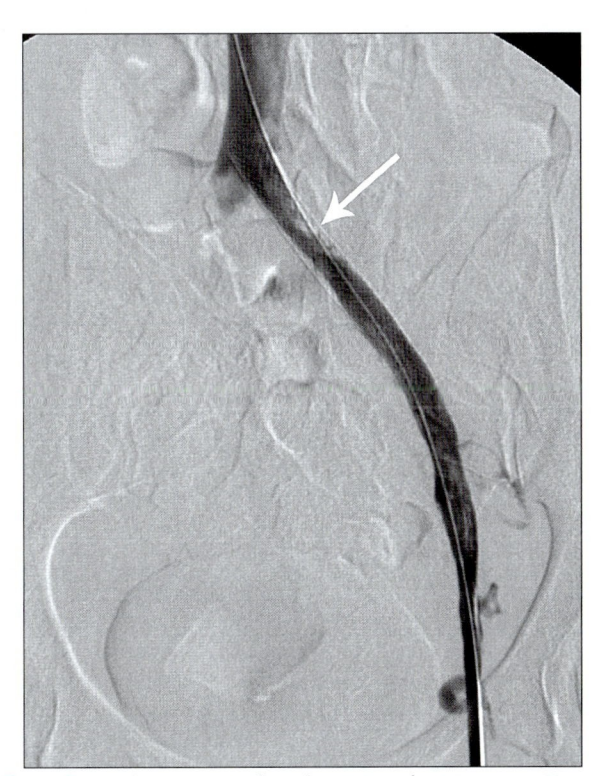

Figure 3. Final venogram after placement of a 12-mm × 60-mm Wallstent. A small filling defect is present within the stent *(arrow)*, and there is continued irregularity of the external iliac vein. The patient's symptoms improved for several months after the stent was placed.

Case 187

DEMOGRAPHICS/CLINICAL HISTORY

An 18-year-old woman with a prior left common iliac vein stent placement presents with new left lower extremity pain and swelling.

DISCUSSION

History/Indications for Procedure

An 18-year-old woman with a known hypercoagulable condition presents with increasing left lower extremity pain and swelling. The patient has undergone prior left common iliac vein stenting following thrombolysis of a left lower extremity deep venous thrombosis.

Procedure

Recanalization of chronically occluded venous stent

Pre-procedure Imaging

Left lower extremity venous ultrasound shows abnormal venous waveforms, suggesting a central venous obstruction.

Intraprocedural Findings

The left common iliac venous stent is occluded (Figs. 1 and 2); conventional attempts to recannulate the stent were unsuccessful. Following sharp recanalization, the guidewire was snared from a right internal jugular vein access and through-and-through guidewire access was obtained; the occluded stent was angioplastied with a 10-mm balloon, and additional stents were placed, stenting the entire left common and external iliac veins (Figs. 3 and 4).

Follow-up and Complications

The patient's pain and swelling resolved following the procedure. However, the symptoms recurred, and the patient underwent repeat venography that showed the stents to remain patent; chronic change from prior deep venous thrombosis of the femoral vein was treated with segmental angioplasties.

Suggested Readings

Neglen P, Hollis KC, Olivier J, et al: Stenting of the venous outflow in chronic venous disease: Long-term stent-related outcome, clinical, and hemodynamic result. J Vasc Surg 46:979-990, 2007.

Neglen P, Raju S: In-stent recurrent stenosis in stents placed in the lower extremity venous outflow tract. J Vasc Surg 39:181-187, 2004.

O'Sullivan G: Endovascular management of chronic iliac vein occlusion. Tech Vasc Intervent Radiol 3:45-53, 2000.

Raju S, Owen S, Neglen P: The clinical impact of iliac venous stents in the management of chronic venous insufficiency. J Vasc Surg 35:8-14, 2002.

Case 187   375

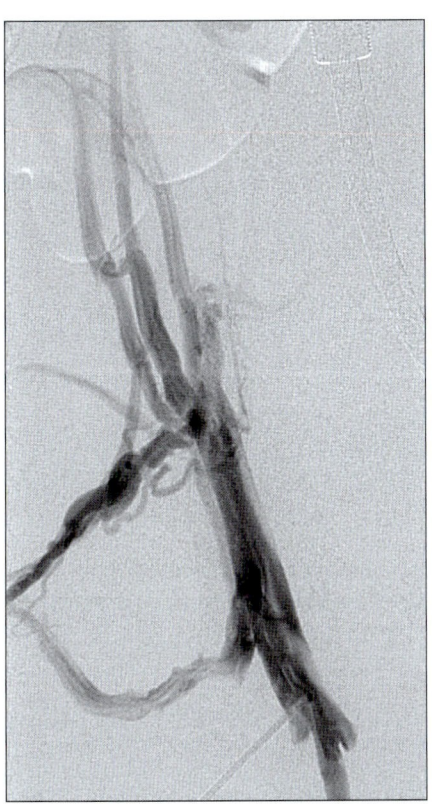

Figure 1. Ascending left lower extremity venogram from a left common femoral vein approach shows occlusion of the left external iliac vein. There is filling of several well-developed venous collaterals.

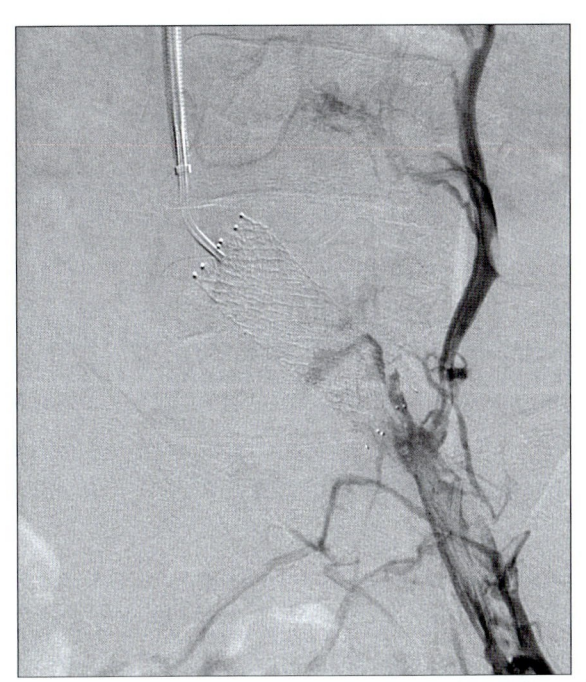

Figure 2. Ascending venogram performed from catheter advanced into the occluded external iliac vein shows complete occlusion of the previously placed common iliac venous stent. Attempts to cross the obstructed stent from either the femoral access or an IJ access using conventional methods were not successful.

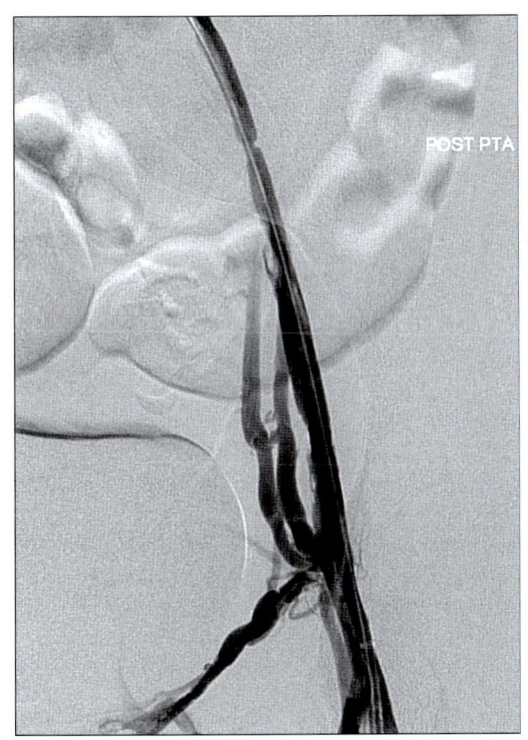

Figure 3. Follow-up venogram after recanalization and angioplasty of the occluded common iliac vein stent and external iliac vein shows improved flow with persistent diffuse narrowing of the external iliac vein.

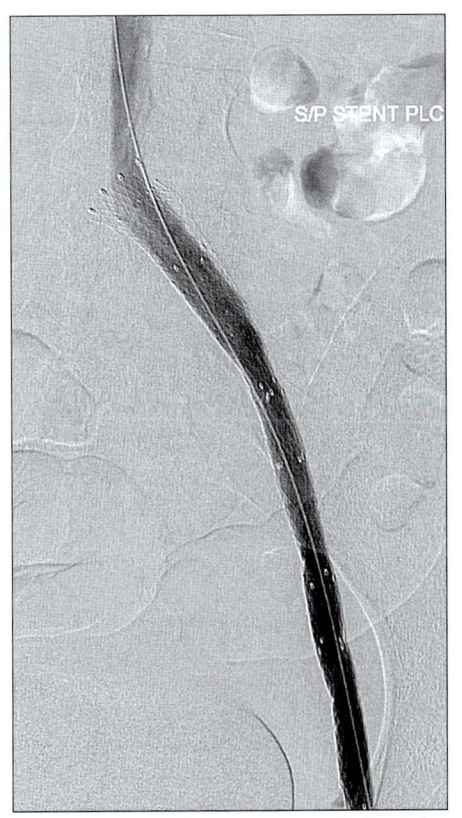

Figure 4. Final venogram. Stents were placed from the common iliac vein to the common femoral vein. After stent placement there is brisk flow through the stents, and the prominent pelvic venous collaterals no longer fill.

Case 188

DEMOGRAPHICS/CLINICAL HISTORY

A 22-year-old woman with right upper extremity swelling.

DISCUSSION

History/Indications for Procedure
A 22-year-old woman volleyball player presents with 1-day history of right upper extremity swelling. She reports intermittent right upper extremity swelling and right hand "tingling" over the past couple of years.

Procedure
Management for acute upper extremity deep venous thrombosis

Pre-procedure Imaging
Contrast-enhanced MR venogram shows occlusion of the right subclavian and axillary veins (Fig 1).

Intraprocedural Findings
Right upper extremity venogram shows a large filling defect in the right axillary and subclavian veins consistent with acute thrombus (Fig. 2). An infusion catheter was placed across the clot, and thrombolysis with urokinase was initiated.

Follow-up and Complications
The patient underwent 48 hours of catheter-directed thrombolysis with near-complete clot lysis; a chronic stenosis was uncovered and angioplastied with a 10-mm balloon (Figs. 3 and 4). The patient went on to right anterior scalenectomy, and she has had no further episodes of upper extremity venous thrombosis in the 3 years since the surgery.

Suggested Readings
Adelman MA, Stone DH, Riles TS, et al: A multidisciplinary approach to the treatment of Paget-Schroetter syndrome. Ann Vasc Surg 11:149-154, 1997.

Baarslag HJ, Kooopman MM, Reekers JA, et al: Diagnosis and management of deep vein thrombosis of the upper extremity: A review. Eur Radiol 14:1263-74, 2004.

Nemchk AA: Jr: Upper extremity deep venous thrombosis: Interventional management. Tech Vasc Intervent Radiol 7:86-90, 2004.

Sharafuddin MJ, Sun S, Hoballah JJ: Endovascular management of venous thrombotic diseases of the upper torso and extremities. J Vasc Intervent Radiol 13:975-90, 2002.

Case 188   377

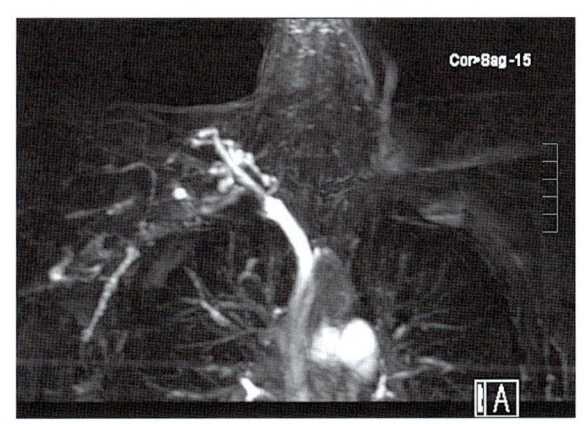

Figure 1. Post-contrast coronal image from MR venogram shows occlusion of the right subclavian and axillary veins. The brachiocephalic vein and SVC are patent.

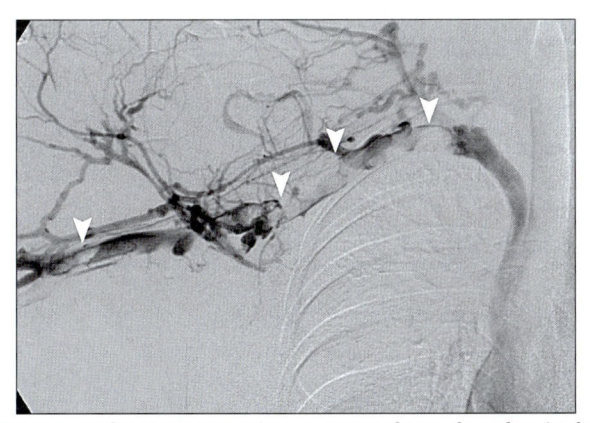

Figure 2. Right upper extremity venogram shows thrombus in the right axillary and subclavian veins *(arrowheads)*.

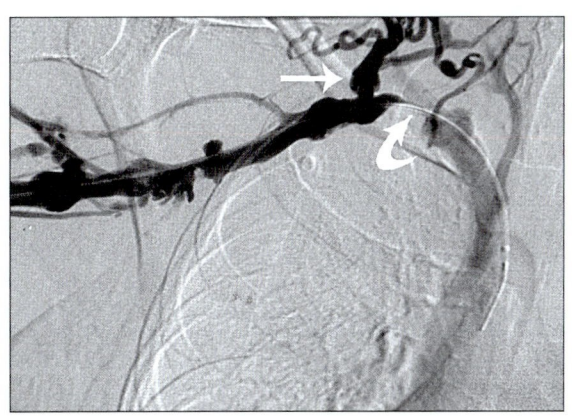

Figure 3. Right upper extremity venogram after 48 hours of thrombolysis. There is near-complete lysis of the axillary and subclavian vein thrombus. A focal stenosis is uncovered at the level of the thoracic outlet *(curved arrow)* with well-developed thyrocervical venous collaterals *(arrow)*.

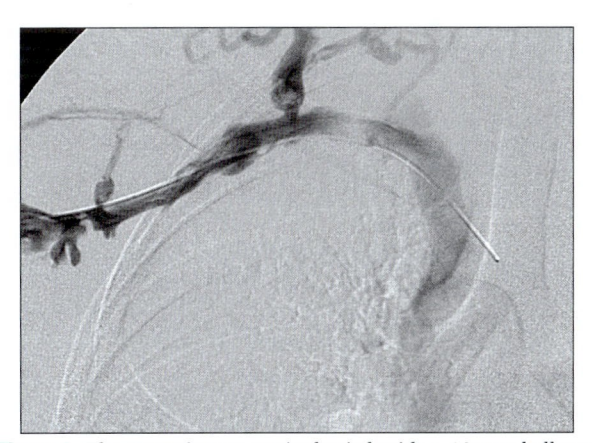

Figure 4. The stenosis was angioplastied with a 10-mm balloon. Follow-up venogram shows a good angiographic result.

Case 189

DEMOGRAPHICS/CLINICAL HISTORY

An 82-year-old man with end-stage renal disease and facial swelling, undergoing venography.

DISCUSSION

History/Indications for Procedure
An 82-year-old man with end-stage renal disease and facial swelling has been dialyzed through a left internal jugular venous catheter for the past 10 months.

Procedure
Endovascular management of catheter-related superior vena cava stenosis

Pre-procedure Imaging
None

Intraprocedural Findings
Superior venacavogram shows a high-grade stenosis of the superior vena cava (SVC) just below the confluence of the brachiocephalic veins (Fig. 1). Angioplasty with a 10-mm balloon was performed on the lesion (Fig. 2), and there was significant elastic recoil on follow-up venogram; a 12-mm × 40-mm, self-expanding, nitinol stent was placed with the top of the stent carefully positioned below the confluence of the brachiocephalic veins (Fig. 3).

Follow-up and Complications
The dialysis catheter was replaced through the SVC stent (Fig. 4). The patient's facial swelling had significantly improved by the next day.

Suggested Readings
Antonucci F, Salomonowitz E, Stuckmann G, et al: Hemodialysis related venous stenoses: Treatment with self-expanding endovascular prostheses. Eur J Radiol 15:328-333, 1992.

Dondelinger RF, Kurdziel JC, Gathy C: Expandable metal stents for stenoses of the venal cava and large veins. Semin Intervent Radiol 8:252-263, 1991.

Trerotola SO: Interventional radiology in central venous stenosis and occlusion. Semin Intervent Radiol 11:291-304, 1994.

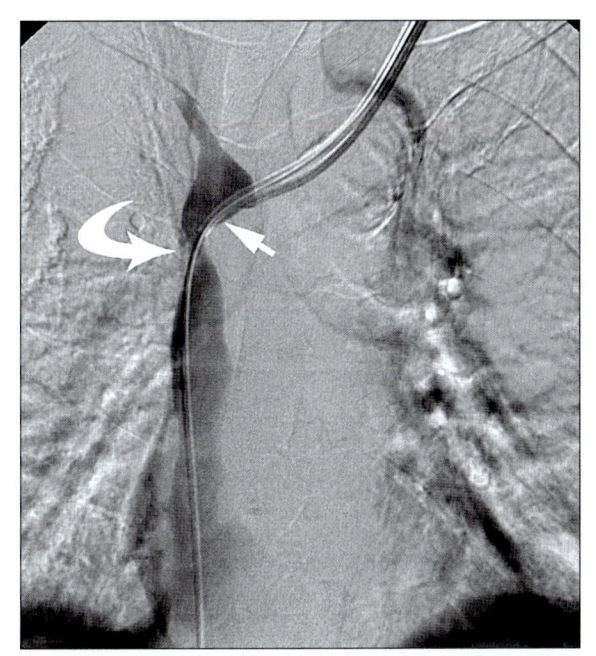

Figure 1. Superior venacavogram performed through the dialysis catheter that has been pulled back to the confluence of the left brachiocephalic vein and SVC *(arrow)*. There is a focal, high-grade stenosis of the SVC just below the confluence of the brachiocephalic veins *(curved arrow)*.

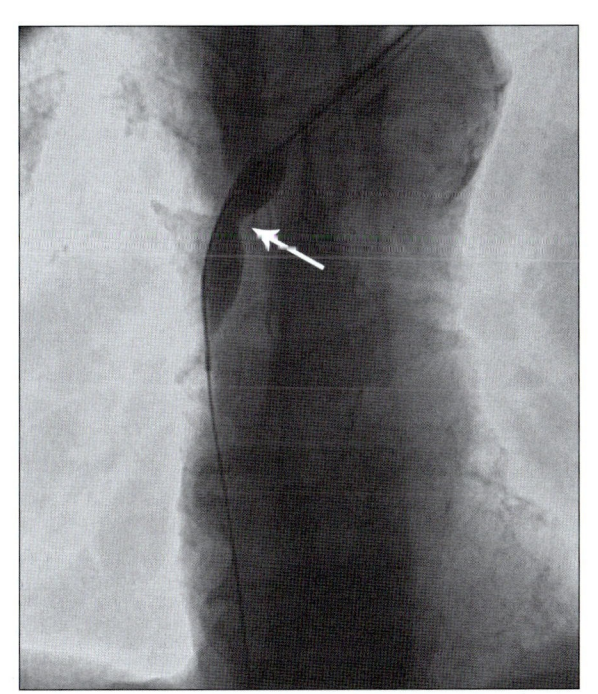

Figure 2. The lesion was dilated with a 10-mm balloon. A focal waist in the balloon is identified at the level of the stenosis *(arrow)*.

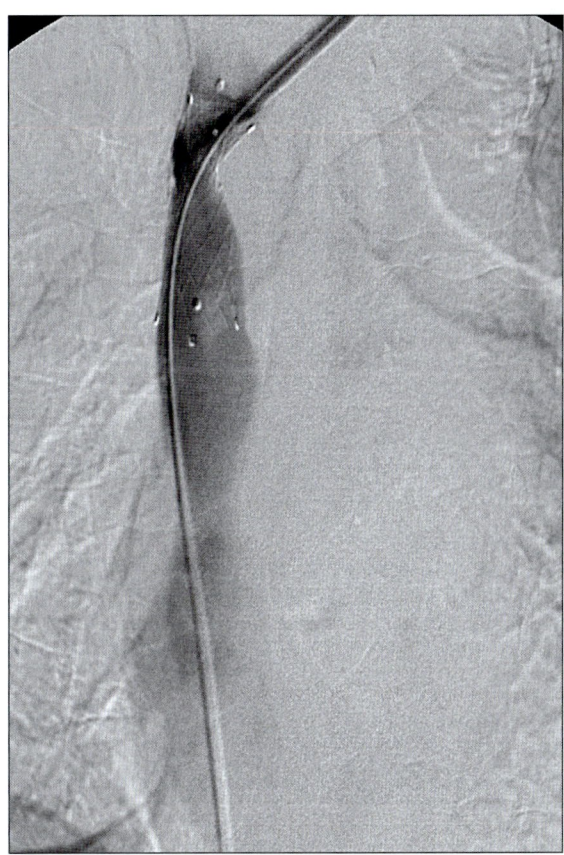

Figure 3. A 12-mm × 40-mm, self-expanding, nitinol stent has been deployed across the lesion. The follow-up cavogram shows improved flow through this region despite the continued narrowing of the stent at the level of the stenosis.

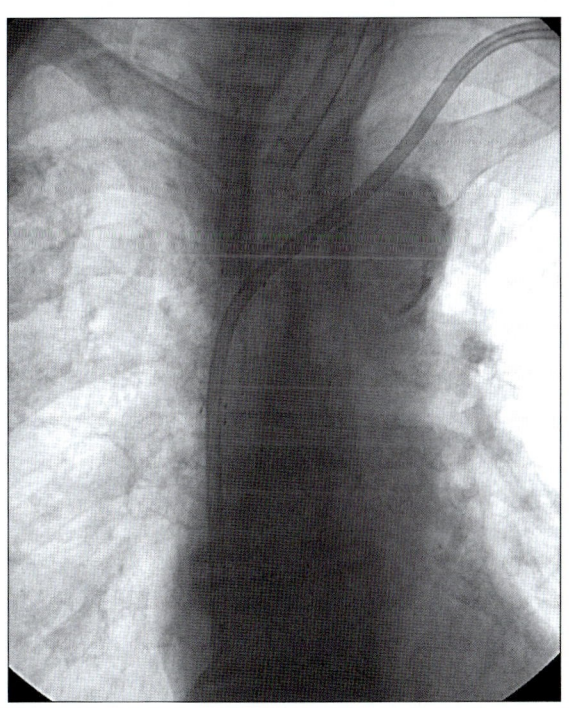

Figure 4. The dialysis catheter has been replaced through the stent.

Case 190

DEMOGRAPHICS/CLINICAL HISTORY

A 69-year-old man with recurrent superior vena cava (SVC) stenosis and facial swelling, undergoing superior venacavography.

DISCUSSION

History/Indications for Procedure
A 69-year-old man had recurrent SVC stenosis and facial swelling. The stenosis most likely resulted from an indwelling venous port catheter.

Procedure
Percutaneous stent for superior vena cava stenosis

Pre-procedure Imaging
The superior venacavogram shows a focal stenosis of the SVC (Fig. 1). A left subclavian venous port is in place.

Intraprocedural Findings
The port catheter was snared from a right internal jugular venous access and pulled into the right brachiocephalic vein (Fig. 2). A 15-mm × 5-cm Gianturco stent was deployed across the stenosis from a right common femoral vein approach (Figs. 2 and 3).

Follow-up and Complications
Surveillance venography was performed 8 months after the stent was placed. The stent remained widely patent (Fig. 4), and the patient has not returned with recurrent symptoms in the 7 years since the stent was placed.

Suggested Readings
Dondelinger RF, Goffette P, Kurdziel JC, Roche A: Expandable metal stents for stenoses of the venae cavae and large veins. Semin Intervent Radiol 8:252-263, 1991.
Gaines PA, Belli AM, Anderson PB, et al: Superior vena caval obstruction managed by the Gianturco Z stent. Clin Radiol 49:202-208, 1994.
Rösch J, Uchida BD, Hall LD, et al: Gianturco-Rösch expandable Z stents in the treatment of superior vena cava syndrome. Cardiovasc Intervent Radiol 15:319-327, 1992.

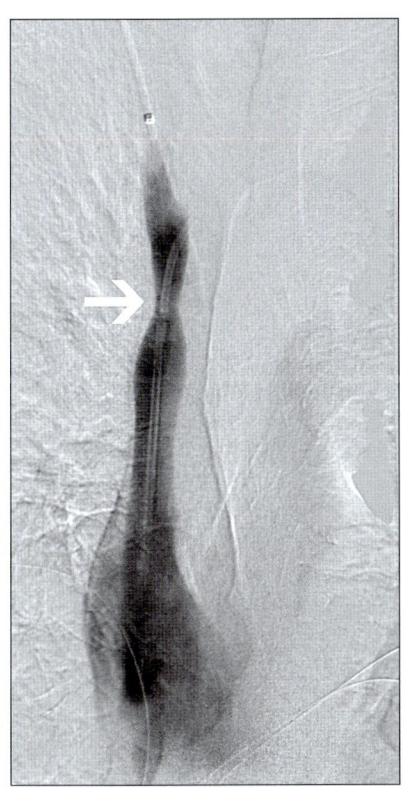

Figure 1. A superior venacavogram performed from right internal jugular vein access shows a focal stenosis of the SVC just below the confluence of the brachiocephalic veins *(arrow)*.

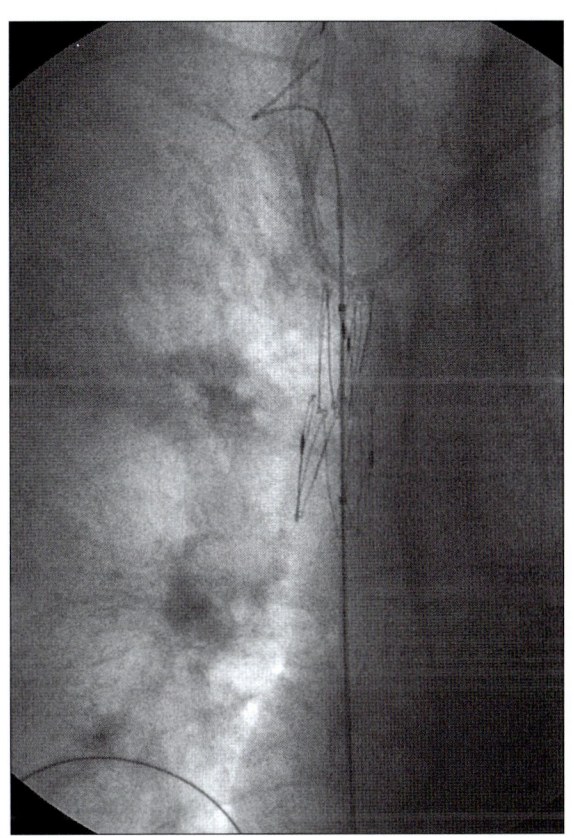

Figure 2. The port catheter has been snared and pulled up and out of the way. A 15-mm × 5-cm Gianturco stent has been placed across the stenosis.

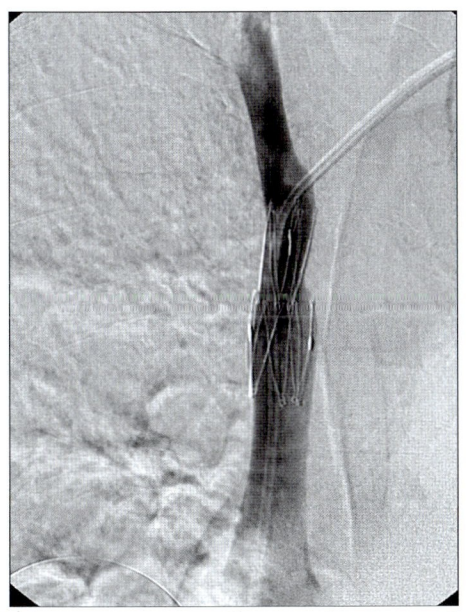

Figure 3. After stent placement, the port catheter was replaced into the right atrium. Follow-up contrast injection shows the stent in an appropriate position and full expansion at the site of stenosis.

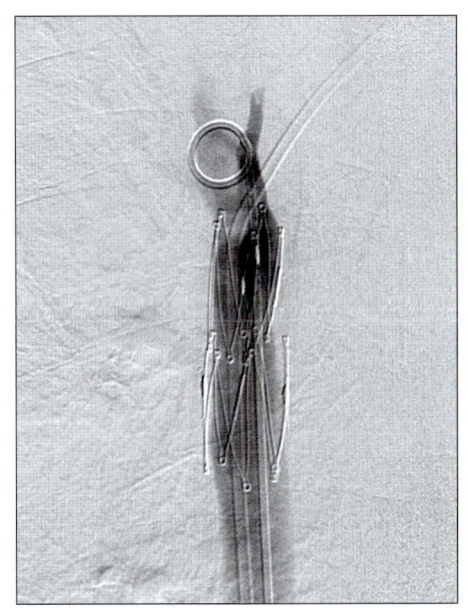

Figure 4. A superior venacavogram performed 8 months after stent placement shows that the stent remains widely patent. The patient has remained asymptomatic since stent placement.

Case 191

DEMOGRAPHICS/CLINICAL HISTORY

A 15-year-old girl with 4- to 5-week history of left upper extremity pain and swelling, undergoing ultrasound, venography, angioplasty, and thoracic outlet decompression.

DISCUSSION

History/Indications for Procedure
A 15-year-old girl has a 4- to 5-week history of left upper extremity pain and swelling. The symptoms are worse after intensive exercise, such as swimming.

Procedure
Upper extremity deep venous thrombosis

Pre-procedure Imaging
Doppler ultrasound revealed acute thrombus in the left subclavian vein.

Intraprocedural Findings
Left upper extremity venogram demonstrates a 3-cm occlusion of the left subclavian vein (Fig. 1). This was treated with balloon angioplasty; only modest improvement was seen on follow-up venogram (Fig. 2).

Follow-up and Complications
After the venoplasty, the patient underwent thoracic outlet decompression with anterior scalenectomy and patch venoplasty. The patient returned with recurrent symptoms and underwent repeat venoplasty (Fig. 3).

Suggested Readings
AbuRahma AF, Robinson PA: Effort subclavian vein thrombosis: Evolution of management. J Endovasc Ther 7:302-308, 2000.

Kreienberg PB, Chang BB, Darling RC 3rd, et al: Long-term results in patients treated with thrombolysis, thoracic inlet decompression, and subclavian vein stenting for Paget-Schroetter syndrome. J Vasc Surg 33:S100-S105, 2001.

Melby SJ, Vedantham S, Narra VR, et al: Comprehensive surgical management of the competitive athlete with effort thrombosis of the subclavian vein (Paget-Schroetter syndrome). J Vasc Surg 47:809-820, 2008.

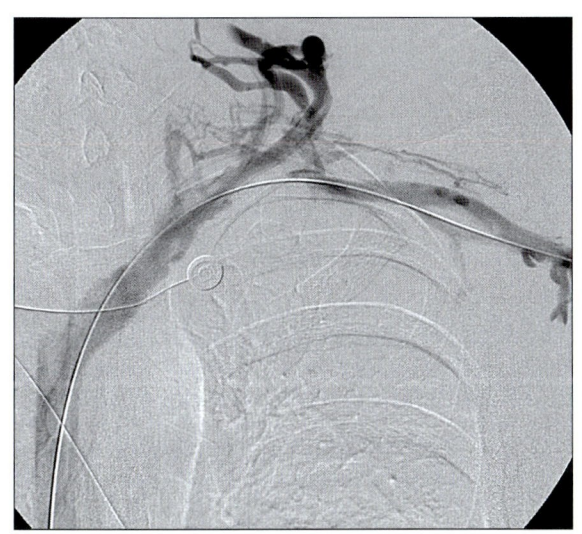

Figure 1. Single image from the left upper extremity venogram demonstrates a 3-cm occlusion of the left subclavian vein and well-developed collaterals.

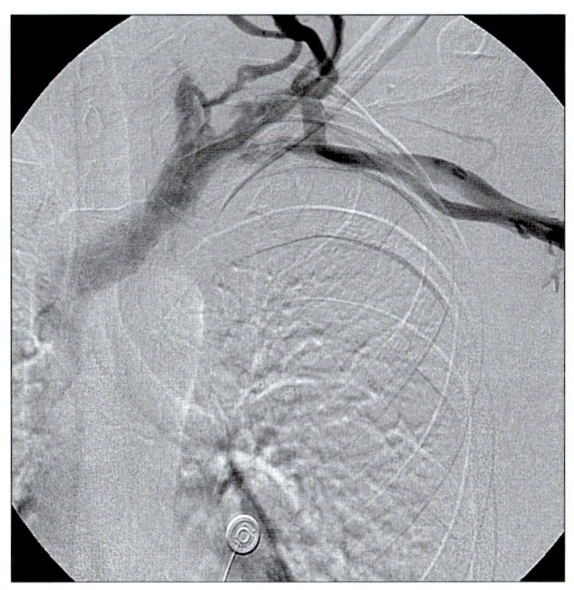

Figure 2. There is persistent stenosis and irregularity of the previously occluded segment after venoplasty.

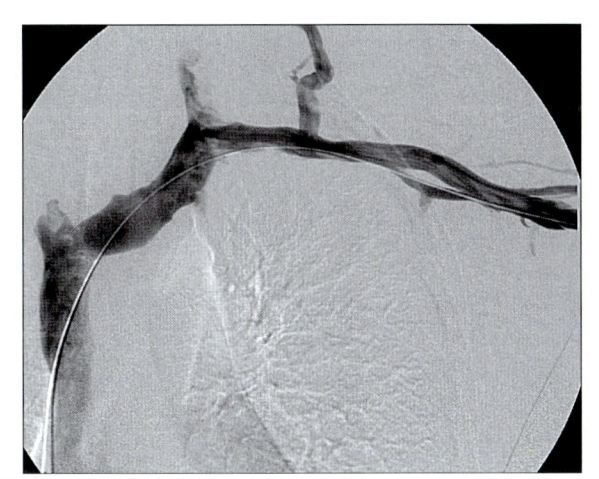

Figure 3. The patient returned with recurrent symptoms after a thoracic outlet decompression procedure. At this point, repeat venoplasty had a significantly better result.

Case 192

DEMOGRAPHICS/CLINICAL HISTORY

A 29-year-old woman with chronic thrombosis of the right internal jugular vein and increasing facial swelling, undergoing venography.

DISCUSSION

History/Indications for Procedure
A 29-year-old woman has antiphospholipid antibody syndrome and chronic occlusion of the right internal jugular vein. She has worsening facial swelling despite adequate anticoagulation.

Procedure
Chronic right upper extremity venous occlusion management

Pre-procedure Imaging
Doppler ultrasound shows chronic occlusion of the right internal jugular vein with suspected obstruction of the right brachiocephalic vein.

Intraprocedural Findings
The right internal jugular and brachiocephalic veins are occluded, with prominent collateral veins seen in the right neck and chest (Fig. 1). The occlusion was crossed (Fig. 2), serially dilated to 12 mm, and stented with a 12-mm × 40-mm, self-expanding, nitinol stent (SMART, Cordis, Miami Lakes, FL) (Figs. 3 and 4).

Follow-up and Complications
The patient's symptoms improved after stent placement. She was again started on anticoagulation, and follow-up ultrasound 1 month later confirmed continued patency of the stent.

Suggested Readings
Rajan DK, Saluja JS: Use of nitinol stents following recanalization of central venous occlusions in hemodialysis patients. Cardiovasc Intervent Radiol 30:662-667, 2007.

Rizvi AZ, Kalra M, Bjarnason H, et al: Benign superior vena cava syndrome: Stenting is now the first line of treatment. J Vasc Surg 47:372-380, 2008.

Trerotola SO: Interventional radiology in central venous stenosis and occlusion. Semin Intervent Radiol 11:291-304, 1994.

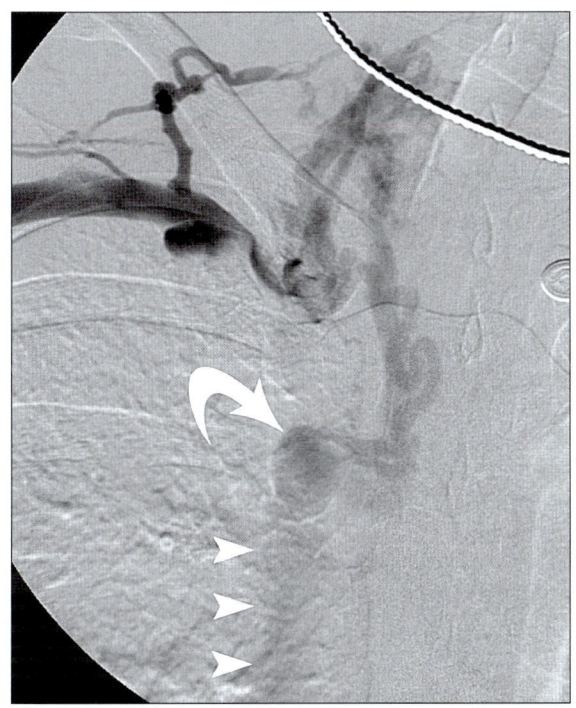

Figure 1. Right upper extremity venogram shows occlusion of the right brachiocephalic vein. Collateral veins drain into the azygous vein *(curved arrow)*, which then empties into the SCV *(arrowheads)*.

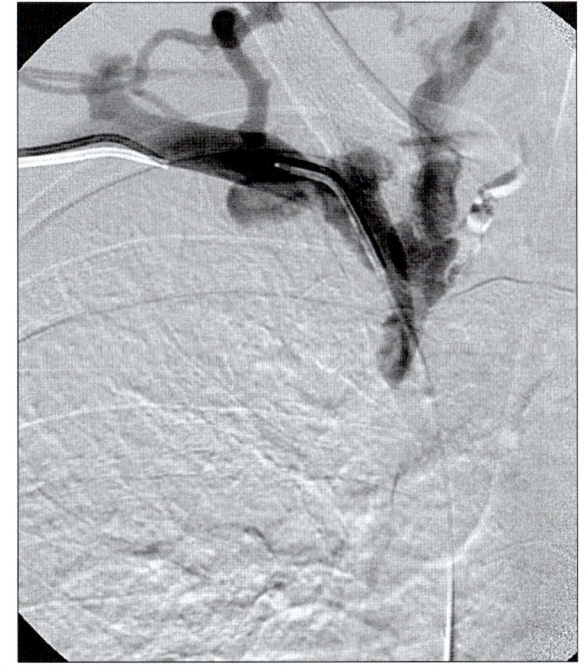

Figure 2. Attempts to cross the obstruction from the upper extremity access were unsuccessful. The right common femoral vein was accessed, and the obstruction was successfully crossed from this approach.

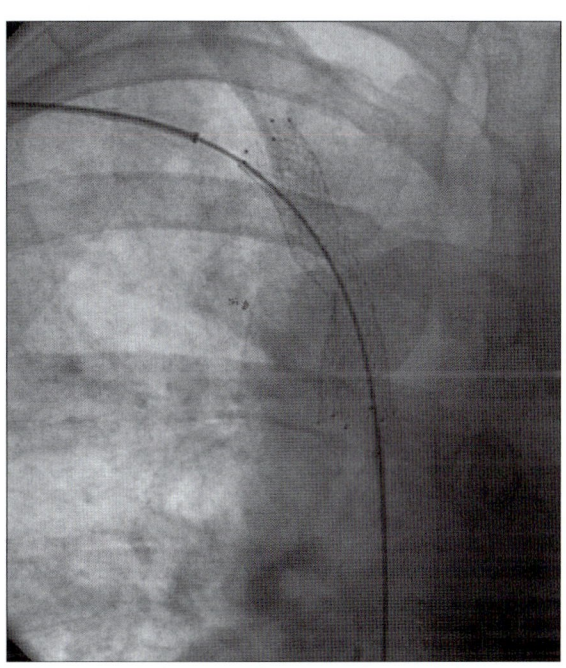

Figure 3. After serial balloon dilatations, the occluded segment was stented with a 12-mm × 40-mm, self-expanding, nitinol stent.

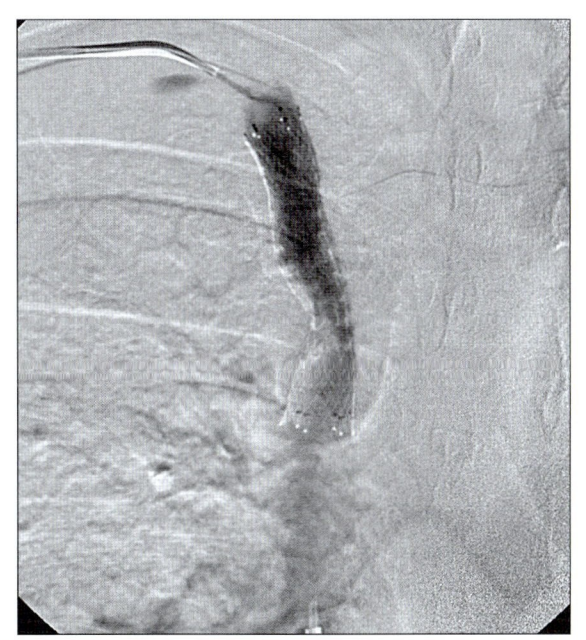

Figure 4. Final venogram shows brisk flow through the stent. The venous collaterals are no longer seen.

Case 193

DEMOGRAPHICS/CLINICAL HISTORY

A 42-year-old man with left upper extremity swelling.

DISCUSSION

History/Indications for Procedure
A 42-year-old man with left upper extremity swelling. The patient has end-stage renal disease and multiple previous upper extremity dialysis grafts, including a left upper extremity arc graft that is currently functional.

Procedure
Endovascular management of chronic upper extremity deep venous thrombosis

Intraprocedural Findings
The left brachiocephalic vein is occluded (Fig. 1). The occluded segment was angioplastied with a 10-mm balloon followed by placement of a 12-mm × 60-mm self-expanding stent (Figs. 2 and 3).

Follow-up and Complications
The patient returned 10 months later for poor flows through the left upper extremity dialysis graft. Follow-up venogram shows a high-grade intrastent stenosis that was successfully treated with repeat balloon angioplasty.

Suggested Readings
Antonucci F, Salomonowitz E, Stuckmann G, et al: Hemodialysis related venous stenosis: Treatment with self-expanding endovascular prostheses. Eur J Radiol 14:195-200, 1992.

Bakken AM, Protack CD, Saad WE, et al: Long-term outcomes of primary angioplasty and primary stenting of central venous stenosis in hemodialysis patients. J Vasc Surg 45:776-783, 2007.

Surowiec SM, Fegley AJ, Tanski WJ, et al: Endo vascular management of central venous stenoses in the hemodialysis patient: Results of percutaneous therapy. Vasc Endovascular Surg 38:349-354, 2004.

Trerotola SO: Interventional radiology in central venous stenosis and occlusion. Semin Intervent Radiol 11:291-304, 1994.

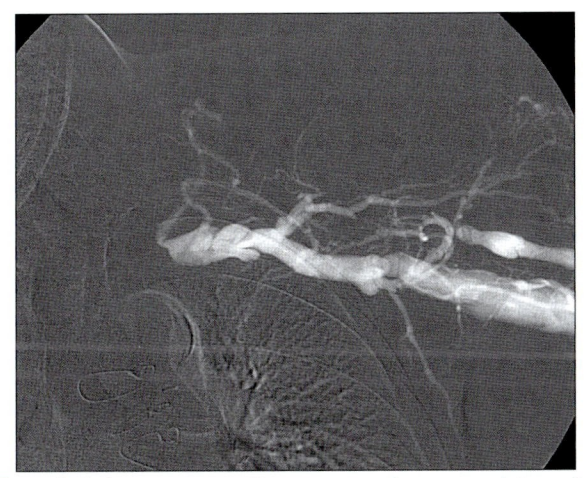

Figure 1. Left upper extremity venogram shows complete occlusion of the left brachiocephalic vein.

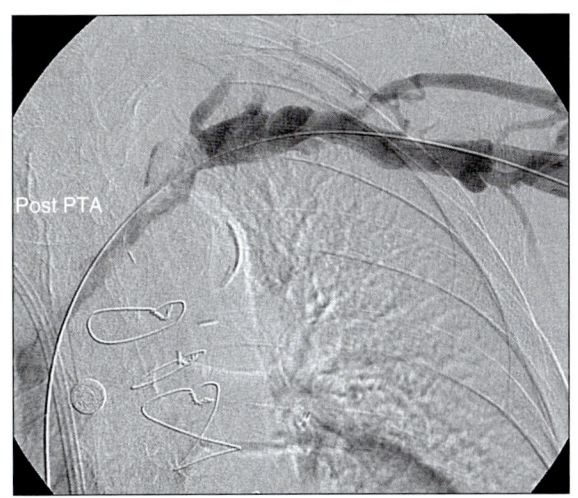

Figure 2. Follow-up venogram after balloon angioplasty shows significant residual narrowing.

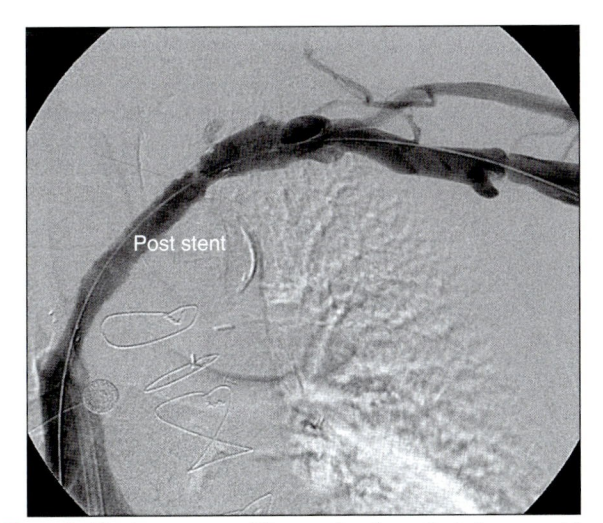

Figure 3. Final venogram. The previously occluded segment has been stented with a 12-mm × 60-mm self-expanding stent.

Case 194

DEMOGRAPHICS/CLINICAL HISTORY

A 28-year-old man with abdominal pain, undergoing magnetic resonance imaging (MRI) and venography.

History/Indications for Procedure

A 28-year-old man had 1 week of worsening abdominal pain, which increased after eating and was associated with vomiting and diarrhea.

Procedure

Portal-mesenteric venous thrombosis

Pre-procedure Imaging

Contrast-enhanced MRI shows extensive occlusive thrombus in the portal vein, splenic vein, and superior mesenteric vein (Fig. 1). There is soft tissue stranding in the mesentery, but the bowel appears normal.

Intraprocedural Findings

Transhepatic venography shows extensive thrombosis of the superior mesenteric vein and portal vein (Fig. 2). Thrombolysis was performed using the power-pulse spray technique with the AngioJet catheter (Possis Medical, Minneapolis, MN) (Fig. 3).

Follow-up and Complications

The patient underwent 3 days of thrombolysis, which produced marked improvement in abdominal pain. The final venogram shows near-complete restoration of flow through the portal-mesenteric venous system (Fig. 4).

Suggested Readings

Hollingshead M, Burke CT, Mauro MA, et al: Transcatheter thrombolytic therapy for acute mesenteric thrombosis. J Vasc Intervent Radiol 16:651-661, 2005.

Kim HS, Patra A, Khan J, et al: Transhepatic catheter-directed thrombectomy and thrombolysis of acute superior mesenteric venous thrombosis. J Vasc Intervent Radiol 16:1685-1691, 2005.

Uflacker R: Applications of percutaneous mechanical thrombectomy in transjugular intrahepatic portosystemic shunt and portal vein thrombosis. Tech Vasc Intervent Radiol 6:59-69, 2003.

Valla DC, Condat B: Portal vein thrombosis in adults: Pathophysiology, pathogenesis and management. J Hepatol 32:865-871, 2000.

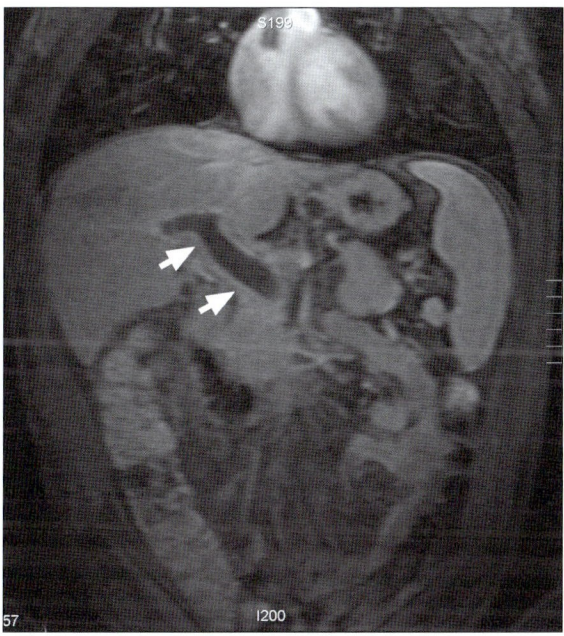

Figure 1. Coronal, T1-weighted, post-contrast MRI shows complete occlusion of the main portal vein, with the thrombus extending into the right and left portal veins *(arrows)*.

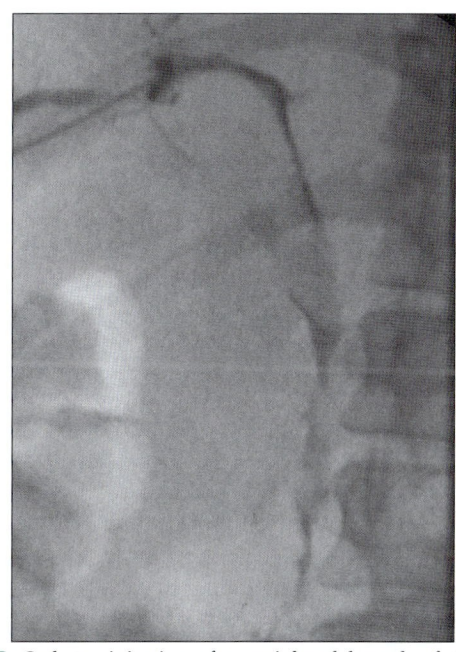

Figure 2. Catheter injection of a peripheral branch of the right portal vein confirms minimal flow in the portal-mesenteric venous system.

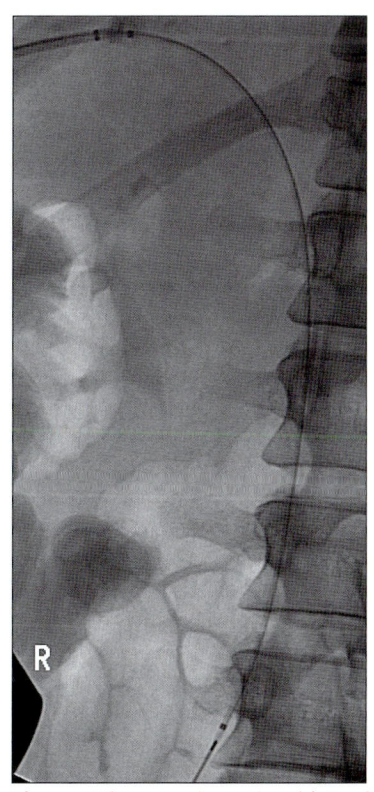

Figure 3. An infusion catheter has been placed for catheter-directed thrombolysis. The patient underwent 3 days of thrombolysis with tissue plasminogen activator (tPA) at a rate of 0.5 mg/hr.

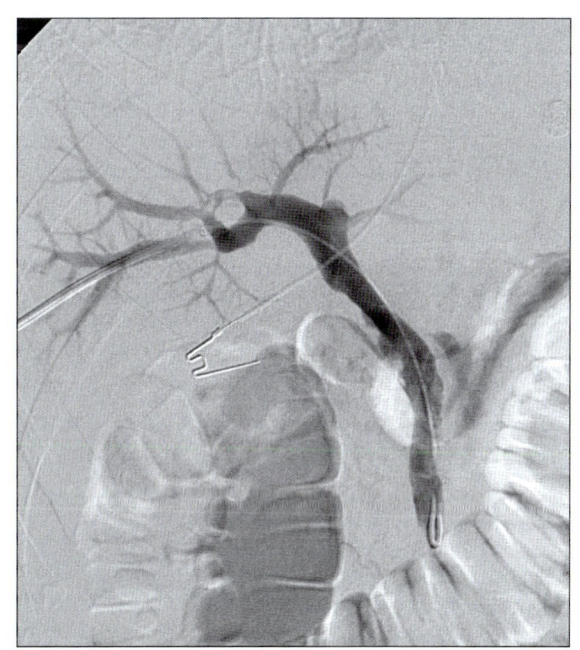

Figure 4. After thrombolysis, flow was restored through the superior mesenteric vein and portal vein. Some mural irregularity indicates a small amount of residual thrombus.

Case 195

DEMOGRAPHICS/CLINICAL HISTORY

A 57-year-old man with portal vein thrombosis after right hepatic lobectomy.

DISCUSSION

History/Indications for Procedure
A 57-year-old man who underwent right hepatic lobectomy for poorly differentiated adenocarcinoma 9 days earlier.

Procedure
Percutaneous management for portal vein thrombosis after hepatectomy

Pre-procedure Imaging
Doppler ultrasound shows no blood flow within the main or left portal vein (Fig. 1). Contrast-enhanced MRI confirms the presence of thrombus in the main portal vein, extending to the confluence of the superior mesenteric vein (SMV) and splenic veins.

Intraprocedural Findings
Transhepatic portal venogram shows thrombus extending from the confluence of the SMV and splenic veins to the intrahepatic portal veins (Fig. 2). Mechanical thrombectomy was performed using the Trerotola (Arrow International, Reading, PA) mechanical thrombectomy device, and catheter-directed thrombolysis was initiated (Figs. 3 and 4).

Follow-up and Complications
The patient underwent 40 hours of catheter-directed thrombolysis, after which time there was no visible thrombus in the main portal vein (Fig. 4). The patient was anticoagulated with intravenous argatroban, which was transitioned to warfarin at the time of discharge from the hospital.

Suggested Readings
Adani GL, Baccarani U, Risaliti A, et al: Percutaneous transhepatic portography for the treatment of early portal vein thrombosis after surgery. Cardiovasc Intervent Radiol 30:1222-1226, 2007.

Hidajat N, Stobbe H, Griesshaber V, et al: Imaging and radiological interventions of portal vein thrombosis. Acta Radiol 46:336-343, 2005.

Valla DC, Condat B: Portal vein thrombosis in adults: Patholphysiology, pathogenesis and management. J Hepatol 32:865-871, 2000.

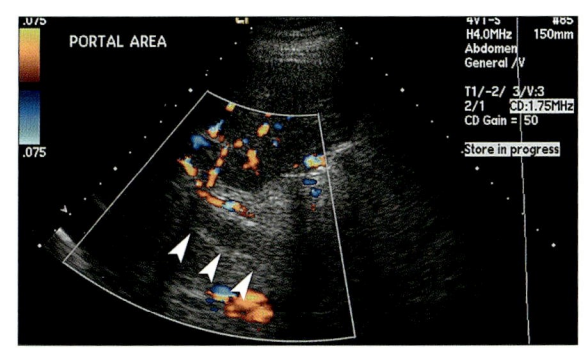

Figure 1. Color Doppler ultrasound of the abdomen. No flow is seen in the main portal vein *(arrowheads)*.

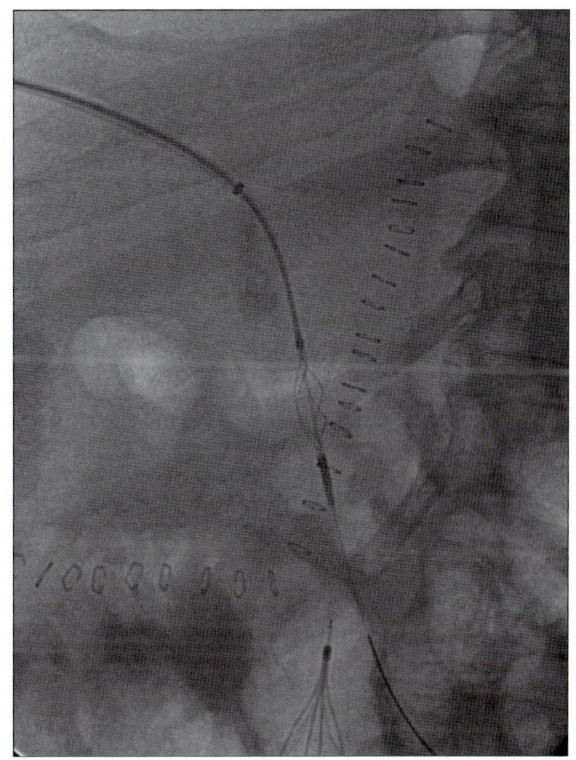

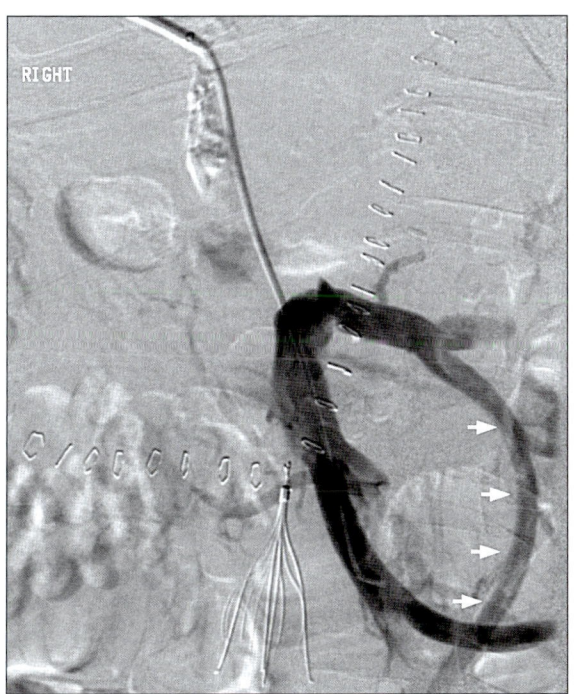

Figure 2. The portal vein was accessed directly through a transhepatic approach. A 5-French catheter has been advanced into the SMV. Mesenteric venogram shows complete occlusion of the main portal vein and reflux of contrast in the inferior mesenteric vein *(arrows)*.

Figure 3. Mechanical thrombectomy was performed using the Trerotola PTD.

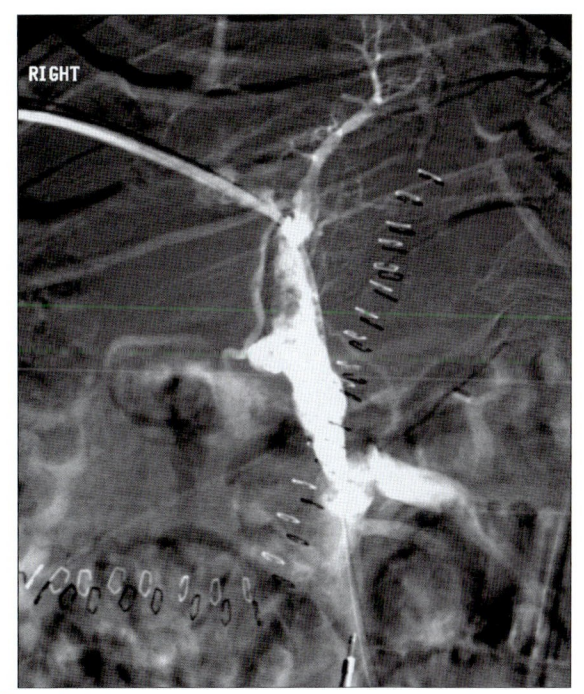

Figure 4. Follow-up venogram after mechanical thrombectomy shows restoration of flow through the main portal vein. The residual thrombus was treated with catheter-directed thrombolysis.

Case 196

DEMOGRAPHICS/CLINICAL HISTORY

A 34-year-old woman with Budd-Chiari syndrome.

DISCUSSION

History/Indications for Procedure
A 34-year-old woman with Budd-Chiari syndrome, antiphospholipid antibody syndrome, and severe ascites.

Procedure
Transjugular intrahepatic portosystemic shunt (TIPSS) placement

Pre-procedure Imaging
Hepatic venogram shows occlusion of a previously placed hepatic vein stent and opacification of intrahepatic venous collaterals (Fig. 1).

Intraprocedural Findings
The hepatic vein was accessed through the hepatic vein stent, and a wedged CO_2 portogram was performed to locate the position of the portal vein (Fig. 2). The right portal vein was accessed approximately 1 cm from the junction with the main portal vein (Fig. 3), a 10-mm covered stent (Viatorr, Gore and assoc, flagstaff, AZ) was deployed from the portal vein to the inferior vena cava (IVC), and an additional covered stent (Fluency, Bard Peripheral Vascular, Tempe, AZ) was deployed to the right atrium (Fig. 4).

Follow-up and Complications
The portosystemic gradient was reduced from 20 mmHg to 7 mmHg. The patient's ascites remained controlled in follow-up, and she was placed on aggressive anticoagulation for her hypercoaguable condition.

Suggested Readings
Beckett D, Olliff S: Interventional radiology in the management of Budd Chiari syndrome. Cardiovasc Intervent Radiol 31:839-847, 2008.

Garcia-Pagan JC, Heydtmann M, Raffa S, et al: TIPS for Budd-Chiari syndrome: Long-term results and prognostics factors in 124 patients. Gastroenterology 135:808-815, 2008.

Olliff SP: Transjugular intrahepatic portosystemic shunt in the management of Budd-Chiari syndrome. Eur J Gastroenterol Hepatol 18:1151-1154, 2006.

Case 196   393

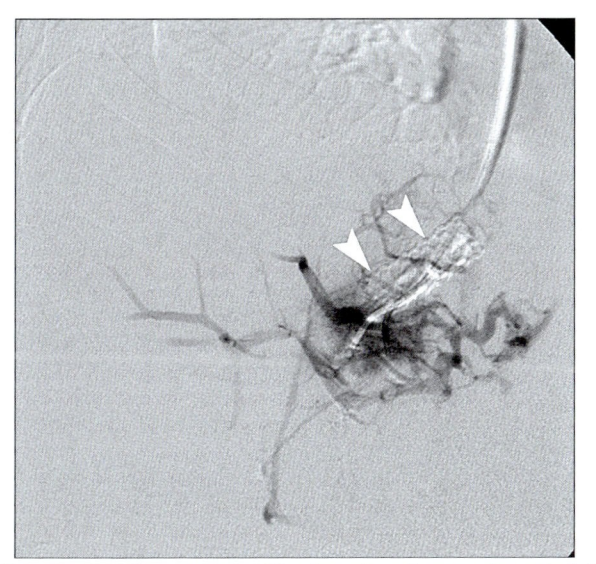

Figure 1. Hepatic venogram. The hepatic vein stent is occluded (arrowheads). Contrast injection opacifies multiple intrahepatic collaterals.

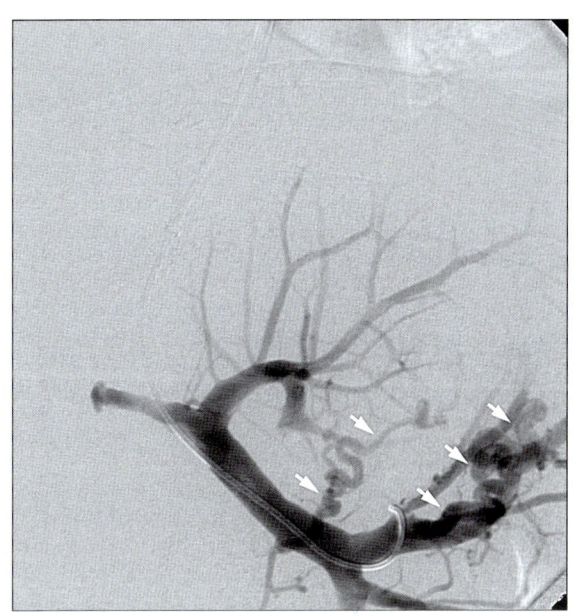

Figure 3. The right portal vein was accessed approximately 1 cm from the portal vein bifurcation. Portal venogram shows filling of the coronary vein and gastric varices (arrows).

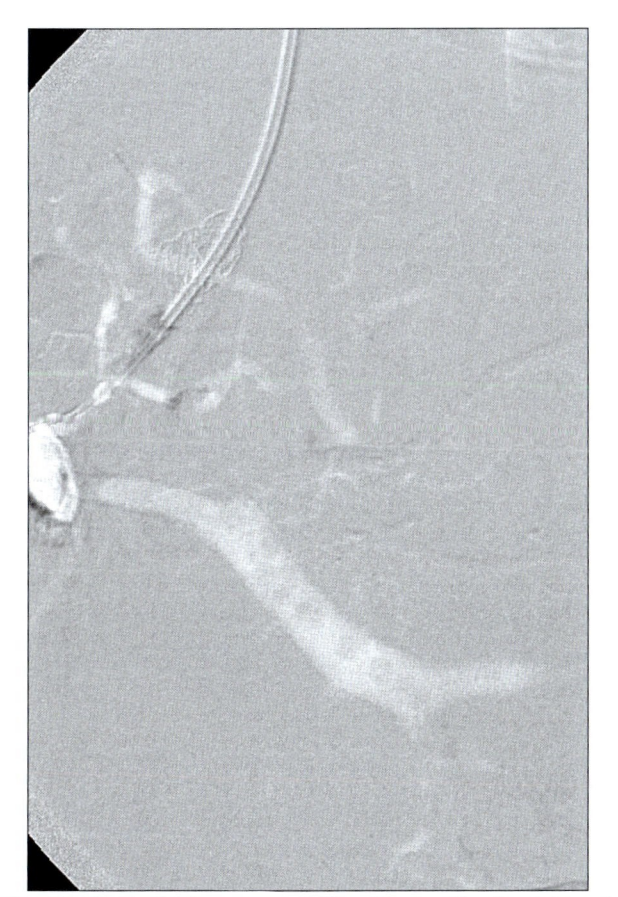

Figure 2. Wedged CO$_2$ portogram. The CO$_2$ opacifies the right and main portal vein.

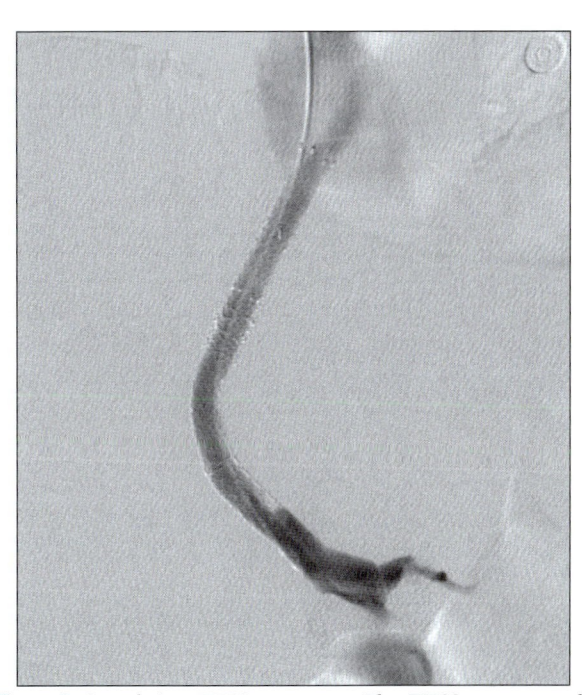

Figure 4. Completion TIPSS venogram. The TIPSS stent extends from the main portal vein to the right atrium. The previously seen collaterals no longer fill.

Case 197

DEMOGRAPHICS/CLINICAL HISTORY

A 56-year-old man with refractory encephalopathy after TIPSS placement, undergoing venography and TIPSS revision.

DISCUSSION

History/Indications for Procedure
A 56-year-old man with alcohol-related liver disease underwent TIPSS placement for intractable ascites. After TIPSS placement, the patient developed refractory encephalopathy.

Procedure
Transjugular intrahepatic portosystemic shunt (TIPSS) reduction

Pre-procedure Imaging
Before TIPSS revision, an occlusion balloon was inflated within the stent, and the patient was monitored for improvement. The encephalopathy did improve with temporary TIPSS occlusion.

Intraprocedural Findings
The TIPSS stent remained patent despite 2 days of balloon occlusion (Fig. 1). A 5-mm × 15-mm, balloon-expandable stent was deployed within the TIPSS stent (Fig. 2), and a 10-mm × 6-cm, covered, self-expanding stent was then deployed within the smaller stent, reducing the flow through the TIPSS (Fig. 3).

Follow-up and Complications
The patient's mental function remained clear after the TIPSS reduction. However, the liver function continued to worsen, and the patient was discharged to hospice because of liver failure.

Suggested Readings
Charon JP, Alaeddin FH, Pimpalwar SA, et al: Results of a retrospective multicenter trial of the Viatorr expanded polytetrafluoroethylene-covered stent-graft for transjugular intrahepatic portosystemic shunt creation. J Vasc Intervent Radiol 15:1219-1230, 2004.

Kochar N, Tripathi D, Ireland H, et al: Transjugular intrahepatic portosystemic stent shunt (TIPSS) modification in the management of post-TIPSS refractory hepatic encephalopathy. Gut 55:1617-1623, 2006.

Maleux G, Heye S, Verslype C, Nevens F: Management of transjugular intrahepatic portosystemic shunt induced refractory hepatic encephalopathy with the parallel technique: Results of a clinical follow-up study. J Vasc Intervent Radiol 18:986-992, 2007.

Maleux G, Verslype C, Heye S, et al: Endovascular shunt reduction in the management of transjugular portosystemic shunt-induced hepatic encephalopathy: Preliminary experience with reduction stents and stent-grafts. AJR Am J Roentgenol 188:659-664, 2007.

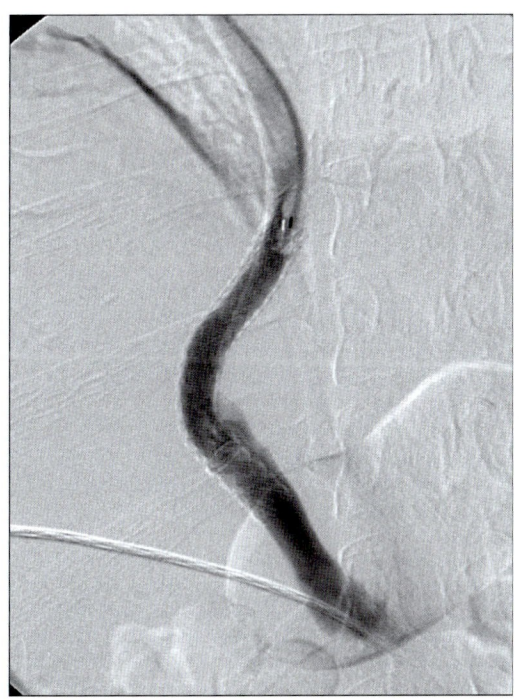

Figure 1. TIPSS venogram after 2 days of balloon occlusion demonstrates that the TIPSS stent remains widely patent.

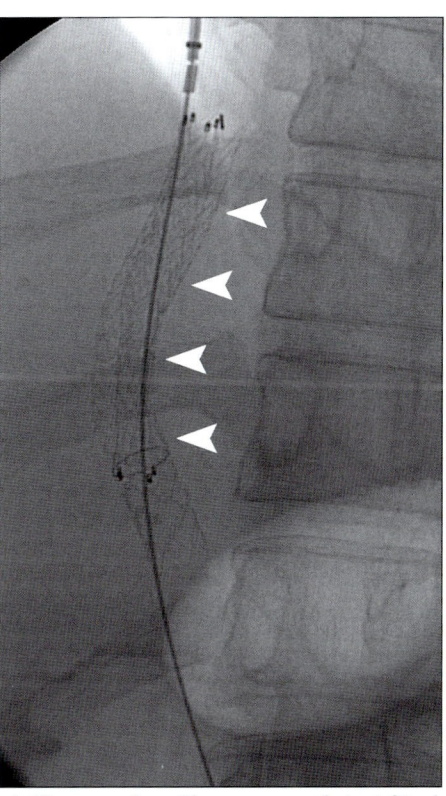

Figure 2. A 10-mm × 6-cm Fluency covered stent (Bard, Tempe, AZ) *(arrowheads)* was placed within a 5-mm × 15-mm, balloon-expandable stent.

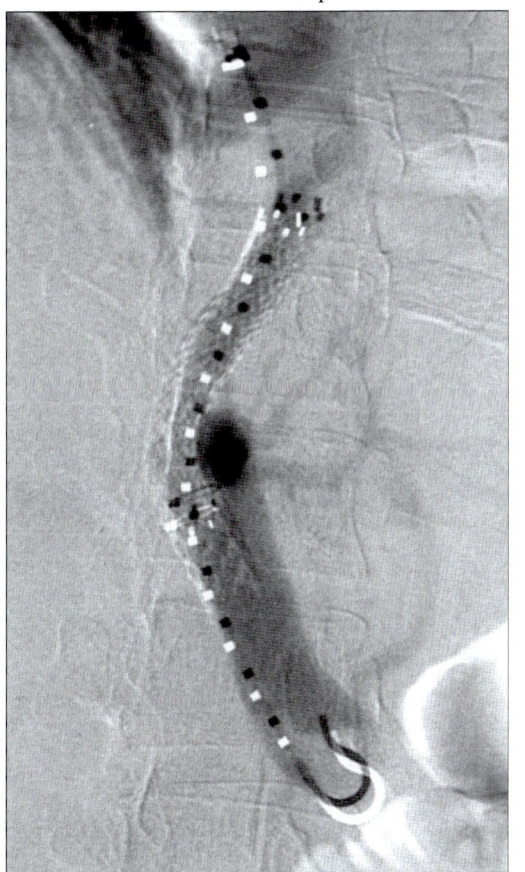

Figure 3. Follow-up TIPSS venogram demonstrates reduction of flow through the middle portion of the TIPSS stent.

Case 198

DEMOGRAPHICS/CLINICAL HISTORY

A 56-year-old man with hepatopulmonary syndrome, undergoing venography and angiography.

DISCUSSION

History/Indications for Procedure
This patient underwent TIPSS placement as a bridge to liver transplantation. After the TIPSS procedure, the patient experienced a decrease in blood pressure and hematocrit.

Procedure
Embolization of hepatic artery as a complication of transjugular intrahepatic portosystemic stent shunt (TIPSS) placement

Intraprocedural Findings
No hemorrhage was identified from the portal venous system (Fig. 1). Active contrast extravasation was identified from a branch of the right hepatic artery (Figs. 2 and 3); this artery was selectively embolized with a combination of platinum coils and absorbable gelatin sponge (Gelfoam) (Fig. 4).

Follow-up and Complications
After the embolization, the patient was hemodynamically stable for approximately 2 hours. The patient then became hypotensive; further resuscitation efforts were unsuccessful, and the patient died.

Suggested Readings

Chevallier P, Novelli L, Motamedi JP, et al: Hepatopulmonary syndrome successfully treated with transjugular intrahepatic portosystemic shunt: A three-year follow-up. J Vasc Intervent Radiol 15:647-648, 2004.

Freedman AM, Sanyal AJ, Tisnado J, et al: Complications of transjugular intrahepatic portosystemic shunt: A comprehensive review. RadioGraphics 13:1185-1210, 1993.

Haskal ZJ, Cope C, Shlansky-Goldberg RD, et al: Transjugular intrahepatic portosystemic shunt-related arterial injuries: Prospective comparison of large- and small-gauge needle systems. J Vasc Intervent Radiol 6:911-915, 1995.

Haskal ZJ, Martin L, Cardella JF, et al: Society of Cardiovascular & Interventional Radiology, Standards of Practice Committee: Quality improvement guidelines for transjugular intrahepatic portosystemic shunts. SCVIR Standards of Practice Committee. J Vasc Intervent Radiol 12:131-136, 2001.

Haskal ZJ, Pentecost MJ, Rubin RA, et al: Hepatic arterial injury after transjugular intrahepatic portosystemic shunt placement: Report of two cases. Radiology 188:85-88, 1993.

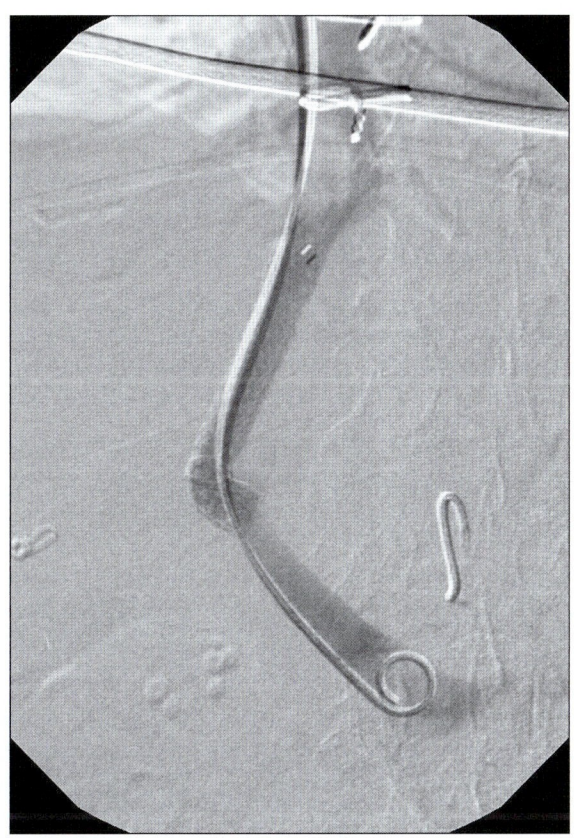

Figure 1. Portal venogram through the TIPSS shows the stent to be patent; there is no evidence of hemorrhage from the portal vein.

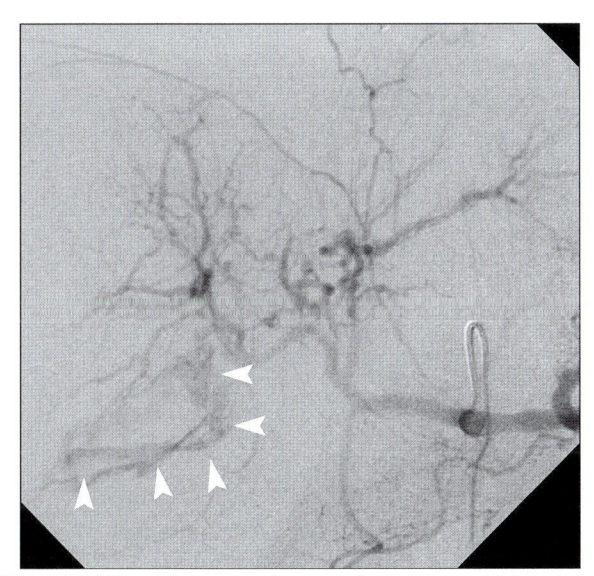

Figure 2. Celiac angiogram shows active contrast extravasation from a branch of the right hepatic artery *(arrowheads)*.

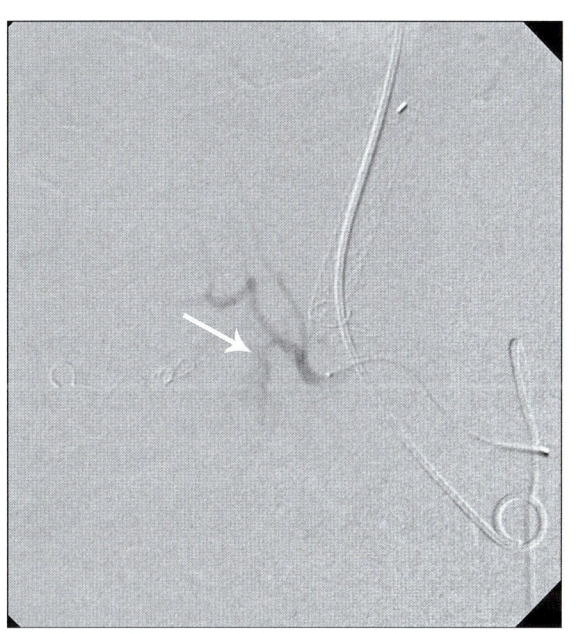

Figure 3. Selective catheterization of the right hepatic artery localizes the site of hemorrhage *(arrow)*.

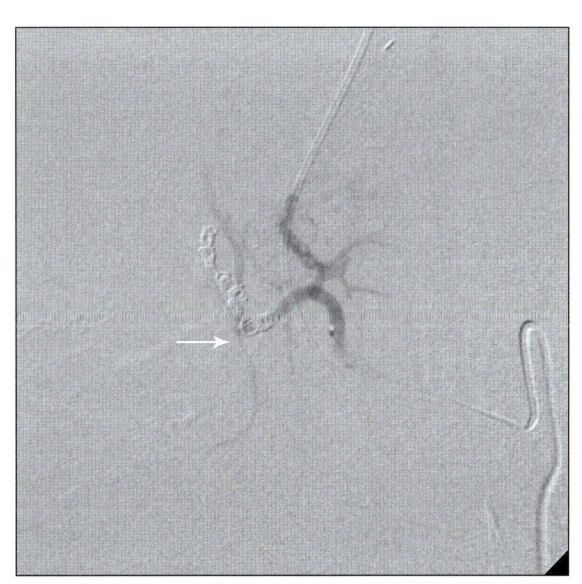

Figure 4. The branch of the right hepatic artery was embolized with coils from distal to proximal across the site of injury. Despite the placement of coils, there continues to be a small amount of extravasation *(arrow)*; Gelfoam was used to complete the embolization.

Case 199

DEMOGRAPHICS/CLINICAL HISTORY
An 82-year-old man, with history of hepatic cirrhosis and variceal bleeding, undergoing MRI.

DISCUSSION

History/Indications for Procedure
This patient had acute upper gastrointestinal bleeding secondary to gastric varices. Bleeding persisted despite endoscopic banding.

Procedure
Retrograde balloon occlusion variceal ablation

Pre-procedure Imaging
MRI shows a cirrhotic liver. A left gastric vein is identified, but no large gastric varicies are seen (Fig. 1).

Intraprocedural Findings
Retrograde balloon occlusion of the left adrenal vein shows filling of numerous prominent varices along the greater and the lesser curvatures of the stomach (Fig. 2). The varices were sclerosed with sodium tetradecyl sulfate opacified with ethiodized oil (Ethiodol) (Fig. 3).

Follow-up and Complications
The patient showed no further evidence of bleeding during his hospital stay. He was discharged home 3 days after the variceal ablation procedure.

Suggested Readings
Hirota S, Matsumoto S, Tomita M, et al: Retrograde transvenous obliteration of gastric varices. Radiology 211:349-356, 1999.

Kanagawa H, Mima S, Kouyama H, et al: Treatment of gastric fundal varices by balloon-occluded retrograde transvenous obliteration. J Gastroenterol Hepatol 11:51-58, 1996.

Kato T, Uematsu T, Nishigaki Y, et al: Therapeutic effect of balloon-occluded retrograde transvenous obliteration on portal-systemic encephalopathy in patients with liver cirrhosis. Intern Med 40: 688-691, 2001.

Takahashi K, Yamada T, Hyodoh H, et al: Selective balloon-occluded retrograde sclerosis of gastric varices using a coaxial microcatheter system. AJR Am J Roentgenol 117:1091-1093, 2001.

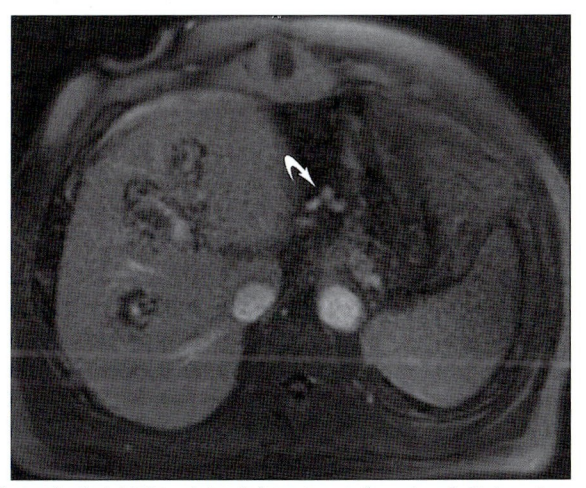

Figure 1. Axial T1-weighted fat-saturated post-gadolinium image shows a prominent left gastric vein *(curved arrow)*.

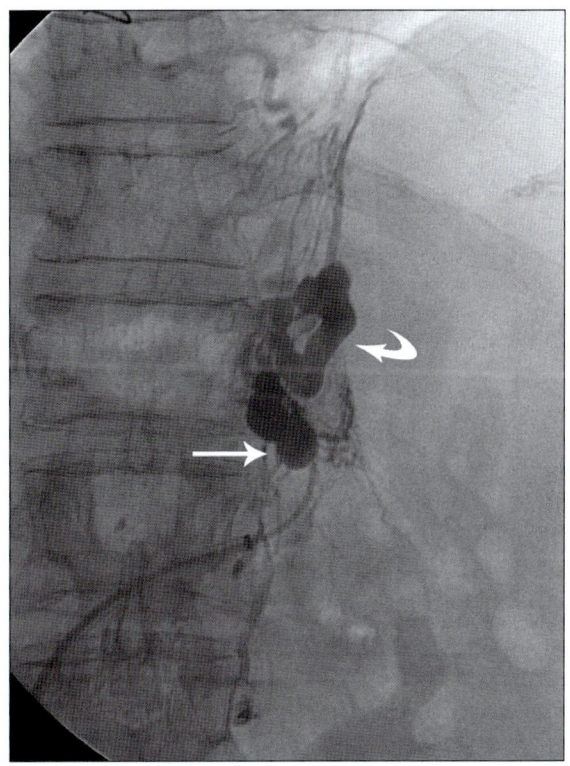

Figure 2. Contrast injection through occlusion balloon catheter *(straight arrow)* positioned in the left adrenal vein shows filling of a prominent gastric varix *(curved arrow)*.

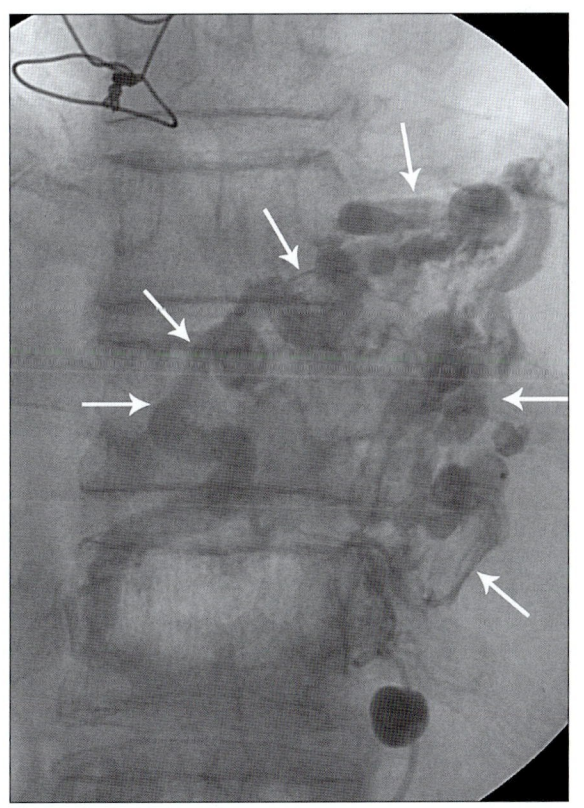

Figure 3. Image obtained after administration of sodium tetradecyl sulfate opacified with ethiodized oil (Ethiodol) shows filling of numerous large gastric varices *(arrows)*.

Case 200

DEMOGRAPHICS/CLINICAL HISTORY

A 51-year-old woman with end-stage liver disease secondary to primary sclerosing cholangitis presents with bleeding gastric varices.

DISCUSSION

History/Indications for Procedure
A 51-year-old woman with end-stage liver disease secondary to primary sclerosing cholangitis presents with bleeding gastric varices.

Procedure
Balloon-occluded retrograde transvenous obliteration of gastric varices

Pre-procedure Imaging
Contrast-enhanced MRI shows a small nodular liver with ascites, splenomegaly, and moderate-sized varices in the gastric fundus (Fig. 1).

Intraprocedural Findings
Retrograde balloon occlusion of the left inferior phrenic vein shows opacification of large gastric varices (Figs. 2 and 3). The varices were sclerosed with a total of 7 mL of 3% sodium tetradecyl sulphate opacified with a small amount of Ethiodol (Fig. 4).

Follow-up and Complications
The patient was discharged from the hospital the day after the procedure. She has had no further episodes of variceal hemorrhage and is currently being evaluated for liver transplant.

Suggested Readings
Fukuda T, Hirota S, Sugimura K: Long-term results of balloon-occluded retrograde transvenous obliteration for the treatment of gastric varices and hepatic encephalopathy. J Vasc Intervent Radiol 12:327-336, 2001.

Kiyosue H, Mori H, Matsumoto S, et al: Transcatheter obliteration of gastric varices: Part 2: Strategy and techniques based on hemodynamic features. Radiographics 23:921-937, 2003.

Ninoi T, Nishida N, Kaminou T, et al: Balloon-occluded retrograde transvenous obliteration of gastric varices with gastrorenal shunt: Long-term follow-up in 78 patients. AJR Am J Roentgenol 184:1340-1346, 2005.

Case 200   401

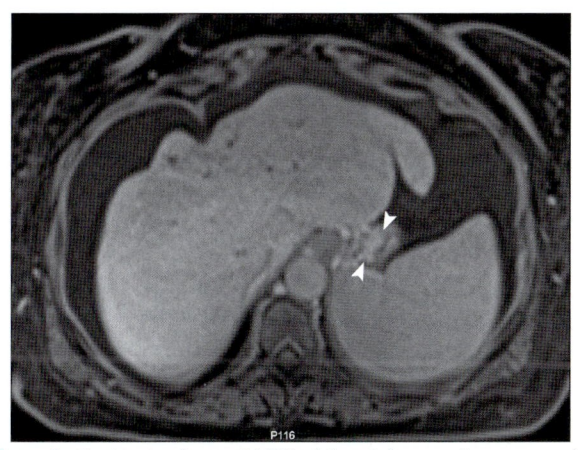

Figure 1. Contrast-enhanced MRI of the abdomen shows a small, cirrhotic-appearing liver. There is splenomegally and ascites. Multiple moderate-sized varices are seen in the gastric fundus *(arrowheads)*.

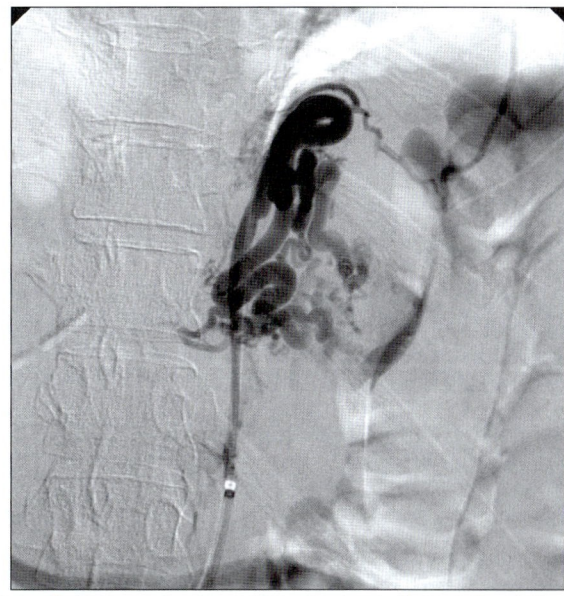

Figure 3. Repeat injection with occlusion balloon inflated shows filling of large gastric varices.

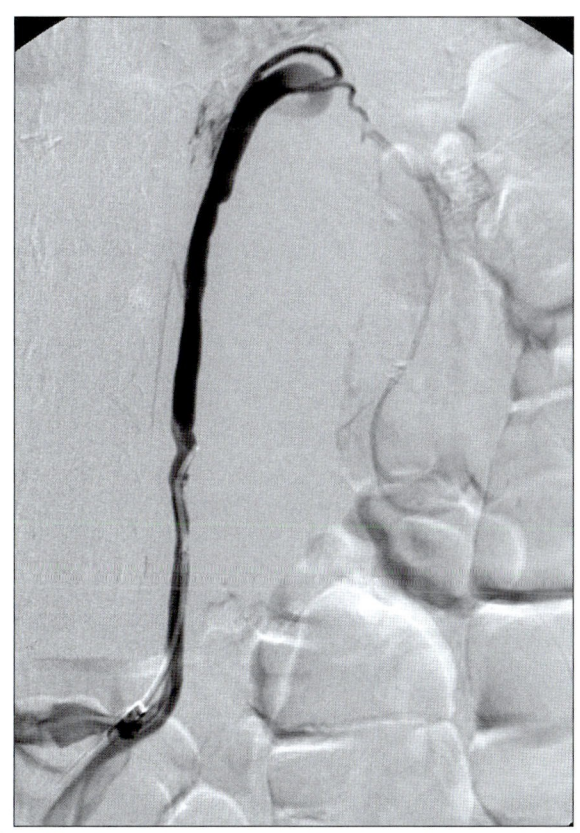

Figure 2. Selective injection of the left inferior phrenic vein shows the vein to be enlarged; no varices are identified.

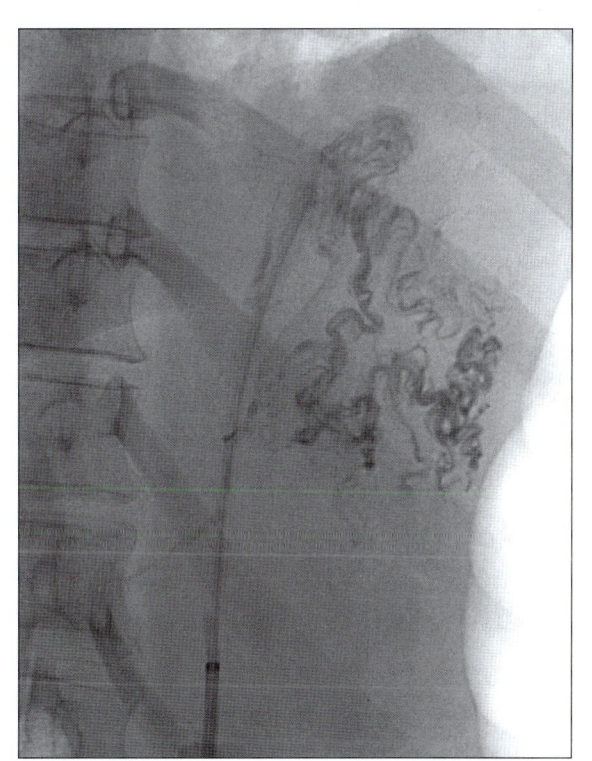

Figure 4. In a final image after sclerotherapy, the 3% sodium tetradecyl sulphate opacified with a small volume of Ethiodol is seen within the gastric varices.

Case 201

DEMOGRAPHICS/CLINICAL HISTORY

A 56-year-old man with prior colectomy and stomal varices.

DISCUSSION

History/Indications for Procedure
A 56-year-old man with prior colectomy secondary to ulcerative colitis. The patient has portal hypertension from primary sclerosing cholangitis and recurrent hemorrhage from stomal varices.

Procedure
Retrograde occlusion of stomal varices

Pre-procedure Imaging
MRI of the abdomen shows a cirrhotic liver with occlusion and cavernous transformation of the main portal vein (Fig. 1). Small varices are seen along the greater curvature of the stomach and adjacent to the ileostomy.

Intraprocedural Findings
A peristomal varix was accessed directly with ultrasound guidance, and venography shows filling of several large peristomal varices (Figs. 2 and 3). While compressing the ostomy to occlude the outflow veins, the peristomal varices were sclerosed with 3% Sotradecol opacified with a small volume of Ethiodol (Fig. 4).

Follow-up and Complications
The patient was observed overnight, and the stoma remained pink and showed no evidence of venous congestion. In the 4 months since the procedure, the patient has shown no further evidence of bleeding.

Suggested Readings
Minami S, Okada K, Matsuo M, et al: Treatment of bleeding stomal varices by balloon-occluded retrograde transvenous obliteration. J Gastroenterol 42:91-95, 2007.

Spier BJ, Fayyad AA, Lucey MR, et al: Bleeding stomal varices: Case series and systematic review of the literature. Clin Gastroenterol Hepatol 6:346-352, 2008.

Thouveny F, Aube C, Konate A, et al: Direct percutaneous approach for endoluminal glue embolization of stomal varices. J Vasc Intervent Radiol 19:774-777, 2008.

Case 201   403

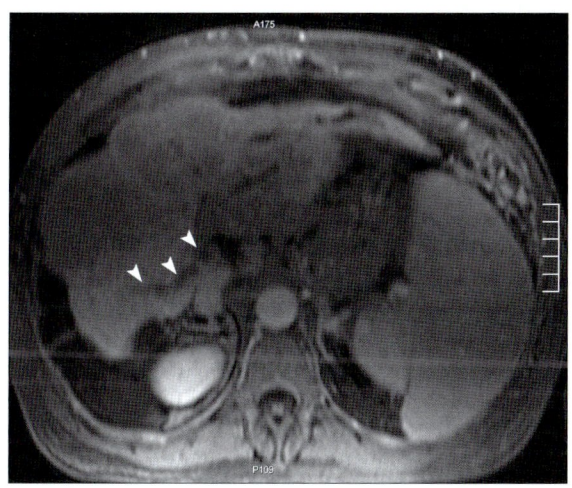

Figure 1. Contrast-enhanced MRI shows a nodular, fibrotic-appearing liver consistent with cirrhosis. There is chronic occlusion of the right and main portal vein *(arrowheads)*.

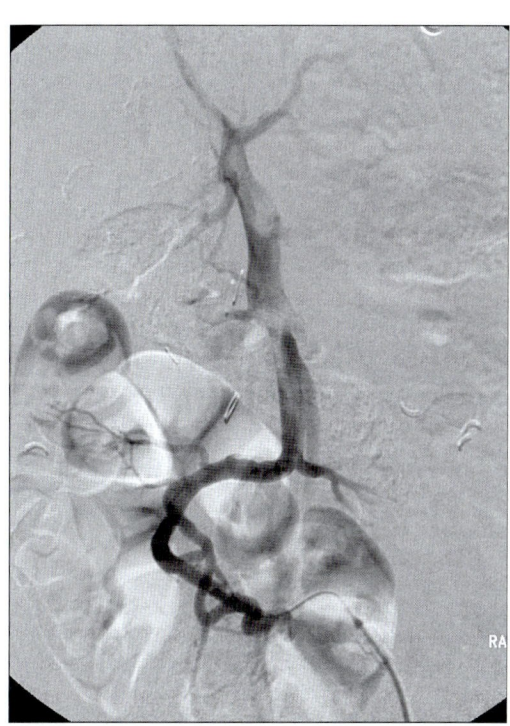

Figure 2. Stomal venogram. A peristomal varix has been directly punctured under ultrasound guidance. Venogram shows filling of prominent right lower quadrant varices and communication with the superior mesenteric vein.

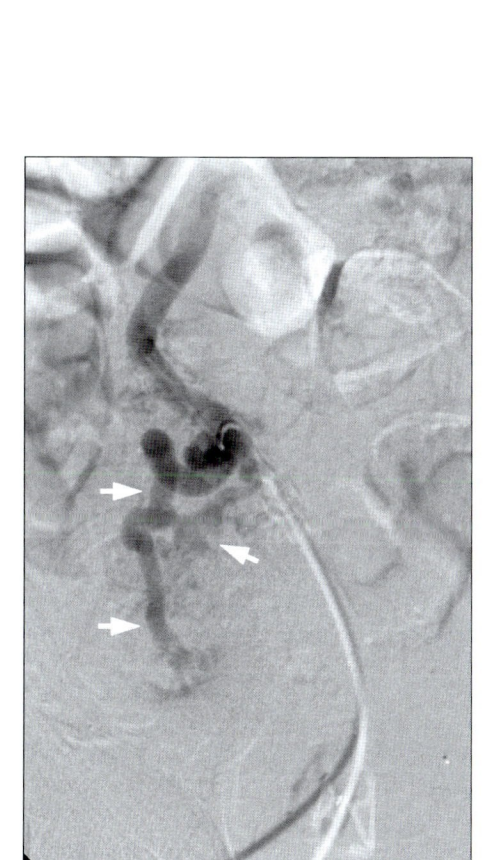

Figure 3. Selective injection of right lower quadrant varix shows communication with multiple prominent stomal varices *(arrows)*.

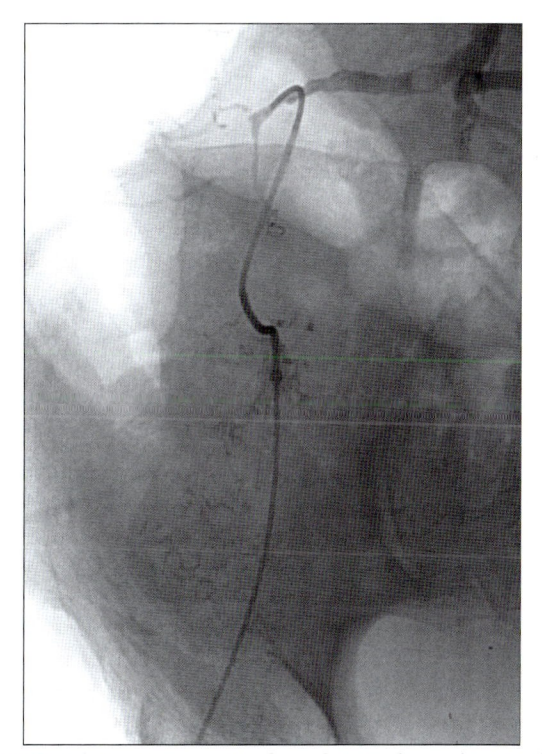

Figure 4. Follow-up venogram after sclerosis shows the opacified Sotradecol filling multiple small stomal varices.

Case 202

DEMOGRAPHICS/CLINICAL HISTORY

A 57-year-old woman with poorly controlled hypertension, undergoing computed tomography (CT), renal vein sampling, and laparoscopic nephrectomy.

DISCUSSION

History/Indications for Procedure
A 57-year-old woman has poorly controlled hypertension despite the use of four antihypertensive medications. The patient has undergone prior bilateral renal artery stenting, and the right renal artery stent has become occluded.

Procedure
Renal vein sampling

Pre-procedure Imaging
Contrast-enhanced CT demonstrates a small hypoenhancing right kidney (Fig. 1).

Intraprocedural Findings
Renal vein sampling was performed (Figs. 2 and 3). Renal vein renin levels from the right kidney were approximately six times higher than levels from the left renal vein and inferior vena cava.

Follow-up and Complications
The patient underwent laparoscopic right nephrectomy. After surgery, the patient's blood pressure was controlled with two antihypertensive medications.

Suggested Readings
Korobkin M, Glickman MG, Schambelan M: Segmental renal vein sampling for renin. Radiology 118:307-313, 1876.

Martin LG, Cork RD, Wells JO: Renal vein renin analysis: Limitations of its use in predicting benefit from percutaneous angioplasty. Cardiovasc Intervent Radiol 16:76-80, 1993.

Case 202   405

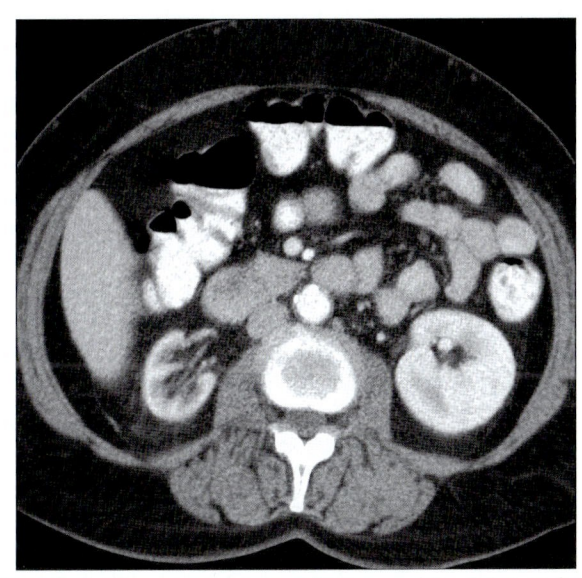

Figure 1. Axial, contrast-enhanced CT image of the abdomen demonstrates a small poorly enhancing right kidney.

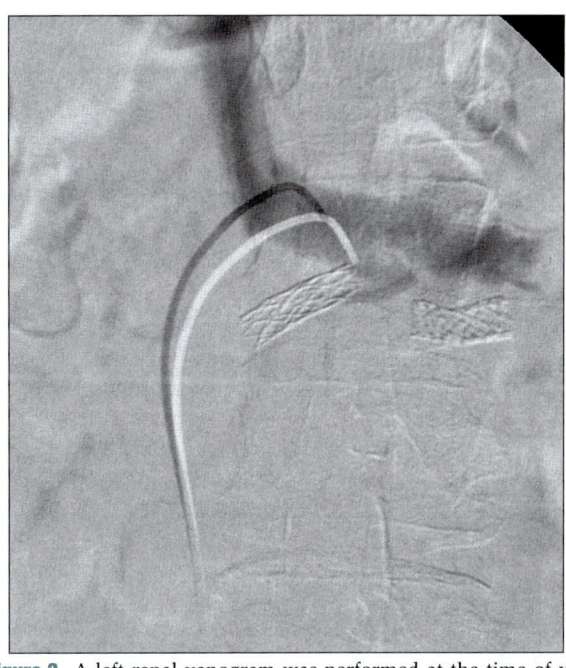

Figure 2. A left renal venogram was performed at the time of venous sampling.

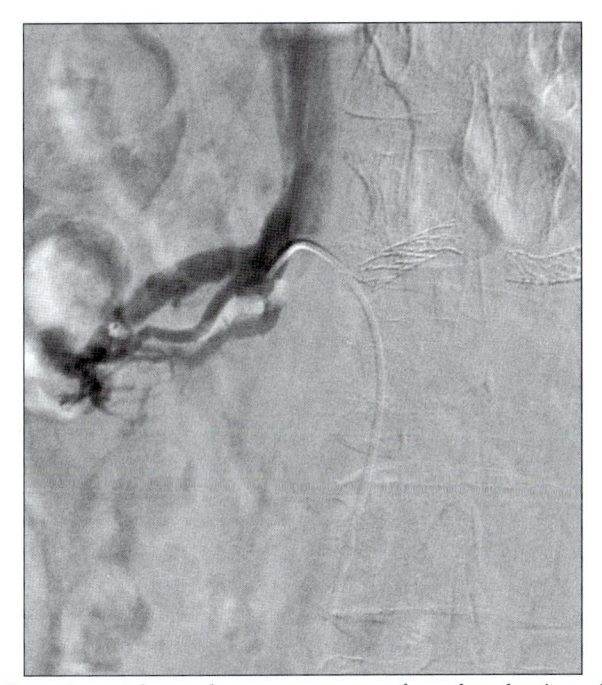

Figure 3. A right renal venogram was performed at the time of venous sampling.

Case 203

DEMOGRAPHICS/CLINICAL HISTORY

A 37-year-old woman with hypertension, undergoing magnetic resonance imaging (MRI), adrenal vein sampling, and laparoscopic adrenalectomy.

DISCUSSION

History/Indications for Procedure
A 37-year-old woman had poorly controlled hypertension and elevated serum aldosterone levels.

Procedure
Adrenal vein sampling

Pre-procedure Imaging
MRI of the abdomen demonstrates a 1-cm nodule in the right adrenal gland (Fig. 1). This nodule does drop in signal on out-of-phase imaging, which is consistent with a lipid-rich nodule.

Intraprocedural Findings
Bilateral adrenal vein sampling was performed for cortisol and aldosterone assays (Fig. 2). The aldosterone level of the right adrenal vein sample measured 2044 ng/dL (normal, 1 to 21 ng/dL) (Fig. 3).

Follow-up and Complications
The patient underwent laparoscopic right adrenalectomy with removal of a 1.5-cm adrenal adenoma. The patient's blood pressure continued to be labile after the surgery, although the patient could be managed with a single antihypertensive medication.

Suggested Readings
Stowasser M, Gordon RD, Gunasekera TG, et al: High rate of detection of primary aldosteronism, including surgically treatable forms, after 'non-selective' screening of hypertensive patients. J Hypertens 21:2149-2157, 2003.

Wheeler MH, Harris DA: Diagnosis and management of primary aldosteronism. World J Surg 27:627-631, 2003.

Young WF, Stanson AW, Thompson GB, et al: Role for adrenal venous sampling in primary aldosteronism. Surgery 136:1227-1235, 2004.

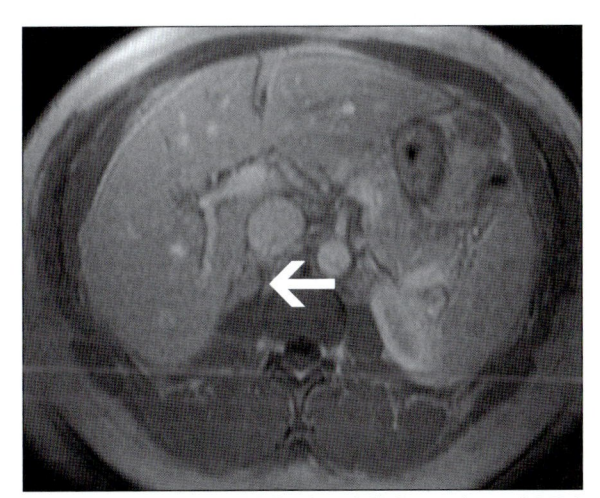

Figure 1. Axial view, T1-weighted, gadolinium-enhanced MR image of the abdomen demonstrates a 1-cm nodule in the right adrenal gland *(arrow)*.

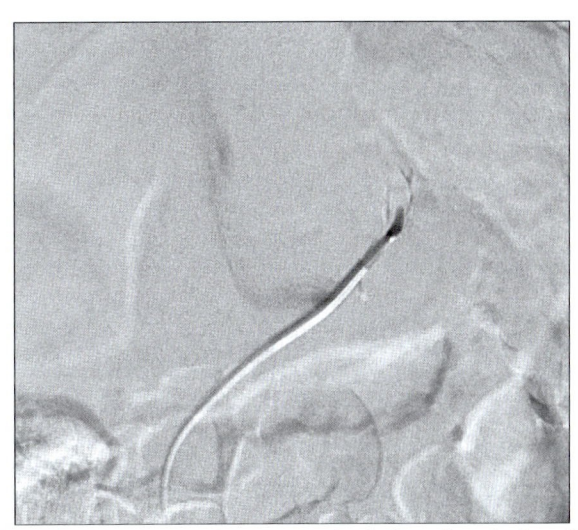

Figure 2. The left adrenal vein was selectively catheterized, and a sample was obtained through a coaxial microcatheter.

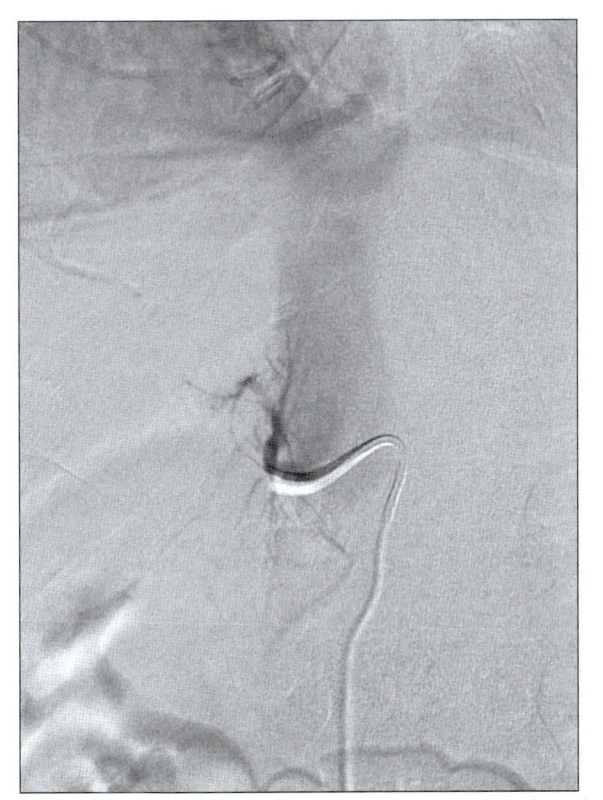

Figure 3. Right adrenal venogram was performed just before obtaining a sample. The aldosterone levels from this sample were significantly elevated, confirming that the adenoma was actively producing aldosterone.

Case 204

DEMOGRAPHICS/CLINICAL HISTORY

A 38-year-old man with hypertension and hyperkalemia.

DISCUSSION

History/Indications for Procedure
A 38-year-old man with hypertension and hypokalemia.

Procedure
Adrenal venous sampling

Intraprocedural Findings
A systemic blood sample was obtained, and a reverse-curve catheter was used to selectively catheterize the right renal vein (Figs. 1 and 2). A microcatheter was needed to catheterize the left adrenal vein (Fig. 3), and samples were obtained bilaterally.

Follow-up and Complications
The aldosterone level from the left adrenal vein measured 280 ng/dL (normal ≤ 21 ng/dL), a finding consistent with a hyperfunctioning adrenal adenoma.

Suggested Readings
Daunt N: Adrenal vein sampling: How to make it quick, easy, and successful. Radiographics 25 Suppl 1:S143-S158, 2005.

Minami I, Yoshimoto T, Hirono Y, et al: Diagnostic accuracy of adrenal venous sampling in comparison with other parameters in primary aldosteronism. Endocr J 55:839-846, 2008.

Rossi GP, Seccia TM, Pessina AC: Primary aldosteronism—part I: Prevalence, screening, and selection of cases for adrenal vein sampling. J Nephrol 21:447-454, 2008.

Case 204   409

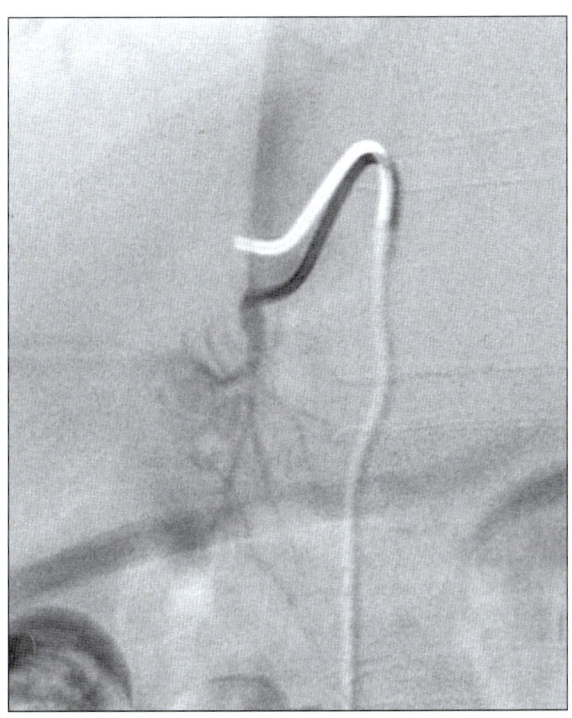

Figure 1. Normal right adrenal venogram.

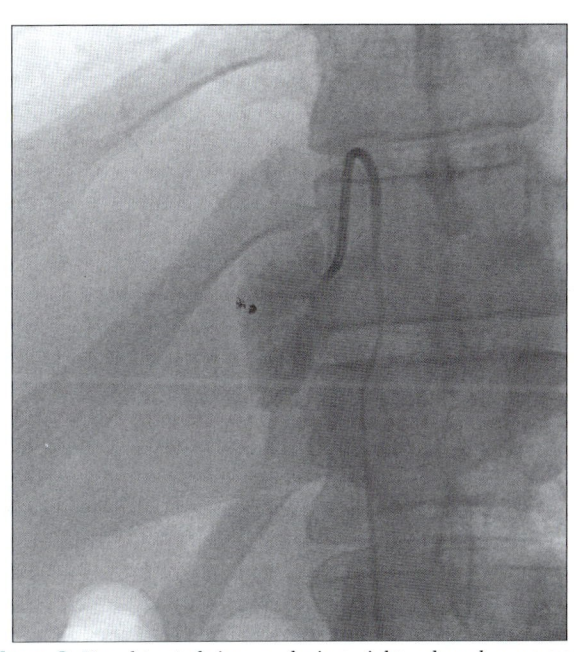

Figure 2. Unsubtracted image during right adrenal venogram showing normal parenchymal blush.

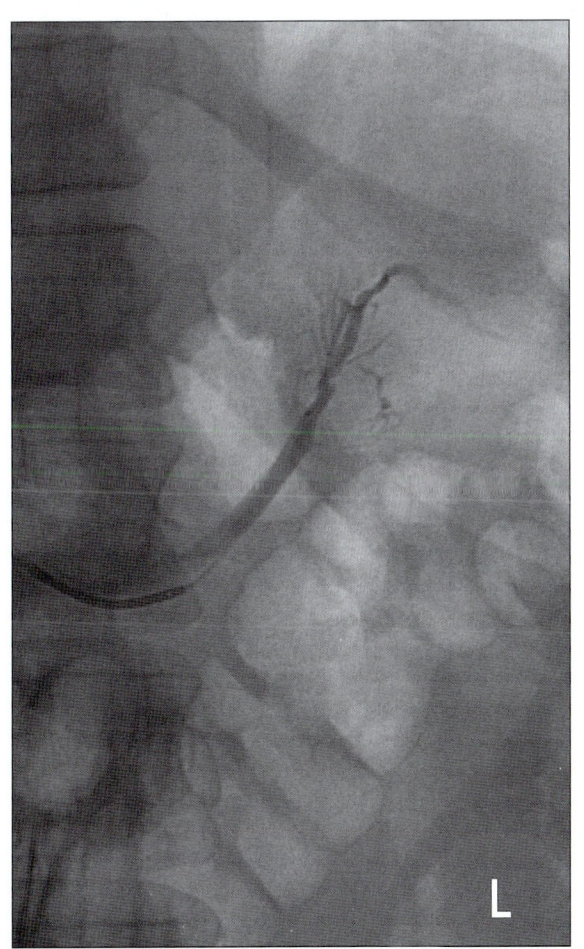

Figure 3. Normal left adrenal venogram. The left adrenal vein has been accessed using a coaxial 3-French microcatheter.

Case 205

DEMOGRAPHICS/CLINICAL HISTORY

A 50-year-old woman with hypercalcemia and hyperparathyroidism.

DISCUSSION

History/Indications for Procedure
A 50-year-old woman with hypercalcemia and hyperparathyroidism.

Procedure
Parathyroid venous sampling

Pre-procedure Imaging
Nuclear medicine parathyroid scan with Sestamibi was normal. No abnormal masses were identified on contrast-enhanced CT of the neck and chest.

Intraprocedural Findings
Parathyroid venous sampling was performed with samples obtained from multiple veins within both sides of the neck (Figs. 1, 2, 3, and 4). Samples were sent for PTH levels, with levels ranging from 85 to 215 pg/mL; a sample obtained from a small left mid thyroidal vein measured >5000 pg/mL.

Follow-up and Complications
Based on the results of the venous sampling, the patient underwent exploration of the left neck. A left superior parathyroid adenoma was identified and resected; the patient's systemic calcium levels returned to normal.

Suggested Readings
Jones JJ, Brunaud L, Dowd CF, et al: Accuracy of selective venous sampling for intact parathyroid hormone in difficult patients with recurrent or persistent hyperparathyroidism. Surgery 132:944-950, 2002.

Reidel MA, Schilling T, Graf S, et al: Localization of hyperfunctioning parathyroid glands by selective venous sampling in reoperation for primary or secondary hyperparathyroidism. Surgery 140:907-913, 2006.

Seehofer D, Steinmuller T, Rayes N, et al: Parathyroid hormone venous sampling before reoperative surgery in renal hyperparathyroidism: Comparison with noninvasive localization procedures and review of the literature. Arch Surg 139:1331-1338, 2004.

Case 205   411

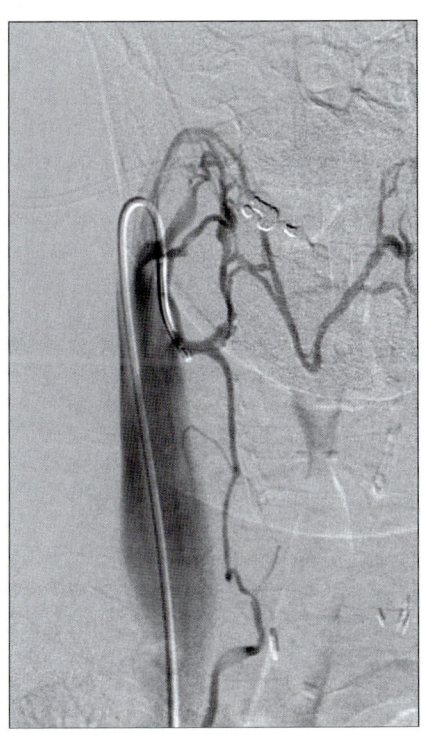

Figure 1. Selective injection of the right middle thyroidal vein. There is also opacification of the right superior thyroidal vein and right inferior thyroidal vein.

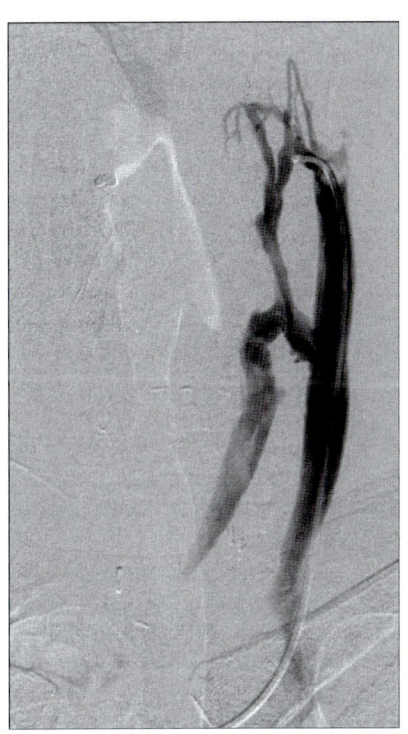

Figure 2. Selective injection of the left superior thyroidal vein. There is filling of an enlarged collateral vein that emptied into the right brachiocephalic vein.

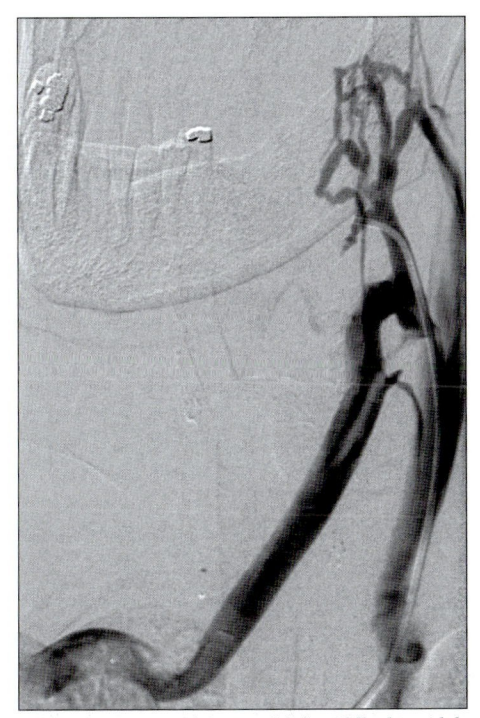

Figure 3. Selective injection of the small left middle thyroidal vein. The sample obtained from this location measured over 5000 pg/mL PTH.

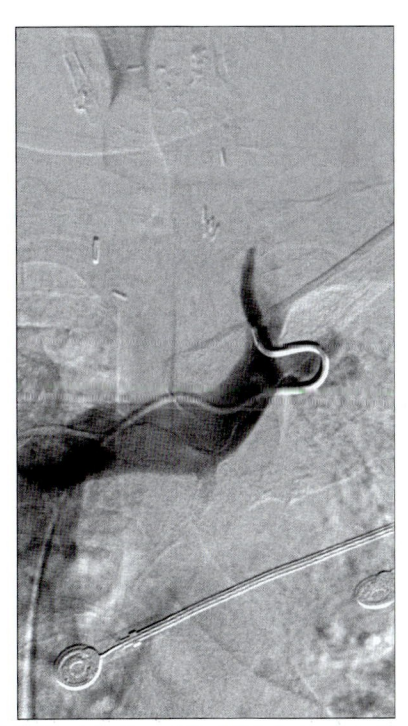

Figure 4. Selective injection of the left inferior thyroidal vein.

Case 206

DEMOGRAPHICS/CLINICAL HISTORY

A 68-year-old woman with persistently elevated parathyroid hormone levels after parathyroidectomy, undergoing venous sampling and parathyroidectomy.

DISCUSSION

History/Indications for Procedure
A 68-year-old woman with persistently elevated parathyroid hormone levels after parathyroidectomy. The patient's calcium levels normalized after the surgery but then became elevated.

Procedure
Parathyroid venous sampling

Intraprocedural Findings
Venous samples were obtained from many locations, including the superior, middle, and inferior thyroidal veins bilaterally (Figs. 1 and 2). Parathyroid hormone levels from the right middle thyroidal vein measured more than 5000 pg/mL (normal, 12 to 72 pg/mL).

Follow-up and Complications
Based on the findings of the venous sampling, the patient underwent a right superior parathyroidectomy. A parathyroid adenoma was discovered during pathologic examination.

Suggested Readings
Seehofer D, Steinmüller T, Rayes N, et al: Parathyroid hormone venous sampling before reoperative surgery in renal hyperparathyroidism: Comparison with noninvasive localization procedures and review of the literature. Arch Surg 139:1331-1338, 2004.

Case 206   413

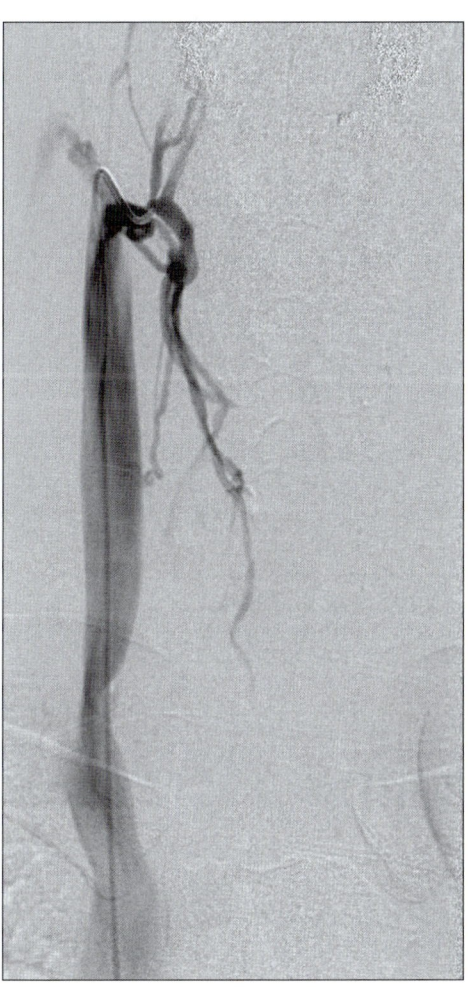

Figure 1. Single image from injection of the right superior thyroidal vein.

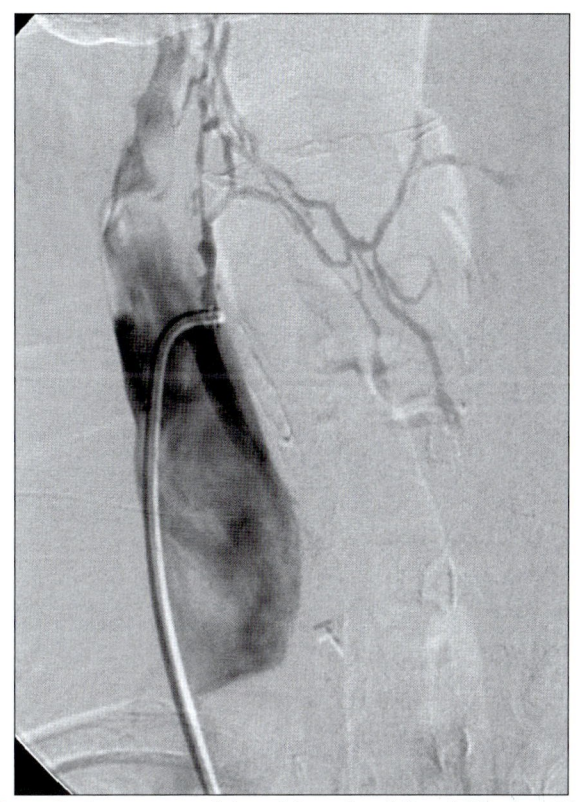

Figure 2. Contrast was injected into the right middle thyroidal vein. Samples from this vein were found have significantly elevated levels of parathyroid hormone.

Case 207

DEMOGRAPHICS/CLINICAL HISTORY

A 57-year-old man with end-stage renal disease and decreasing flows through his left upper arm dialysis graft, undergoing angioplasty.

DISCUSSION

A 57-year-old man has end-stage renal disease. He had a left upper extremity arc graft placed approximately 1 year before presentation.

Procedure
Hemodialysis graft management

Intraprocedural Findings
Graft study demonstrated a stenosis of the brachial vein just beyond the venous anastomosis (Fig. 1), and it was dilated using a 7-mm-diameter angioplasty balloon (Fig. 2). Flow rates increased from 590 mL/min before intervention to 1030 mL/min after intervention (Figs. 3 and 4).

Follow-up and Complications
The patient has been able to undergo dialysis through the graft successfully since the angioplasty, and no further intervention has been required.

Suggested Readings
Funaki B, Kim R, Lorenz J, et al: Using pullback pressure measurements to identify venous stenoses persisting after successful angioplasty in failing hemodialysis grafts. AJR Am J Roentgenol 178:1161-1165, 2002.

Gray RJ: Angioplasty and stents for peripheral and central venous lesions. Tech Vasc Intervent Radiol 2:189-198, 1999.

Murray BM, Herman A, Mepani B, Rajczak S: Access flow after angioplasty predicts subsequent arteriovenous graft survival. J Vasc Intervent Radiol 17:303-308, 2006.

Trerotola SO, Kwak A, Clark TWI, et al: Prospective study of balloon inflation pressures and other technical aspects of hemodialysis access angioplasty. J Vasc Intervent Radiol 16:1613-1618, 2005.

Case 207   415

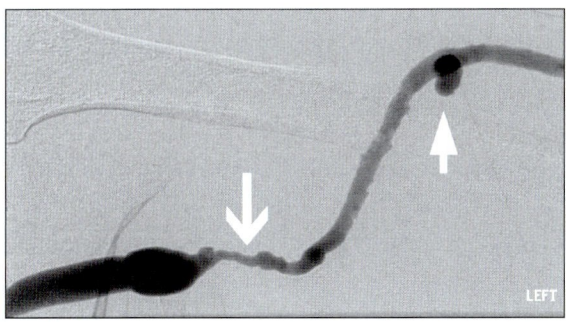

Figure 1. There is a 2.5- to 3-cm-long stenosis of the brachial vein just beyond the venous anastomosis *(arrow)*. Filling of a small pseudoaneurysm *(short arrow)* is indicated.

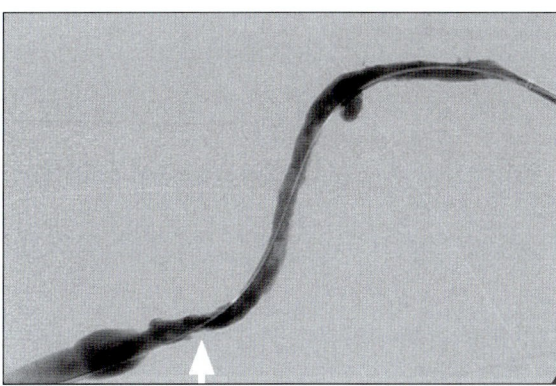

Figure 3. Follow-up contrast injection demonstrates significantly improved venographic appearance of the stenosis. Only a mild irregularity persists *(arrow)*.

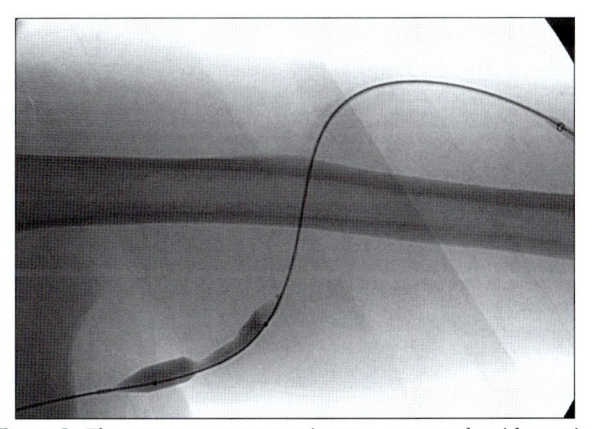

Figure 2. The venous anastomosis was corrected with angioplasty using a 7-mm balloon until the waist of the balloon fully resolved.

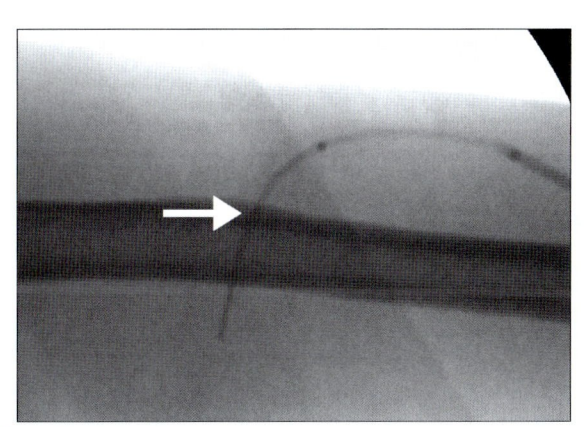

Figure 4. After angioplasty, a functional assessment of the intervention *(arrow)* was performed using the Angioflow catheter (Angiodynamics, Queensbury, NY). This study confirmed appropriate physiologic and anatomic responses to the intervention.

Case 208

DEMOGRAPHICS/CLINICAL HISTORY

A 58-year-old woman with end-stage renal disease secondary to diabetes and chronic hypertension presents with decreased flows in the right upper extremity dialysis graft.

DISCUSSION

History/Indications for Procedure

A 58-year-old woman with end-stage renal disease secondary to diabetes and chronic hypertension. The patient has had multiple failed surgical accesses; currently, she dialyzes through a right upper extremity arc graft placed 1 year earlier.

Procedure

Management of recurrent dialysis graft stenosis

Pre-procedure Imaging

Dialysis graft study performed 4 months earlier shows a focal, high-grade stenosis at the venous anastomosis (Fig. 1). This was successfully dilated with a 7-mm balloon (Fig. 2).

Intraprocedural Findings

Dialysis graft study shows recurrent stenosis at the venous anastamosis. There was significant elastic recoil following balloon angioplasty (Fig. 3), so an 8-mm x 6-cm self-expanding nitinol stent was placed (Fig. 4).

Suggested Readings

Gallego Beuter JJ, Hernandez Lezana A, Herrero Calvo J, et al: Early detection and treatment of hemodialysis access dysfunction. Cardiovasc Intervent Radiol 23:40-46, 2000.

Vesely TM, Amin MZ, Pilgram T: Use of stents and stent grafts to salvage angioplasty failures in patients with hemodialysis grafts. Semin Dial 21:100-104, 2008.

Vogel PM, Parise C: Comparison of SMART stent placement for arteriovenous graft salvage versus successful graft PTA. J Vasc Intervent Radiol 16:1619-1626, 2005.

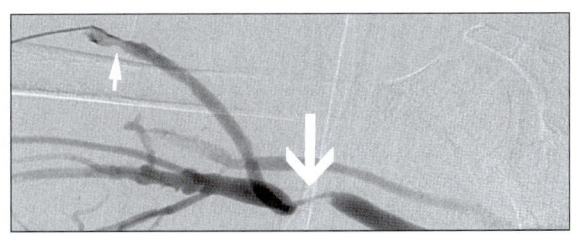

Figure 1. There is a high-grade stenosis of the brachial vein at the venous anastamosis *(arrow)*. In addition, there is a focal intragraft stenosis *(short arrow)*.

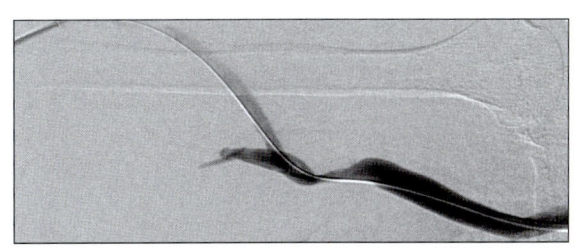

Figure 3. The patient returned 4 months later with recurrent stenosis at the venous anastamosis. Following balloon angioplasty, there is persistent narrowing of the brachial vein.

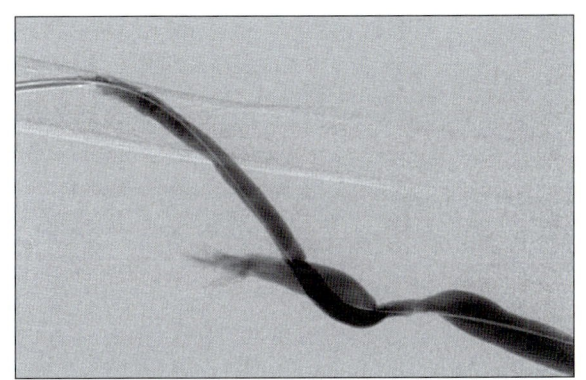

Figure 2. Both lesions were successfully treated with balloon angioplasty. There is mild residual stenosis of the brachial vein at the venous anastamosis.

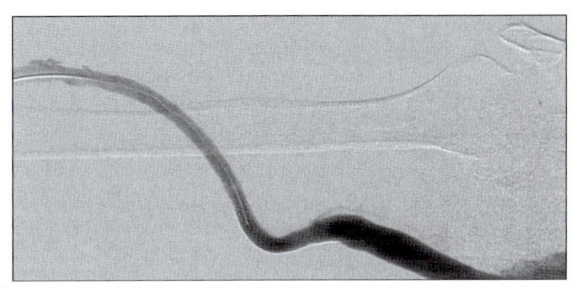

Figure 4. Final shunt study following stent placement shows no residual stenosis following the placement of a self-expanding stent.

Case 209

DEMOGRAPHICS/CLINICAL HISTORY

A 54-year-old man with decreased clearance during dialysis.

DISCUSSION

History/Indications for Procedure
A 54-year-old man with end-stage renal disease secondary to hypertension and diabetes. He has been dialyzed through a left upper-extremity arc graft for the past 8 months; he is now referred for graft evaluation because of decreasing clearance during dialysis.

Procedure
Dialysis graft maintenance

Intraprocedural Findings
There is a high-grade stenosis of the outflow vein that was successfully treated with balloon angioplasty (Figs. 1, 2, and 3). Also identified were two pseudoaneurysms arising from the arterial limb of the graft; these were treated with percutaneous injection of thrombin under direct ultrasound observation until pseudoaneurysm thrombosis.

Follow-up and Complications
The patient was able to undergo successful dialysis following the procedure.

Suggested Readings
Kang SS, Labropoulos N, Mansour MA, et al: Expanded indications for ultrasound-guided thrombin injection of pseudoaneurysms. J Vasc Surg 31:289-298, 2000.

Keeling AN, Naughton PA, McGrath FP, et al: Successful endovascular treatment of a hemodialysis graft pseudoaneurysm by covered stent and direct percutaneous thrombin injection. Semin Dialysis : [e-pub ahead of print].

Trerotola SO, Kwak A, Clark TWI, et al: Prospective study of balloon inflation pressures and other technical aspects of hemodialysis access angioplasty. J Vasc Intervent Radiol 16:1613-1618, 2005.

Turmel-Rodrigues L, Pengloan J, Bourquelot P: Interventional radiology in hemodialysis fistulae and grafts: A multidisciplinary approach. Cardiovasc Intervent Radiol 25:3-16, 2002.

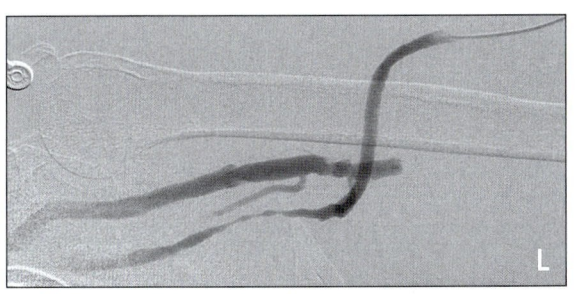

Figure 1. Contrast injection into the left upper extremity arc graft shows a stenosis of the outflow vein, just beyond the venous anastamosis.

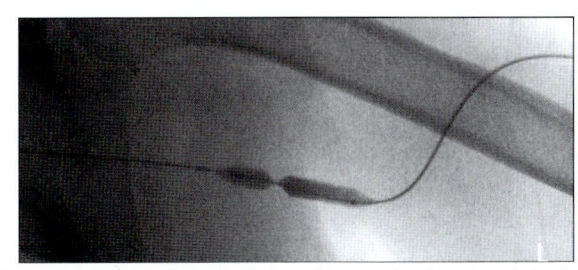

Figure 2. Initial balloon inflation shows a focal waist of the balloon. This opened on repeat balloon inflation.

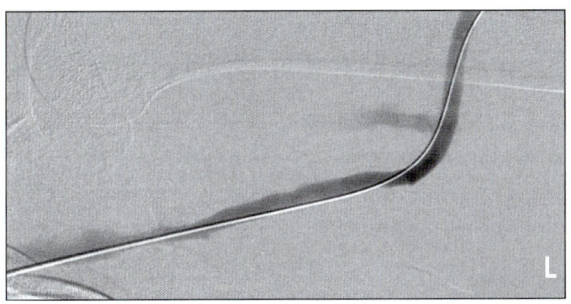

Figure 3. Follow-up venogram shows no residual stenosis after angioplasty.

Case 210

DEMOGRAPHICS/CLINICAL HISTORY

A 32-year-old man with end-stage renal disease, undergoing angioplasty and embolization.

DISCUSSION

History/Indications for Procedure
A 32-year-old man has a nonmaturing, right radiocephalic dialysis fistula.

Procedure
Nonmaturing fistula

Intraprocedural Findings
There is a 70% stenosis of the cephalic vein adjacent to the arteriovenous anastomosis and a large, competitive collateral vein (Fig. 1). The stenosis was treated with angioplasty using a 4-mm balloon (Fig. 2), and the large collateral vein was embolized with coils (Fig. 3).

Follow-up and Complications
The fistula matured and became usable for dialysis. However, the patient has returned several times for repeat balloon dilatation of the cephalic vein stenosis near the arteriovenous anastomosis (Fig. 4).

Suggested Readings
Kian K, Vassalotti JA: The new arteriovenous fistula: The need for earlier evaluation and intervention. Semin Dialysis 18:3-7, 2005.

Nassar GM, Nguyen B, Rhee E, Achkar K: Endovascular treatment of the failing-to-mature arteriovenous fistula. Clin J Am Soc Nephrol 1:275-280, 2006.

Shin SW, Do YS, Choo SW, et al: Salvage of immature arteriovenous fistulas with percutaneous transluminal angioplasty. Cardiovasc Intervent Radiol 28:434-438, 2005.

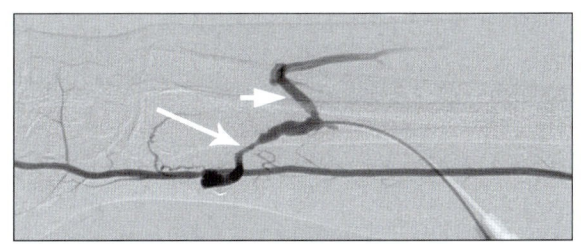

Figure 1. The fistula study demonstrates a stenosis of the cephalic vein just distal to the arteriovenous anastomosis *(long arrow)*. There also is a large, competitive collateral vein *(short arrow)*.

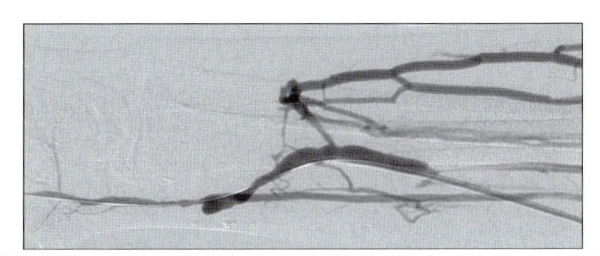

Figure 2. The stenosis was opened with angioplasty to 4 mm, with a good angiographic result.

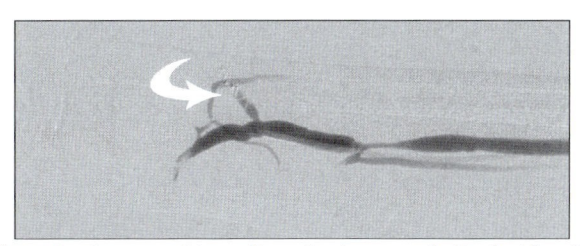

Figure 3. The competitive collateral vein was embolized with coils *(arrow)*.

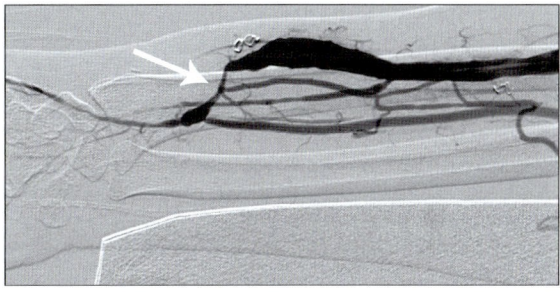

Figure 4. A follow-up fistula study 1 year later shows the cephalic vein has matured. There is recurrent stenosis of the cephalic vein *(arrow)* that was treated with repeat angioplasty.

Case 211

DEMOGRAPHICS/CLINICAL HISTORY

A 60-year-old woman with end-stage renal disease and reduced clearance from the left upper extremity dialysis fistula, undergoing balloon angioplasty, stent placement, and venography.

DISCUSSION

History/Indications for Procedure

A 60-year-old woman with end-stage renal disease dialyzes through a left brachiocephalic fistula placed approximately 18 months earlier. Recently, there has been reduced clearance through the fistula during dialysis.

Procedure

Cephalic vein stent placement for hemodialysis fistula maintenance

Intraprocedural Findings

The arteriovenous anastomosis is patent; there is a more than 90% stenosis of the arch of the cephalic vein (Figs. 1 and 2). The cephalic vein stenosis was treated with balloon angioplasty complicated by rupture (Fig. 3).

Follow-up and Complications

An 8-mm × 4-cm, self-expanding nitinol stent was placed across the stenosis (Fig. 4). There was no further contrast extravasation, and the patient was able to undergo successful hemodialysis through the fistula.

Suggested Readings

Clark TW, Hirsch DA, Jindal KJ, et al: Outcome and prognostic factors of restenosis after percutaneous treatment of native hemodialysis fistulas. J Vasc Intervent Radiol 13:51-59, 2002.

Jaberi A, Schwartz D, Marticorena R, et al: Risk factors for the development of cephalic arch stenosis. J Vasc Access 8:287-295, 2007.

Rajan DK, Clark TW, Patel NK, et al: Prevalence and treatment of cephalic arch stenosis in dysfunctional autogenous hemodialysis fistulas. J Vasc Intervent Radiol 14:567-573, 2003.

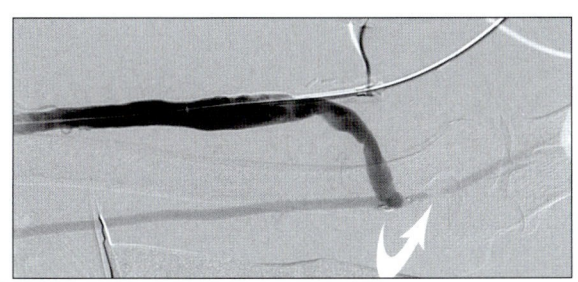

Figure 1. In a dialysis fistula study, the cephalic vein was accessed in an antegrade direction, and contrast was refluxed back across the arteriovenous anastomosis. The anastomosis is patent, but there is a focal, near-occlusive stenosis of the brachial artery that is just distal to the anastomosis *(curved arrow)*.

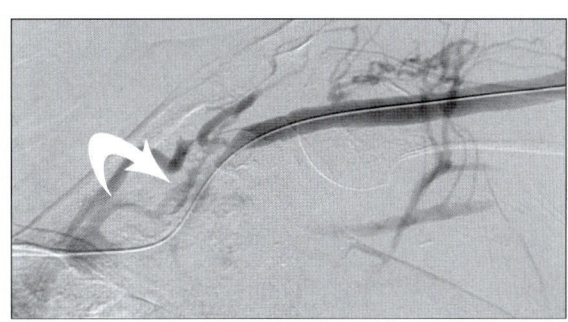

Figure 3. After angioplasty with a 7-mm balloon, extravasation indicates venous rupture *(curved arrow)*. This was initially treated with prolonged balloon inflation.

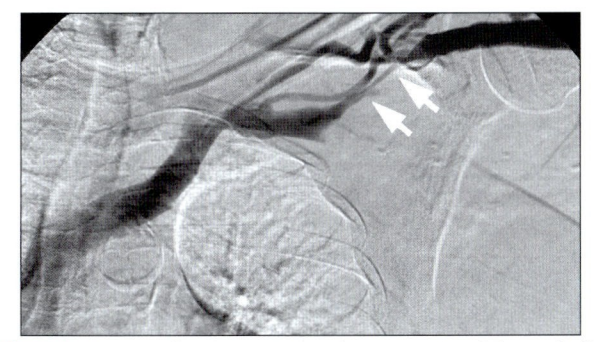

Figure 2. Venography shows a 3-cm-long stenosis of the cephalic arch *(arrows)*.

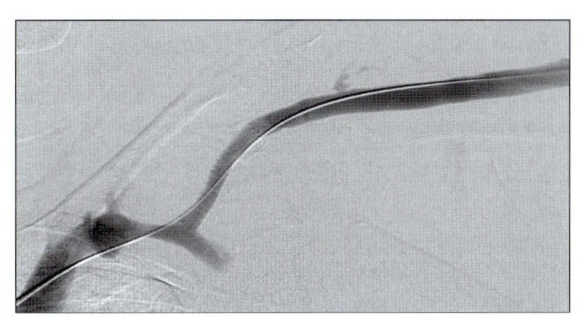

Figure 4. Because there was persistent luminal narrowing after balloon angioplasty, the cephalic arch was stented with a self-expanding nitinol stent. After stent placement, no residual stenosis is observed on venography, and there was no further extravasation.

Case 212

DEMOGRAPHICS/CLINICAL HISTORY

A 53-year-old woman with end-stage renal disease and a thrombosed transposed basilic vein dialysis fistula, undergoing declotting using tissue plasminogen activator (tPA), thrombectomy, and angioplasty and stent placement.

DISCUSSION

History/Indications for Procedure
A 53-year-old woman has end-stage renal disease and is on hemodialysis. The patient has been dialyzed the previous 2 years through a right upper extremity transposed basilic vein fistula that is now thrombosed.

Procedure
Clotted hemodialysis fistula

Intraprocedural Findings
The transposed basilic vein was declotted using a combination of tPA, rheolytic thrombectomy, and balloon angioplasty and maceration. A venous outflow stenosis was identified (Fig. 1) and treated with angioplasty; a self-expanding stent was placed because of significant elastic recoil (Fig. 2).

Follow-up and Complications
The patient has been able to undergo dialysis successfully for the past 1 year since the declotting procedure (Fig. 3), and she has required no further intervention for her dialysis fistula.

Suggested Readings

Haage P, Vorwerk D, Wildberger JE, et al: Percutaneous treatment of thrombosed primary arteriovenous hemodialysis access fistulae. Kidney Int 57:1169-1175, 2000.

Poulain F, Raynaud A, Bourquelot P, et al: Local thrombolysis and thromboaspiration in the treatment of acutely thrombosed arteriovenous hemodialysis fistulas. Cardiovasc Intervent Radiol 14:98-101, 1991.

Rajan DK, Clark TW, Simons ME, et al: Procedural success and patency after percutaneous treatment of thrombosed autogenous arteriovenous dialysis fistulas. J Vasc Intervent Radiol 13:1211-1218, 2002.

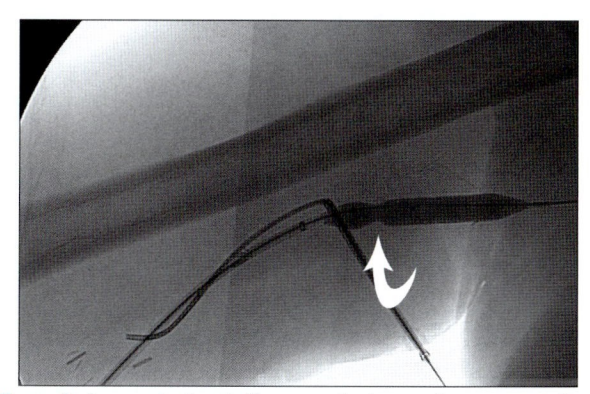

Figure 1. Image during balloon angioplasty of venous outflow stenosis demonstrates a focal waist in the angioplasty balloon *(arrow)*.

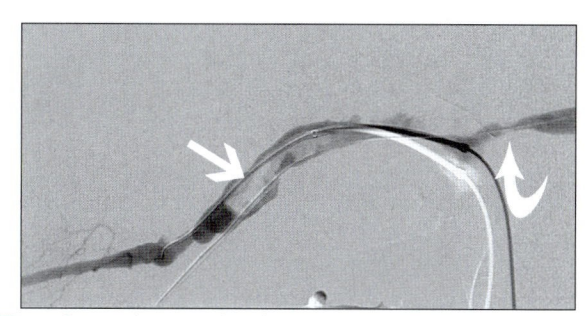

Figure 2. Fistulogram after flow was restored demonstrates the continued presence of acute thrombus with the basilic vein *(arrow)*. There is elastic recoil of the outflow vein stenosis *(curved arrow)*.

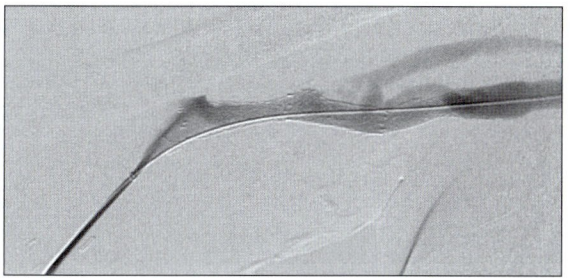

Figure 3. The outflow vein was stented with two 10-mm × 6-cm, self-expanding nitinol stents, resulting in marked improvement in outflow. At this point, a palpable thrill returned to the fistula.

Case 213

DEMOGRAPHICS/CLINICAL HISTORY

An 86-year-old man with a thrombosed left upper extremity brachiocephalic dialysis fistula, undergoing fistulography.

DISCUSSION

History/Indications for Procedure
An 86-year-old man presents with a thrombosed left upper extremity brachiocephalic dialysis fistula.

Procedure
Dialysis fistula declot

Pre-procedure Imaging
A diagnostic fistulogram shows a moderate stenosis of the cephalic vein adjacent to the arteriovenous anastomosis; a long segment of cephalic vein in the upper arm is thrombosed (Fig. 1).

Intraprocedural Findings
Mechanical thrombectomy was performed with the AngioJet thrombectomy catheter (Possis, Minneapolis, MN), uncovering a high-grade stenosis at the cephalic arch (Fig. 2). The cephalic arch stenosis was dilated with a 10-mm angioplasty balloon, and the stenosis at the arteriovenous anastomosis was dilated with a 6-mm angioplasty balloon.

Follow-up and Complications
After balloon angioplasty and additional mechanical thrombectomy, flow was restored in the fistula with minimal residual thrombus (Figs. 3 and 4); a thrill was palpable. The patient was able to go on to successful dialysis after the procedure.

Suggested Readings
Clark TW, Hirsch DA, Jindal KJ, et al: Outcome and prognostic factors of restenosis after percutaneous treatment of native hemodialysis fistulas. J Vasc Intervent Radiol 13:51, 2002.

Rajan DK, Clark TW, Simons ME, et al: Procedural success and patency after percutaneous treatment of thrombosed autogenous arteriovenous dialysis fistulas. J Vasc Intervent Radiol 13:1211, 2002.

Turmel-Rodrigues L: Application of percutaneous mechanical thrombectomy in autogenous fistulae. Tech Vasc Intervent Radiol 6:42, 2003.

Case 213   427

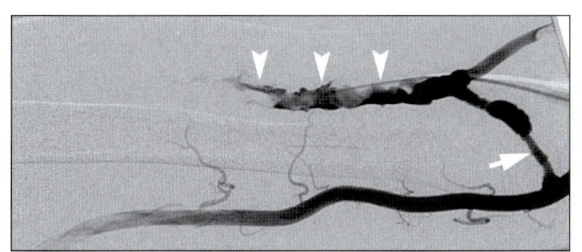

Figure 1. Cephalic vein has been accessed with 5-French micropuncture catheter (Cook, Bloomington, IN), and contrast injection shows acute thrombus in cephalic vein *(arrowheads)*. Contrast material refluxes across arteriovenous anastomosis revealing perianastomotic stricture of cephalic vein *(arrow)*.

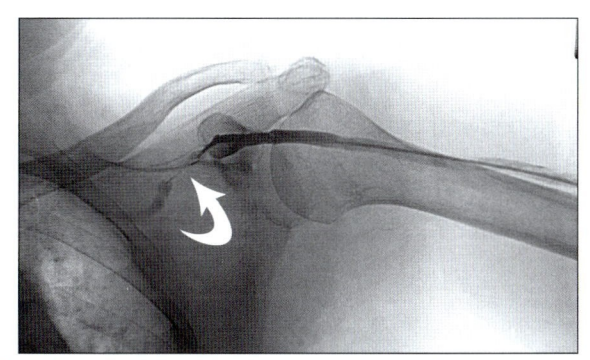

Figure 2. Follow-up contrast injection after mechanical thrombectomy shows focal, high-grade stenosis at cephalic arch *(arrow)*.

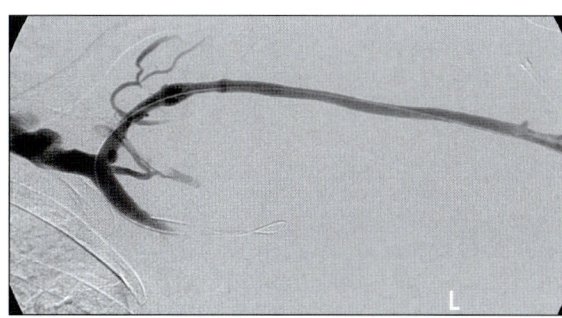

Figure 3. There is mild residual narrowing after balloon angioplasty, and flow through the fistula is brisk.

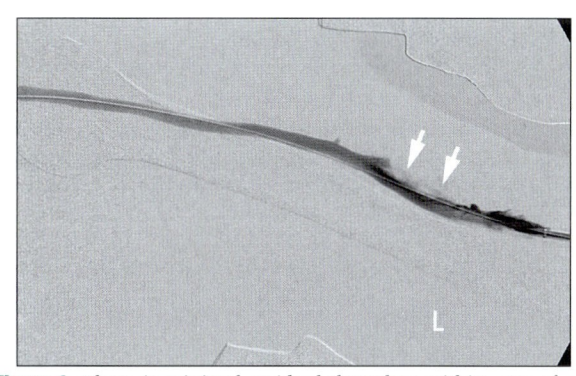

Figure 4. There is minimal residual thrombus within area of venous dilatation *(arrows)*. Despite multiple passes with the mechanical thrombectomy catheter, this thrombus could not be removed.

Case 214

DEMOGRAPHICS/CLINICAL HISTORY

A 75-year-old woman on hemodiaysis with enlarging dialysis graft pseudoaneurysms.

History/Indications for Procedure
A 75-year-old woman with end-stage renal disease, secondary to diabetes and hypertension, on hemodialysis. The patient has received dialysis through a left upper extremity forearm loop graft for the past 7 years and now has enlarging pseudoaneurysms within the graft.

Procedure
Management of dialysis graft pseudoaneurysms

Intraprocedural Findings
There is a large pseudoaneurysm of the venous limb of the graft (Fig. 1); two overlapping covered stents (Viabahn, Gore and Assoc., Flagstaff, AZ) were deployed across the pseudoaneurysm. Follow-up venogram shows successful exclusion of the pseudoaneurysm (Fig. 2).

Follow-up and Complications
Three weeks after exclusion of the pseudoaneurysm on the venous limb, the patient presented with enlargement of the pseudoaneurysm over the arterial limb with overlying skin ulceration (Fig. 3). This pseudoaneurysm was treated with the placement of a 14-mm × 5-cm Wallgraft (Boston Scientific, Natick, MA) (Fig. 4).

Suggested Readings
Barshes NR, Annambhotla S, Bechara C, et al: Endovascular repair of hemodialysis graft-related pseudoaneurysm: An alternative treatment strategy in salvaging failing dialysis access. Vasc Endovasc Surg 42:228-234, 2008.

Lin PH, Johnson CK, Pullium JK, et al: Transluminal stent graft repair with Wallgraft endoprosthesis in a porcine arteriovenous graft pseudoaneurysm model. J Vasc Surg 37:175-181, 2003.

Ryan JM, Dumbleton SA, Doherty J, et al: Using a covered stent (Wallgraft) to treat pseudoaneurysms of dialysis grafts and fistulas. AJR Am J Roentgenol 180:1067-1071, 2003.

Vesely TM: Use of stent grafts to repair hemodialysis graft-related pseudoaneurysms. J Vasc Intervent Radiol 16:1301-1307, 2005.

Case 214   429

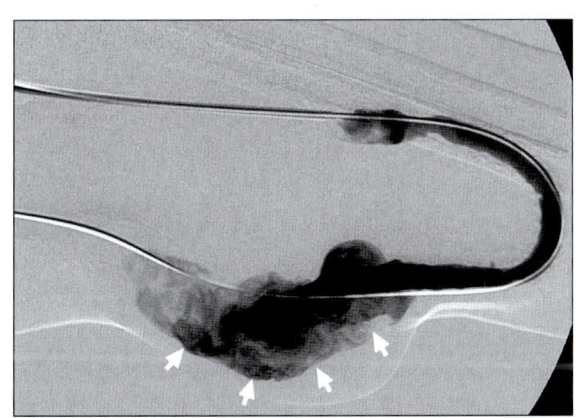

Figure 1. The forearm loop graft has been accessed in the arterial limb in an antegrade direction. There is opacification of a large pseudoaneurysm of the venous limb of the graft *(arrows)*.

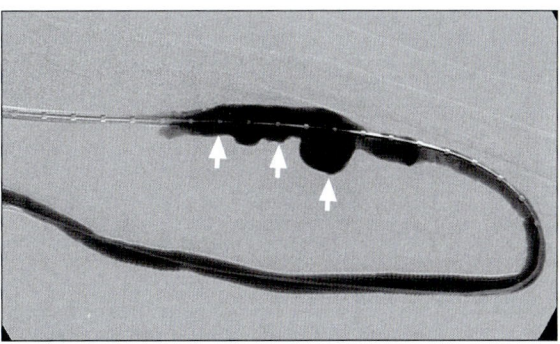

Figure 3. Shunt study 3 weeks later. The pseudoaneurysm of the venous limb remains excluded. There has been interval enlargement of a pseudoaneurysm of the arterial limb *(arrows)*. This was accompanied by overlying skin ulceration.

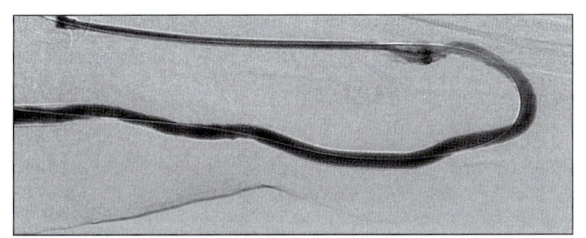

Figure 2. Follow-up shunt study after the placement of two overlapping covered stents shows complete exclusion of the pseudoaneurysm.

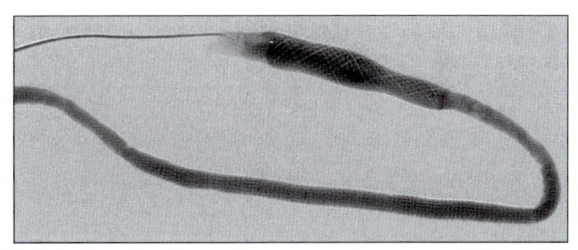

Figure 4. The second pseudoaneurysm was successfully excluded with the placement of a 14-mm × 5-cm Wallgraft.

Case 215

DEMOGRAPHICS/CLINICAL HISTORY

A 69-year-old woman on hemodialysis with a thrombosed left upper extremity dialysis graft, undergoing arteriography.

DISCUSSION

History/Indications for Procedure
In this patient, the graft was placed approximately 18 months earlier and has required no previous intervention.

Procedure
Shunt declot

Intraprocedural Findings
The graft was declotted with 2 mg of tissue plasminogen activator, and angioplasty of the venous anastomosis was performed with a 7-mm Conquest balloon (Bard, Tempe, AZ) (Figs. 1 and 2). After restoration of flow within the graft, a flow rate of 390 mL/min was obtained with the AngioFlow catheter (Angiodynamics, Queensbury, NY).

Follow-up and Complications
The venous anastomosis was dilated further, to 8 mm (Fig. 3), and the flow within the graft increased to 720 mL/min (Fig. 4). The patient has since undergone successful dialysis and required no additional intervention.

Suggested Readings
Patel AA, Tuite CM, Trerotola SO, et al: Mechanical thrombectomy of hemodialysis fistulae and grafts. Cardiovasc Intervent Radiol 28:704-713, 2005.

Turmel-Rodrigues L, Pengloan J, Bourquelot P: Interventional radiology in hemodialysis fistulae and grafts: A multidisciplinary approach. Cardiovasc Intervent Radiol 25:3-16, 2002.

Turmel-Rodrigues L, Pengloan J, Baudin S, et al: Treatment of stenosis and thrombosis in haemodialysis fistulas and grafts by interventional radiology. Nephrol Dial Transplant 15:2029-2036, 2000.

Vesely TM, Gherardini D, Gleed RD, et al: Use of a catheter-based system to measure blood flow in hemodialysis grafts during angioplasty procedures. J Vasc Intervent Radiol 13:371-378, 2002.

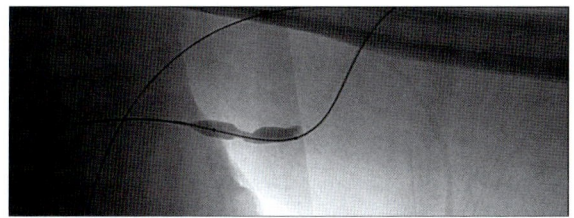

Figure 1. Stenosis at the venous anastomosis was the likely culprit in the graft thrombosis. Angioplasty of the stenosis was initially performed with a 7-mm × 4-cm balloon. A waist in the balloon is evident at the location of the stenosis.

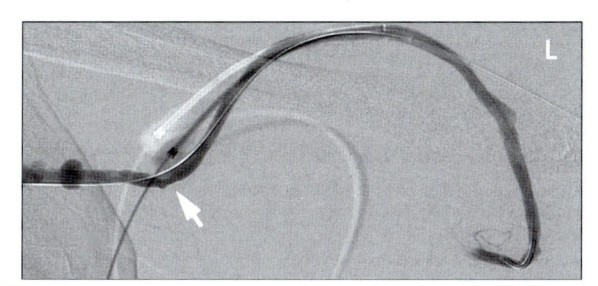

Figure 2. The graft was opened with 2 mg of tissue plasminogen activator administered with pulse-spray technique. Shunt study shows persistent narrowing at the venous anastomosis *(arrow)*. At this point, the flow through the graft measured only 390 mL/min.

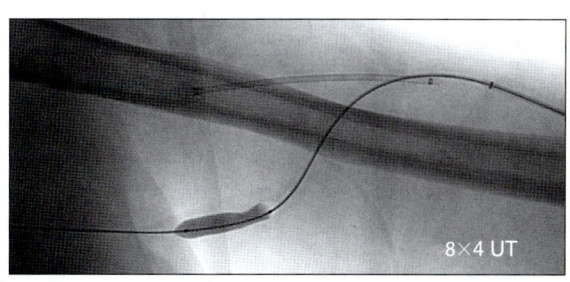

Figure 3. Angioplasty of the venous anastomosis was performed again, this time using an 8-mm × 4-cm balloon.

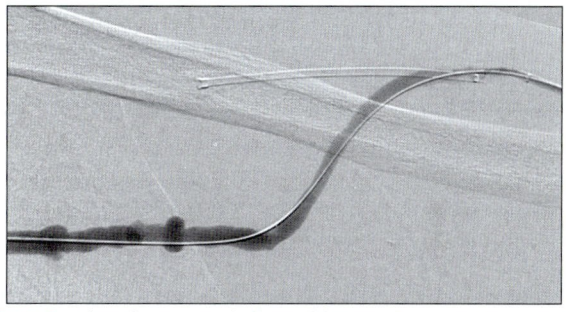

Figure 4. After the second balloon dilation, there continues to be mild narrowing at the venous anastomosis. The flow rate had increased to an acceptable 720 mL/min, however.

Case 216

DEMOGRAPHICS/CLINICAL HISTORY

A 71-year-old woman with end-stage renal disease and thrombosed left femoral dialysis graft.

DISCUSSION

History/Indications for Procedure

A 71-year-old woman with end-stage renal disease requiring dialysis for the past 7 years. She had a left thigh loop graft placed 4 years ago for dialysis access.

Procedure

Management of thrombosed femoral dialysis graft

Intraprocedural Findings

The intragraft thrombus was treated with 4 mg tPA, administered using pulse-spray technique through an infusion catheter (Fig. 1). Following venoplasty at the venous anastomosis (Fig. 2), the arterial plug was removed using a 5.5-French Fogarty balloon (Fig. 3).

Follow-up and Complications

Flow was restored through the graft, but there was significant elastic recoil at the venous anastomosis, for which a self-expanding stent was placed (Fig. 4). The patient was able to dialyze successfully after the procedure.

Suggested Readings

Clark TW: Nitinol stents in hemodialysis access. J Vasc Intervent Radiol 15:1037-1040, 2004.

Gibbens DT, Triolo J, Yu T, et al: Contemporary treatment of thrombosed hemodialysis grafts. Tech Vasc Intervent Radiol 4:122-126, 2001.

Peirce RM, Funaki B, Van Ha TG, et al: Percutaneous declotting of virgin femoral hemodialysis grafts. AJR Am J Roentgenol 185: 1615-1619, 2005.

Case 216   433

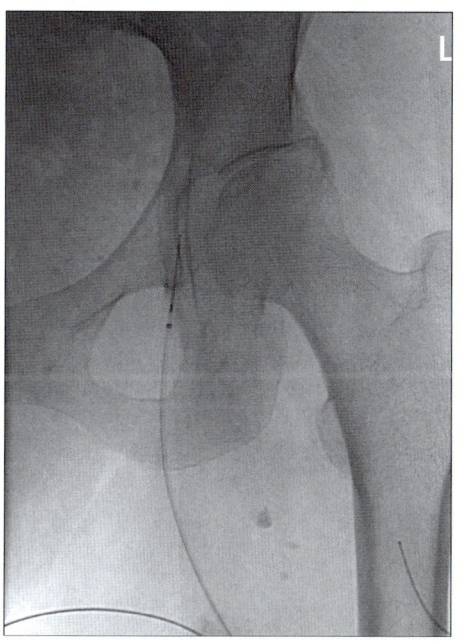

Figure 1. An infusion catheter has been placed across the venous side of the graft, through which 4 mg of tPA was administered using pulse-spray technique.

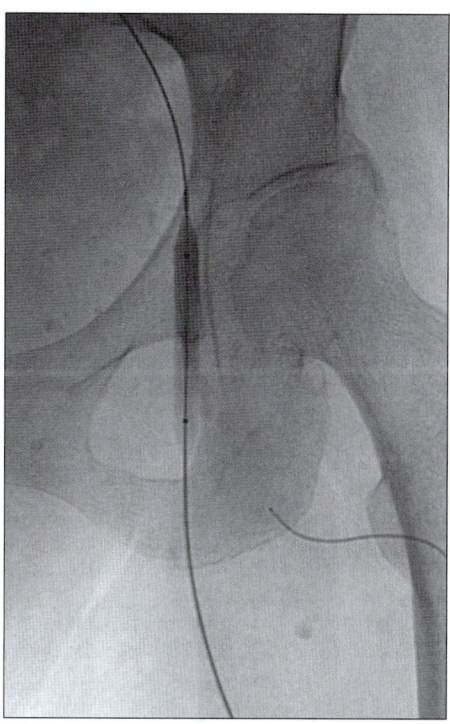

Figure 2. The venous anastomosis was dilated using a 7-mm balloon.

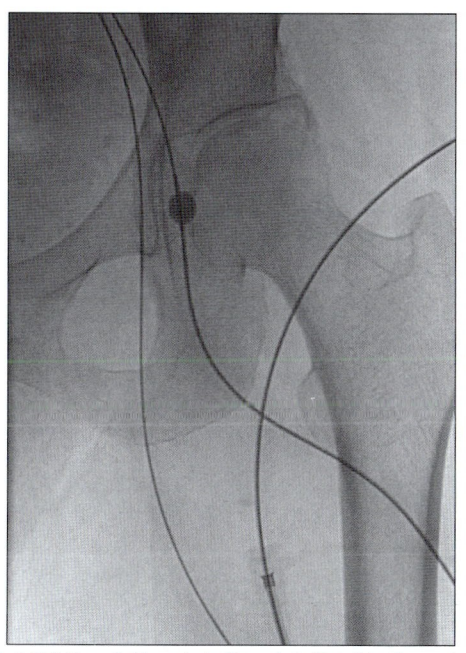

Figure 3. A 5.5-French Fogarty balloon is inflated in the native artery and pulled back across the arterial anastomosis to "pull the plug."

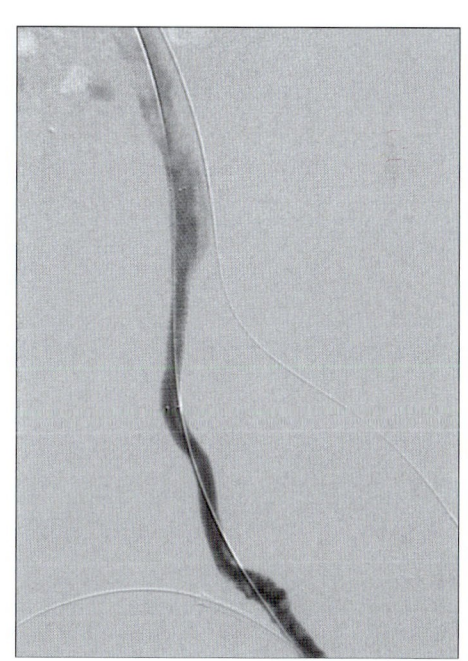

Figure 4. Final venogram after stent placement. There is brisk flow through the stent; a thrill in the graft was palpable following stent placement.

Case 217

DEMOGRAPHICS/CLINICAL HISTORY

A 55-year-old woman with thrombosed necklace hemodialysis graft, undergoing pulse-spray thrombolysis and balloon thrombectomy.

DISCUSSION

History/Indications for Procedure

A 55-year-old woman had end-stage renal disease resulting from hypertension and diabetes. She was dialyzed using an axillary artery-to–axillary vein hemodialysis graft for the past 13 months, and during this time, the graft required many interventions.

Procedure

Clotted necklace hemodialysis graft

Intraprocedural Findings

The graft was declotted using a combination of pulse-spray thrombolysis and balloon thrombectomy (Figs. 1 and 2). After restoration of flow, an irregular stenosis of the axillary vein around the venous anastomosis was uncovered (Fig. 3).

Follow-up and Complications

Two overlapping, self-expanding nitinol stents were deployed across the venous anastomosis into the subclavian vein (Fig. 4). The patient was able to undergo dialysis successfully for the next month, at which time the graft rethrombosed.

Suggested Readings

Fidelman N, Allen D, Bloom AI, et al: Percutaneous interventions in subclavian artery-to-contralateral vein "necklace" hemodialysis grafts: Experience in five patients. J Vasc Intervent Radiol 18:597-601, 2007.

Patel AA, Tuite CM, Trerotola SO: Mechanical thrombectomy of hemodialysis fistulae and grafts. Cardiovasc Intervent Radiol 28:704-713, 2005.

Turmel-Rodrigues L, Pengloan J, Baudin S, et al: Treatment of stenosis and thrombosis in haemodialysis fistulas and grafts by interventional radiology. Nephrol Dial Transplant 15:2029-2036, 2000.

Vesely TM, Gherardini D, Gleed RD, et al: Use of a catheter-based system to measure blood flow in hemodialysis grafts during angioplasty procedures. J Vasc Intervent Radiol 13:371-378, 2002.

Vogel PM, Parise C: SMART stent for salvage of hemodialysis access grafts. J Vasc Intervent Radiol 15:1051-1060, 2004.

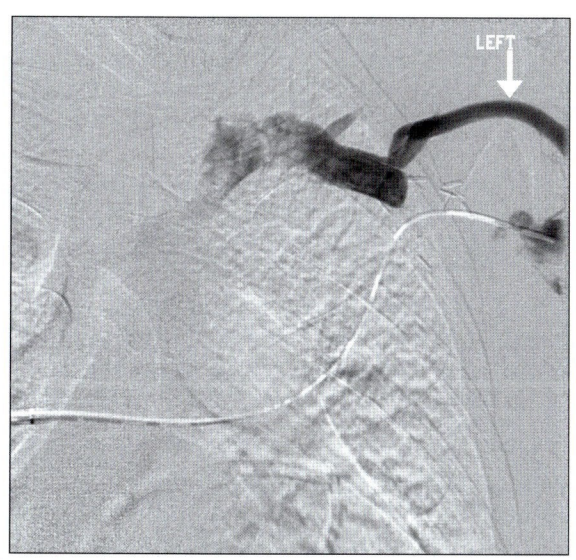

Figure 1. Left upper extremity venogram demonstrates occlusion of the axillary vein around the venous anastomosis. There is a prominent collateral vein around the occluded segment *(arrow)*.

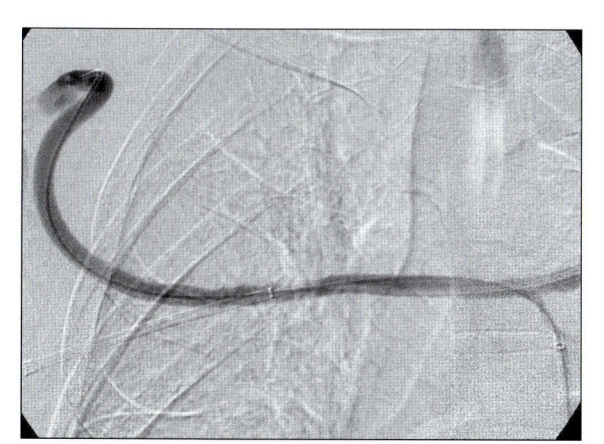

Figure 2. Shunt study performed after flow was restored shows the arterial anastomosis is widely patent.

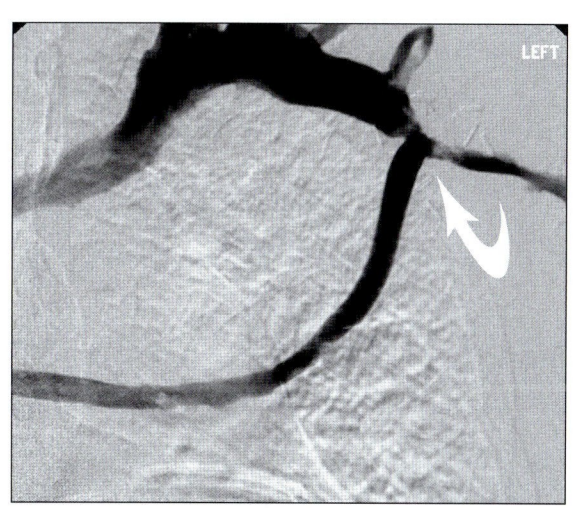

Figure 3. There is persistent narrowing and irregularity *(arrow)* of the axillary vein around the site of the venous anastomosis.

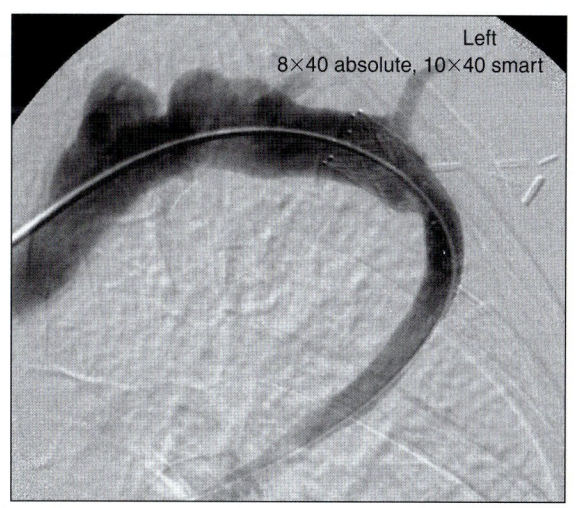

Figure 4. The venous anastomosis was treated with two overlapping, self-expanding nitinol stents.

Case 218

DEMOGRAPHICS/CLINICAL HISTORY

A 25-year-old man with end-stage renal disease with limited venous access for dialysis, undergoing venography, ultrasound, and dialysis catheter placement.

DISCUSSION

History/Indications for Procedure
A 25-year-old man has end-stage renal disease and limited venous access. His previous femoral dialysis catheter was removed because of catheter-related sepsis.

Procedure
Placement of transhepatic dialysis catheter

Pre-procedure Imaging
Upper extremity venography revealed chronic occlusion of the brachiocephalic veins and superior vena cava (Fig. 1). Inferior vena cavogram demonstrates occlusion of the intrahepatic inferior vena cava (Fig. 2).

Intraprocedural Findings
A hepatic vein was accessed with ultrasound (Fig. 3), and a 15-French dialysis catheter was placed with the tip positioned in the right atrium (Fig. 4).

Follow-up and Complications
The patient continues to use this access for hemodialysis. He has returned once to have the catheter exchanged because of possible catheter-related infection.

Suggested Readings
Bagul A, Brook NR, Kaushik M, Nicholson ML: Tunnelled catheters for the haemodialysis patient. Eur J Vasc Endovasc Surg 33: 105-112, 2007.

Smith TP, Ryan JM, Reddan DN: Transhepatic catheter access for hemodialysis. J Vasc Intervent Radiol 232:246-251, 2003.

Stavropoulos SW, Pan JJ, Clark TW, et al: Percutaneous transhepatic venous access for hemodialysis. J Vasc Intervent Radiol 14(Pt 1):1187-1190, 2003.

Trerotola SO: Hemodialysis catheter placement and management. Radiology 215:651-658, 2000.

Case 218   437

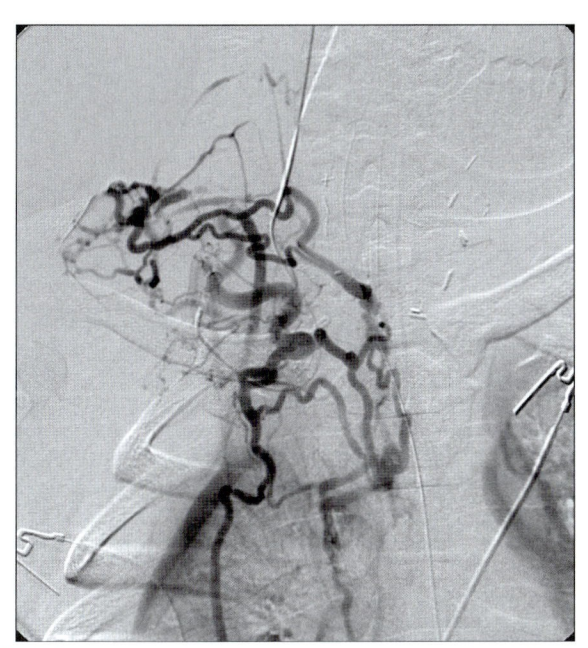

Figure 1. Contrast injection into collateral vein in the right neck shows filling of numerous, small collateral veins in the right neck and chest. The internal jugular vein is chronically occluded.

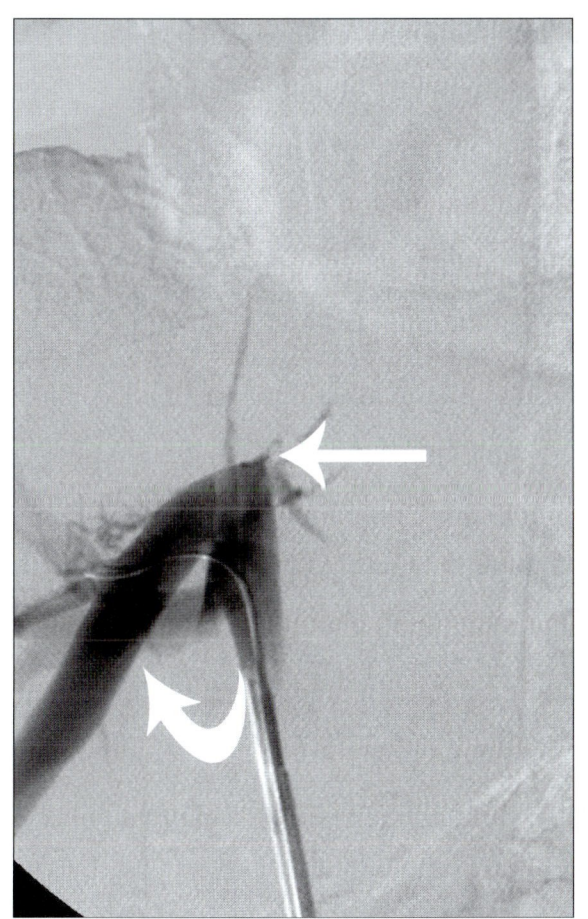

Figure 2. Inferior vena cavogram shows focal occlusion of the intrahepatic inferior vena cava *(arrow)* with reflux of contrast into a large accessory hepatic vein *(curved arrow)*.

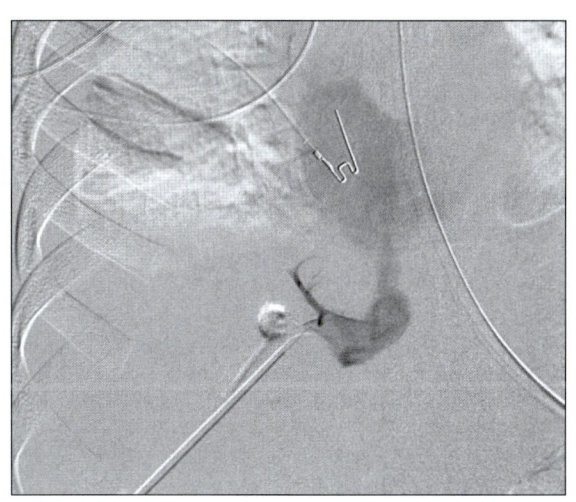

Figure 3. A hepatic vein was accessed using ultrasound guidance.

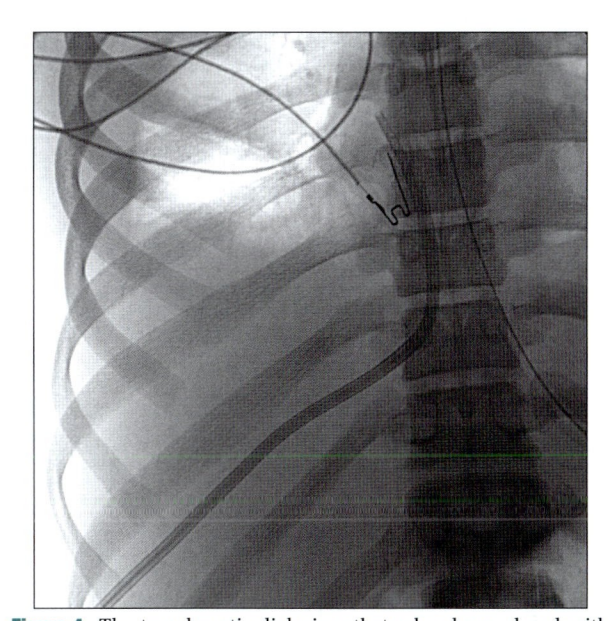

Figure 4. The transhepatic dialysis catheter has been placed with the tip positioned in the right atrium.

Case 219

DEMOGRAPHICS/CLINICAL HISTORY

A 37-year-old woman with Down syndrome and renal failure.

DISCUSSION

History/Indications for Procedure
A 37-year-old woman with Down syndrome and renal failure; the patient has had multiple prior hemodialysis catheters and failed upper extremity fistulas in the past. Attempts at placement of a femoral dialysis catheter at an outside hospital were not successful.

Procedure
Placement of transhepatic dialysis catheter

Pre-procedure Imaging
The left external jugular vein was accessed and contrast venography shows that the superior vena cava (SVC) is occluded. The azygous vein is patent and fills multiple upper abdominal collateral veins; the inferior vena cava (IVC) is not visualized and appears occluded (Fig. 1).

Intraprocedural Findings
A peripheral hepatic vein branch was accessed with ultrasound, and an hepatic venogram shows a stenosis between the hepatic vein and IVC (Fig. 2). The stenosis was angioplastied with a 10-mm balloon (Fig. 3), and a cuffed dialysis catheter was placed, with both tips positioned in the right atrium (Fig. 4).

Follow-up and Complications
On the following day, the patient became hypotensive and tachycardic; CT of the abdomen was performed and showed a perihepatic hematoma. The patient was given a blood transfusion and the hemoglobin level stabilized; the patient was able to go on to successful dialysis through the transhepatic catheter.

Suggested Readings
Smith TP, Ryan JM, Reddan DN: Transhepatic catheter access for hemodialysis. Radiology 232:246-251, 2004.
Stavropoulos SW, Pan JJ, Clark TW, et al: Percutaneous transhepatic venous access for hemodialysis. J Vasc Intervent Radiol 14:1187-1190, 2003.
Weeks SM: Unconventional venous access. Tech Vasc Intervent Radiol 5:114-120, 2002.

Case 219   439

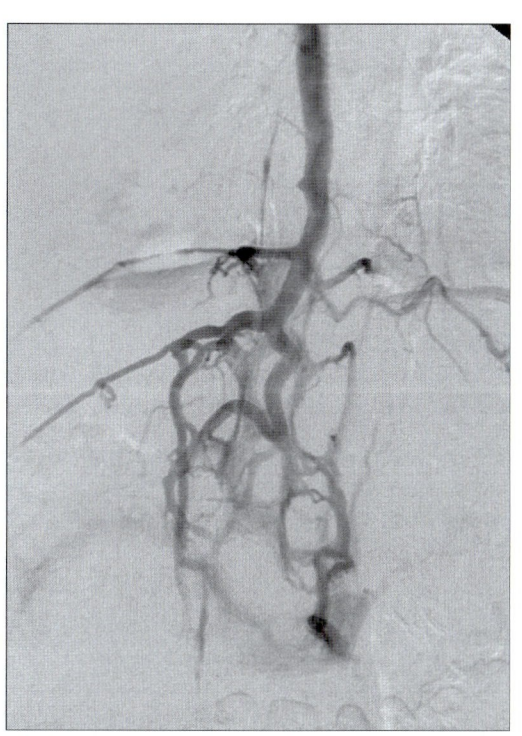

Figure 1. Contrast venogram through a left external jugular vein access. There is filling of the azygous vein, which drains into multiple collaterals in the upper abdomen. The IVC was not visualized and was thought to be occluded.

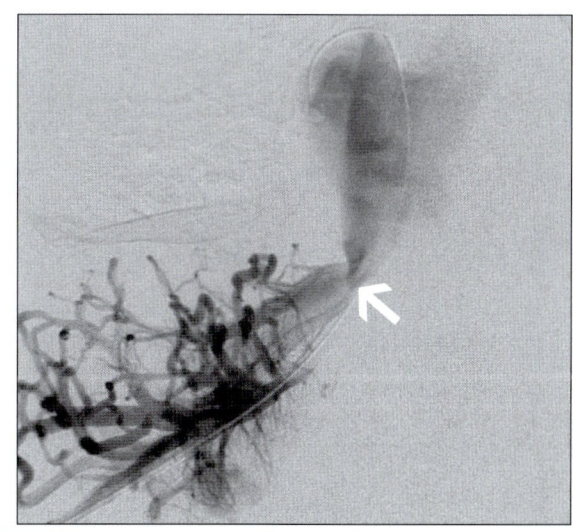

Figure 2. Hepatic venogram. There is filling of numerous intrahepatic venous collaterals, and a stenosis is seen at the junction of the hepatic vein and IVC *(arrow)*.

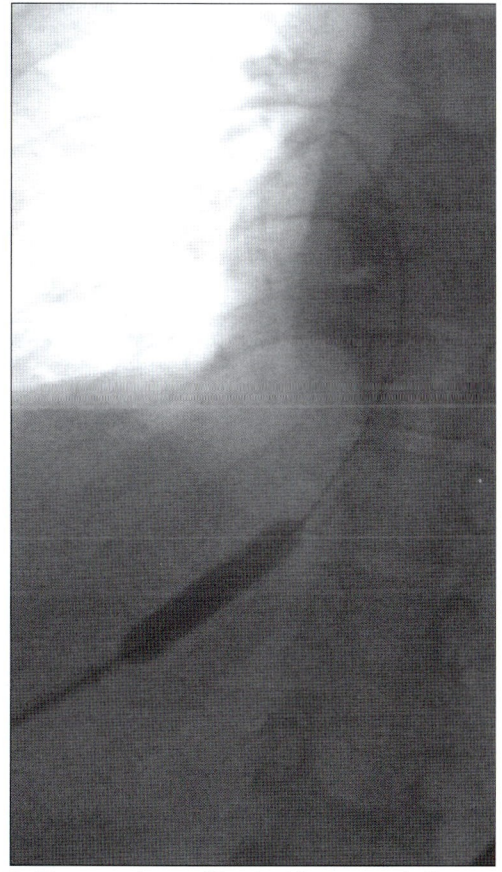

Figure 3. The stenosis was dilated with a 10-mm balloon.

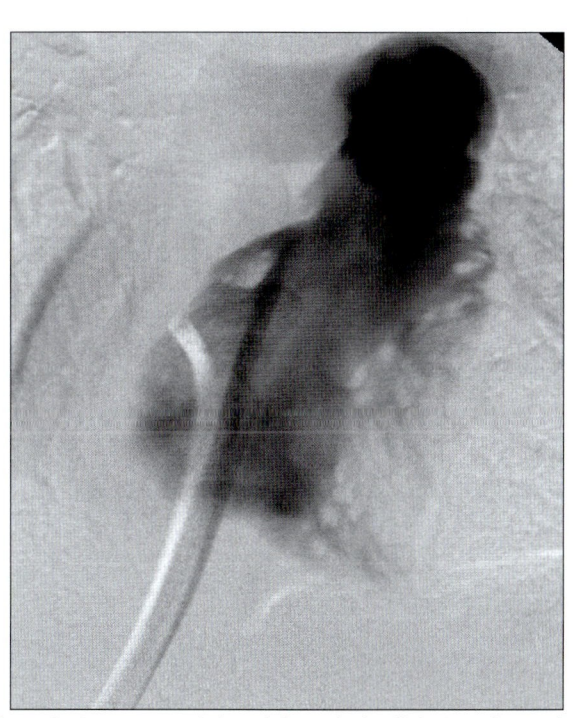

Figure 4. Contrast was injected through the dialysis catheter after placement. The catheter tips are positioned within the small right atrium.

Case 220

DEMOGRAPHICS/CLINICAL HISTORY

A 42-year-old woman with end-stage renal disease and limited venous access sites, undergoing venography and dialysis catheter placement.

DISCUSSION

History/Indications for Procedure
A 42-year-old woman has end-stage renal disease. Her previous internal jugular venous catheter was removed because of a catheter-related infection, and she requires new hemodialysis access.

Procedure
Translumbar dialysis catheter placement

Pre-procedure Imaging
Upper and lower extremity venography demonstrates chronic occlusion of the brachiocephalic and iliac veins.

Intraprocedural Findings
The location of the inferior vena cava (IVC) was marked by placement of a guidewire using a transhepatic approach (Fig. 1). The IVC was accessed under fluoroscopy, the tract was dilated, and a 31-cm dialysis catheter was placed (Figs. 2 and 3).

Follow-up and Complications
The patient was able to undergo dialysis successfully with the translumbar catheter. However, she did return several times during the next 3 months to have the catheter exchanged because of poor flow.

Suggested Readings
Biswal R, Nosher JL, Siegel RL, Bodner LJ: Translumbar placement of paired hemodialysis catheters (Tesio catheters) and follow-up in 10 patients. Cardivasc Intervent Radiol 23:75-78, 2000.

Rajan DK, Croteau DL, Sturza SG, et al: Translumbar placement of inferior vena caval catheters: A solution for challenging hemodialysis access. Radiographics 18:1155-1167, 1998.

Weeks SM: Unconventional venous access. Tech Vasc Intervent Radiol 5:114-120, 2002.

Case 220   441

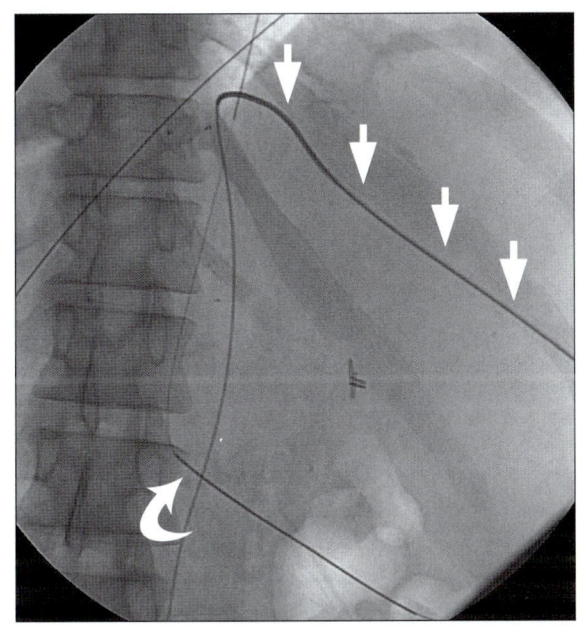

Figure 1. A transhepatic catheter has been placed *(arrows)* to allow placement of a guidewire in the IVC. The guidewire is then used as a target for IVC puncture under fluoroscopy *(curved arrow)*.

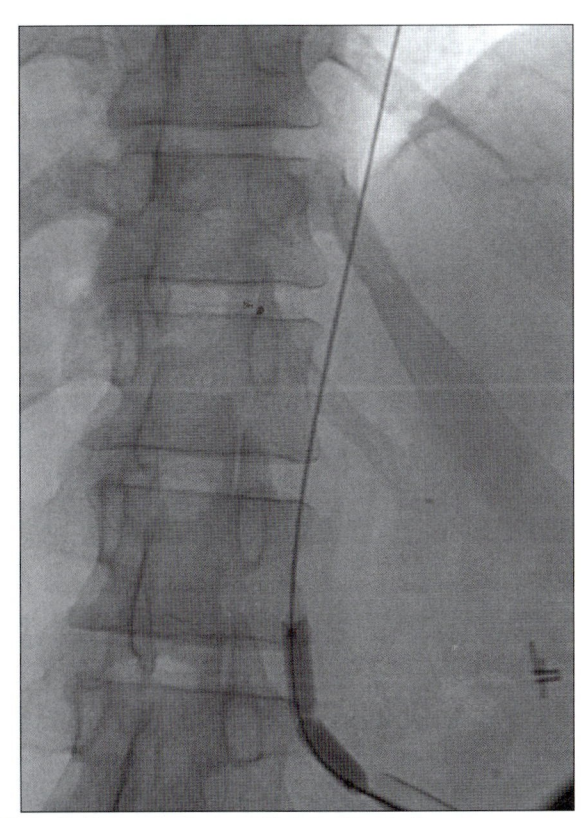

Figure 2. The entry site was dilated with a balloon.

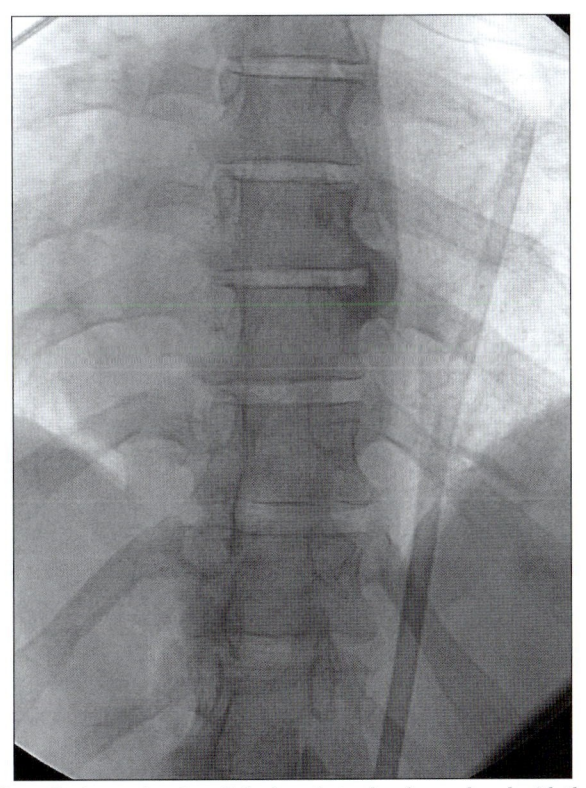

Figure 3. A translumbar dialysis catheter has been placed with the catheter tip positioned in the right atrium.

Case 221

DEMOGRAPHICS/CLINICAL HISTORY

A 26-year-old woman with cystic fibrosis and right middle lobe pneumonia, undergoing chest radiography.

DISCUSSION

History/Indications for Procedure
This patient required central venous access for a 2-week course of intravenous antibiotics.

Procedure
Peripherally inserted central catheter (PICC) placement with left-sided superior vena cava (SVC)

Pre-procedure Imaging
A chest radiograph showed pulmonary hyperinflation and bronchiectasis consistent with the patient's known history of cystic fibrosis. There was a new focal, confluent airspace opacity in the right middle lobe.

Intraprocedural Findings
The guidewire repeatedly took an unusual course, so a left upper extremity venogram was performed. The venogram showed a left-sided SVC (Fig. 1).

Follow-up and Complications
The PICC was placed through the left SVC (Fig. 2). The patient was discharged home to complete her antibiotic therapy.

Suggested Readings
Cardella JF, Cardella K, Bacci N, et al: Cumulative experience with 1,273 peripherally inserted central catheters at a single institution. J Vasc Intervent Radiol 7:5-13, 1996.

Danielpour PJ, Aalberg JK, El-Ramey M, et al: Persistent left superior vena cava: An incidental finding during central venous catheterization—a case report. Vasc Endovascular Surg 39:109-111, 2005.

Sarodia BD, Stoller JK: Persistent left superior vena cava: Case report and literature review. Respir Care 45:411-416, 2000.

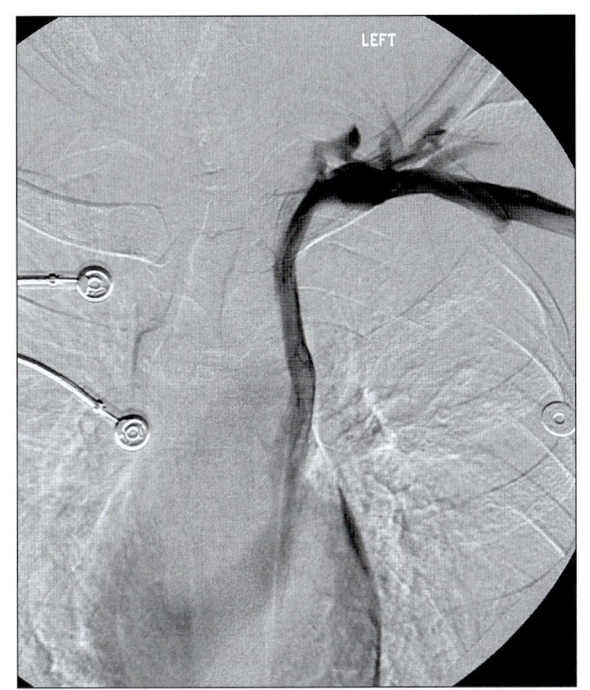

Figure 1. Left upper extremity venogram shows a left-sided SVC. The left SVC drains into the coronary sinus, then to the right atrium.

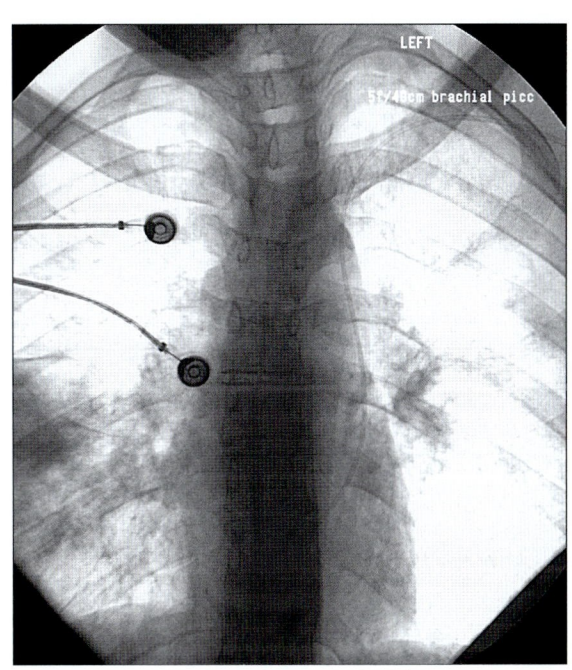

Figure 2. The PICC was placed through the left SVC.

Case 222

DEMOGRAPHICS/CLINICAL HISTORY

A 47-year-old man with inadvertent intra-arterial placement of central venous catheter, undergoing radiography, arteriography, and catheter removal.

DISCUSSION

History/Indications for Procedure
A 47-year-old man in the burn intensive care unit had a subclavian central venous catheter placed at the bedside using anatomic landmarks.

Procedure
Intra-arterial central venous catheter removal

Pre-procedure Imaging
Portable chest radiograph shows the right subclavian central venous catheter taking an abnormal course, crossing to the left of the spine (Fig. 1).

Intraprocedural Findings
Right subclavian arteriogram confirms the presence of the catheter in the right subclavian artery (Fig. 2). The catheter was removed while inflating a balloon across the site of injury (Fig. 3).

Follow-up and Complications
The balloon remained inflated for 10 minutes. After balloon deflation, there was no further evidence of injury to the subclavian artery (Fig. 4), and the patient had no further complication from the line placement.

Suggested Readings
McGee DC, Gould MK: Preventing complications of central venous catheterization. N Engl J Med 348:1123-1133, 2003.

Case 222   445

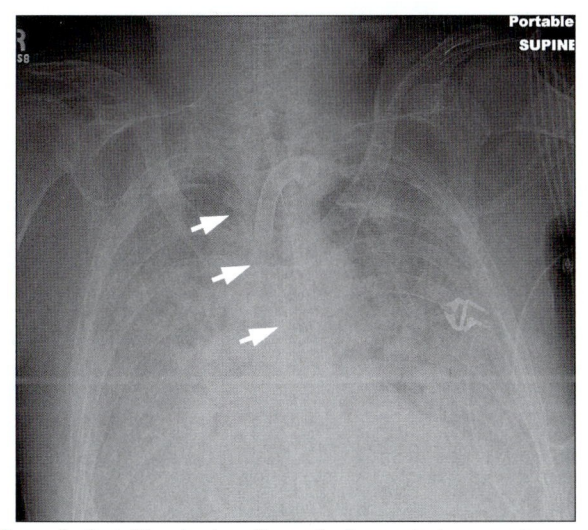

Figure 1. Portable chest radiograph demonstrates an abnormal course of the right subclavian central venous catheter *(arrows)*.

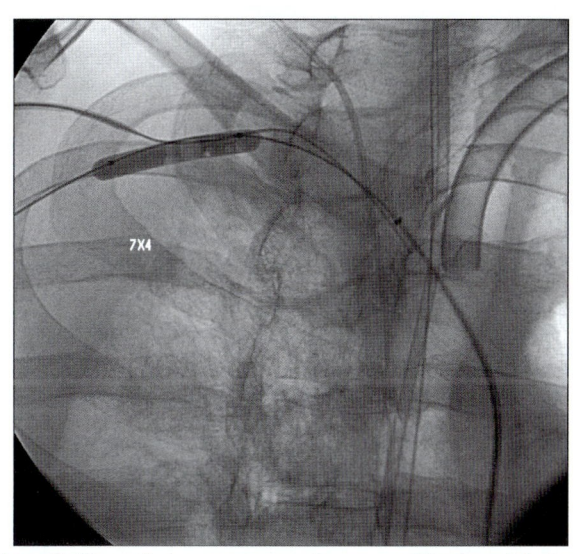

Figure 3. The catheter was removed over a guidewire while tamponading the site with a 7-mm balloon.

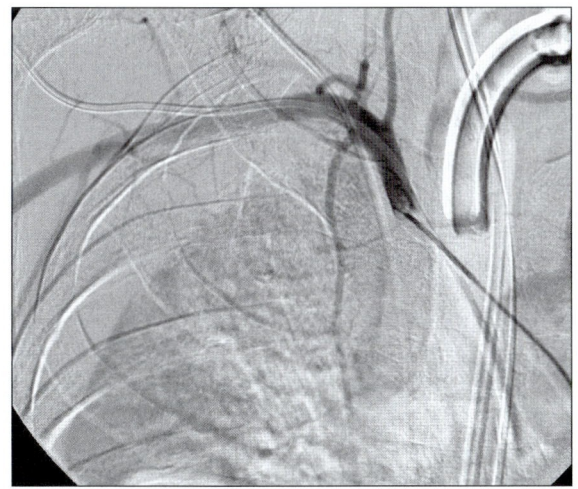

Figure 2. Selective subclavian arteriogram confirms intra-arterial placement of the central venous catheter.

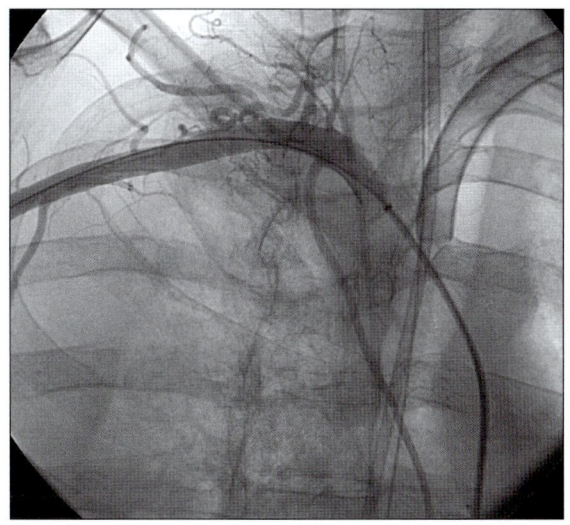

Figure 4. Follow-up subclavian artery injection shows no further extravasation from the arterial injury.

Case 223

DEMOGRAPHICS/CLINICAL HISTORY

A 68-year-old woman, involved in a grease fire, with central venous catheter placed for fluid resuscitation and medications.

DISCUSSION

History/Indications for Procedure
A 68-year-old woman in the burn ICU for management of burns suffered in a grease fire. A triple-lumen central venous catheter was placed at the bedside.

Procedure
Management of inadvertent placement of central venous catheter in the vertebral artery

Pre-procedure Imaging
Chest radiograph shows the tip of the central venous catheter as overlying the descending thoracic aorta. Contrast-enhanced chest CT shows the catheter entering the left vertebral artery and descending into the thoracic aorta (Fig. 1).

Intraprocedural Findings
Left subclavian arteriogram shows the central venous catheter entering the left vertebral artery (Fig. 2). The patient was given an intravenous bolus of heparin, and the catheter was removed over an 0.018-inch guidewire; the vertebral artery injury was treated with the placement of two overlapping covered stents (Jomed International AB, Helsingborg, Sweden) (Fig. 3).

Follow-up and Complications
Arteriogram following stent-graft placement shows successful sealing of the puncture site within the vertebral artery (Fig. 4).

Suggested Readings
Guilbert MC, Elkouri S, Bracco D, et al: Arterial trauma during central venous catheter insertion: Case series, review and proposed algorithm. J Vasc Surg, 2008 [e-pub ahead of print].

Herrera DA, Vargas SA, Dublin AB: Endovascular treatment of traumatic injuries of the vertebral artery. AJNR Am J Neuroradiol 29:1585-1589, 2008.

Nicholson T, Ettles D, Robinson G: Managing inadvertent arterial catheterization during central venous access procedures. Cardiovasc Intervent Radiol 27:21-25, 2004.

Case 223   447

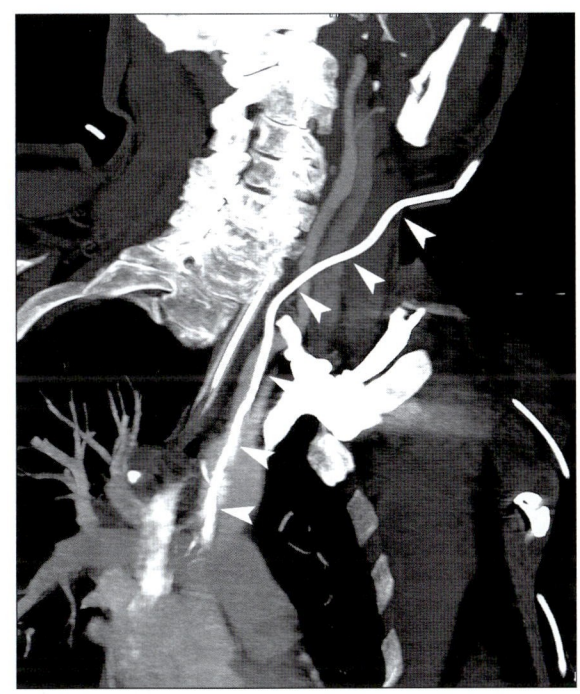

Figure 1. Reformatted image from contrast-enhanced chest CT shows the central venous catheter *(arrowheads)* entering the left vertebral artery and coursing into the thoracic aorta.

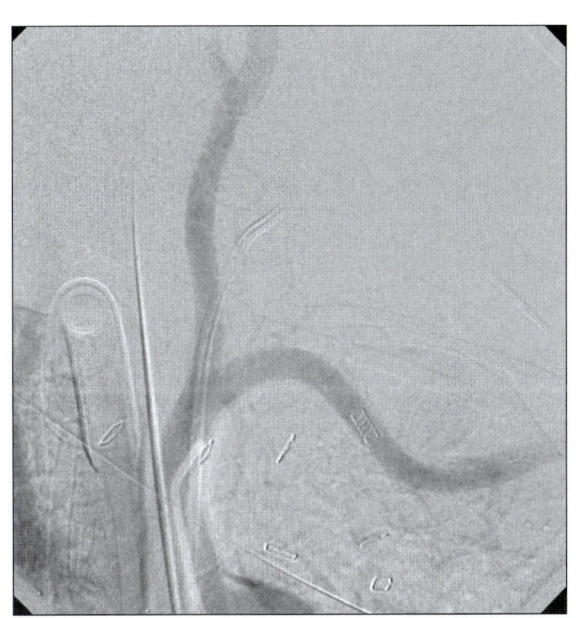

Figure 2. Left subclavian arteriogram confirms the placement of the central venous catheter in the vertebral artery.

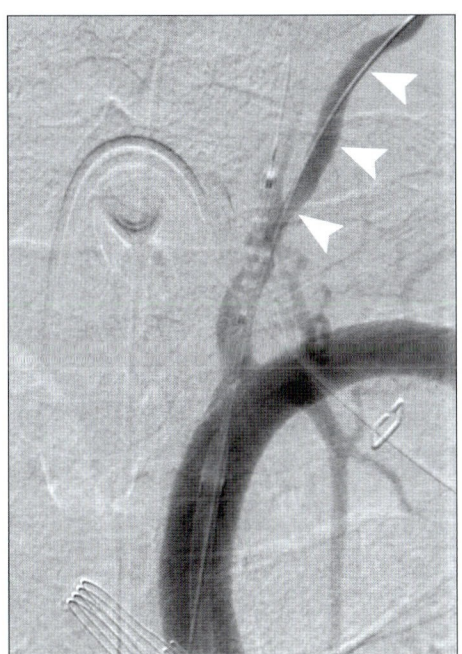

Figure 3. The central venous catheter has been removed over an 0.018-inch guidewire. Contrast injected through catheter in left subclavaian artery briskly extravasates along the tract of the central venous line *(arrowheads)*.

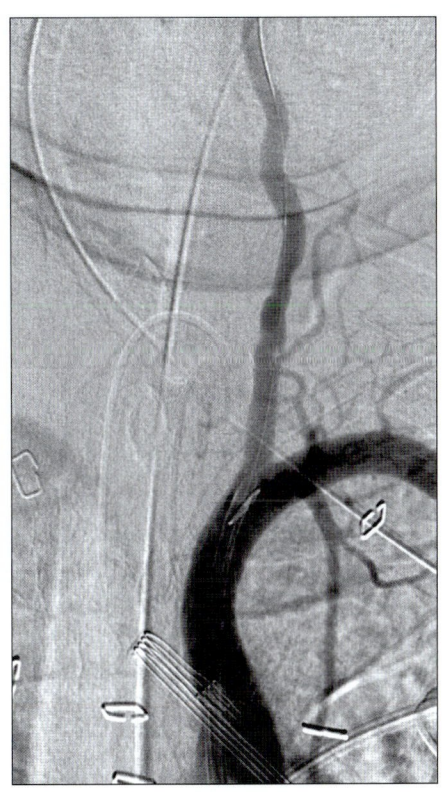

Figure 4. Following placement of two overlapping covered stents, there is no further extravasation from the site of injury. There is good antegrade flow within the vertebral artery.

Case 224

DEMOGRAPHICS/CLINICAL HISTORY

A 50-year-old woman with locally advanced right breast carcinoma, undergoing ultrasound and subcutaneous port insertion.

DISCUSSION

History/Indications for Procedure
A 50-year-old woman with locally advanced right breast carcinoma has a left-sided ventriculoperitoneal shunt that was placed 10 years earlier.

Procedure
Subclavian vein port insertion

Intraprocedural Findings
The ventriculoperitoneal shunt precluded internal jugular vein access. The subclavian vein was accessed with ultrasound (Fig. 1), and the port was positioned lateral to the shunt (Figs. 2 and 3).

Follow-up and Complications
The patient has had no complications from the port and has begun chemotherapy treatments.

Suggested Readings
Denny DF: Placement and management of long-term central venous access catheters and ports. AJR Am J Roentgenol 161:385-393, 1993.

Jaques PF, Mauro MA, Keefe B: US guidance for vascular access. Technical note. J Vasc Intervent Radiol 3:427-430, 1992.

Mauro MA, Jaques PF: Radiologic placement of long-term central venous catheters: A review. J Vasc Intervent Radiol 4:127-137, 1993.

Case 224   449

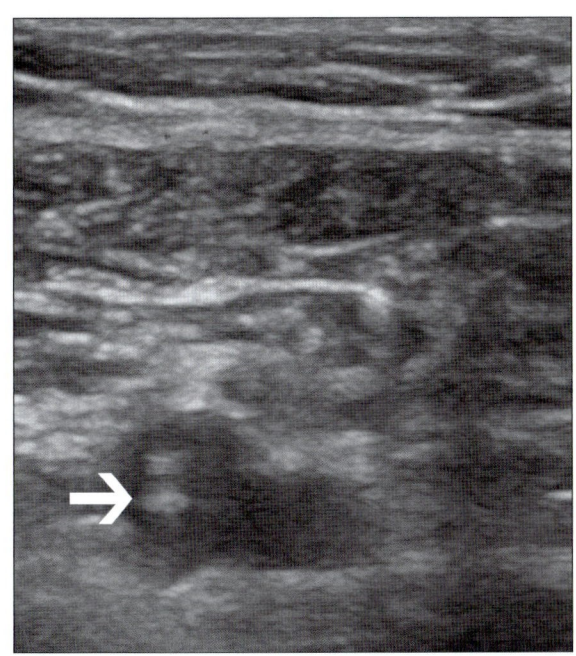

Figure 1. Ultrasound image of the left chest during venous access demonstrates the tip of the needle in the subclavian vein (*arrow*).

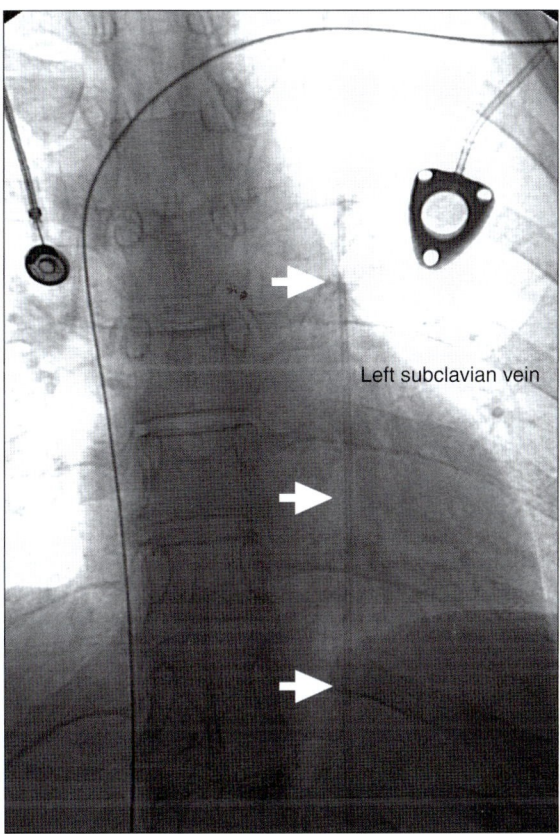

Figure 2. The port pocket was created lateral to the ventriculoperitoneal shunt (*arrows*). A guidewire was advanced into the inferior vena cava.

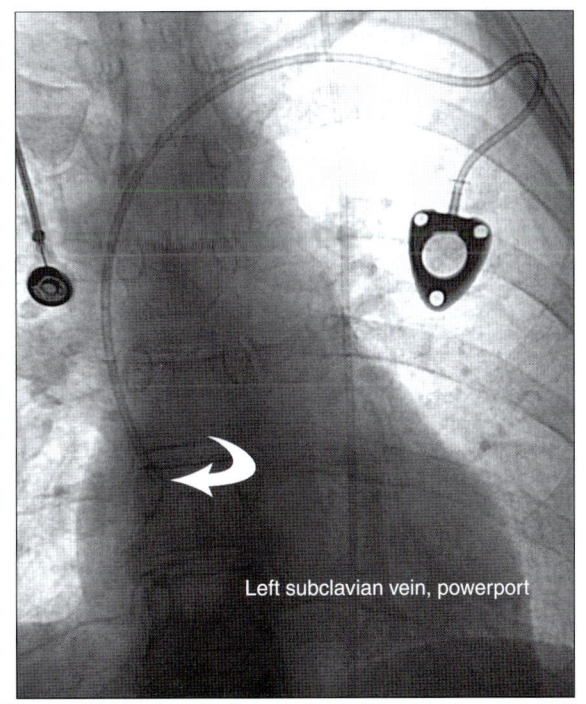

Figure 3. The final image demonstrates the port catheter extending to the upper right atrium (*arrow*).

Case 225
Robert G. Dixon, MD

DEMOGRAPHICS/CLINICAL HISTORY
A 48-year-old man with history of chronic pancreatitis and seizures.

DISCUSSION

History/Indications for Procedure
The patient had the subcutaneous port placed approximately 1 year prior at an outside institution because of his multiple admissions for pancreatitis and poor peripheral access. The port had not functioned properly for approximately 2 months.

Procedure
"Pinch-off syndrome"—foreign body retrieval

Pre-procedure Imaging
Chest x-ray identified the left chest port placed via a left subclavian vein approach; however, the catheter has fractured (Fig. 1) secondary to "pinch-off syndrome" (repeated compression within the costoclavicular space). This can be avoided by entering the axillary/subclavian vein more laterally at the time of port placement.

Intraprocedural Findings
From a right common femoral vein approach the catheter was successfully snared and removed (Fig. 2). The port and proximal catheter fragment were also successfully removed.

Follow-up and Complications
The patient tolerated the procedure well and sustained no immediate complications.

Suggested Readings
Hinke DH, Zandt-Stastny DA, Goodman LR, Quebbeman EJ, Krzywda EA, Andris DA: Pinch-off syndrome: A complication of implantable subclavian venous access devices. Radiology 177:353-356, 1990.

Funaki B: Central venous access: A primer for the diagnostic radiologist. AJR Am J Roentgenol 179:309-318, 2002.

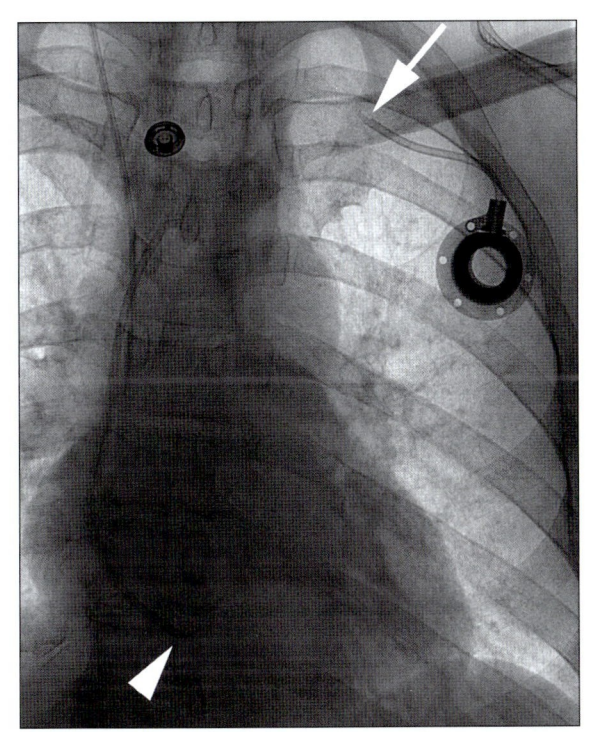

Figure 1. Frontal chest radiograph demonstrates the left subclavian port with a fractured catheter *(arrow)* secondary to pinch-off syndrome. The distal fragment has migrated and is positioned with the tip in the region of the tricuspid valve *(arrowhead)*. Incidental note is made of a recently placed right internal jugular triple lumen catheter.

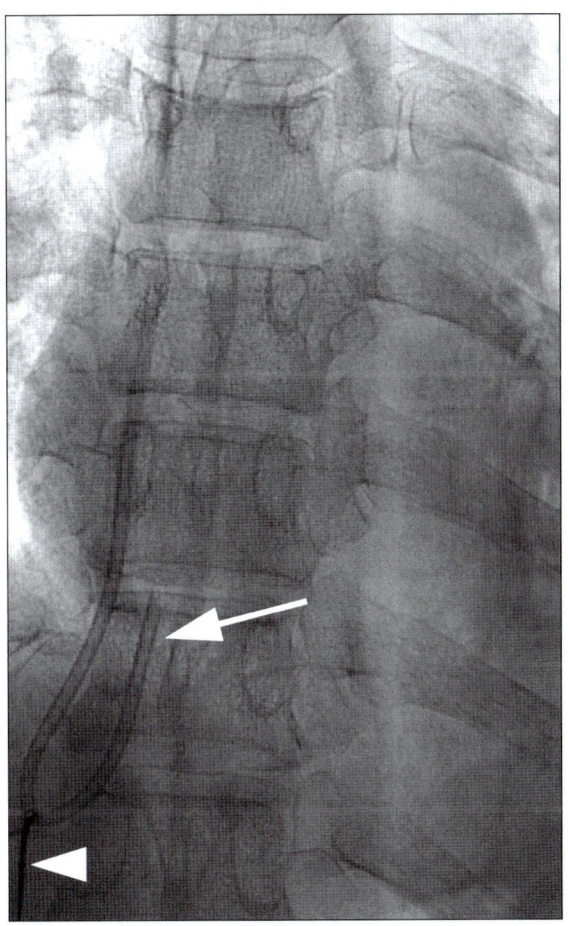

Figure 2. Magnified radiograph identifies the snare *(arrowhead)* successfully capturing the distal catheter fragment *(arrow)*, which was removed without incident.

Case 226

DEMOGRAPHICS/CLINICAL HISTORY

A 22-year-old man with lost guidewire after subclavian central venous catheter placement, undergoing radiography.

DISCUSSION

History/Indications for Procedure
This patient had multiple injuries following a motor vehicle accident. A guidewire was lost during placement of a right subclavian central venous catheter at the bedside.

Procedure
Retrieval of lost guidewire

Pre-procedure Imaging
An anteroposterior chest radiograph shows the guidewire to be extending from the distal tip of the venous catheter, looping in the right atrium, and extending below the hemidiaphragm (Fig. 1).

Intraprocedural Findings
The subclavian catheter had been removed before the procedure. From a right internal jugular venous approach, the tip of the lost guidewire was grasped with a T-Rex forceps device (Fig. 2); the guidewire was removed; and the sheath was exchanged for a new central venous catheter (Fig. 3).

Follow-up and Complications
After a long hospital course, the patient recovered from his extensive injuries sustained in the motor vehicle collision. There were no clinical sequelae as a result of the lost guidewire.

Suggested Readings
Egglin TK, Dickey KW, Rosenblatt M, et al: Retrieval of intravascular foreign bodies: Experience in 32 cases. AJR Am J Roentgenol 164:1259-1264, 1995.
Gabelmann A, Krämer S, Görich J: Percutaneous retrieval of lost or misplaced intravascular objects. AJR Am J Roentgenol 176: 1509-1513, 2001.
Uflacker R, Lima S, Melichar AC: Intravascular foreign bodies: Percutaneous retrieval. Radiology 160:731-735, 1986.

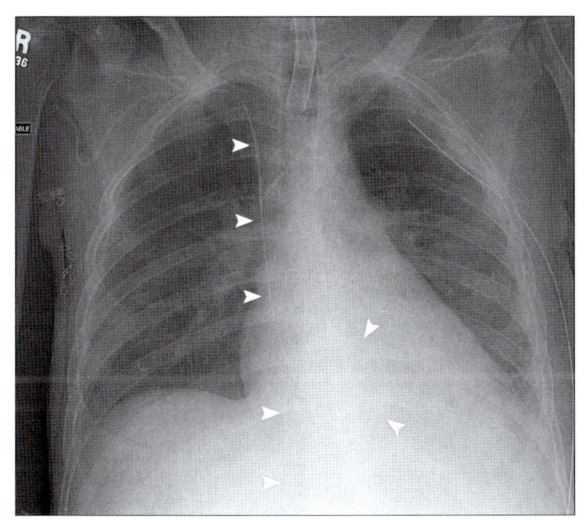

Figure 1. Anteroposterior chest radiograph shows a right subclavian venous catheter. A guidewire is seen extending from the distal tip of the catheter, coiling in the right atrium, and passing beneath the hemidiaphragm *(arrowheads)*.

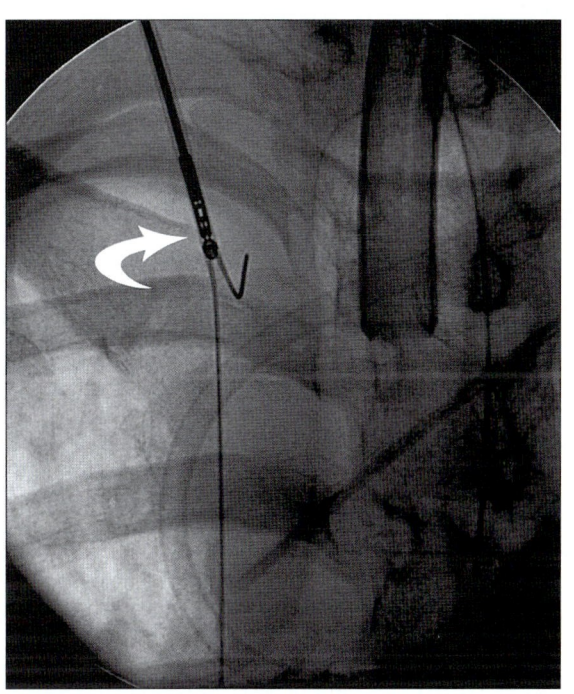

Figure 2. From a right internal jugular vein access, forceps were used to grasp the end of the guidewire *(arrow)*.

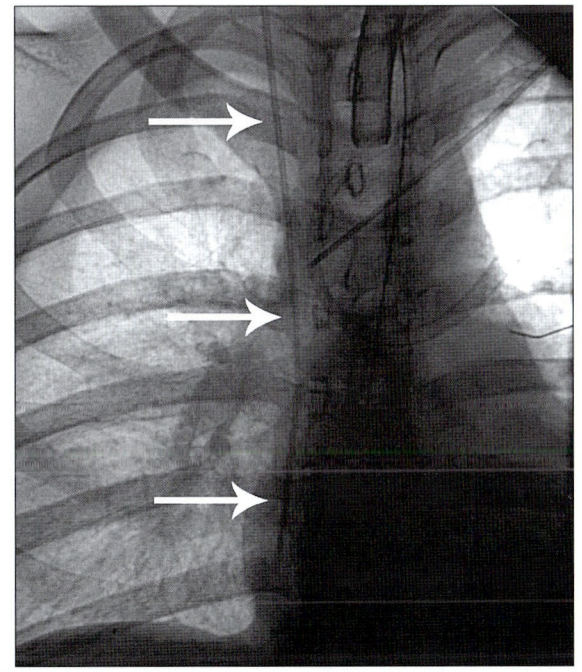

Figure 3. A right internal jugular central venous catheter was placed *(arrows)* after removal of the lost guidewire.

Case 227

DEMOGRAPHICS/CLINICAL HISTORY

A 63-year-old man after orthotopic liver transplantation with a hepatic venous stenosis, undergoing angioplasty and venography.

DISCUSSION

History/Indications for Procedure
A 63-year-old man underwent liver transplantation 2 days before this procedure. The hepatic veins were anastomosed to the patient's native inferior vena cava (IVC) using the piggyback technique.

Procedure
Management of malpositioned intravascular stent

Pre-procedure Imaging
Doppler ultrasound showed narrowing at the confluence of the hepatic veins and IVC, with monophasic waveforms in the hepatic veins.

Intraprocedural Findings
A focal stenosis at the confluence of the hepatic veins and IVC was identified (Fig. 1) and treated with balloon angioplasty. An expandable stent using a 10-mm × 25-mm balloon was then deployed across the stenosis to remedy significant residual stenosis.

Follow-up and Complications
Immediately after stent deployment, the stent migrated into the IVC (Fig. 2). The stent was captured with a 15-mm gooseneck snare (Fig. 3). The stent was pulled down and the balloon dilated in the right external iliac vein (Fig. 4).

Suggested Readings
Gabelmann A, Kramer S, Gorich J: Percutaneous retrieval of lost or misplaced intravascular objects. AJR Am J Roentgenol 176: 1509-1513, 2001.

Gabelmann A, Kramer S, Tomczak R, Gorich J: Percutaneous technique for managing maldeployed or migrated stents. J Endovasc Ther 8:291-302, 2001.

Hartnell GG, Jordan SJ: Percutaneous removal of a misplaced Palmaz stent with a coaxial snare technique. J Vasc Radiol 6:799-801, 1995.

Slonim SM, Dake MD, Razavi MK, et al: Management of misplaced or migrated endovascular stents. J Vasc Intervent Radiol 10:851-859, 1999.

Case 227   455

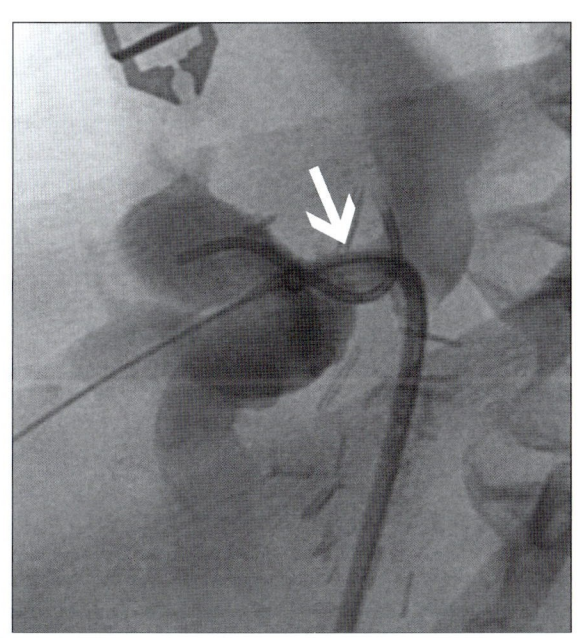

Figure 1. Hepatic venogram shows a focal stenosis at the confluence of the hepatic veins and IVC *(arrow)*. This stenosis was associated with a pressure gradient of 12 mm Hg.

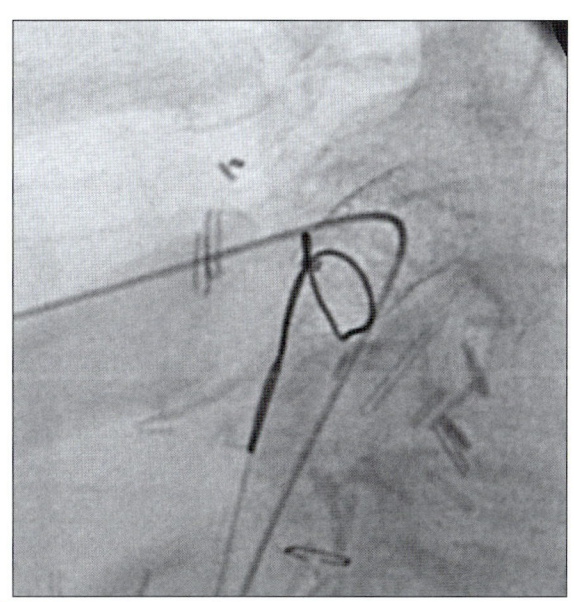

Figure 3. The bottom of the stent was grasped with a 15-mm gooseneck snare.

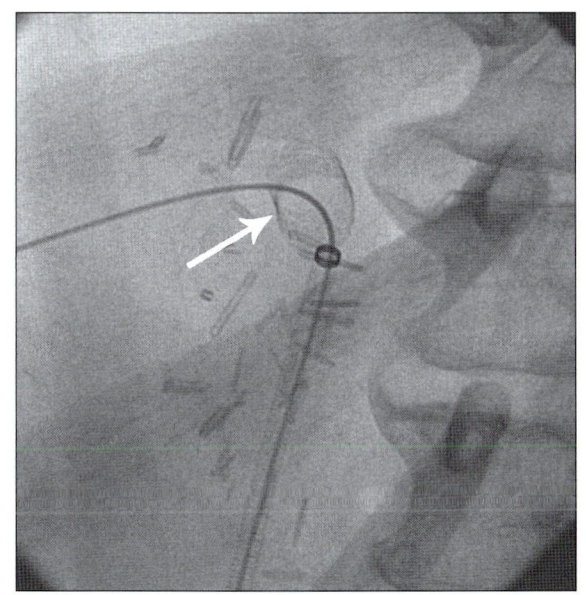

Figure 2. Immediately after stent deployment, the stent migrated back into the IVC *(arrow)*. Leaving the guidewire in place prevented further migration of the stent.

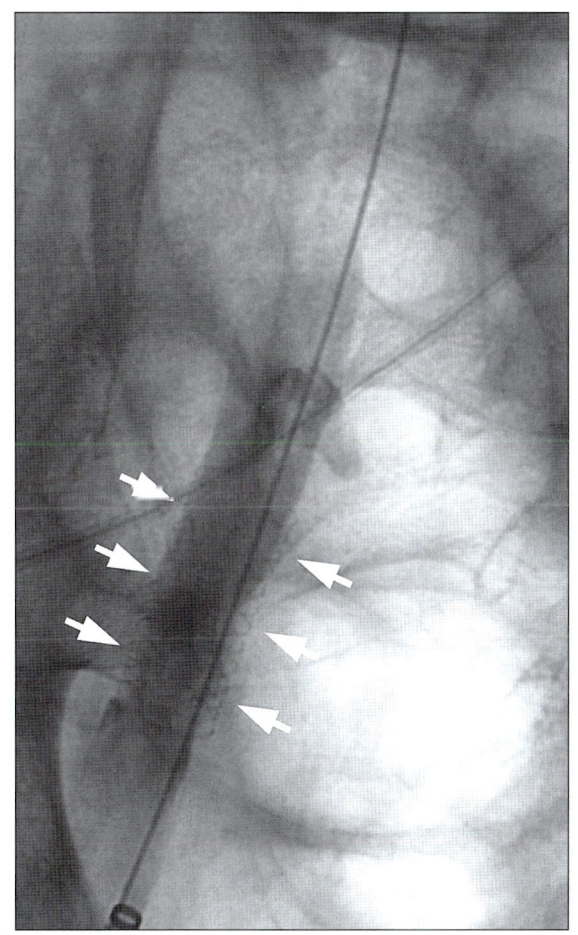

Figure 4. The stent was pulled down into the right external iliac vein *(arrows)*. The stent was then balloon dilated to stabilize its position.

Case 228

DEMOGRAPHICS/CLINICAL HISTORY

A 23-year-old woman with non-target coil embolization during splenic artery embolization.

DISCUSSION

History/Indications for Procedure
A 23-year-old woman with hematemesis secondary to gastric varices. The varices are the result of compression of the splenic vein by a large left upper quadrant solid pseudopapillary pancreatic tumor.

Procedure
Retrieval of lost embolization coil

Pre-procedure Imaging
MRI of the abdomen shows a 15-cm mass arising from the pancreatic tail (not shown). Multiple varices are present in the gastrohepatic ligament.

Intraprocedural Findings
The splenic artery was embolized with coils; final contrast injection caused one of the coils to dislodge and to migrate to the distal right hepatic artery (Fig. 1). The coil was retrieved with a 5-mm gooseneck snare (Figs. 2 and 3).

Follow-up and Complications
Following coil retrieval, repeat hepatic arteriogram shows mild vasospasm in the right hepatic artery (Fig. 4). The hepatic artery remained patent.

Suggested Readings

Dondelinger RF, Lepoutre B, Kurdziel JC: Percutaneous vascular foreign body retrieval: Experience of an 11-year period. Eur J Radiol 12:4-10, 1991.

Gabelmann A, Kramer S, Gorich J: Percutaneous retrieval of lost or misplaced intravascular objects. AJR Am J Roentgenol 176: 1509-1513, 2001.

Uflacker R, Lima S, Melichar AC: Intravascular foreign bodies: Percutaneous retrieval. Radiology 160:731-735, 1986.

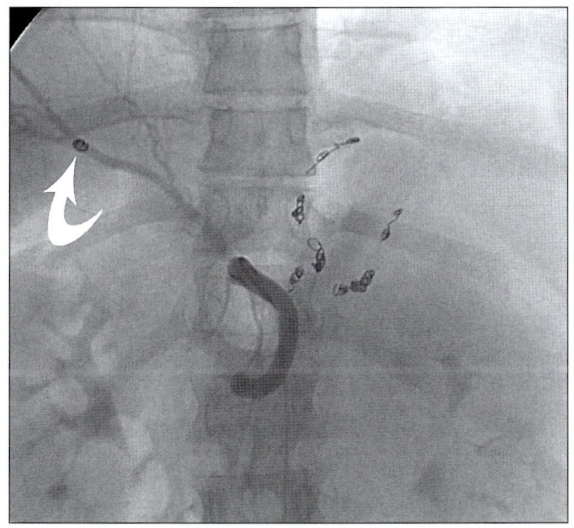

Figure 1. Celiac arteriogram after splenic artery embolization. A coil has embolized to the right hepatic artery *(curved arrow)*.

Figure 2. The right hepatic artery was catheterized, and the coil was snared.

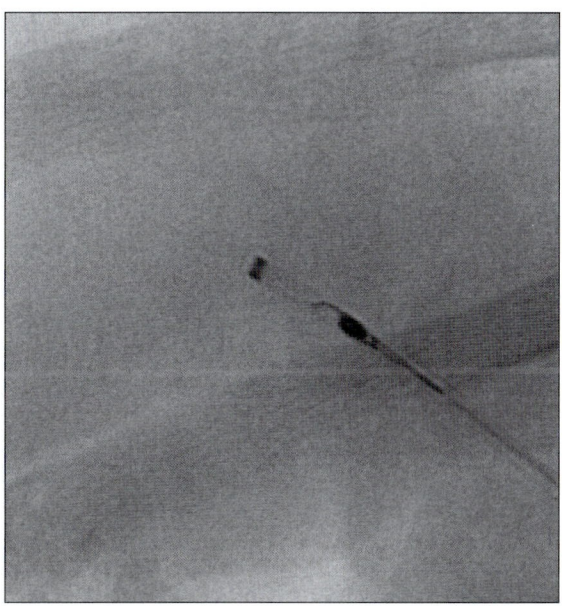

Figure 3. The snared coil was withdrawn into the guiding sheath.

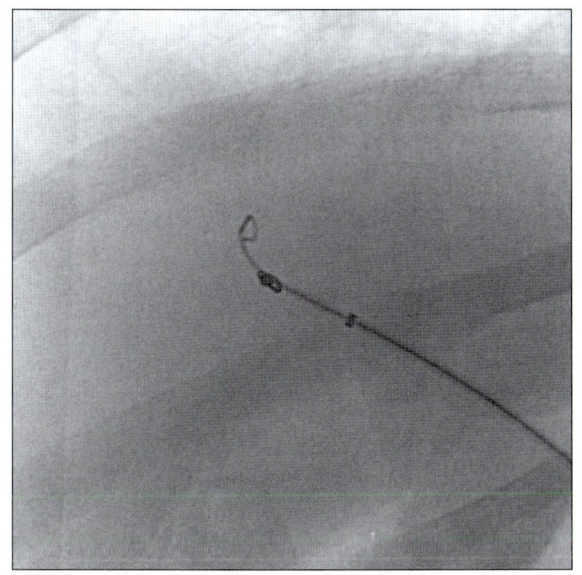

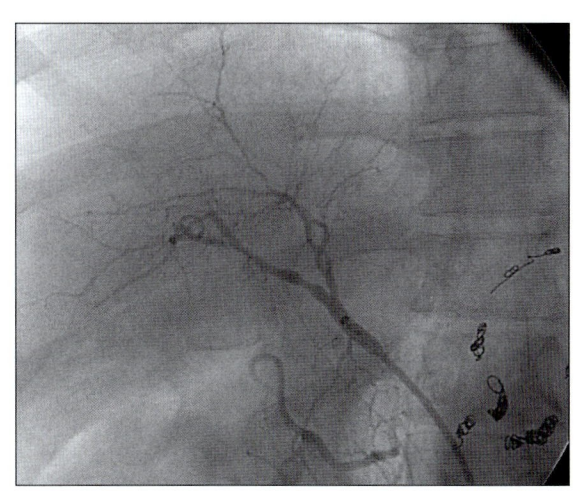

Figure 4. Follow-up angiogram after coil removal shows continued patency of the right hepatic artery.

Case 229

DEMOGRAPHICS/CLINICAL HISTORY

A 17-year-old boy with recurrent, left-sided varicocele, undergoing embolization.

DISCUSSION

History/Indications for Procedure
A 17-year-old boy has an asymptomatic, recurrent, left-sided varicocele. He underwent surgical ligation 1 year before presentation.

Procedure
Varicocele embolization

Intraprocedural Findings
The valves of the left testicular vein are incompetent, allowing for free reflux (Fig. 1). The left testicular vein was embolized with coils starting at the level of the inguinal canal (Figs. 2 to 4).

Follow-up and Complications
The patient recovered uneventfully from the procedure and has had no evidence of varicocele recurrence in the 3 years since the embolization.

Suggested Readings
Demas BE, Hricak H, McClure RD: Varicoceles: Radiologic diagnosis and treatment. Radiol Clin North Am 29:619-627, 1991.
Evers JLH, Collins JA: Assessment of efficacy of varicocele repair for male subfertility: A systematic review. Lancet 361:1849-1852, 2003.
Kass EJ: Adolescent varicocele. Pediatr Clin North Am 48:1559-1569, 2001.
Zuckerman AM, Michell SE, Venbrux AC: Percutaneous varicocele occlusion: Long-term follow-up. J Vasc Intervent Radiol 5:315-319, 1994.

Case 229   459

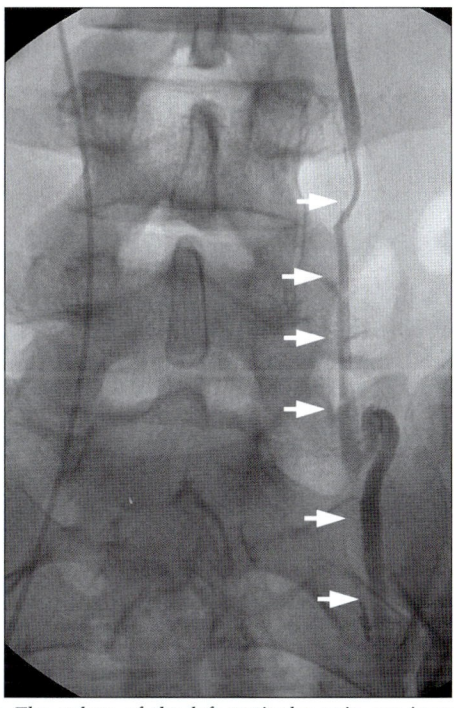

Figure 1. The valves of the left testicular vein are incompetent, allowing for free reflux *(arrows)*.

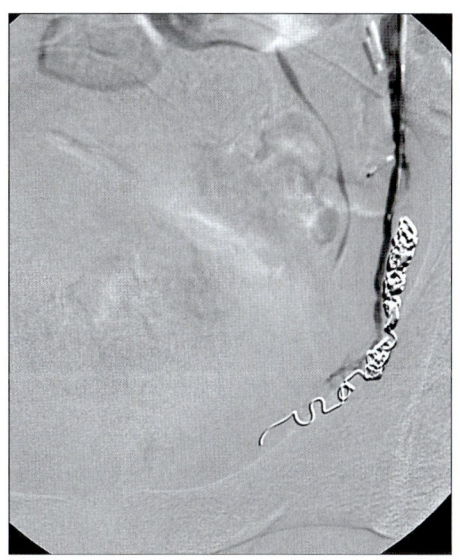

Figure 2. The left testicular vein was embolized with coils, starting at about the level of the inguinal canal.

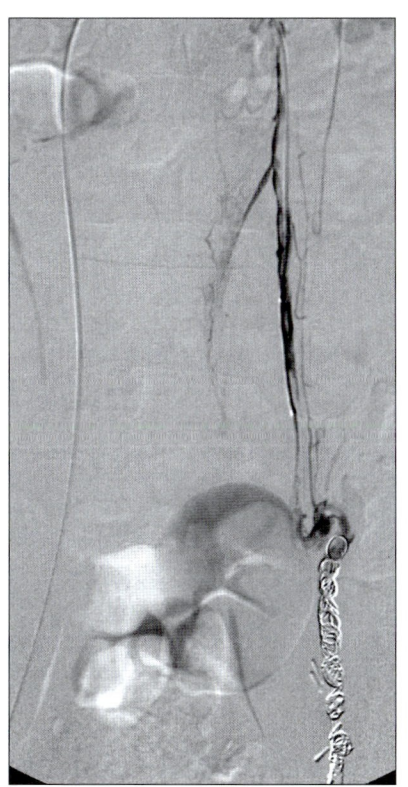

Figure 3. As the testicular vein is embolized, several small collateral veins are visualized.

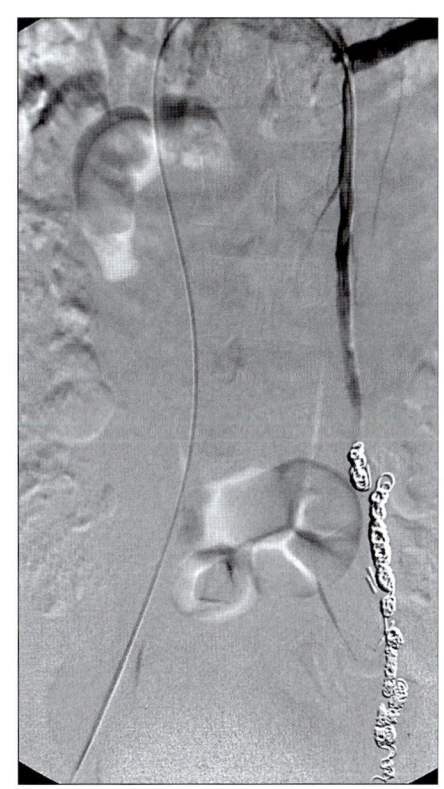

Figure 4. The left testicular vein was packed with coils.

Case 230

DEMOGRAPHICS/CLINICAL HISTORY

A 14-year-old boy with persistent varicocele despite surgical intervention, undergoing ultrasonography and venography.

DISCUSSION

History/Indications for Procedure
A 14-year-old boy has a grade 3 left varicocele. The dilated veins have persisted despite undergoing laparoscopic varicocelectomy 2 years earlier.

Procedure
Varicocele embolization

Pre-procedure Imaging
Testicular ultrasound demonstrates a dilated pampiniform plexus on the left. The veins prominently distend with Valsalva maneuvers (Fig. 1).

Intraprocedural Findings
Left gonadal venography shows reflux to the level of the surgical clips in the pelvis (Fig. 2). The entire length of the left gonadal vein was embolized with coils from the level of the inguinal canal to the left renal vein (Fig. 3).

Follow-up and Complications
At the 1-week follow-up examination, the patient had returned to normal activity. The varicocele had significantly diminished (Fig. 4), and the patient has not had any evidence of recurrence 1 year since the procedure.

Suggested Readings
Chalmers N, Hufton AP, Jackson RW, Conway B: Radiation risk in varicocele embolization. Br J Radiol 73:293-297, 2000.

Demas BE, Hricak H, McClure RD: Varicoceles: Radiologic diagnosis and treatment. Radiol Clin North Am 29:619-627, 1991.

Zuckerman AM, Mitchell SE, Venbrux AC, et al: Percutaneous varicocele occlusion: Long-term follow-up. J Vasc Intervent Radiol 5:315-319, 1994.

Venbrux AC, Tretotola SO: Transcatheter embolotherapy of varicoceles. Semin Intervent Radiol 11:305-311, 1994.

Case 230   461

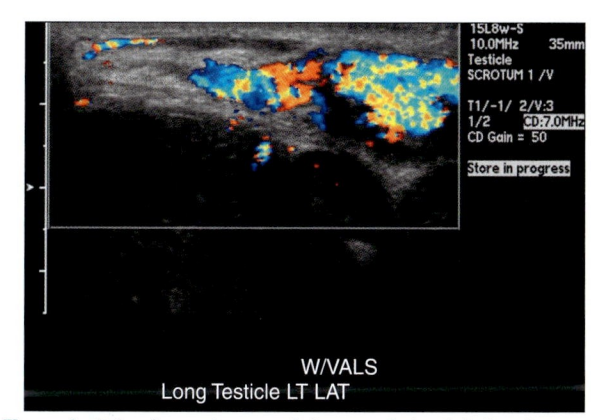

Figure 1. Color-flow ultrasound image of the left hemiscrotum during a Valsalva maneuver shows filling of multiple prominent veins.

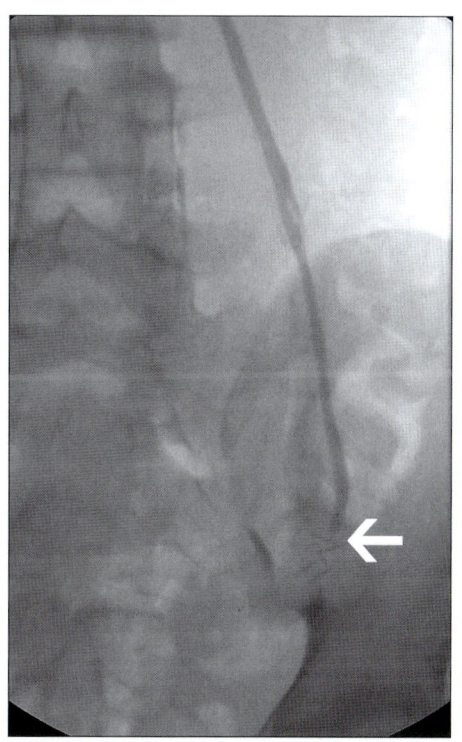

Figure 2. Left gonadal venogram shows reflux to the level of the surgical clips *(arrow)*.

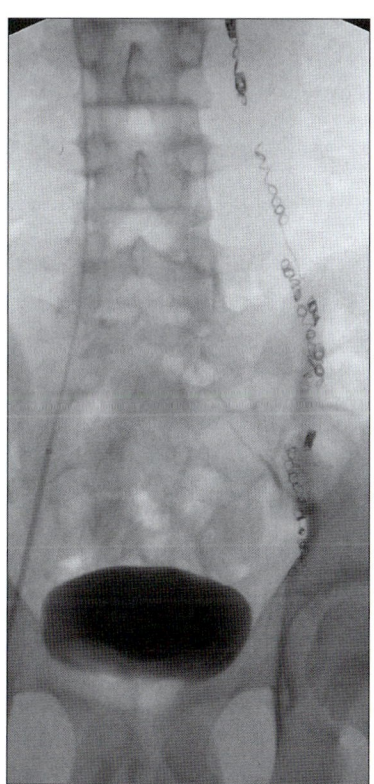

Figure 3. The left gonadal vein was embolized with coils starting at the level of the inguinal canal.

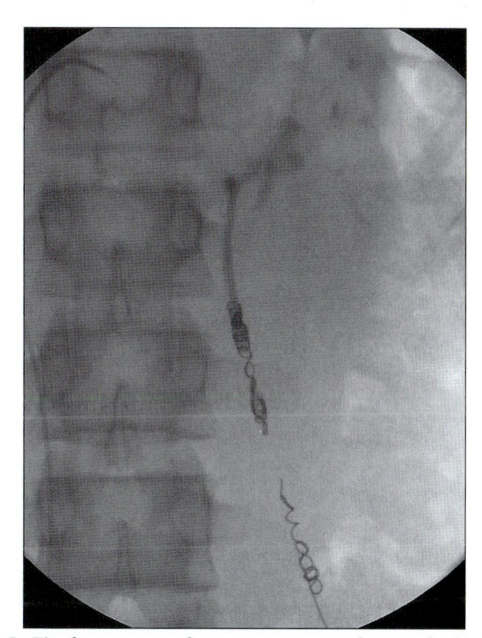

Figure 4. Final venogram demonstrates complete occlusion of the left gonadal vein.

Case 231

DEMOGRAPHICS/CLINICAL HISTORY
A 33-year-old man with infertility.

DISCUSSION

History/Indications for Procedure
A 33-year-old man with infertility. The patient has a palpable varicocele on physical exam.

Procedure
Gonadal vein embolization for the treatment of a left-sided varicocele

Pre-procedure Imaging
Scrotal ultrasound shows multiple prominent veins in the left hemiscrotum consistent with a varicocele (Fig. 1).

Intraprocedural Findings
There is reflux in the left gonadal vein, filling a dilated venous plexus in the left hemiscrotum (Figs. 2, 3). The left gonadal vein was embolized with coils from the level of the inguinal canal to the left renal vein (Fig. 4).

Follow-up and Complications
The patient recovered uneventfully from the embolization, and the varicocele was palpably smaller on physical exam 3 weeks after the embolization.

Suggested Readings
Evers JLH, Collins JA: Assessment of efficacy of varicocele repair for male subfertility: A systematic review. Lancet 361:1849-1852, 2003.

Demas BE, Hricak H, McClure RD: Varicoceles: Radiologic diagnosis and treatment. Radiol Clin North Am 29:619-627, 1991.

Jarow JP: Effects of varicocele on male infertility. Hum Reprod Update 7:59-64, 2001.

Zuckerman AM, Michell SE, Venbrux AC: Percutaneous varicocele occlusion: Long-term follow-up. J Vasc Intervent Radiol 5:315-319, 1994.

Case 231   463

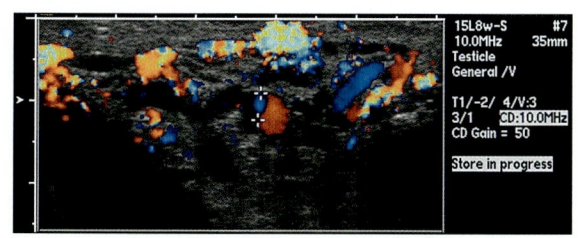

Figure 1. Color Doppler ultrasound shows multiple dilated veins in the left hemiscrotum consistent with a varicocele.

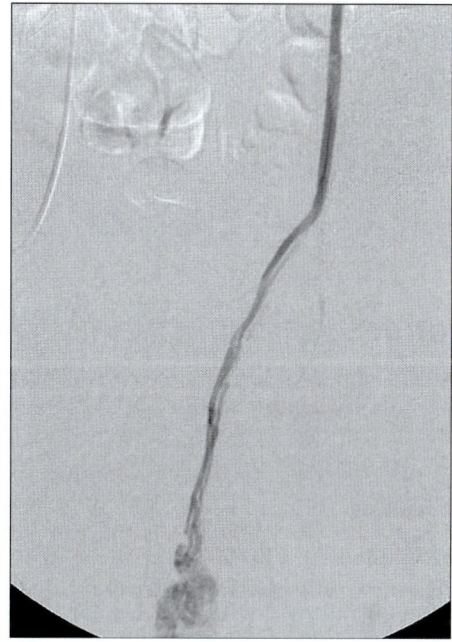

Figure 2. Selective injection of the left gonadal vein shows reflux to the scrotum with partial visualization of the dilated pampiniform plexus.

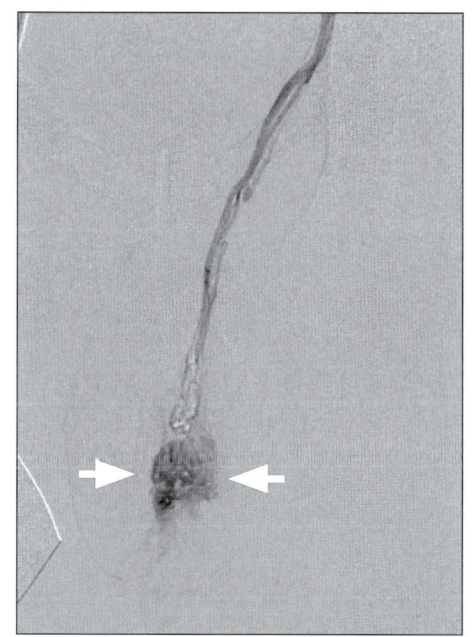

Figure 3. Slightly more caudal image again shows filling of the dilated pampiniform plexus *(arrows)*.

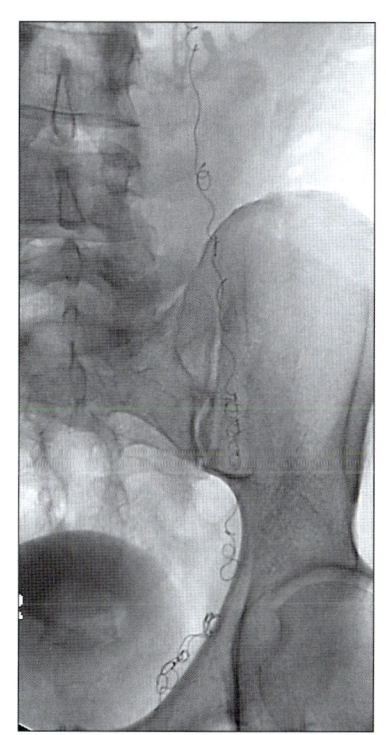

Figure 4. The left gonadal vein was embolized with coils from the level of the pubic symphysis to the left renal vein.

Case 232

DEMOGRAPHICS/CLINICAL HISTORY

A 36-year-old woman with pelvic pain and vulvar varices, undergoing venography.

DISCUSSION

History/Indications for Procedure
A 36-year-old woman presents with an 8-month history of significant pelvic pain that is of sufficient severity to limit her ability to work, and occasionally requires high-dose narcotics for pain relief. On physical examination, vaginal and labial varicose veins are identified.

procedure
Gonadal vein embolization, pelvic varicosities

Intraprocedural Findings
The gonadal veins are enlarged and incompetent bilaterally, and large pelvic varicosities are identified (Figs. 1-3). The pelvic varicosities were sclerosed with 3% sodium tetradecyl sulfate, and the entire length of both gonadal veins was embolized with coils (Fig. 4).

Follow-up and Complications
The patient's symptoms were improved on follow-up. The labial varicosities were significantly reduced on follow-up physical examination.

Suggested Readings
Ganeshan A, Upponi S, Hon LQ, et al: Chronic pelvic pain due to pelvic congestion syndrome: The role of diagnostic and interventional radiology. Cardiovasc Intervent Radiol 30:1105, 2007.

Kim HS, Malhotra AD, Rowe PC, et al: Embolotherapy for pelvic congestion syndrome: Long-term results. J Vasc Intervent Radiol 17:289, 2006.

Maleux G, Stockx L, Wilms G, et al: Ovarian vein embolization for the treatment of pelvic congestion syndrome: Long-term technical and clinical results. J Vasc Intervent Radiol 11:859, 2000.

Venbrux AC, Chang AH, Kim HS, et al: Pelvic congestion syndrome (pelvic venous incompetence): Impact of ovarian and internal iliac vein embolotherapy on menstrual cycle and chronic pelvic pain. J Vasc Intervent Radiol 13:171, 2002.

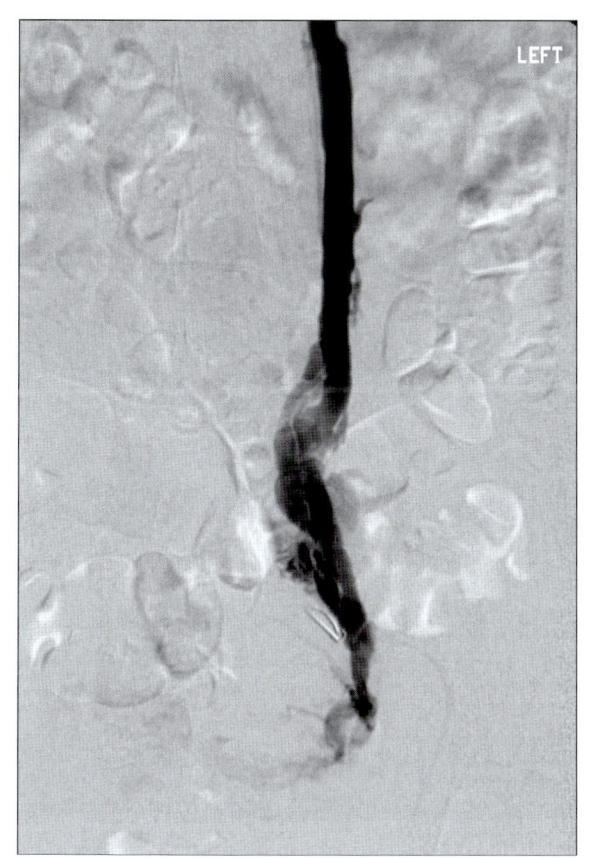

Figure 1. Left gonadal venogram. Direct injection of left gonadal vein shows vein to be enlarged and incompetent.

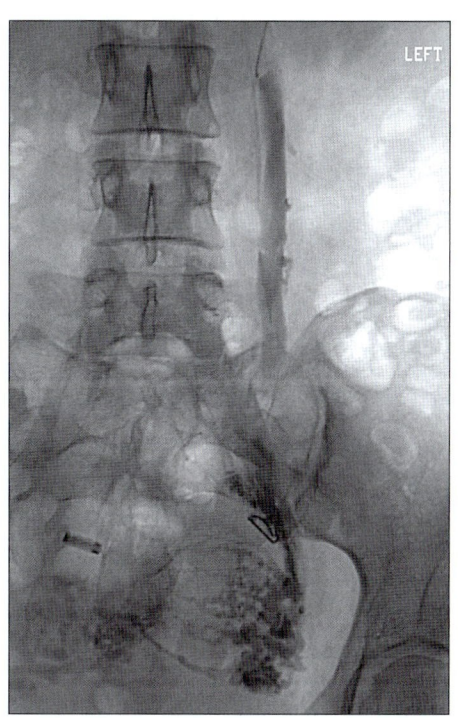

Figure 2. Delayed image left gonadal venogram. There is filling of numerous pelvic varicosities supplied by left ovarian vein.

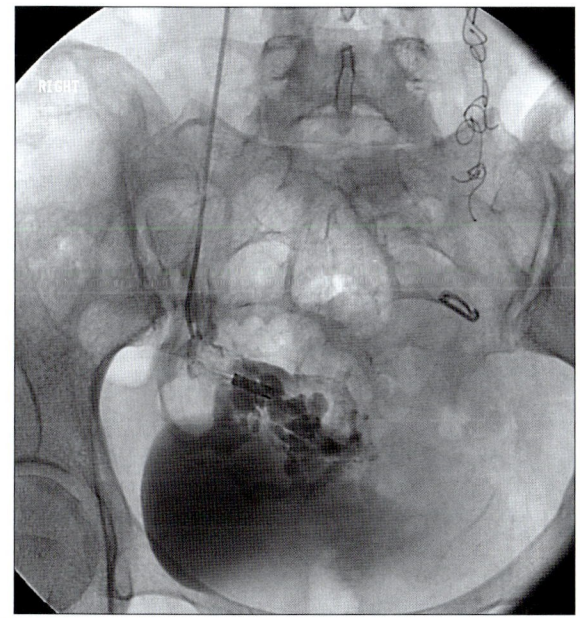

Figure 3. Selective injection of caudal right gonadal vein. There is opacification of numerous large pelvic varicosities.

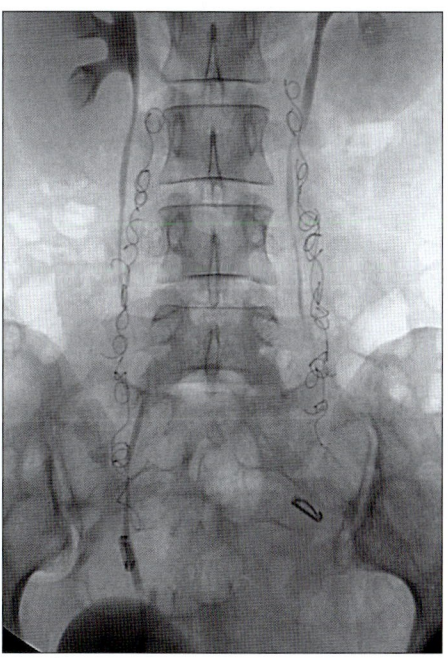

Figure 4. Final image. Entire length of both gonadal veins was embolized with coils.

Case 233

DEMOGRAPHICS/CLINICAL HISTORY

A 53-year-old woman with pelvic congestion syndrome.

DISCUSSION

History/Indications for Procedure
A 53-year-old woman with painful pelvic and buttock varicose veins since her pregnancy 20 years earlier. She reports pelvic heaviness and aching while standing.

Procedure
Bilateral ovarian vein embolization for pelvic congestion syndrome

Pre-procedure Imaging
Contrast-enhanced CT of the abdomen and pelvis shows enlarged ovarian veins bilaterally with pelvic varicosities.

Intraprocedural Findings
The ovarian veins are enlarged and incompetent bilaterally with filling of large pelvic varicose veins (Figs. 1, 2, and 3). The pelvic varicosities were sclerosed with a mixture of 3% Sotradecol and Gelfoam, and the entire length of the ovarian veins was embolized with coils (Fig. 4).

Follow-up and Complications
The patient's symptoms significantly improved after the embolization. She reported continued discomfort from an enlarged gluteal varix that was treated with direct injection of 1.5% Sotradecol.

Suggested Readings
Kim HS, Malhotra AD, Rowe PC, et al: Embolotherapy for pelvic congestion syndrome: Long-term results. J Vasc Intervent Radiol 17:289-297, 2006.

Maleux G, Stockx L, Wilms G, Marchal G: Ovarian vein embolization for the treatment of pelvic congestion syndrome: Long-term technical and clinical results. J Vasc Intervent Radiol 11:859-864, 2000.

Venbrux AC, Chang AH, Kim HS, et al: Pelvic congestion syndrome (pelvic venous incompetence): Impact of ovarian and internal iliac vein embolotherapy on menstrual cycle and chronic pelvic pain. J Vasc Intervent Radiol 13:171-178, 2002.

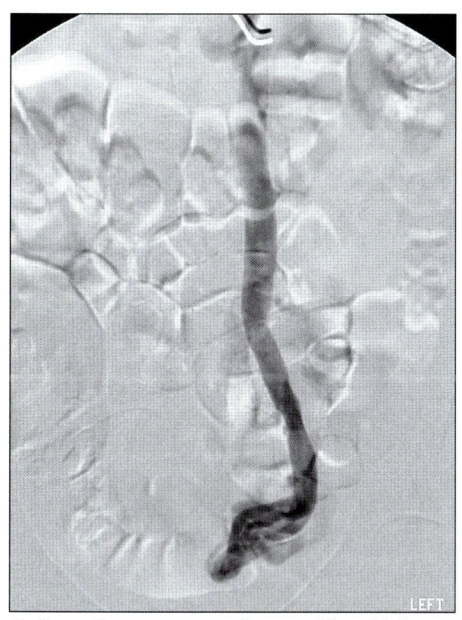

Figure 1. Left ovarian venogram shows a dilated left ovarian vein with filling of pelvic varices.

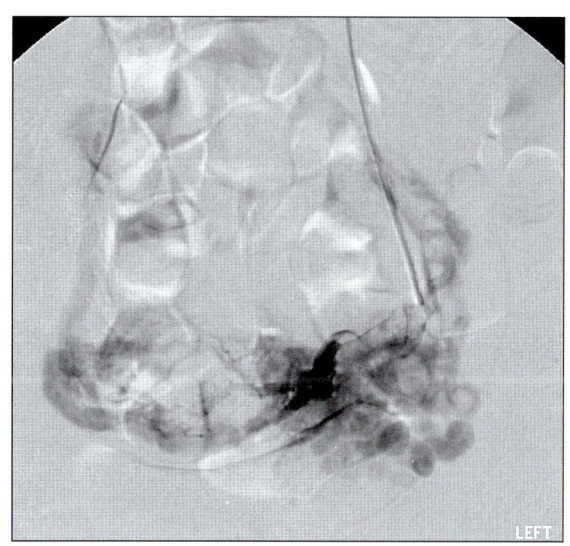

Figure 2. Selective injection of the left ovarian vein at the level of the pelvis shows filling of large bilateral pelvic varicosities.

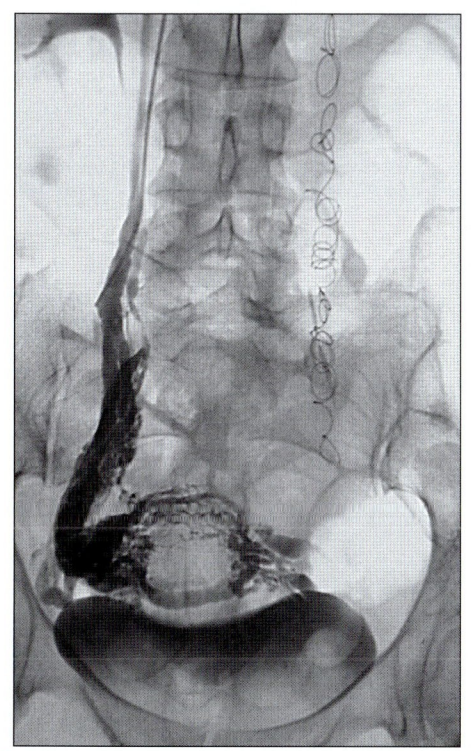

Figure 3. Selective right ovarian venogram also shows filling of multiple pelvic varicosities.

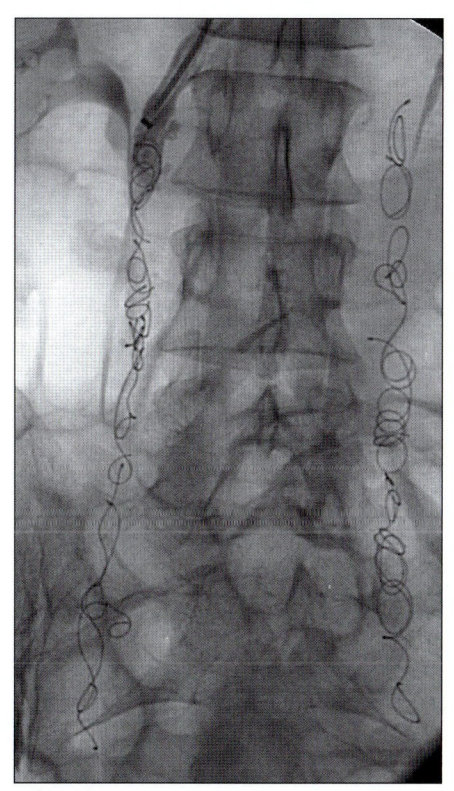

Figure 4. Bilateral ovarian veins were embolized with coils. The embolization was performed from the level of the SI joints to the origin of the ovarian veins.

Case 234

Susan Weeks, MD

DEMOGRAPHICS/CLINICAL HISTORY

A 55-year-old woman with a 10-year history of painful, heavy lower extremities.

DISCUSSION

History/Indications for Procedure
A 55-year-old woman with a 10-year history of painful, heavy lower extremities.

Procedure
Endovenous laser ablation of the great saphenous vein

Pre-procedure Imaging
Ultrasound examination demonstrates a normal deep venous system, without deep vein thrombosis or reflux, and significant reflux in the great saphenous vein (GSV) peripheral to the subterminal valve (Fig. 1).

Intraprocedural Findings
Following ultrasound-guided access to the GSV at the level of the knee, the tip of laser fiber (Angiodynamics, Queensbury, NY) was advanced to approximately 1.5 cm peripheral to the saphenofemoral junction (SFJ) (Fig. 2), and 250 mL of tumescent anesthetic was administered circumferentially around the vein along the entire length of the vein to be treated (Fig. 3). Following ablation of the vein, repeat ultrasound was performed, demonstrating patency of the saphenofemoral junction and no flow within the treated GSV.

Follow-up and Complications
The patient returned one week later with some mild bruising and tightness in the medial thigh (not unexpected), and repeat ultrasound demonstrated no deep vein thrombosis, patency of the SFJ, and occlusion of the treated GSV (Fig. 4). One month later, she reported notable improvement in her symptoms.

Suggested Readings
Min RJ: Interventional radiology of venous insufficiency. In Baum S, Pentecost MJ, editors. Abrams' Angiography Interventional Radiology. Philadelphia: Lippincott Williams & Wilkins, 2006: 1099-1109.

Min RJ, Khilnani N, Zimmet SE: Endovenous laser treatment of saphenous vein reflux: Long-term results. J Vasc Intervent Radiol 14:991-996, 2003.

Tipperman PE: Endovenous laser treatment of incompetent below-knee great saphenous veins. J Vasc Intervent Radiol 18:1495-1499, 2007.

Case 234   469

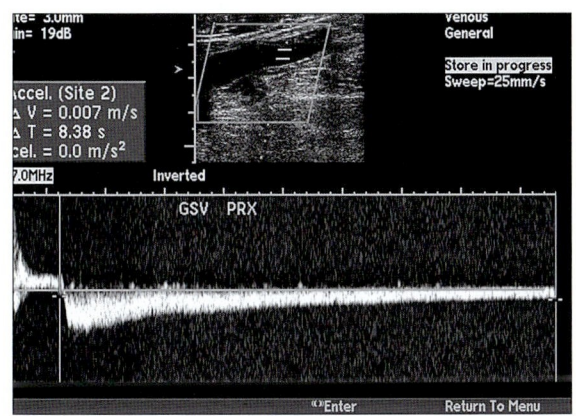

Figure 1. Abnormal reflux greater than 8 seconds within the central aspect of the great saphenous vein.

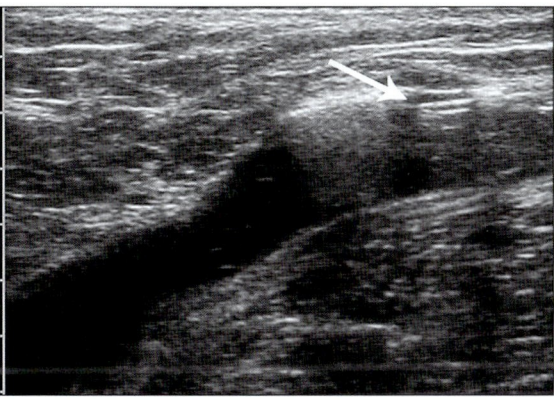

Figure 2. Laser fiber tip *(arrow)* placement approximately 1.5 cm peripheral to the SFJ.

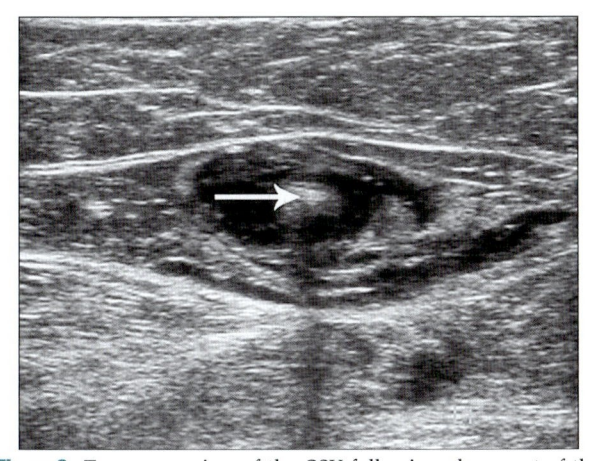

Figure 3. Transverse view of the GSV following placement of the laser fiber *(arrow)* and administration of tumescent anesthetic. Note the spasm of the vein around the catheter.

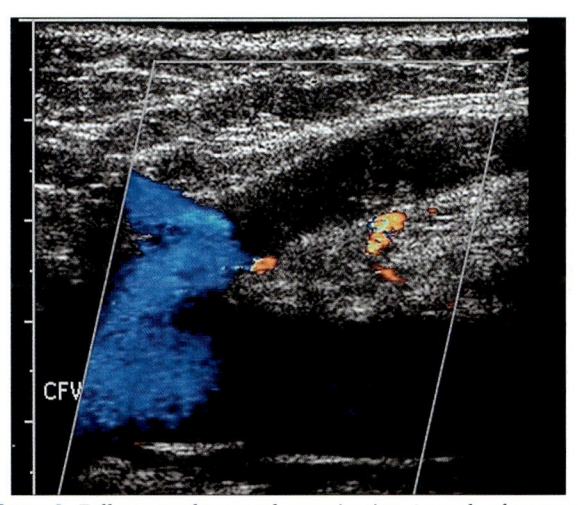

Figure 4. Follow-up ultrasound examination 1 week after treatment, demonstrating patency of the SFJ and occlusion of the treated GSV.

Case 235

DEMOGRAPHICS/CLINICAL HISTORY

A 77-year-old woman with cirrhosis of unknown origin, undergoing magnetic resonance imaging (MRI) and transjugular liver biopsy.

DISCUSSION

History/Indications for Procedure
A 77-year-old woman with cirrhosis of unknown origin.

Procedure
Transjugular liver biopsy

Pre-procedure Imaging
MRI demonstrated a small, nodular liver with gastroesophageal, perisplenic, and paraumbilical varices.

Intraprocedural Findings
Pressure measurements were obtained, and the corrected sinusoidal gradient measured 20 mm Hg. A transjugular liver biopsy was performed from a right internal jugular approach, and because of the acute angle between the inferior vena cava and hepatic vein, a 9-French transjugular intrahepatic portosystemic shunt (TIPSS) sheath was needed to advance the biopsy cannula into the hepatic vein (Figs. 1 to 4).

Follow-up and Complications
Pathologic analysis of the specimen revealed chronic hepatitis, but the caused was not determined.

Suggested Readings
McAfee JH, Keeffe EB, Lee RG, Rösch J: Transjugular liver biopsy. Hepatology 15:726-732, 1992.

Miraglia R, Luca A, Gruttadauria S, et al: Contribution of transjugular liver biopsy in patients with the clinical presentation of acute liver failure. Cardiovasc Intervent Radiol 29:1008-1010, 2006.

Velt PM, Choy OG, Shimkin PM, Link RJ: Transjugular liver biopsy in high-risk patients with hepatic disease. Radiology 153:91-93, 1984.

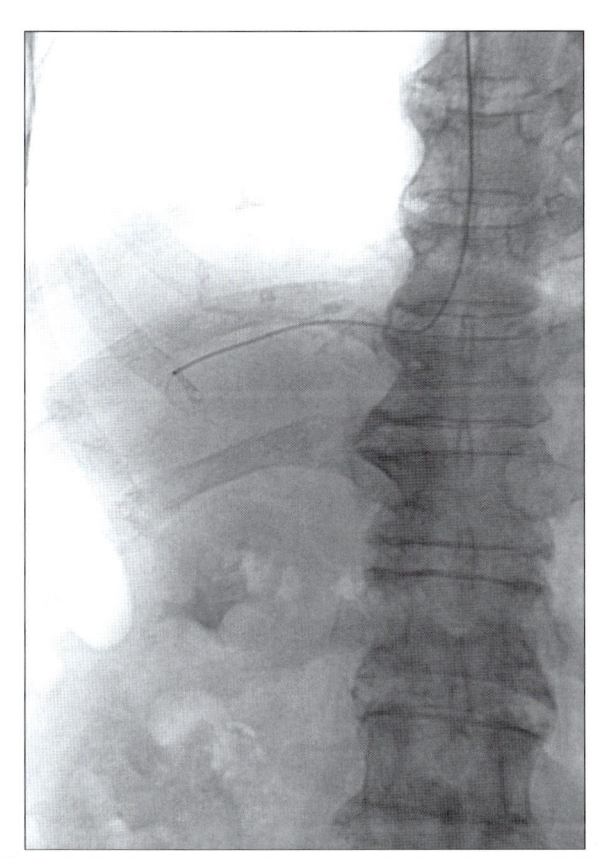

Figure 1. Single image from the transjugular liver biopsy with the guidewire positioned in the hepatic vein. Notice the acute angle between the hepatic vein and inferior vena cava. The biopsy cannula could not be advanced into the hepatic vein, despite the use of stiff guidewires.

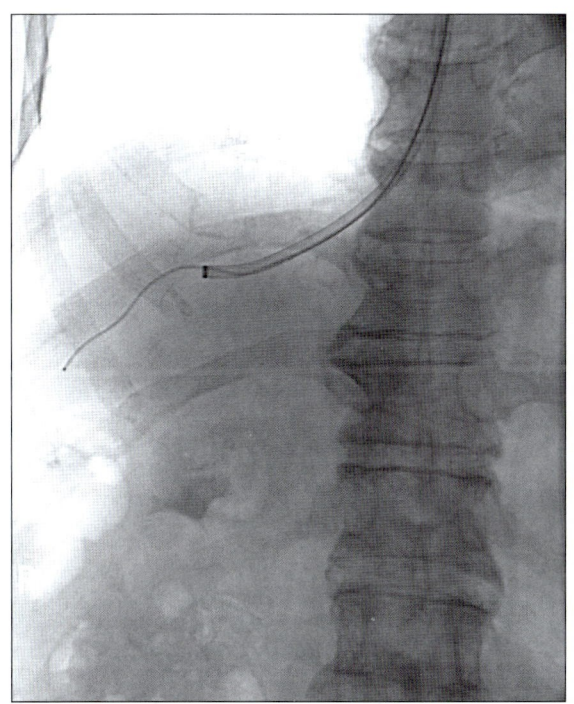

Figure 2. A 9-French TIPSS sheath was advanced into the hepatic vein.

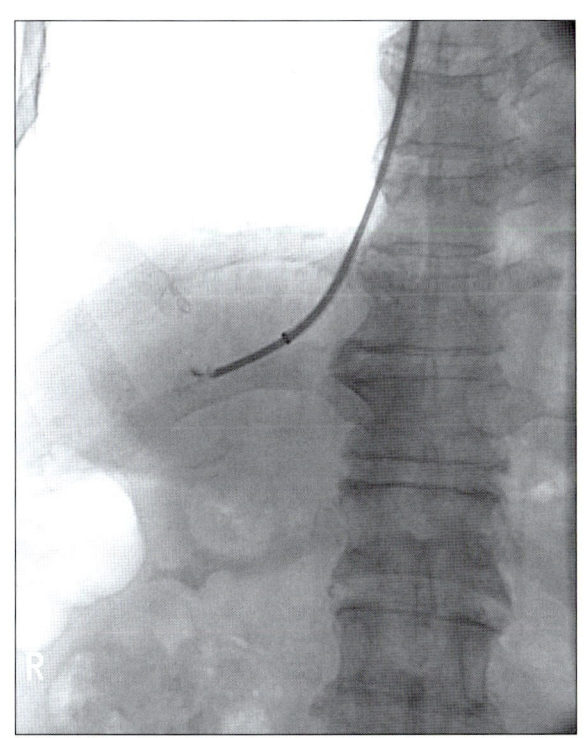

Figure 3. The biopsy cannula was then advanced through the TIPSS sheath into the hepatic vein.

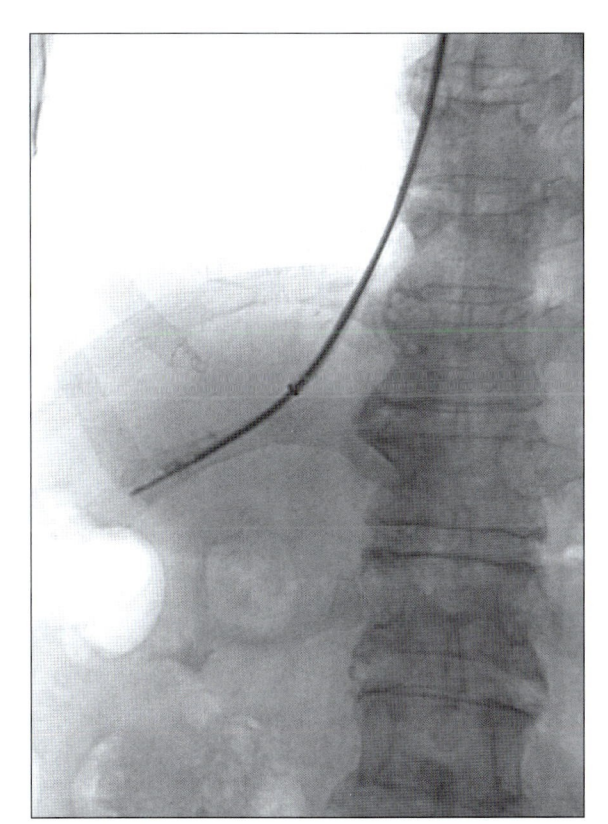

Figure 4. A spot fluoroscopic image was obtained while taking a specimen. The needle has been advanced into the middle third of the hepatic parenchyma.

Case 236

DEMOGRAPHICS/CLINICAL HISTORY

A 43-year-old woman who previously underwent resection of a malignant adrenal gland mass presents with new mass in the inferior vena cava.

DISCUSSION

History/Indications for Procedure
A 43-year-old woman with a history of prior resection of a 16-cm adrenal cortical carcinoma. Two months after resection, the patient presents with an asymptomatic mass in the inferior vena cava (IVC).

Procedure
Transvenous biopsy of inferior vena cava mass

Pre-procedure Imaging
Contrast-enhanced MRI shows a large mass in the suprarenal IVC that is hyperintense on precontrast T1 and T2 sequences (Fig. 1). PET scan shows intense fluorodeoxyglucose (FDG) uptake within the mass (Fig. 2).

Intraprocedural Findings
Inferior vena cavogram performed from a right common femoral venous approach shows a large filling defect within the suprarenal IVC (Fig. 3). The mass was biopsied using an 18-gauge transvenous biopsy needle (Quick-core, Cook, Bloomington, IN) (Fig. 4).

Follow-up and Complications
Histologic examination of the specimen confirmed recurrent adrenal cortical carcinoma.

Suggested Readings
Krieves D, Keller FS, Dotter CT, et al: Percutaneous intravenous biopsy. Diagn Imaging 49:297-302, 1980.

Withers CE, Casola G, Herba MJ, et al: Intravascular tumors: Transvenous biopsy. Radiology 167:713-715, 1988.

Case 236   473

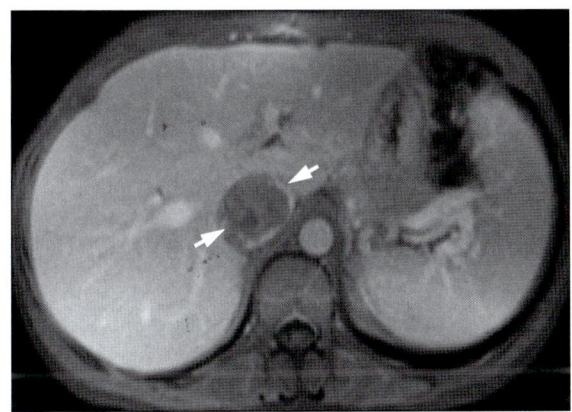

Figure 1. T1, post-contrast, fat-saturated MR image through the upper abdomen shows a large, heterogeneous mass in the inferior vena cava (arrows).

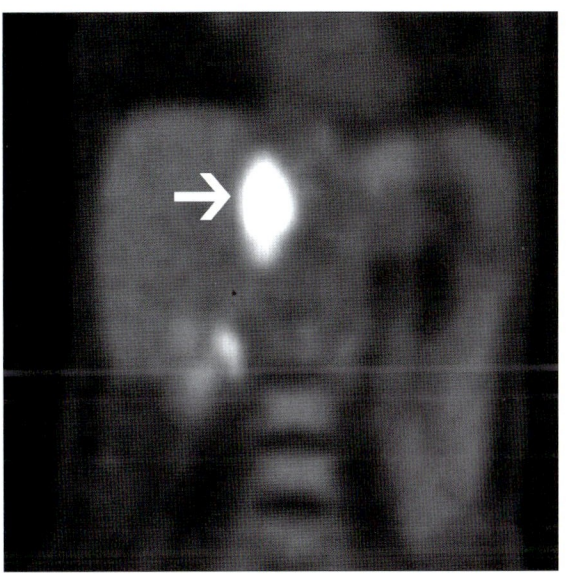

Figure 2. Coronal image from FDG-PET scan shows intense radiotracer uptake in the suprarenal IVC (arrow).

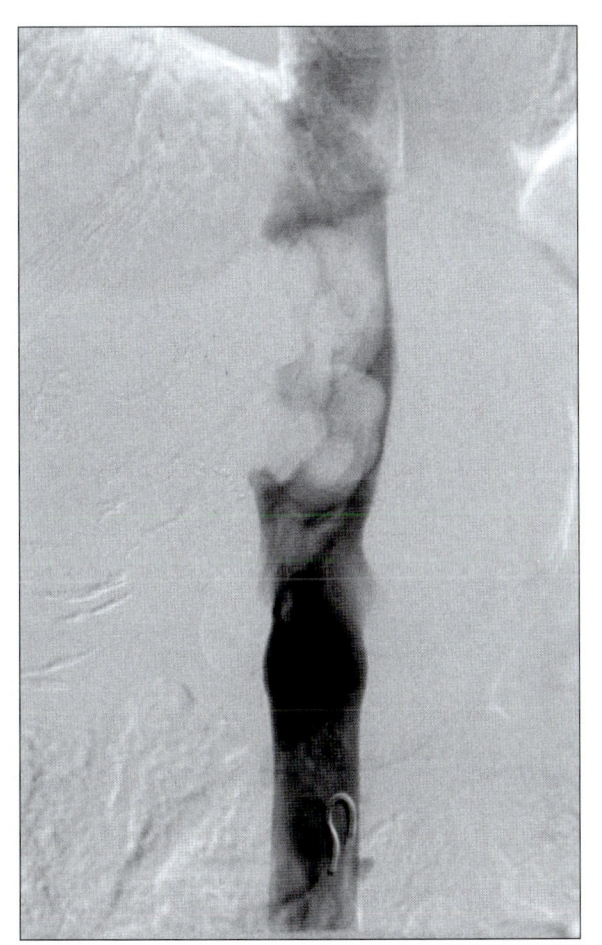

Figure 3. Inferior vena cavogram shows a large lobulated filling defect in the suprarenal IVC.

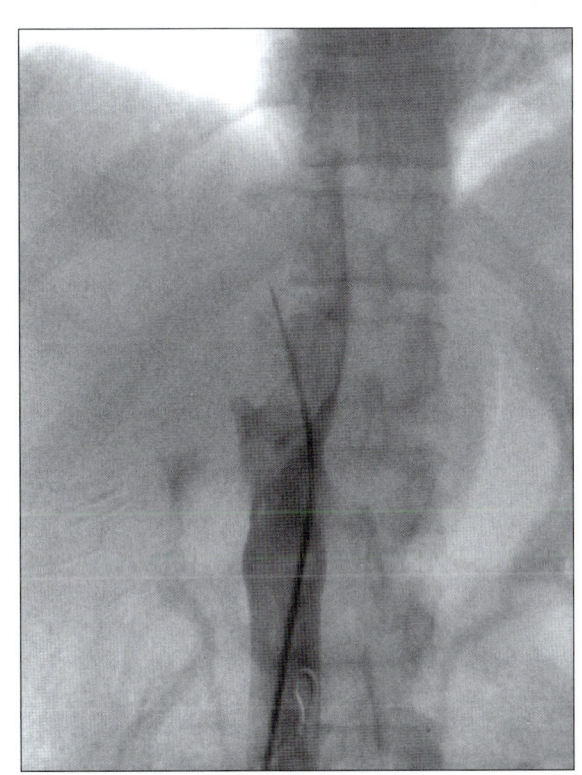

Figure 4. An 18-gauge transvenous biopsy needle is used to obtain tissue samples. The location of the mass is identified by an image overlay from the earlier venogram.

Case 237

DEMOGRAPHICS/CLINICAL HISTORY

A 71-year-old woman with a liver mass, undergoing MRI and ultrasound.

DISCUSSION

History/Indications for Procedure
A 71-year-old woman had idiopathic hepatic cirrhosis diagnosed 2 years earlier. A mass was identified on surveillance MRI, and α-fetoprotein levels are mildly elevated.

Procedure
Ultrasound-guided liver biopsy

Pre-procedure Imaging
Contrast-enhanced MR image of the abdomen shows a small, nodular liver with a 6.5-cm × 5-cm mass in the lateral segment of the left hepatic lobe (Fig. 1). A moderate volume of ascites is also present.

Intraprocedural Findings
A paracentesis was performed to reduce the volume of fluid around the liver. The mass was identified with ultrasound (Fig. 2), a 17-gauge coaxial needle was advanced to the edge of the mass (Fig. 3), and multiple core biopsy samples were obtained using an 18-guage automatic biopsy device (Fig. 4).

Follow-up and Complications
The specimen was sent to surgical pathology. Moderately differentiated hepatocellular carcinoma arising in a background of primary biliary cirrhosis was diagnosed.

Suggested Readings
Cardella JF, Bakal CW, Bertino RE, et al: Quality improvement guidelines for image-guided percutaneous biopsy in adults. J Vasc Intervent Radiol 14:S227, 2003.

Gupta S: New techniques in image-guided percutaneous biopsy. Cardiovasc Intervent Radiol 27:91, 2004.

Case 237   475

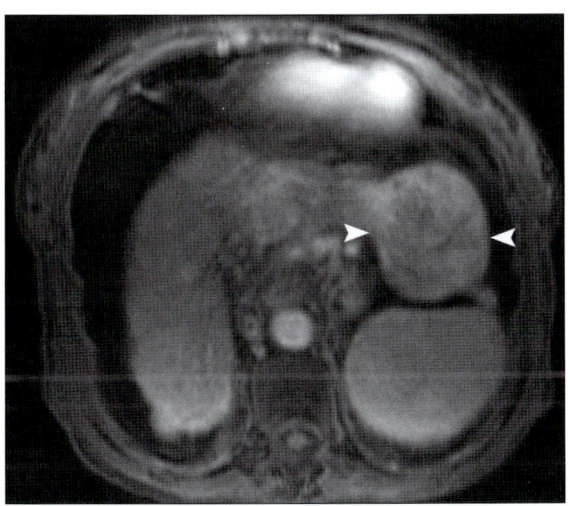

Figure 1. T1-weighted, fat-saturated, post-contrast MR image through liver shows 6.5-cm × 5-cm mass arising in lateral segment of left hepatic lobe *(arrowheads)*. The liver is small and nodular, and there is a moderate volume of perihepatic ascites.

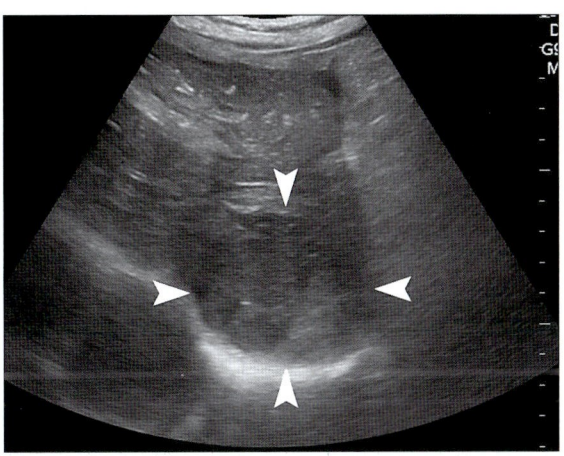

Figure 2. Ultrasound of liver performed at time of biopsy shows mass in lateral aspect of left hepatic lobe *(arrowheads)*. The mass is slightly hypoechoic relative to hepatic parenchyma.

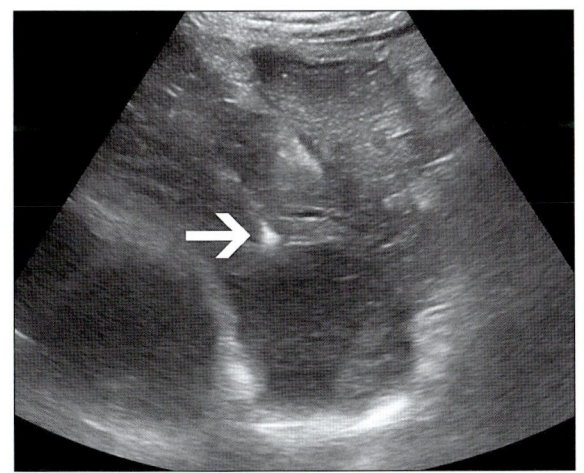

Figure 3. Ultrasound shows coaxial introducer needle has been advanced to edge of mass *(arrow)*.

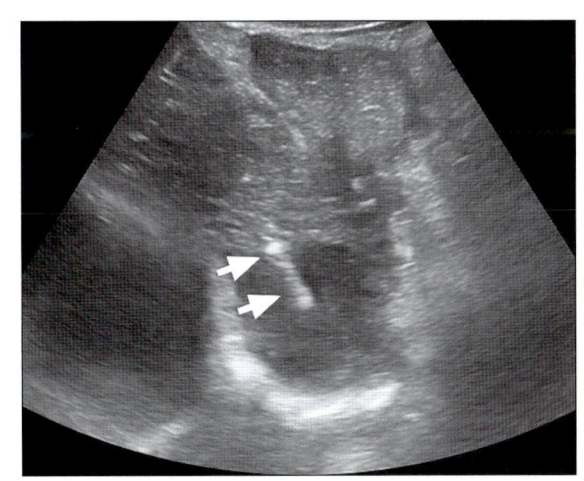

Figure 4. Multiple biopsy specimens were obtained through coaxial needle. This image shows biopsy device obtaining a sample of the periphery of mass *(arrows)*.

Case 238

DEMOGRAPHICS/CLINICAL HISTORY

A 55-year-old woman with left retroperitoneal mass, undergoing computed tomography (CT) and biopsy of a mass.

DISCUSSION

History/Indications for Procedure
A 55-year-old woman has increasing discomfort in the left lower quadrant.

Procedure
CT-guided pelvic mass biopsy

Pre-procedure Imaging
Contrast-enhanced CT demonstrates a 3.7-cm × 3.2-cm, low-density lesion abutting the left iliacus muscle (Fig. 1).

Intraprocedural Findings
Using CT guidance, several core biopsy samples were obtained using an 18-gauge, spring-loaded biopsy device (Fig. 2).

Follow-up and Complications
After the biopsy, the patient complained of pain in the biopsy site (Fig. 3) that extended into the anterior thigh, and a CT scan confirmed the presence of an intramuscular hematoma (Fig. 4). The pathologic examination result was most consistent with a schwannoma, and no intervention was required.

Suggested Readings
Cardella JF, Bakal CW, Bertino RE, et al: Quality improvement guidelines for image-guided percutaneous biopsy in adults. J Vasc Intervent Radiol 14(Pt 2):S227-S230, 2003.

Gupta S: New techniques in image-guided percutaneous biopsy. Cardiovasc Intervent Radiol 27:91-104, 2004.

Case 238   477

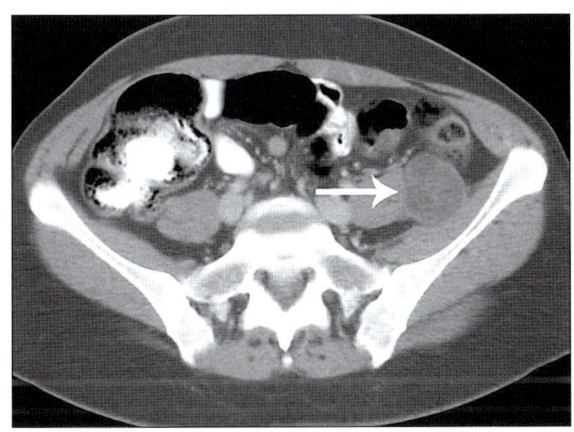

Figure 1. Contrast-enhanced, axial CT image through the pelvis shows a hypodense mass *(arrow)* adjacent to the left iliacus muscle.

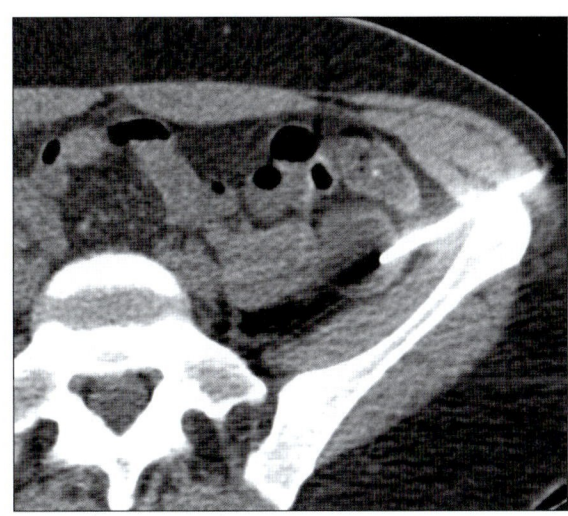

Figure 2. Using CT-guidance, a 17-gauge coaxial needle was placed into the mass.

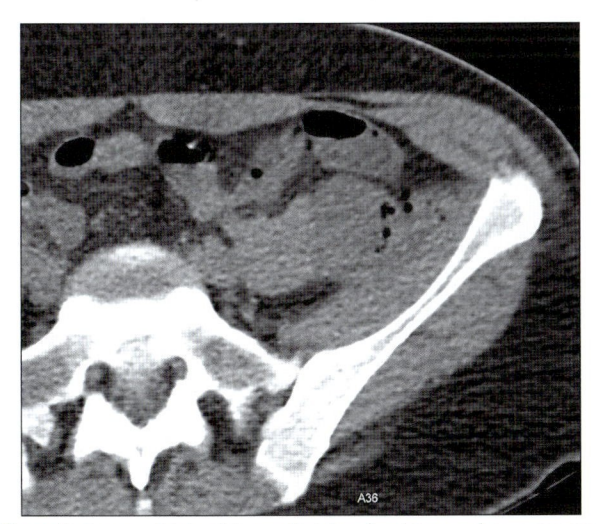

Figure 3. Image obtained immediately after biopsy shows gas and a small amount of fluid in the biopsy site.

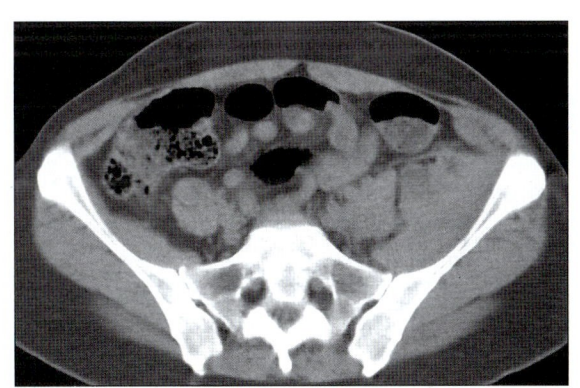

Figure 4. Unenhanced CT-image obtained 2 hours after the biopsy shows a hematoma within the left iliacus muscle.

Case 239

DEMOGRAPHICS/CLINICAL HISTORY

An 81-year-old woman with suspicious calcifications identified on mammography, undergoing mammography and stereotactic biopsy.

DISCUSSION

History/Indications for Procedure
An 81-year-old woman has microcalcifications in the right upper outer quadrant of the breast that have increased in size and number since the previous examination.

Procedure
Stereotactic breast biopsy

Pre-procedure Imaging
Diagnostic mammogram shows pleomorphic, clustered microcalcifications in the right upper outer quadrant of the breast (Fig. 1).

Intraprocedural Findings
A 9-gauge, vacuum-assisted core biopsy device was used (Fig. 2). Specimen radiograph obtained after the biopsy demonstrates many microcalcifications that are of concern in the biopsy specimen (Fig. 3).

Follow-up and Complications
The biopsy revealed ductal carcinoma in situ, grade 2, without an invasive component. The patient had a total mastectomy of the right breast with sentinel lymph node biopsy.

Suggested Readings
Jackman RJ, Burbank F, Parker SH, et al: Stereotactic breast biopsy of nonpalpable lesions: Determinants of ductal carcinoma in situ underestimation rates. Radiology 218:497-502, 2001.

Jackman RJ, Marzoni FA: Stereotactic histologic biopsy with patients prone: Technical feasibility in 98% of mammographically detected lesions. AJR Am J Roentgenol 180:785-794, 2003.

Liberman L: Percutaneous image-guided core breast biopsy. Radiol Clin North Am 40:483-500, 2002.

Case 239   479

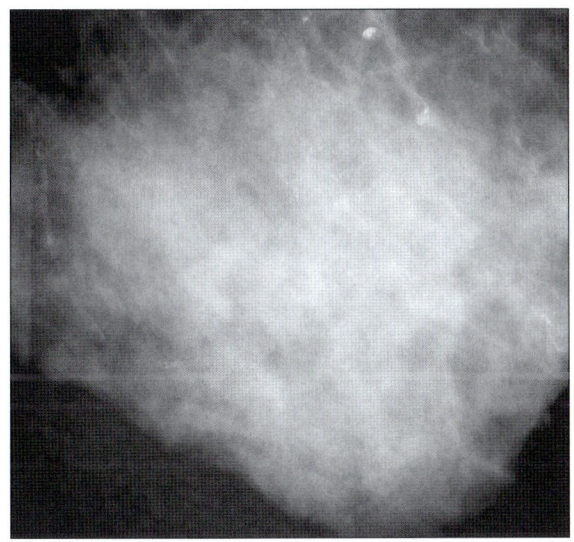

Figure 1. Diagnostic mammogram demonstrates pleomorphic microcalcifications in the upper outer quadrant of the right breast.

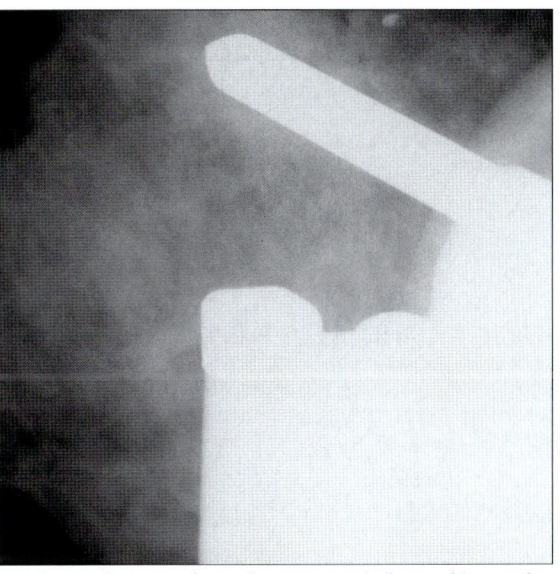

Figure 2. Single image from the stereotactic breast biopsy shows targeting of suspicious microcalcifications.

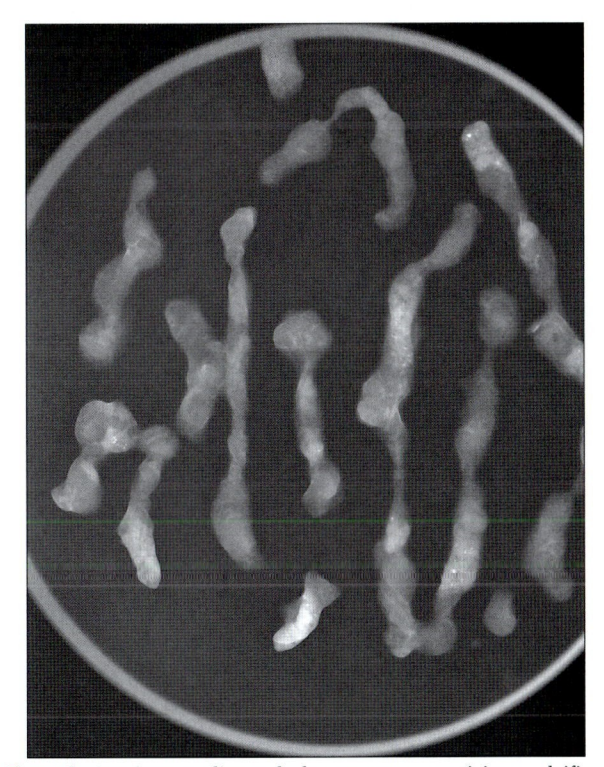

Figure 3. Specimen radiograph demonstrates suspicious calcifications within several of the biopsy specimens.

Case 240

DEMOGRAPHICS/CLINICAL HISTORY

A 66-year-old woman with an abnormal mammogram, undergoing stereotactic core biopsy.

DISCUSSION

History/Indications for Procedure
A 66-year-old woman had an abnormal mammogram result.

Procedure
Stereotactic breast biopsy

Pre-procedure Imaging
A diagnostic mammogram shows suspicious, linear calcifications in the lower outer quadrant of the left breast (Fig. 1). The calcifications are new and were not seen on the mammogram from the previous year.

Intraprocedural Findings
A stereotactic core biopsy of the microcalcifications was performed with a 9-gauge, vacuum-assisted device, and a specimen radiograph was obtained to confirm the presence of the microcalcifications in the biopsy specimen (Fig. 2). A metallic marker clip was placed into the biopsy cavity (Fig. 3).

Follow-up and Complications
Pathological examination of the biopsy specimen revealed ductal carcinoma in situ. The patient subsequently underwent needle-localized surgical excision (Fig. 4).

Suggested Readings
Jackman RJ, Marzoni FA: Stereotactic histologic biopsy with patients prone: Technical feasibility in 98% of mammographically detected lesions. AJR Am J Roentgenol 180:785-794, 2003.

Jackman RJ, Burbank F, Parker SH, et al: Stereotactic breast biopsy of nonpalpable lesions: Determinants of ductal carcinoma in situ underestimation rates. Radiology 218:497-502, 2001.

Liberman L: Percutaneous image-guided core breast biopsy. Radiol Clin North Am 40:483-500, 2002.

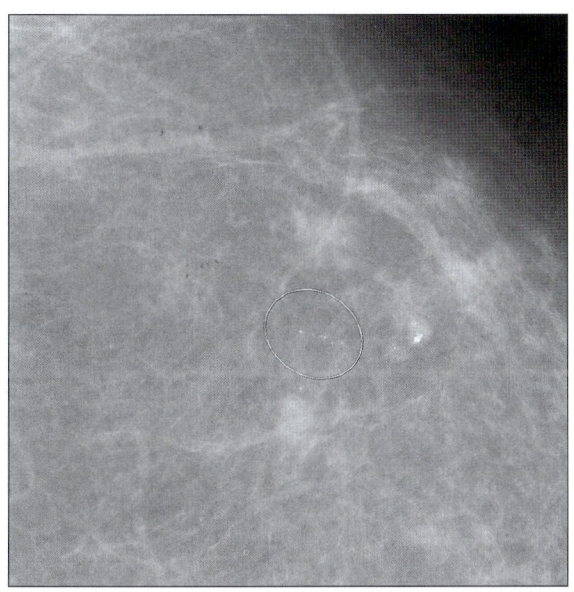

Figure 1. Diagnostic mammogram demonstrates suspicious-appearing linear calcifications in the lower outer quadrant of the left breast.

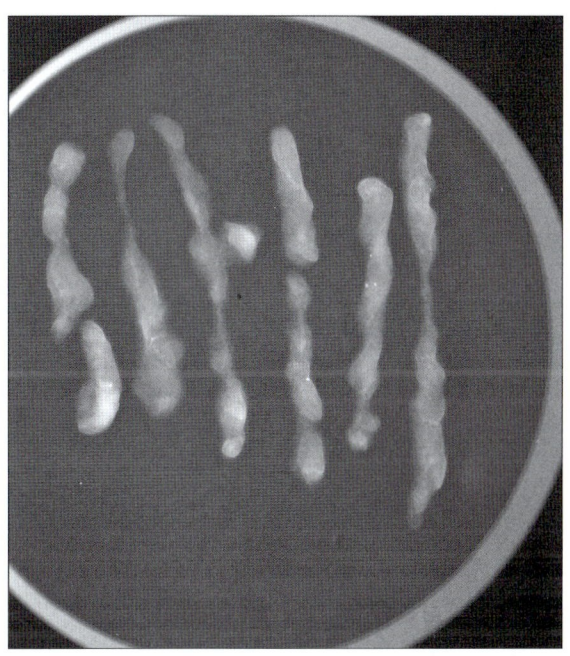

Figure 2. After stereotactic core biopsy, a specimen radiograph confirmed the presence of abnormal calcifications within the biopsy specimen.

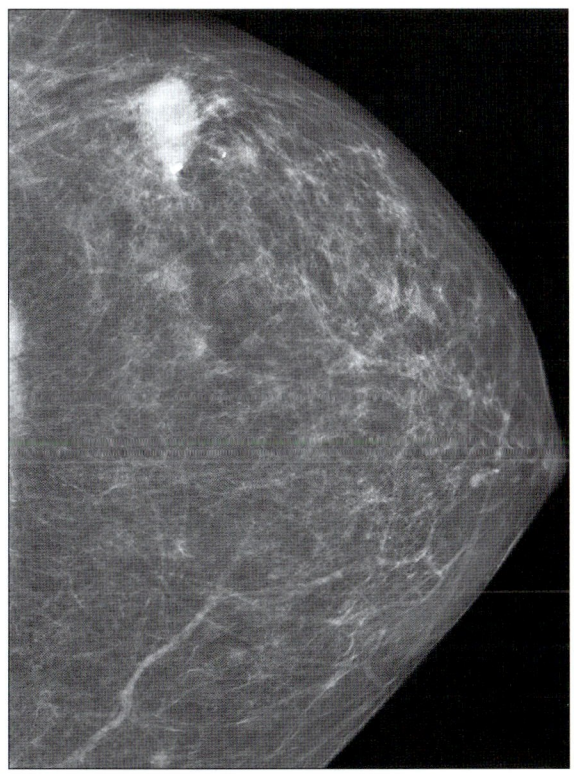

Figure 3. A metallic marker was placed in the biopsy cavity after the biopsy specimen was obtained. Notice the presence of a small hematoma at the site of the biopsy.

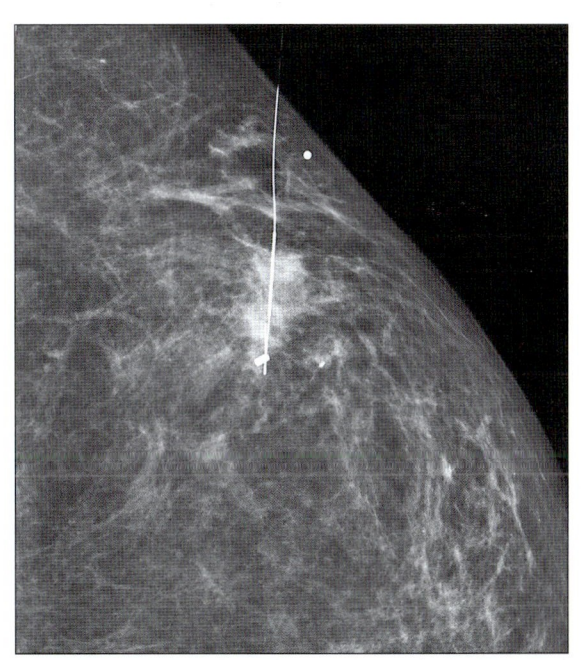

Figure 4. The patient returned for placement of a localizing wire. The wire was placed with the assistance of the metallic marker placed at the time of the biopsy.

Case 241

DEMOGRAPHICS/CLINICAL HISTORY

A 60-year-old woman with right breast mass, undergoing MRI.

DISCUSSION

History/Indications for Procedure
A 60-year-old woman has an abnormal mammogram. The patient has known infiltrating ductal carcinoma in the right breast, diagnosed by ultrasound-guided biopsy; two additional enhancing lesions are seen in the right breast on MRI.

Procedure
Breast biopsy, MRI guidance

Pre-procedure Imaging
Contrast-enhanced MRI shows three enhancing masses in the right breast (Fig. 1). Ultrasound of the right breast shows one of the masses; the other two masses have no ultrasound correlate.

Intraprocedural Findings
The two masses were localized using the DynaCAD intervention system (Invivo, Pewaukee, WI) (Fig. 2). A 9-gauge vacuum-assisted biopsy device was used to obtain core biopsy specimens (Fig. 3).

Follow-up and Complications
Pathologic examination of the mass revealed sclerosing adenosis. Because this diagnosis was believed to be discordant with imaging findings, the mass was localized and excised; infiltrating lobular carcinoma was identified on excision.

Suggested Readings
Eby PR, Lehman CD: Magnetic resonance imaging-guided breast interventions. Top Magn Reson Imaging 19:151, 2008.
Mahoney MC: Initial clinical experience with a new MRI vacuum-assisted breast biopsy device. J Magn Reson Imaging 28:900, 2008.
Perlet C, Heywang-Kobrunner SH, Heinig A, et al: Magnetic resonance-guided, vacuum-assisted breast biopsy: Results from a European multicenter study of 538 lesions. Cancer 106:982, 2006.

Case 241   483

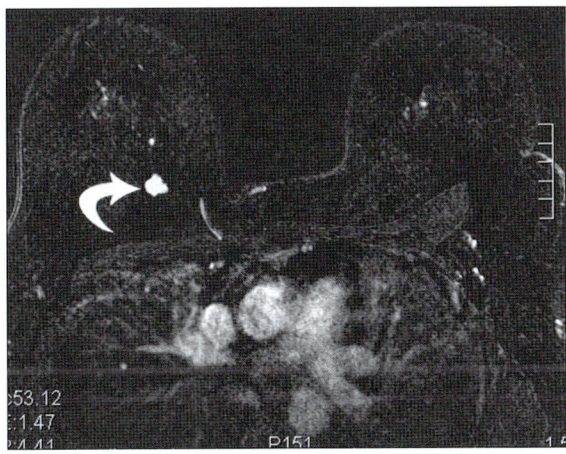

Figure 1. Contrast-enhanced MR image of breast shows enhancing mass in upper inner quadrant of right breast *(curved arrow)*.

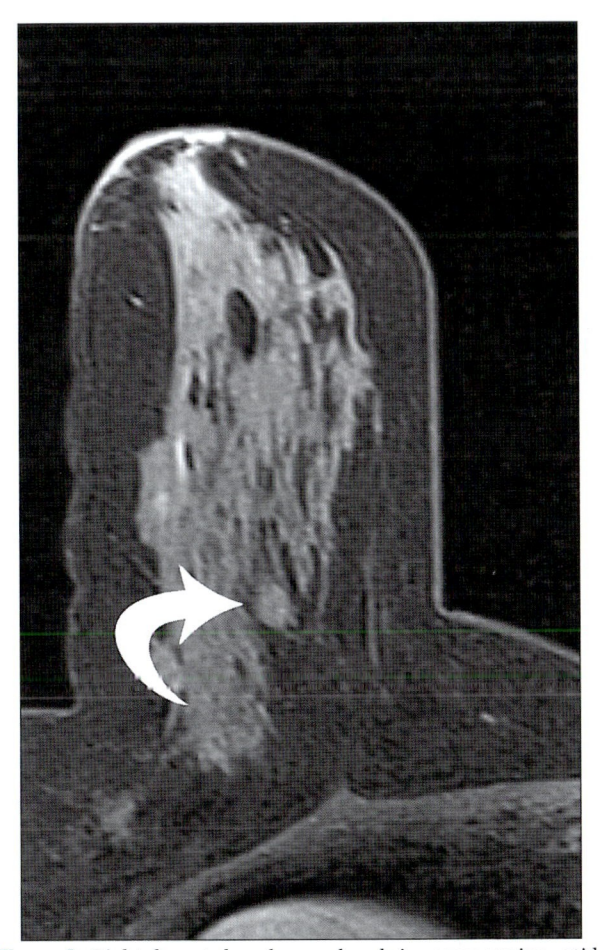

Figure 2. Right breast has been placed in compression grid. *(Curved arrow* indicates mass.)

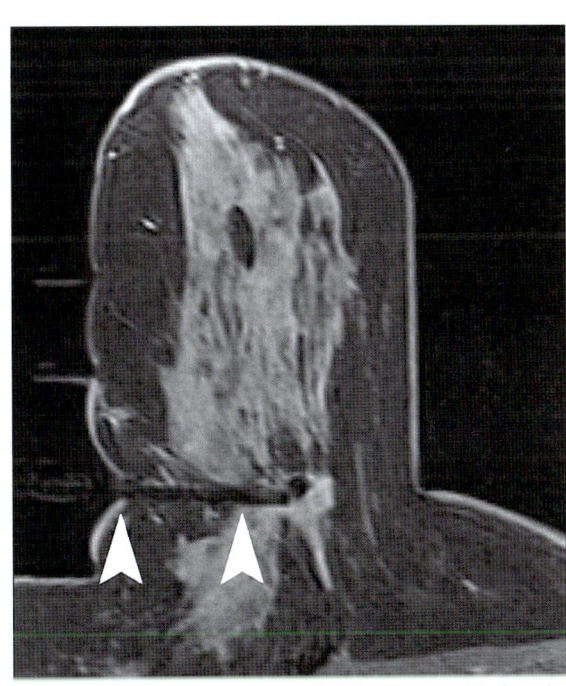

Figure 3. A 9-gauge vacuum-assisted biopsy needle has been placed into mass with MRI guidance *(arrowheads)*.

Case 242

DEMOGRAPHICS/CLINICAL HISTORY

A 69-year-old man with weight loss.

DISCUSSION

History/Indications for Procedure
A 69-year-old man with a 100-pack-year smoking history and left upper lobe mass incidentally discovered on chest radiograph.

Procedure
Percutaneous biopsy of the lung

Pre-procedure Imaging
Unenhanced CT of the chest shows a 1.4-cm spiculated mass in the left upper lobe.

Intraprocedural Findings
An 18-gauge coaxial with a 20-gauge Chiba needle was used for fine-needle aspiration of the mass (Fig. 2). After the second pass, the patient developed chest pain and shortness of breath; further imaging revealed the development of a pneumothorax (Fig. 3).

Follow-up and Complications
A chest tube was placed for persistent air leak. The air leak (Fig. 4) was resolved after several days, at which point the chest tube was removed.

Suggested Readings
Anderson JM, Murchison J, Patel D: CT-guided lung biopsy: Factors influencing diagnostic yield and complication rate. Clin Radiol 58:791-797, 2003.

Geraghty PR, Kee ST, McFarlane G, et al: CT-guided transthoracic needle aspiration biopsy of pulmonary nodules: Needle size and pneumothorax rate. Radiology 229:475-481, 2003.

Heck SL, Blom P, Berstad A: Accuracy and complications in computed tomography fluoroscopy-guided needle biopsies of lung masses. Eur Radiol 16:1387-1392, 2006.

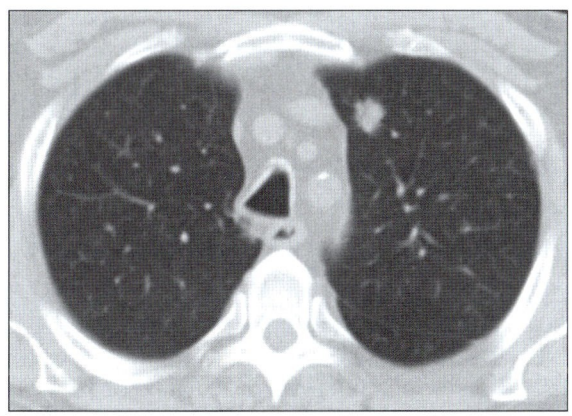

Figure 1. CT of the chest shows a 1.4-cm spiculated mass in the left upper lobe.

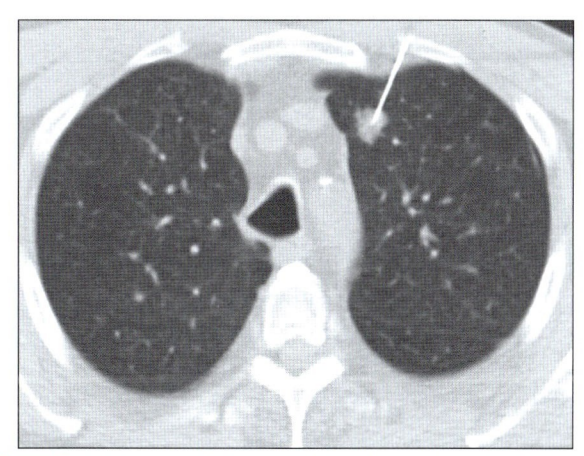

Figure 2. A 20-gauge Chiba needle has been placed in the mass and a fine-needle aspiration was performed.

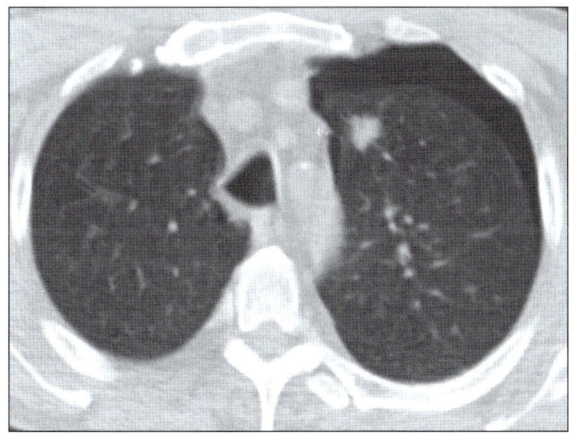

Figure 3. After the second pass, a moderate-sized pneumothorax is present.

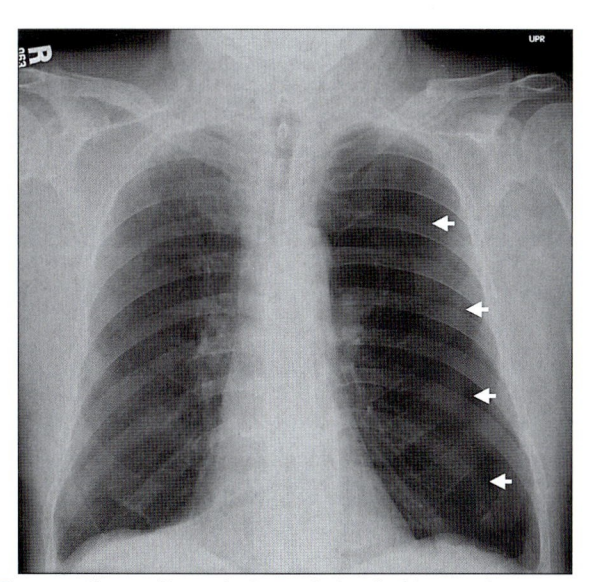

Figure 4. Chest radiograph obtained after the biopsy. The pneumothorax has enlarged since the biopsy, suggesting the presence of an air leak *(arrows indicate pleural edge)*.

Case 243

DEMOGRAPHICS/CLINICAL HISTORY

A 72-year-old man with right upper lobe pulmonary mass.

DISCUSSION

History/Indications for Procedure
A 72-year-old man with severe emphysema presents with a spiculated mass in the right upper lobe.

Procedure
Percutaneous biopsy of the lung

Pre-procedure Imaging
CT of the chest shows a 1.6-cm × 1.5-cm spiculated mass in the medial aspect of the right lung apex (Fig. 1). The mass shows increased uptake on F-18 FDG PET scan.

Intraprocedural Findings
With the patient prone on the CT table, a 15-gauge cannula was inserted into the lesion (Fig. 2). A fine-needle aspiration biopsy was performed using a 22-gauge needle through the cannula.

Follow-up and Complications
The fine-needle aspiration biopsy showed the lesion to be squamous cell carcinoma. At the time of the biopsy, the lesion was treated with radiofrequency ablation (Fig. 3); in the 4 years since the ablation, the lesion has shown no further growth (Fig. 4) and has remained PET-negative.

Suggested Readings

Anderson JM, Murchison J, Patel D: CT-guided lung biopsy: Factors influencing diagnostic yield and complication rate. Clin Radiol 58:791-797, 2003.

Geraghty PR, Kee ST, McFarlane G, et al: CT-guided transthoracic needle aspiration biopsy of pulmonary nodules: Needle size and pneumothorax rate. Radiology 229:475-481, 2003.

Steinke K: Radiofrequency ablation of pulmonary tumours: Current status. Cancer Imaging 8:27-35, 2008.

Zhu JC, Yan TD, Morris DL: A systemic review of radiofrequency ablation for lung tumors. Ann Surg Oncol 15:1765-1774, 2008.

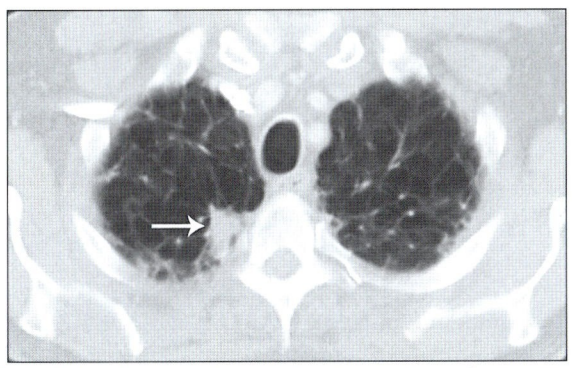

Figure 1. Axial image through the lung apices shows severe emphysematous changes in both lungs. There is a 1.6-cm × 1.5-cm spiculated mass in the posterior segment of the right upper lobe *(arrow)*.

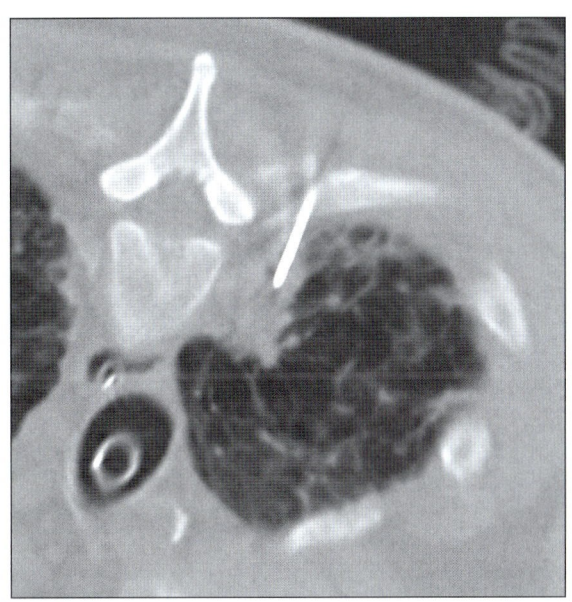

Figure 2. The patient was positioned prone on the CT table. A 15-gauge cannula has been inserted into the mass. Through this cannula, multiple fine-needle aspiration biopsies were obtained.

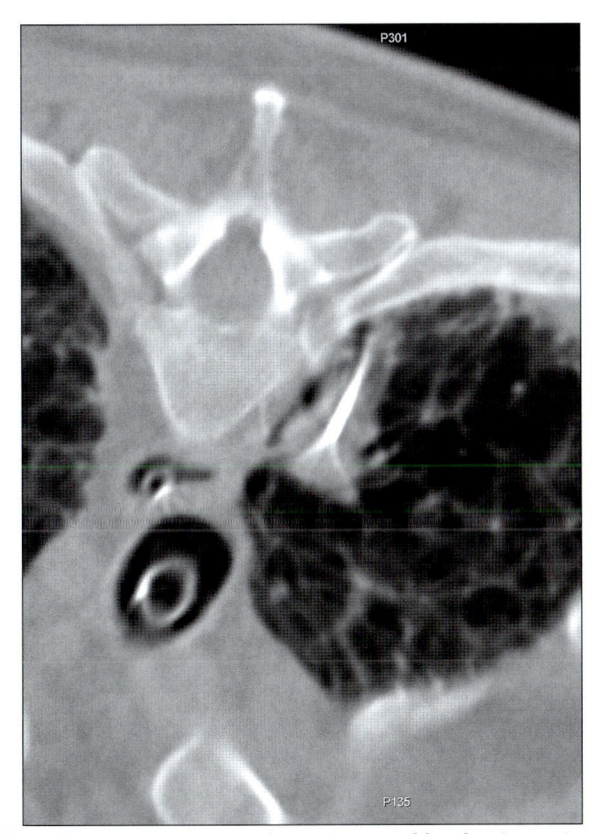

Figure 3. After the biopsy, the mass was ablated using a 3-cm radiofrequency probe (Laveen, Boston Scientific, Nanick, MA).

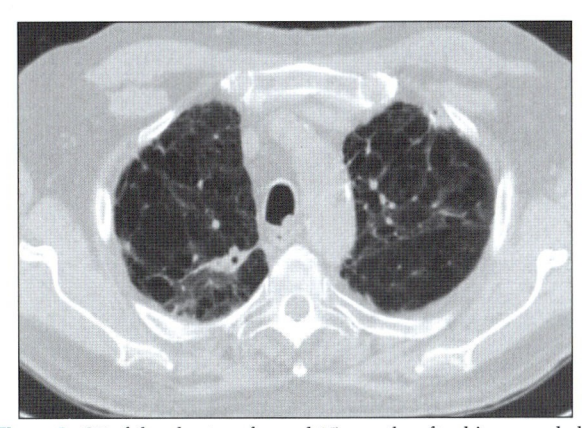

Figure 4. CT of the chest performed 15 months after biopsy and ablation shows residual soft tissue in the region of the mass, which has decreased in size since the ablation. This soft-tissue specimen was PET negative.

Case 244

DEMOGRAPHICS/CLINICAL HISTORY

A 61-year-old woman with multifocal hepatocellular carcinoma, undergoing magnetic resonance imaging (MRI), computed tomography (CT), and radiofrequency ablation (RFA).

DISCUSSION

History/Indications for Procedure
A 61-year-old woman has multifocal hepatocellular carcinoma. The patient has undergone chemoembolization, and she now has a dominant lesion in segment IV of the liver.

Procedure
Radiofrequency ablation of hepatocellular carcinoma

Pre-procedure Imaging
Contrast-enhanced MRI of the abdomen shows a 5.8-cm × 4.8-cm mass in segment 4 of the liver (Fig. 1).

Intraprocedural Findings
The ablation was performed with CT guidance, and sterile water was injected for hydrodissection to displace the stomach and duodenum. Three 4-cm probes were used to perform the ablation (Fig. 2).

Follow-up and Complications
The patient had a moderate amount of hemoperitoneum after the procedure (Fig. 3), although no further intervention was required. On follow-up MRI, the lesion had decreased in size, although nodular peripheral enhancement persisted, suggesting residual viable tumor (Fig. 4).

Suggested Readings
Bleicher RJ, Allegra DP, Nora DT, et al: Radiofrequency ablation in 447 complex unresectable liver tumors: Lessons learned. Ann Surg Oncol 10:52-58, 2003.
Goldberg SN, Gazelle GS, Mueller PR, et al: Thermal ablation therapy for focal malignancies: A unified approach to underlying principles, techniques, and diagnostic imaging guidance. AJR Am J Roentgenol 174:323-331, 2000.
Lencioni R, Della Pina C, Bartolozzi C, et al: Percutaneous image-guided radiofrequency ablation in the therapeutic management of hepatocellular carcinoma. Abdom Imaging 30:401-408, 2005.
Livraghi T, Solbiati L, Meloni MF, et al: Treatment of focal liver tumors with percutaneous radio-frequency ablation: Complications encountered in a multicenter study. Radiology 226:441-451, 2003.

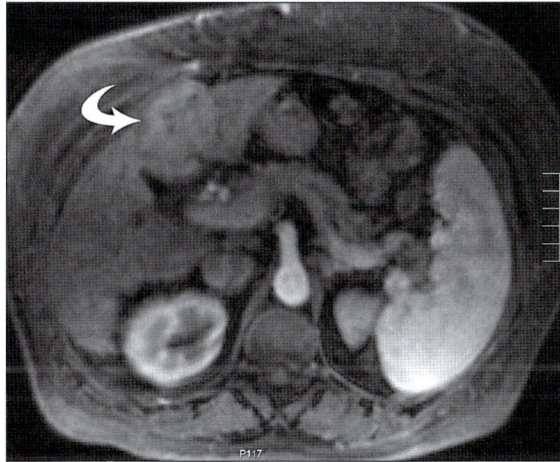

Figure 1. Single axial image from a contrast-enhanced MRI study of the abdomen shows a hypervascular mass within segment IV of the liver *(arrow)*.

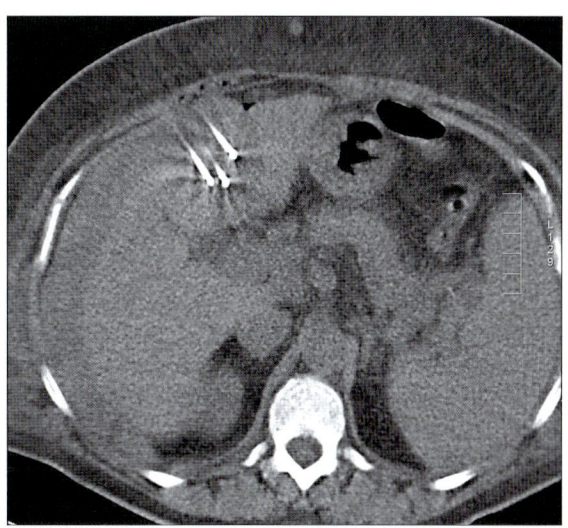

Figure 2. Three 4-cm probes have been placed into the lesion. Notice the new, high-density, perihepatic fluid, which is consistent with hemoperitoneum.

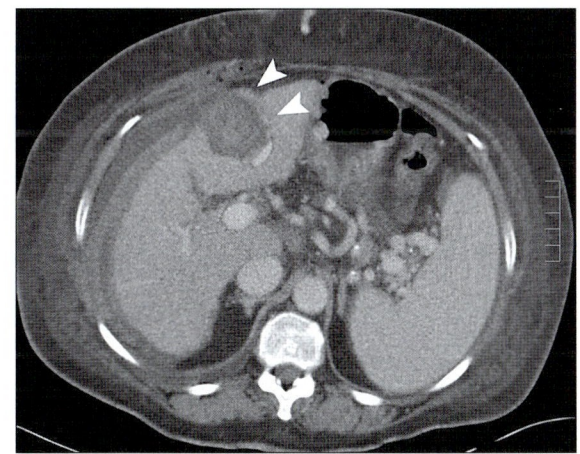

Figure 3. Contrast-enhanced CT performed immediately after the completion of the RFA shows the hemoperitoneum along the surface of the liver. There is residual enhancement along the margin of the tumor, indicating residual disease *(arrowheads)*.

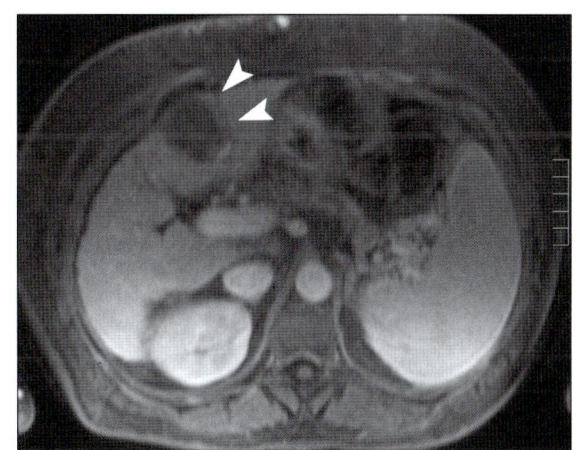

Figure 4. Follow-up MRI was performed 1 month after ablation. T1-weighted, fat-saturated, post-gadolinium MR image shows necrosis of most of the mass. There is persistent enhancing tissue along the margin of the lesion that is consistent with residual disease *(arrowheads)*.

Case 245

DEMOGRAPHICS/CLINICAL HISTORY

A 63-year-old man with hepatic cirrhosis secondary to cryptogenic cirrhosis presents with a 3.2-cm mass in segment 5 of the liver.

DISCUSSION

History/Indications for Procedure
A 63-year-old man with hepatic cirrhosis secondary to cryptogenic cirrhosis presents with a 3.2-cm mass in segment 5 of the liver.

Procedure
Ultrasound and CT-guided microwave ablation of hepatocellular carcinoma

Pre-procedure Imaging
Contrast-enhanced MRI of the liver shows a 3.2-cm lesion in segment 5 that has early arterial enhancement (Fig. 1).

Intraprocedural Findings
Two microwave antennae were placed into the lesion using ultrasound guidance, and the lesion was ablated for 10 minutes (Figs. 2 and 3). Contrast-enhanced CT after the ablation shows no residual enhancement, suggesting complete tumor ablation (Fig. 4).

Follow-up and Complications
One month after the ablation, the patient underwent liver transplantation. Examination of the explant liver revealed poorly differentiated hepatocellular carcinoma with coagulative necrosis and <20% viable tumor.

Suggested Readings
Ahmed M, Goldberg SN: Thermal ablation therapy for hepatocellular carcinoma. J Vasc Intervent Radiol 13(9 Pt 2):S231-S244, 2002.
Iannitti DA, Martin RC, Simon CJ, et al: Hepatic tumor ablation with clustered microwave antennae: The US Phase II Trial. HPB 9:120-124, 2007.
Liang P, Wang Y: Microwave ablation of hepatocellular carcinoma. Oncology 72 (Suppl 1):124-131, 2007.

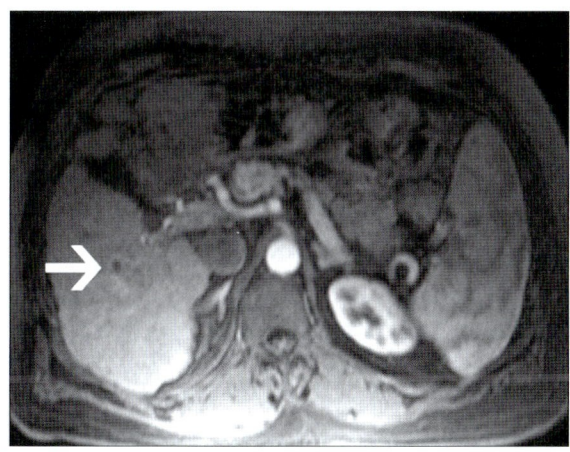

Figure 1. Axial T1, post-contrast MR image of the liver shows a heterogeneous, enhancing mass in segment V *(arrow)*. The lesion had shown interval growth since prior imaging studies.

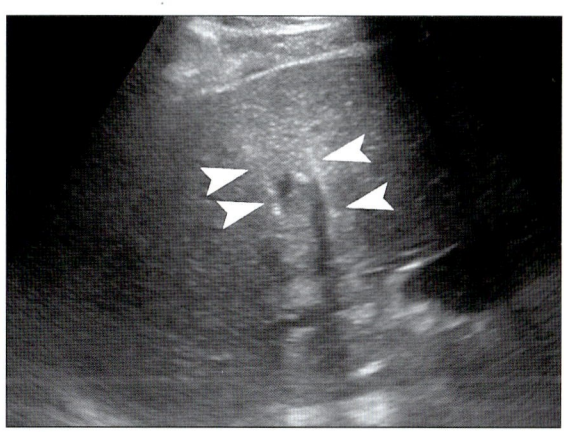

Figure 2. Two microwave antennae were placed into the mass, 1.5 cm apart, with ultrasound guidance *(arrowheads)*.

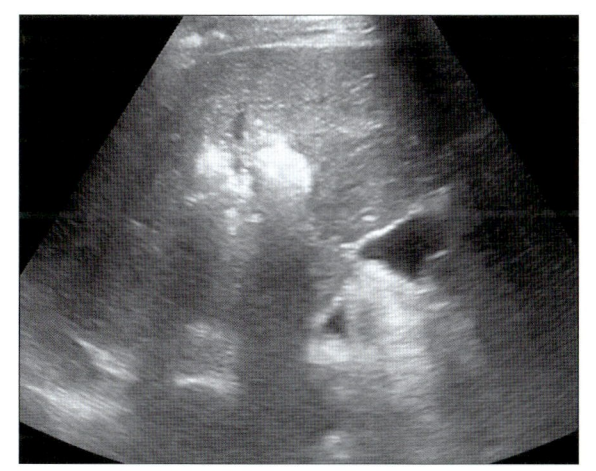

Figure 3. Ultrasound image after tumor ablation shows complete obscuration of the tumor by gas formation in the ablation bed.

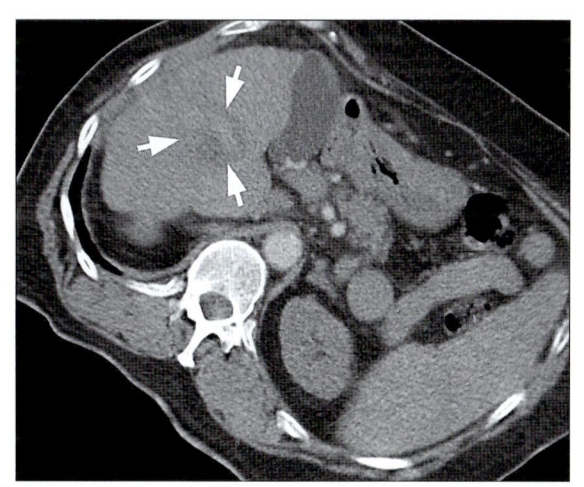

Figure 4. Contrast-enhanced CT after ablation shows mixed attenuation within the ablation bed *(arrows)* consistent with edema and hemorrhage. No enhancement was seen to suggest residual tumor.

Case 246

DEMOGRAPHICS/CLINICAL HISTORY

A 52-year-old man with hepatitis C presents with a new mass in the right hepatic lobe.

DISCUSSION

History/Indications for Procedure

A 52-year-old man with hepatitis C presents with a new mass in the right hepatic lobe and elevated serum α-fetoprotein levels.

Procedure

Ultrasound-guided microwave ablation of hepatocellular carcinoma

Pre-procedure Imaging

Contrast-enhanced MRI shows a 2.8-cm mass in the right hepatic lobe (Fig. 1). The lesion shows early arterial enhancement and early washout.

Intraprocedural Findings

The microwave antenna was placed within the mass under ultrasound guidance (Figs. 2 and 3). The lesion was ablated for 9 minutes, and the antenna was removed while coagulating the tract (Fig. 4).

Follow-up and Complications

The patient recovered uneventfully from the ablation. Follow-up MRI 6 weeks after the ablation showed increased T1 signal in the mass with no visible enhancement or evidence of residual disease.

Suggested Readings

Ahmed M, Goldberg SN: Thermal ablation therapy for hepatocellular carcinoma. J Vasc Intervent Radiol 13(9 Pt 2):S231-S244, 2002.

Liang P, Wang Y: Microwave ablation of hepatocellular carcinoma. Oncology 72 (Suppl 1):124-131, 2007.

Lu MD, Xu HX, Xie XY, et al: Percutaneous microwave and radiofrequency ablation for hepatocellular carcinoma: A retrospective comparative study. J Gastroenterol 40:1054-1060, 2005.

Case 246   493

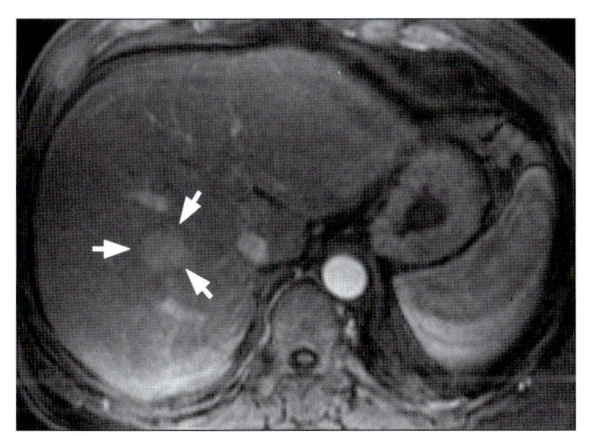

Figure 1. Contrast-enhanced MRI shows an enhancing 2.8-cm mass in the right hepatic lobe *(arrows)*.

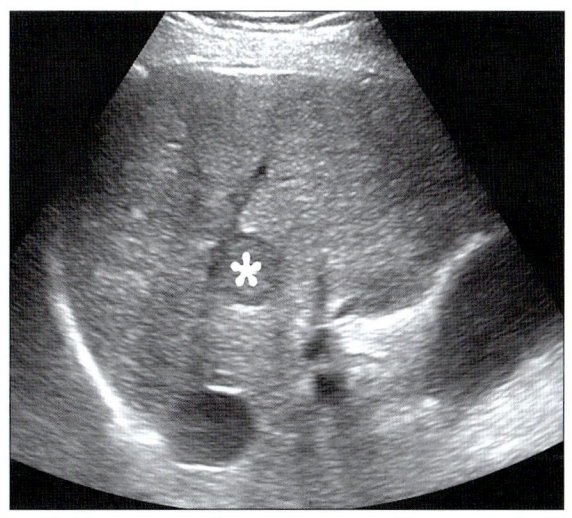

Figure 2. The mass is easily visualized using ultrasound *(asterisk)*.

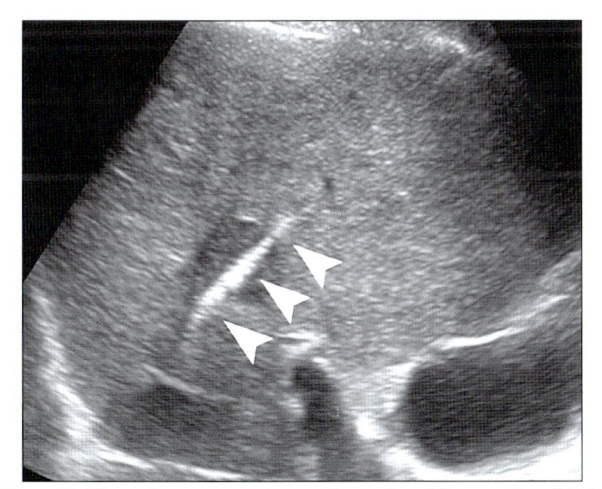

Figure 3. The microwave antenna *(arrowheads)* was placed into the mass with ultrasound guidance.

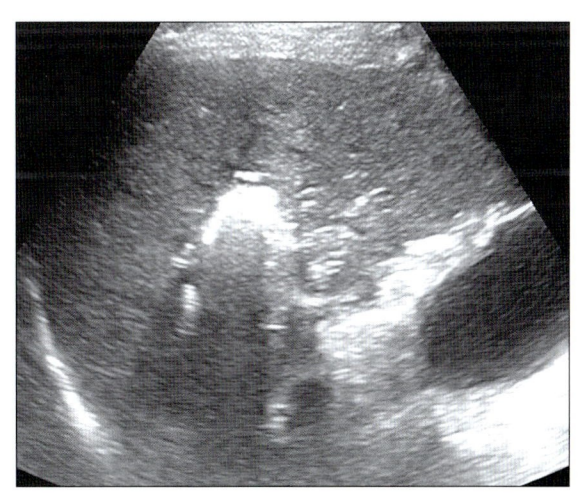

Figure 4. After a 9-minute ablation, the lesion is completely obscured by gas formation in the ablation bed.

Case 247

DEMOGRAPHICS/CLINICAL HISTORY

A 50-year-old woman with hepatic cirrhosis and 2.5-cm hepatocellular carcinoma.

DISCUSSION

History/Indications for Procedure
A 50-year-old woman with hepatic cirrhosis, status post–transjugular intrahepatic portal systemic shunt (TIPSS) placement, with an enlarging mass in segment 3.

Procedure
Cryoablation of hepatocellular carcinoma

Pre-procedure Imaging
Contrast-enhanced MRI shows a 2.5-cm mass in segment 3 (Fig. 1). The mass shows early arterial enhancement with gradual washout and has grown from 1.8 cm 3 months earlier.

Intraprocedural Findings
A 24-mm cryoprobe (Endocare, Irvine, CA) was placed into the mass with CT guidance (Figs. 2 and 3). Three freeze-thaw cycles were performed while monitoring of the freeze zone was performed with CT (Fig. 4).

Follow-up and Complications
MRI performed 3 months after cryoablation shows a small nodule of residual enhancement within the tumor. The lesion continued to grow on subsequent MRIs, and the patient eventually underwent transarterial chemoembolization of the lesion for palliation.

Suggested Readings
Jansen MC, van Hillegersberg R, Chamuleau RA, et al: Outcome of regional and local ablative therapies for hepatocellular carcinoma: A collective review. Eur J Surg Oncol 31:331-347, 2005.

Weber SM, Lee FT Jr: Expanded treatment of hepatic tumors with readiofrequency ablation and cryoablation. Oncology 19(11 Suppl 4):27-32, 2005.

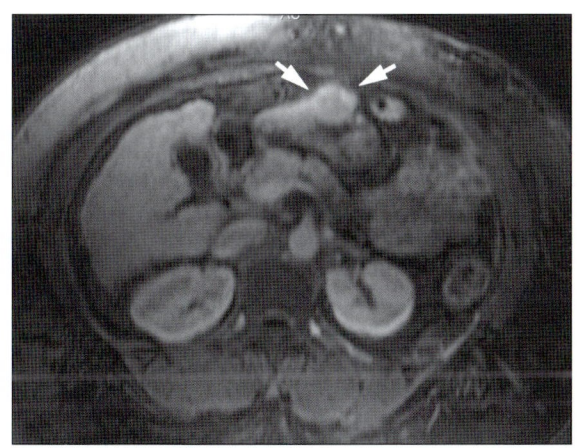

Figure 1. Contrast-enhanced MRI shows a 2.5-cm enhancing mass in segment 3 of the liver *(arrows)*.

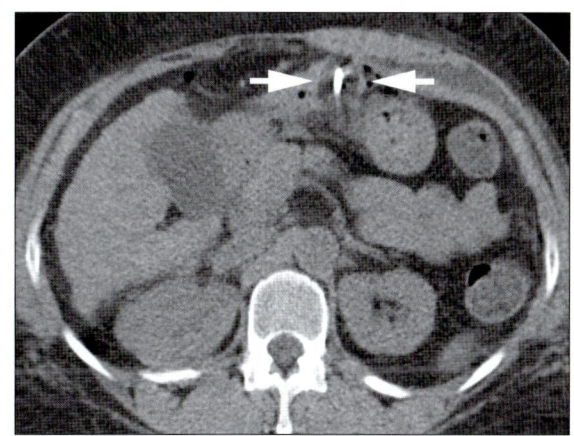

Figure 2. Axial CT during freeze cycle of cryoablation. The probe has been placed in the lesion, and an ice ball is visible *(arrows)*.

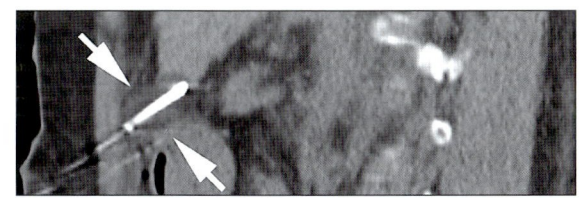

Figure 3. Sagittal reconstructed CT image during freeze cycle. The ice ball is clearly evident around the cryoablation probe *(arrows)*.

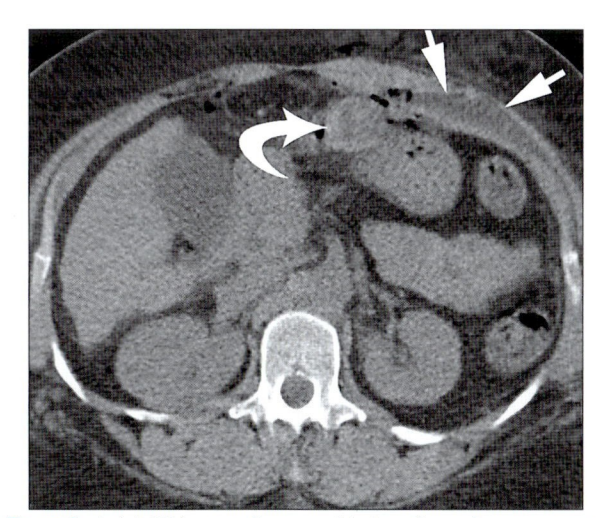

Figure 4. Axial CT image after cryoablation shows heterogeneous attenuation within the mass *(curved arrow)*. Gas and edema within the anterior abdominal wall are from probe placement *(short arrows)*.

Case 248

DEMOGRAPHICS/CLINICAL HISTORY

An 83-year-old woman with a history of colon carcinoma and a new liver lesion, undergoing magnetic resonance imaging (MRI), radiofrequency ablation (RFA), and computed tomography (CT).

DISCUSSION

History/Indications for Procedure
An 83-year-old woman was diagnosed with colon carcinoma 6 months earlier and has a new liver lesion.

Procedure
Radiofrequency ablation of colorectal liver metastasis

Pre-procedure Imaging
Contrast-enhanced MRI shows a peripherally enhancing, 1.3-cm lesion in segment 4a (Fig. 1).

Intraprocedural Findings
A 3.5-cm RFA probe was placed in the lesion with CT guidance (Fig. 2), and the lesion was ablated for 15 minutes.

Follow-up and Complications
Contrast-enhanced MRI performed 1 month after the ablation shows complete necrosis of the lesion and no evidence of residual disease (Fig. 3).

Suggested Readings
Curley SA, Izzo F, Delrio P, et al: Radiofrequency ablation of unresectable primary and metastatic hepatic malignancies: Results in 123 patients. Ann Surg 230:1-8, 1999.

Rhim H, Goldberg SN, Dodd GD 3rd, et al: Essential techniques for successful radio-frequency thermal ablation of malignant hepatic tumors. Radiographics 21:S17-S35; discussion S36-S39, 2001.

Solbiati L, Livraghi T, Goldberg SN, et al: Percutaneous radiofrequency ablation of hepatic metastases from colorectal cancer: Long-term results in 117 patients. Radiology 221:159-166, 2001.

Sørensen SM, Mortensen FV, Nielsen DT, et al: Radiofrequency ablation of colorectal liver metastases: Long-term survival. Acta Radiol 48:253-258, 2007.

Case 248   497

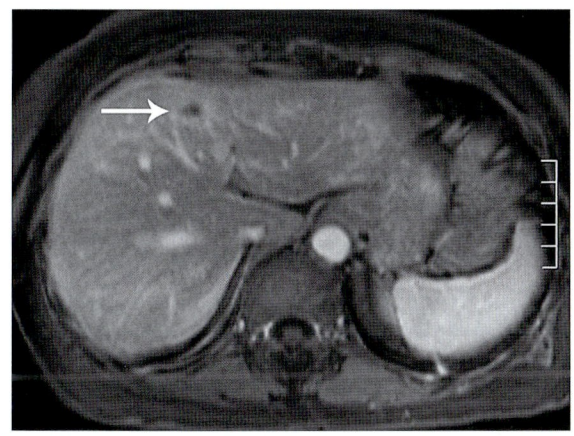

Figure 1. Contrast-enhanced MRI shows a 1.3-cm, peripherally enhancing lesion in segment 4a *(arrow)*.

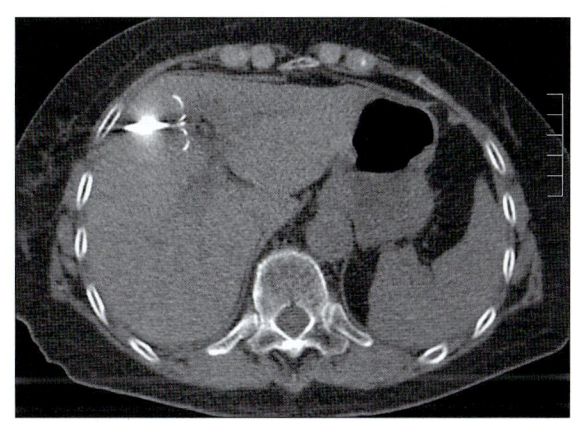

Figure 2. A 3.5-cm probe with extendible tines was deployed in the center of the lesion with CT guidance.

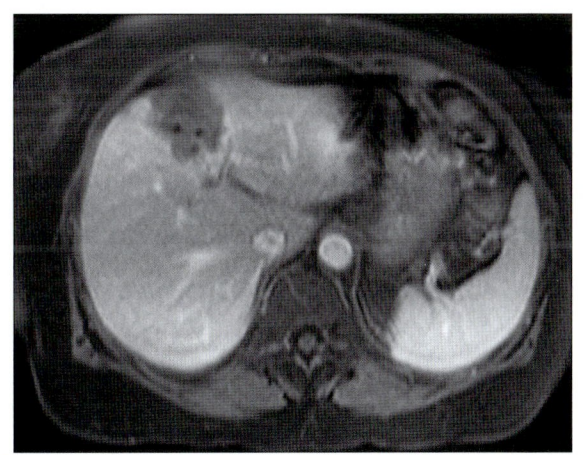

Figure 3. Follow-up MRI performed 1 month after the ablation shows complete necrosis of the lesion. There is no evidence of residual tumor.

Case 249

DEMOGRAPHICS/CLINICAL HISTORY

A 53-year-old woman with leiomyosarcoma metastatic to the liver, undergoing computed tomography (CT) and magnetic resonance imaging (MRI).

DISCUSSION

History/Indications for Procedure
A 53-year-old woman was diagnosed with a T3N0M1 retroperitoneal leiomyosarcoma 10 months earlier. A new liver mass was identified in segment IVb, and subsequent biopsy confirmed metastatic sarcoma.

Procedure
Radiofrequency ablation of metastatic sarcoma to liver

Pre-procedure Imaging
Contrast-enhanced CT shows a hypodense mass in segment IV of the liver that is 2.2 cm in the greatest diameter (Fig. 1).

Intraprocedural Findings
A 3-cm radiofrequency probe (Cool Tip, Valley Lab, Boulder, CO) was inserted into the lesion using CT guidance, and the lesion was heated to 77° C for 10 minutes. Immediately after ablation, unenhanced CT shows hemorrhage and edema within the ablation bed (Fig. 2).

Follow-up and Complications
Contrast-enhanced MRI performed 3 months after ablation shows complete ablation of the lesion, with a thin rim of enhancement that is consistent with granulation tissue (Fig. 3). MRI of the liver 1 year later showed continued local control of the ablated lesions; however, new liver lesions and a thoracic paraspinal metastasis developed in the interim.

Suggested Readings
Curley SA, Izzo F, Delrio P, et al: Radiofrequency ablation of unresectable primary and metastatic hepatic malignancies: Results in 123 patients. Ann Surg 230:1-8, 1999.
Pawlik TM, Vauthey JN, Abdalla EK, et al: Results of a single-center experience with resection and ablation for sarcoma metastatic to the liver. Arch Surg 141:537-543, 2006.
Solbiati L, Goldberg SN, Ierace T, et al: Hepatic metastases: Percutaneous radio-frequency ablation with cooled-tip electrodes. Radiology 205:367-373, 1997.
Solbiati L, Ierace T, Goldberg SN, et al: Percutaneous US-guided radio-frequency tissue ablation of liver metastases: Treatment and follow-up in 16 patients. Radiology 202:195-203, 1997.

Case 249   499

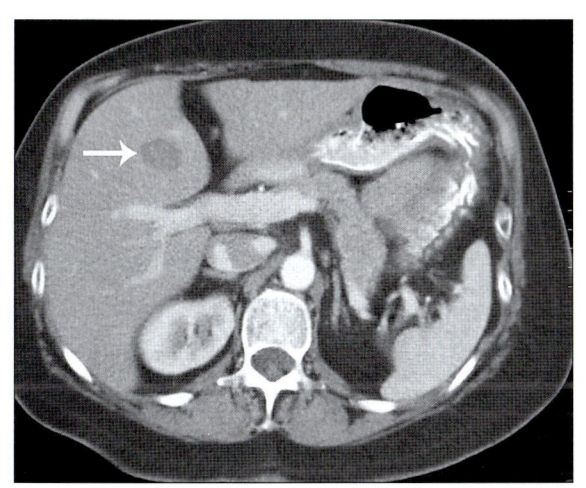

Figure 1. Contrast-enhanced CT of the abdomen at the level of the portal vein shows a 2.2-cm, low-attenuation lesion in segment 4b *(arrow)*.

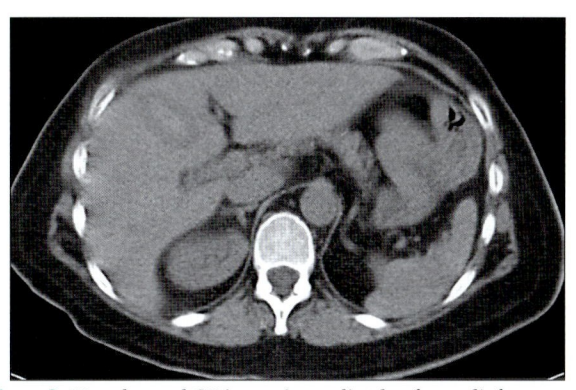

Figure 2. Unenhanced CT image immediately after radiofrequency ablation shows mixed attenuation of the lesion, likely due to hemorrhage within the ablation bed and surrounding edema.

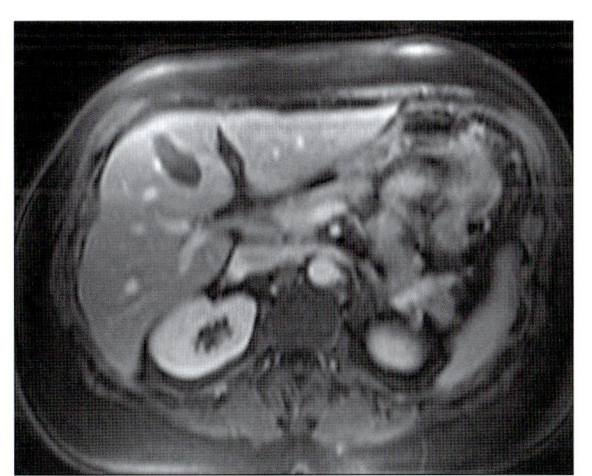

Figure 3. Follow-up contrast MRI performed 3 months after ablation shows homogeneous low signal intensity within the ablation bed and a thin rim of circumferential enhancement caused by granulation tissue. There is no evidence of residual tumor.

Case 250

DEMOGRAPHICS/CLINICAL HISTORY

A 55-year-old woman with recurrent adrenal cortical carcinoma and elevated cortisol levels, undergoing magnetic resonance imaging (MRI), computed tomography (CT), and radiofrequency ablation (RFA).

DISCUSSION

History/Indications for Procedure
A 55-year-old woman had recurrent adrenal cortical carcinoma and elevated cortisol levels. She underwent prior left adrenalectomy and now has a recurrence in the resection bed.

Procedure
Radiofrequency ablation of recurrent adrenal corticocarcinoma

Pre-procedure Imaging
Contrast-enhanced MRI of the abdomen shows a 5.8-cm × 5.6-cm mass in the left adrenalectomy bed (Fig. 1). The many enhancing liver lesions are consistent with metastases.

Intraprocedural Findings
A 3.5-cm RFA probe was placed into the center of the mass, and overlapping ablations of the left adrenal bed were performed (Fig. 2).

Follow-up and Complications
Follow-up MRI shows a significant decrease in enhancement of the mass, with some residual peripheral enhancement (Fig. 3). Six months after the original ablation, the lesion began to enlarge, and the patient was taken to the operating room for surgical debulking.

Suggested Readings
Mayo-Smith WW, Dupuy DE: Adrenal neoplasms: CT-guided radiofrequency ablation—preliminary results. Radiology 231:225-230, 2004.

Ng L, Libertino JM: Adrenocortical carcinoma: Diagnosis, evaluation, and treatment. J Urol 169:5-11, 2003.

Wood BJ, Abraham J, Hvizda JL, et al: Radiofrequency ablation of adrenal tumors and adrenocortical metastases. Cancer 97:554-560, 2003.

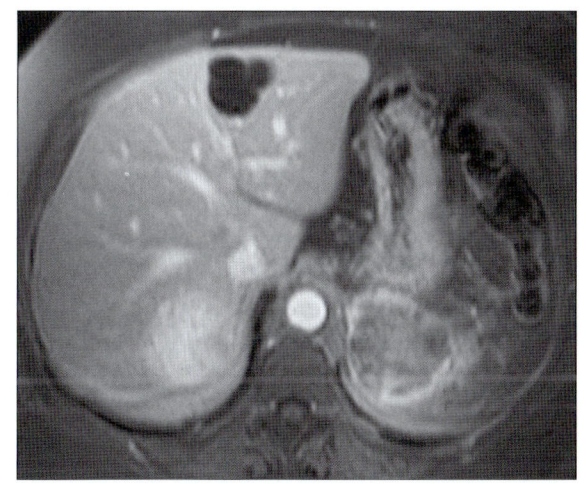

Figure 1. Axial, T1-weighted MRI with fat saturation shows a large, heterogeneously enhancing mass in the left adrenalectomy bed *(arrowheads)*. There is also a large, hyperenhancing mass and a smaller peripherally enhancing mass in the visualized liver that are consistent with metastatic disease *(arrows)*.

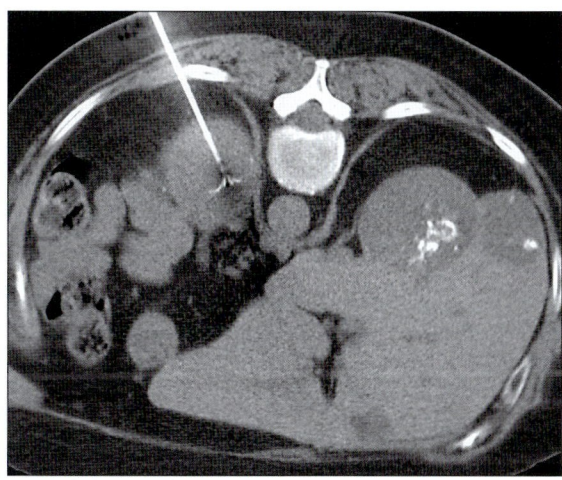

Figure 2. With the patient prone on the CT table, the RFA probe has been inserted from a posterolateral approach.

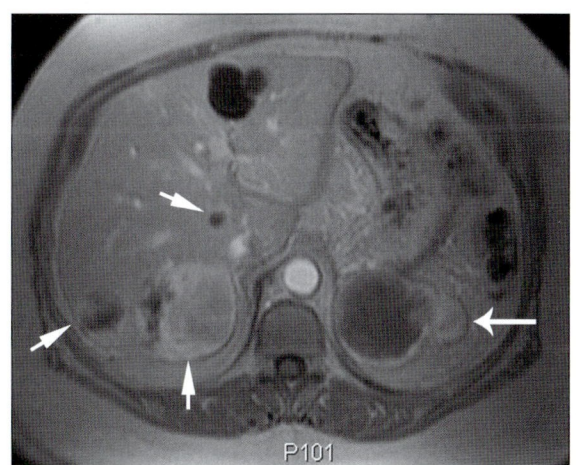

Figure 3. Follow-up MRI performed 6 weeks after the ablation shows the mass to be largely necrotic. There is continued peripheral enhancement with continued nodular enhancement along the lateral wall *(arrow)*, indicating residual disease. There has been interval progression of liver metastases *(short arrows)*.

Case 251

DEMOGRAPHICS/CLINICAL HISTORY

A 44-year-old woman with an incidentally discovered, 1.8-cm renal mass, undergoing computed tomography (CT) and magnetic resonance imaging (MRI).

DISCUSSION

History/Indications for Procedure
A 1.8-cm renal mass was discovered as an incidental finding on abdominal CT after gastric surgery in a 44-year-old woman.

Procedure
Radiofrequency ablation of renal cell carcinoma

Pre-procedure Imaging
Contrast-enhanced CT shows a 1.5-cm × 1.8-cm exophytic mass arising from the upper pole of the left kidney (Fig. 1). The mass shows homogeneous enhancement after contrast administration.

Intraprocedural Findings
Using CT guidance, a 3-cm radiofrequency probe (Cooltip, Valley Lab, Boulder, CO) was angled cephalad into the lesion. Two overlapping ablations were performed: one on the medial side of the mass (Fig. 2) and one on the lateral side of the mass.

Follow-up and Complications
Contrast-enhanced CT performed 3 months after the ablation shows an interval reduction in size of the renal mass and no residual enhancement (Fig. 3). MRI performed 22 months after the ablation shows the lesion's size has remained stable in size and there is no evidence of recurrent tumor (Fig. 4).

Suggested Readings
Gervais DA, McGovern FJ, Arellano RS, et al: Radiofrequency ablation of renal cell carcinoma. I. Indications, results, and role in patient management over a 6-year period and ablation of 100 tumors. AJR Am J Roentgenol 185:64-71, 2005.

Rutherford ED, Cast JE, Breen DJ: Immediate and long-term CT appearances following radiofrequency ablation of renal tumours. Clin Radiol 63:220-230, 2008.

Stone MJ, Venkatesan AM, Locklin J, et al: Radiofrequency ablation of renal tumors. Tech Vasc Intervent Radiol 10:132-139, 2007.

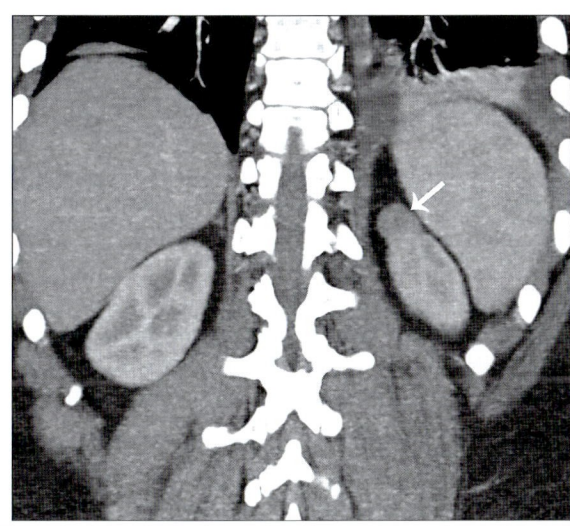

Figure 1. Coronal reconstruction of a contrast-enhanced CT scan shows an exophytic mass arising from the upper pole of the left kidney *(arrow)*.

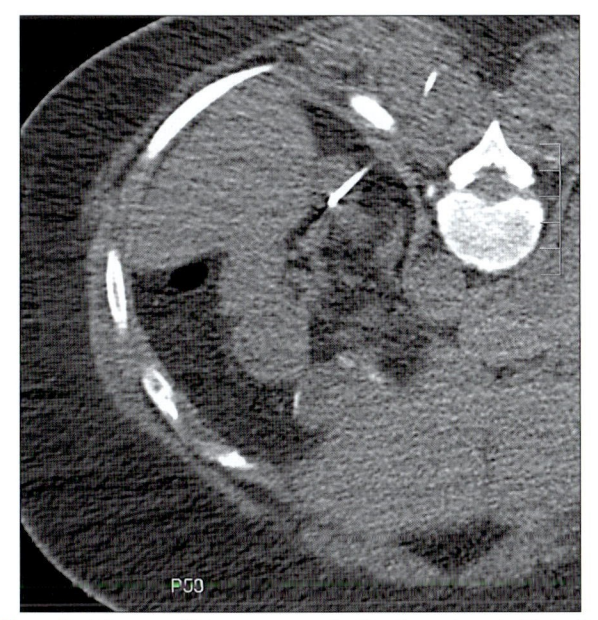

Figure 2. A 3-cm radiofrequency probe has been inserted into the medial aspect of the mass with CT guidance.

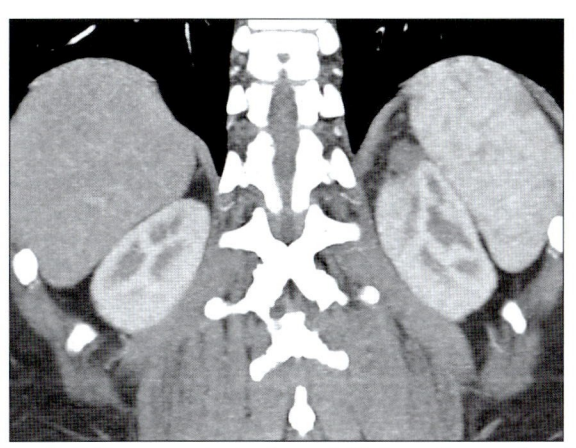

Figure 3. Follow-up contrast-enhanced CT shows the mass has decreased in size. There was no difference in attenuation between images before and after contrast.

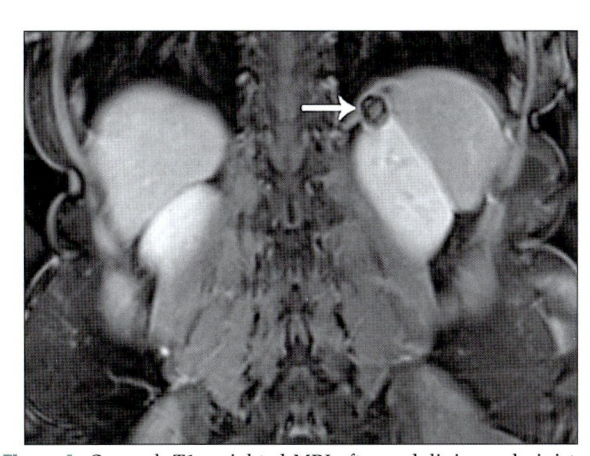

Figure 4. Coronal, T1-weighted MRI after gadolinium administration shows the mass has remained stable in size and has no visible enhancement *(arrow)*.

Case 252

Charles Burke, MD, and Robert G. Dixon, MD

DEMOGRAPHICS/CLINICAL HISTORY

A 30-year-old woman with von Hippel-Lindau disease (VHL), undergoing computed tomography (CT), radiofrequency ablation (RFA), and magnetic resonance imaging (MRI).

DISCUSSION

History/Indications for Procedure
A 30-year-old woman has disease and bilateral renal-cell carcinomas. Because of the history of VHL and prior bilateral, partial nephrectomies, it was decided to proceed with CT-guided RFA in a staged fashion, targeting the right lesion first.

Procedure
Radiofrequency ablation of renal tumors

Pre-procedure Imaging
Prior serial CT scans demonstrated progressive enlargement of bilateral, enhancing, solid lesions consistent with renal cell carcinoma. Before RFA, CT with the patient prone (Fig. 1) identified the exophytic right renal mass.

Intraprocedural Findings
A 21-gauge needle was placed percutaneously to inject sterile water and hydrodissect the adjacent colon away from the exophytic lesion (Fig. 2). A 3-cm Valley Lab probe (Covidien, Boulder, CO) was then placed under CT guidance and successfully used to ablate the tumor (Fig. 3), using two overlapping ablations.

Follow-up and Complications
The bilateral lesions were successfully ablated in a staged fashion, with follow-up MRI at 3, 6, and 12 months demonstrating necrosis of each lesion, and no enhancement was seen. An additional lesion has been ablated since these two initial lesions were treated.

Suggested Readings
Gervais DA, McGovern FJ, Arellano RS, et al: Radiofrequency ablation of renal cell carcinoma. Part 1. Indications, results, and role in patient management over a 6-year period and ablation of 100 tumors. AJR Am J Roentgenol 185:64-71, 2005.

Goldberg SN, Grassi CJ, Cardella JF, et al: Image-guided tumor ablation: Standardization of terminology and reporting criteria. J Vasc Intervent Radiol 16:765-778, 2005.

Gervais DA, Arellano RS, Mueller P: Percutaneous ablation of kidney tumors in nonsurgical candidates. Oncology (Williston Park) 19(Suppl 4):6-11, 2005.

Zagoria RF, Traver MA, Werle DM, et al: Oncologic efficacy of CT-guided percutaneous radiofrequency ablation of renal cell carcinomas. AJR Am J Roentgenol 2007;189:429-436.

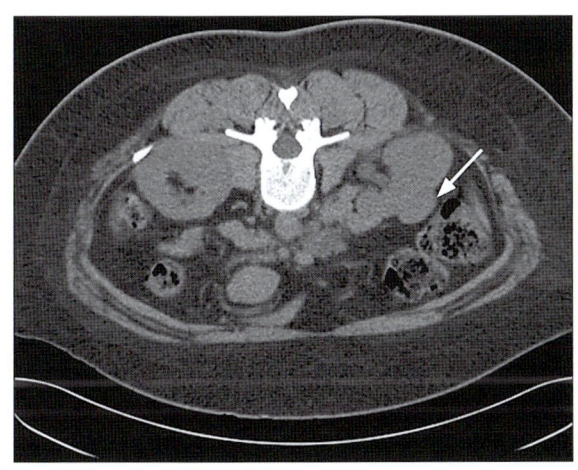

Figure 1. CT before RFA with the patient prone shows the exophytic renal mass *(arrow)*, which measured approximately 1.5 x 3 cm.

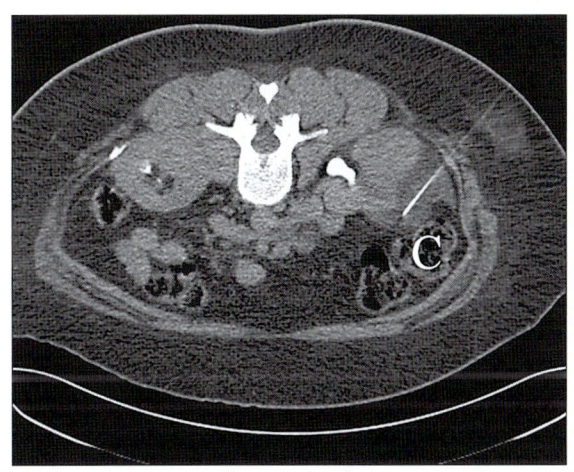

Figure 2. A 21-gauge needle was placed percutaneously under CT guidance and used to hydrodissect the adjacent colon (C) away from the exophytic lesion.

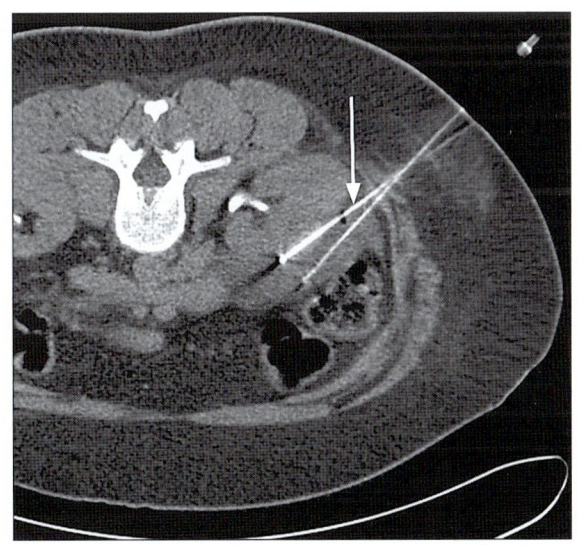

Figure 3. A 3-cm RFA probe *(arrow)* was placed under CT guidance and successfully used to ablate the tumor, using two overlapping ablations.

Case 253

DEMOGRAPHICS/CLINICAL HISTORY

A 64-year-old man with incidentally discovered right renal mass.

DISCUSSION

History/Indications for Procedure
A 64-year-old man with a right renal mass discovered incidentally during a workup for back pain. The patient is considered at high surgical risk because of his history of atrial fibrillation, mitral valve replacement, and recent stroke.

Procedure
Cryoablation for renal cell carcinoma

Pre-procedure Imaging
Contrast-enhanced CT shows a 3.2-cm × 3.7-cm mass in the mid-right kidney (Fig. 1). The mass is central in location and shows marked enhancement following contrast administration.

Intraprocedural Findings
Before ablation, a CT-guided biopsy of the mass was performed with a 20-gauge automatic biopsy device. Three cryoablation probes were inserted into the mass using CT guidance (Fig. 2); two freeze-thaw cycles were performed, and the ice-ball formation was monitored with CT imaging to ensure complete coverage of the tumor (Fig. 3).

Follow-up and Complications
The biopsy confirmed the mass to be a clear-cell renal cell carcinoma. Follow-up serial CT scans show the mass to be decreasing in size with no residual enhancement (Fig. 4).

Suggested Readings
Finley DS, Beck S, Box G, et al: Percutaneous and laparoscopic cryoablation of small renal masses. J Urol 180:492-498, 2008.

Georgiades CS, Hong K, Bizzell C, et al: Safety and efficacy of CT-guided percutaneous cryoablation for renal cell carcinoma. J Vasc Intervent Radiol 19:1302-1310, 2008.

Gill IS, Remer EM, Hasan WA, et al: Renal cryoablation: Outcome at 3 years. J Urol 173:1903-1907, 2005.

Maybody M, Solomon SB: Image-guided percutaneous cryoablation of renal tumors. Tech Vasc Intervent Radiol 10:140-148, 2007.

Case 253   507

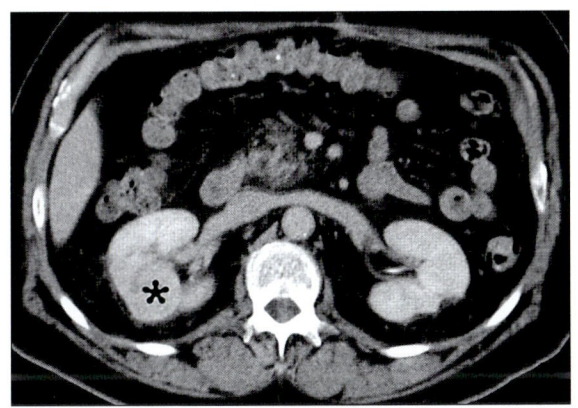

Figure 1. Contrast-enhanced CT shows a centrally located, 3.6-cm enhancing mass in the mid-right kidney *(asterisk)*.

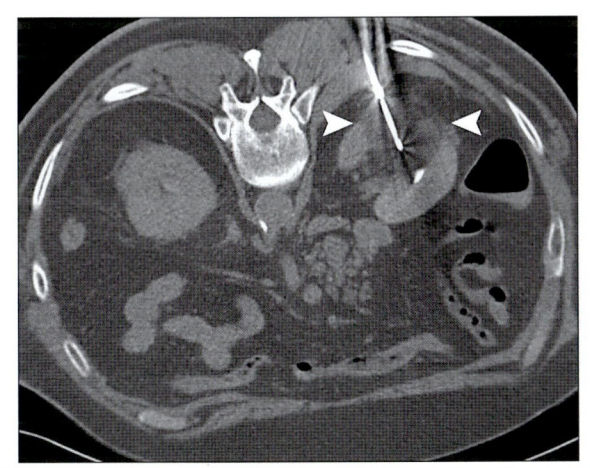

Figure 2. CT image obtained during the cryoablation. The patient has been positioned prone on the CT table, and multiple cryoablation probes have been placed. There is low attenuation in the mass from ice-ball formation *(arrowheads)*.

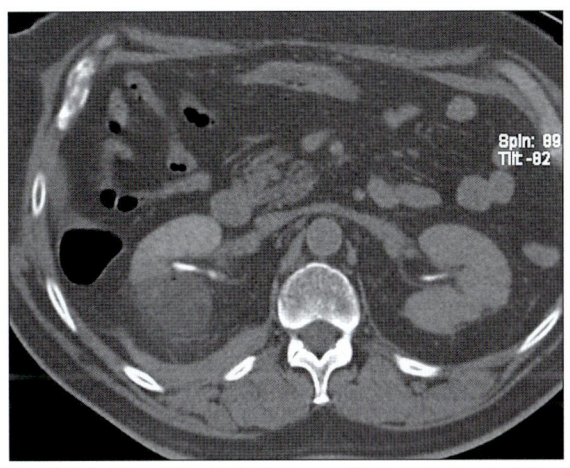

Figure 3. CT image obtained after cryoablation. There is diffusely decreased attenuation within the mass, and a small retroperitoneal hematoma is present.

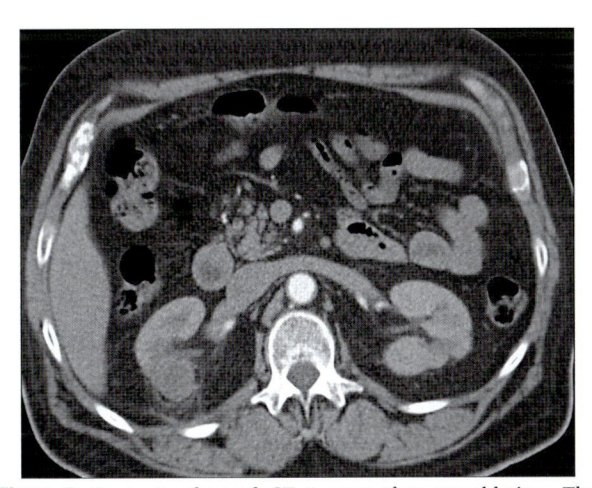

Figure 4. Contrast-enhanced CT 1 year after cryoablation. The mass now measures 2.4 cm × 2.6 cm, and there is no visible enhancement.

Case 254

DEMOGRAPHICS/CLINICAL HISTORY

A 58-year-old man with a 3.3-cm enhancing renal cell carcinoma, undergoing CT.

DISCUSSION

History/Indications for Procedure
This patient had undergone two prior unsuccessful radiofrequency ablation procedures on the mass.

Procedure
Cryoablation of renal cell carcinoma

Pre-procedure Imaging
Contrast-enhanced CT scan of the abdomen shows a well-circumscribed, 3.3-cm × 2.9-cm enhancing mass within the upper pole of the left kidney (Fig. 1).

Intraprocedural Findings
Using CT guidance, four 3-cm cryoablation probes were positioned within the renal mass (Fig. 2). Two freeze-thaw cycles were performed; the mass was frozen to a temperature of −147°C.

Follow-up and Complications
The patient developed a moderate-sized perinephric hematoma after the procedure that did not require any further intervention. On CT performed 9 months after the cryoablation, there is no enhancement of the mass to suggest any residual viable tumor (Fig. 3).

Suggested Readings

Gervais DA, Arellano RS, Mueller P: Percutaneous ablation of kidney tumors in nonsurgical candidates. Oncology (Williston Park) 19(11 Suppl 4):6-11, 2005.

Gill IS, Remer EM, Hasan WA, et al: Renal cryoablation: Outcome at 3 years. J Urol 173:1903-1907, 2005.

Gupta A, Allaf ME, Kavoussi LR, et al: Computerized tomography guided percutaneous renal cryoablation with the patient under conscious sedation: Initial clinical experience. J Urol 175(2):447-452; discussion 452-433, 2006.

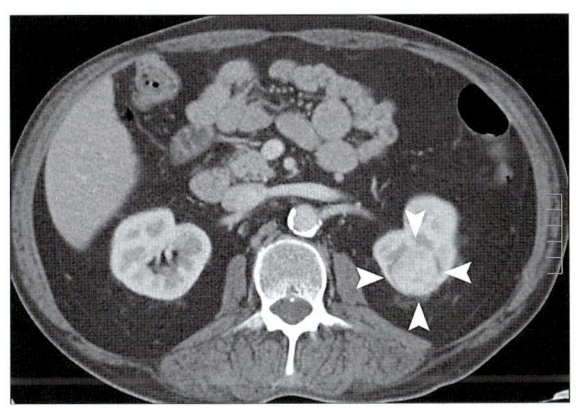

Figure 1. Axial image from contrast-enhanced CT scan shows a 3.3-cm enhancing mass in the upper pole of the left kidney (*arrowheads*).

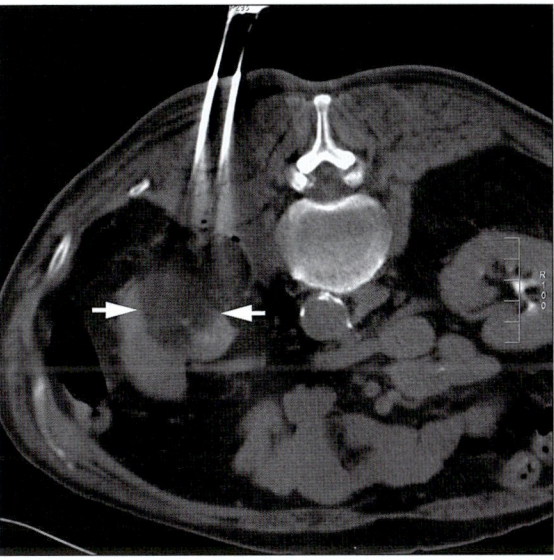

Figure 2. Axial CT image obtained during cryoablation shows the formation of the ice ball within the mass (*arrows*).

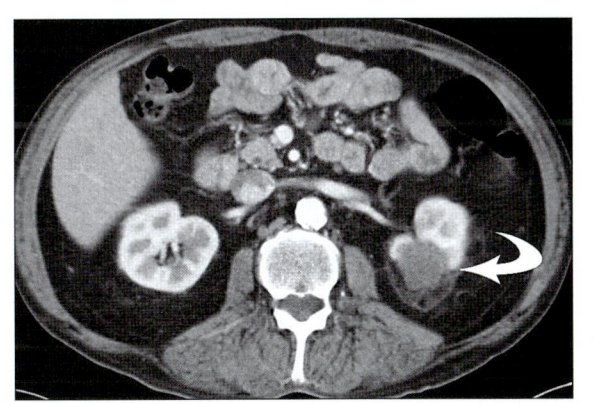

Figure 3. Axial image from contrast-enhanced CT scan 9 months after cryoablation. The mass is slightly smaller (*curved arrow*), and there was no residual enhancement.

Case 255

DEMOGRAPHICS/CLINICAL HISTORY

A 21-year-old man with foot pain secondary to an osteoid osteoma, undergoing CT.

DISCUSSION

History/Indications for Procedure
This patient had a previous surgical resection, with continued pain.

Procedure
Radiofrequency ablation for osteoid osteoma

Pre-procedure Imaging
CT scan of the ankle shows a focus of sclerotic bone in the talar neck corresponding to the bone graft. There is an adjacent, round focal lucency consistent with the residual osteoid osteoma (Figs. 1 and 2).

Intraprocedural Findings
The lesion was approached from the lateral side using a Bonopty system. The osteoid osteoma was ablated at 90°C for 6 minutes (Fig. 3).

Follow-up and Complications
The patient had near-complete relief of symptoms after the radiofrequency ablation procedure.

Suggested Readings
Cantwell CT, Obyrne J, Eustace S: Current trends in the treatment of osteoid osteoma with an emphasis on radiofrequency ablation. Eur Radiol 14:607-617, 2004.

Pinto CH, Taminiau AH, Vanderschueren GM, et al: Technical considerations in CT-guided radiofrequency thermal ablation of osteoid osteoma: Tricks of the trade. AJR Am J Roentgenol 179:1633-1642, 2002.

Case 255   511

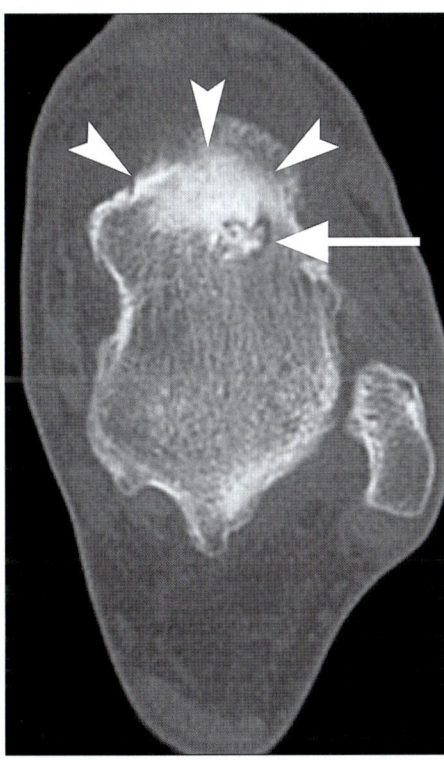

Figure 1. Axial CT scan of the talus shows an area of sclerotic bone *(arrowheads)* corresponding to the patient's prior bone graft. Immediately adjacent to this is a lucent lesion with sclerotic center consistent with residual osteoid osteoma *(arrow)*.

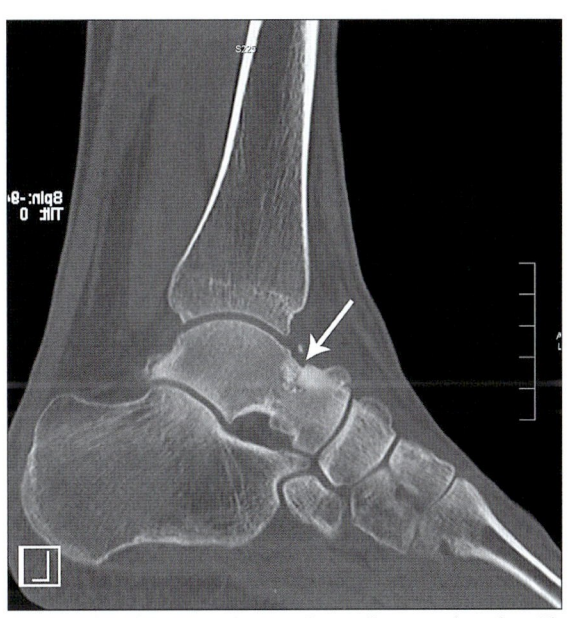

Figure 2. Sagittal CT scan shows sclerotic bone graft and residual osteoid osteoma *(arrow)*.

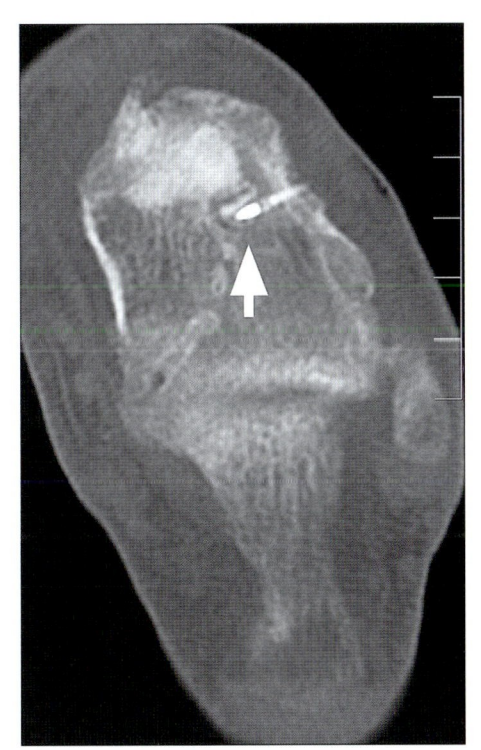

Figure 3. Axial CT scan obtained during the RFA procedure shows the tip of the RFA probe in the center of the lesion *(arrow)*.

Case 256

DEMOGRAPHICS/CLINICAL HISTORY

A 14-year-old boy with right leg pain, undergoing radiography and computed tomography (CT).

DISCUSSION

History/Indications for Procedure
A 14-year-old boy has a 2-year history of right lower leg pain that occurs at rest and is relieved by nonsteroidal anti-inflammatory medications.

Procedure
Radiofrequency ablation of osteoid osteoma

Pre-procedure Imaging
Radiograph of the right lower extremity shows a focal fusiform expansion of the fibular cortex (Fig. 1). CT shows a central radiolucent nidus within the cortical expansion that is compatible with an osteoid osteoma (Fig. 2).

Intraprocedural Findings
Using CT guidance, a cannula was inserted into the nidus using a bone drill (Fig. 3). A 10-mm radiofrequency ablation probe was placed coaxially, and the nidus was ablated for 5 minutes at 95° C.

Follow-up and Complications
The pain completely resolved after radiofrequency ablation.

Suggested Readings
Lindner NJ, Ozaki T, Roedl R, et al: Percutaneous radiofrequency ablation in osteoid osteoma. J Bone Joint Surg Br 83:391-396, 2001.

Martel J, Bueno A, Ortiz E: Percutaneous radiofrequency treatment of osteoid osteoma using cool-tip electrodes. Eur J Radiol 56:403-408, 2005.

Rosenthal DI, Hornicek FJ, Torriani M, et al: Osteoid osteoma: Percutaneous treatment with radiofrequency energy. Radiology 229:171-175, 2003.

Vanbrux AC, Montague BJ, Murphy KP, et al: Image-guided percutaneous radiofrequency ablation for osteoid osteomas. J Vasc Intervent Radiol 14:375-380, 2003.

Woertler K, Vestring T, Boettner F, et al: Osteoid osteoma: CT-guided percutaneous radiofrequency ablation and follow-up in 47 patients. J Vasc Intervent Radiol 12:717-722, 2001.

Case 256   513

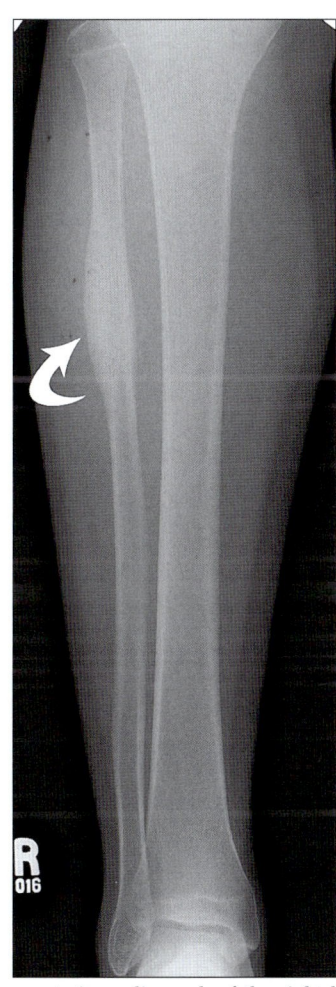

Figure 1. Anteroposterior radiograph of the right lower extremity shows a focal, fusiform, cortical expansion of the proximal fibula (*arrow*).

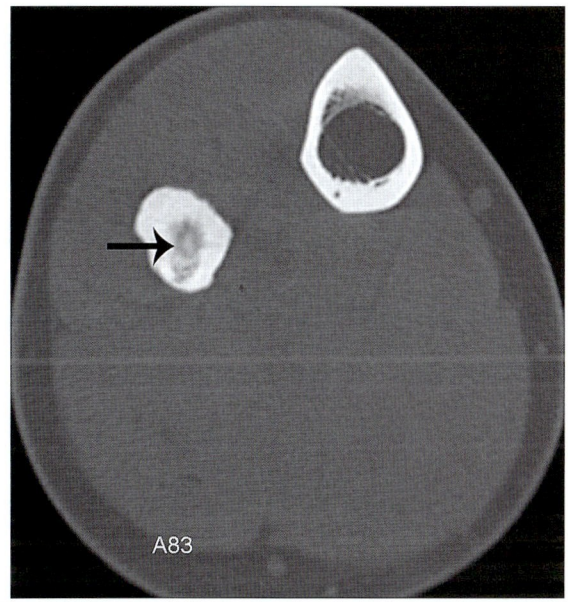

Figure 2. CT of the fibula shows a radiolucent nidus at the level of the cortical expansion (*arrow*).

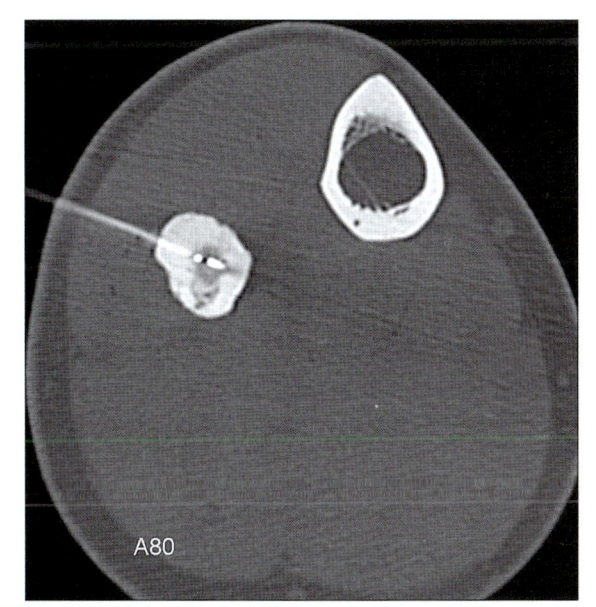

Figure 3. A 10-mm radiofrequency ablation probe was advanced into the nidus, and the lesion was ablated for 5 minutes at 95° C.

Case 257

DEMOGRAPHICS/CLINICAL HISTORY

A 74-year-old man with renal cell carcinoma metastatic to the right acetabulum, undergoing computed tomography (CT), radiofrequency ablation (RFA), and polymethylmethacrylate injection.

DISCUSSION

History/Indications for Procedure
A 74-year-old man has renal cell carcinoma metastatic to the right acetabulum. The patient has a new pathologic fracture that causes significant pain and prevents ambulation.

Procedure
Radiofrequency ablation for painful acetabular metastasis

Pre-procedure Imaging
CT of the pelvis demonstrates a 3-cm, lytic lesion in the right iliac wing. This is associated with a pathologic comminuted fracture that extends into the right superior-anterior acetabulum (Fig. 1).

Intraprocedural Findings
Using CT guidance, a clustered RFA probe was placed into the lytic lesion from a lateral approach (Fig. 2). After RFA, the patient was transferred to a fluoroscopic table, where polymethylmethacrylate was injected into the lesion (Fig. 3).

Follow-up and Complications
After the procedure, the patient continued to have significant pain in the right hip. However, he is able to ambulate with the assistance of a walker.

Suggested Readings
Hoffmann RT, Jakobs TF, Trumm C, et al: Radiofrequency ablation in combination with osteoplasty in the treatment of painful metastatic bone disease. J Vasc Intervent Radiol 19:419-425, 2008.

Nakatsuka A, Yamakado K, Maeda M, et al: Radiofrequency ablation combined with bone cement injection for the treatment of bone malignancies. J Vasc Intervent Radiol 15:707-712, 2004.

Posteraro AF, Dupuy DE, Mayo-Smith WW: Radiofrequency ablation of bony metastatic disease. Clin Radiol 59:803-811, 2004.

Sabharwal T, Salter R, Adam A, Gangi A: Image-guided therapies in orthopedic oncology. Orthop Clin North Am 37:105-112, 2006.

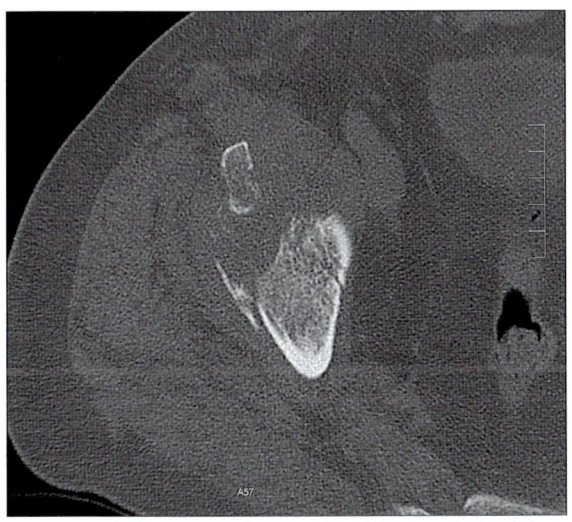

Figure 1. Axial CT through the superior right acetabulum demonstrates a lytic lesion with an associated pathologic comminuted fracture.

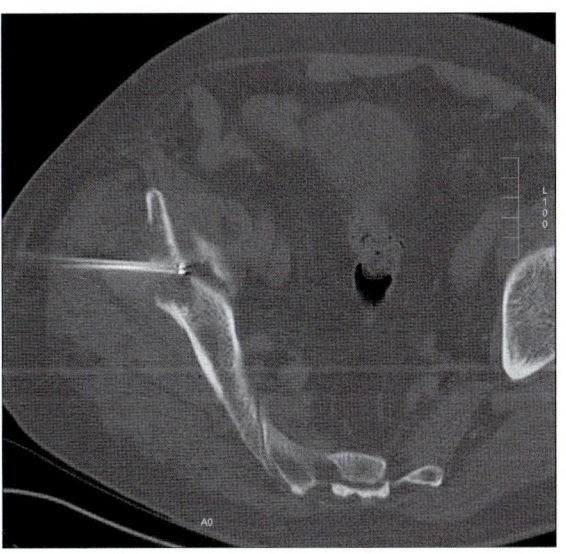

Figure 2. Using CT guidance, a clustered RFA probe was advanced into the lytic metastasis.

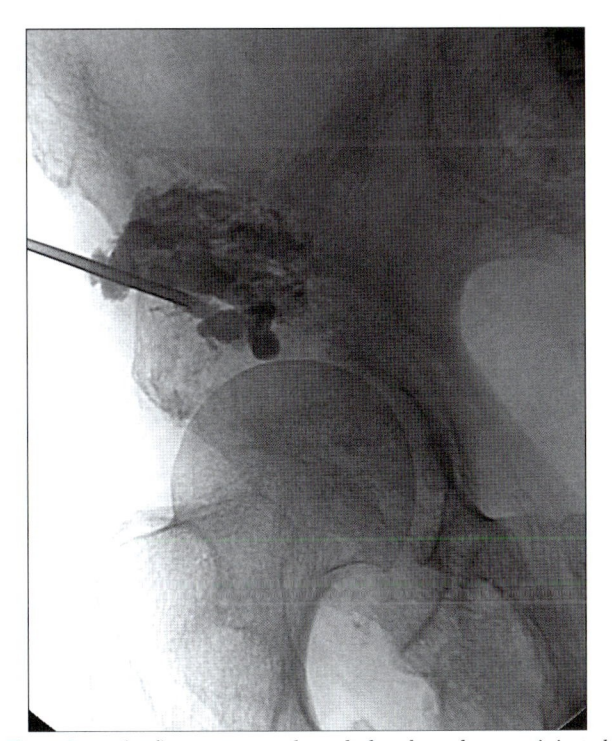

Figure 3. Under fluoroscopy, polymethylmethacrylate was injected into the lytic lesion. The injection was stopped after the cement began to leak into the soft tissues.

Case 258

DEMOGRAPHICS/CLINICAL HISTORY

A 67-year-old man with T7 vertebral compression fracture, undergoing MRI and radiography.

DISCUSSION

History/Indications for Procedure
This patient's history included non–small cell lung carcinoma in addition to a painful T7 compression fracture. The onset of back pain occurred 3 days after a fall.

Procedure
Thoracic vertebroplasty

Pre-procedure Imaging
MRI with contrast agent shows a 30% compression fracture of T7 with marrow edema and vertebral body enhancement (Figs. 1 and 2). No soft-tissue mass or cord compromise was present.

Intraprocedural Findings
A biopsy was done at the time of the vertebroplasty, confirming the benign etiology of the fracture. Vertebroplasty was performed using a bipedicular approach (Figs. 3 and 4).

Follow-up and Complications
The patient reported being pain-free after the procedure. He remained pain-free at last follow-up.

Suggested Readings
Deramond H, Depriester C, Galibert P, et al: Percutaneous vertebroplasty with polymethylmethacrylate: Technique, indications, and results. Radiol Clin North Am 36:533-546, 1998.

Mathis J, et al: Percutaneous vertebroplasty: A therapeutic option for pain associated with vertebral compression fracture. J Back Musculoskel Rehab 13:11-17, 1999.

Weill A, Chiras J, Simon JM, et al: Spinal metastases: Indications for and results of percutaneous injection of acrylic surgical cement. Radiology 199:241-247, 1996.

Case 258   517

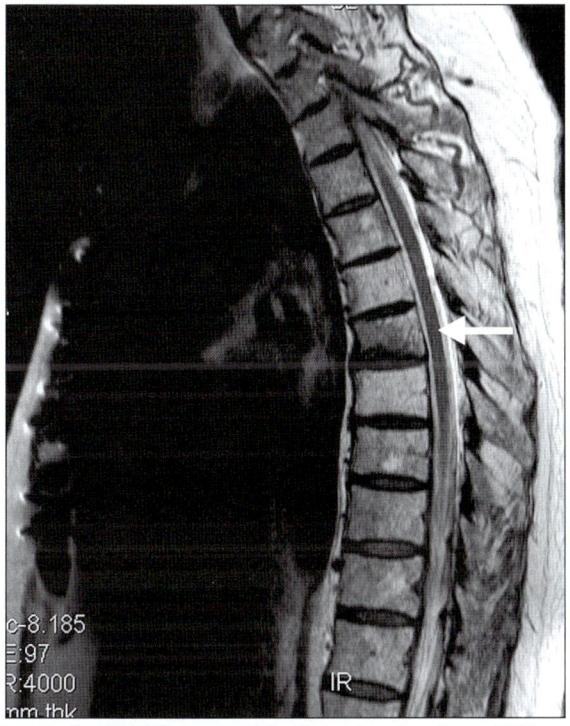

Figure 1. Sagittal MR image of the thoracic spine shows 30% compression of the T7 vertebral body *(arrow)*.

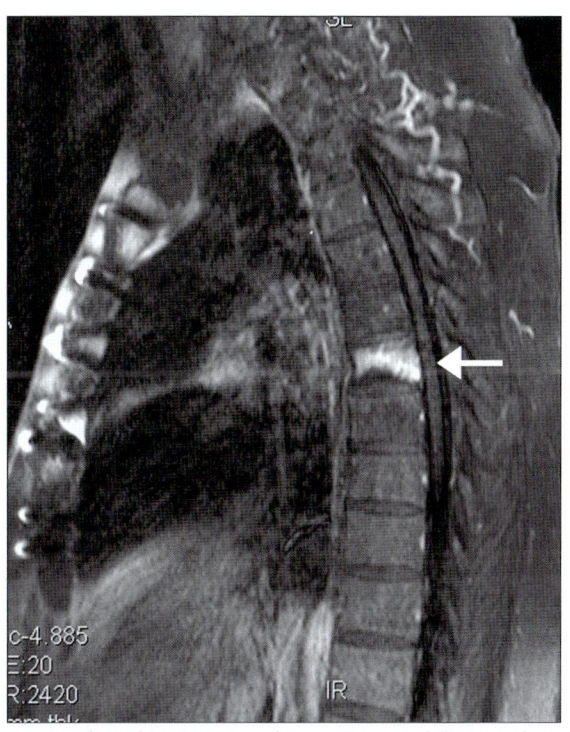

Figure 2. After administration of intravenous gadolinium, the collapsed vertebral body intensely enhances *(arrow)*. No soft-tissue mass is present.

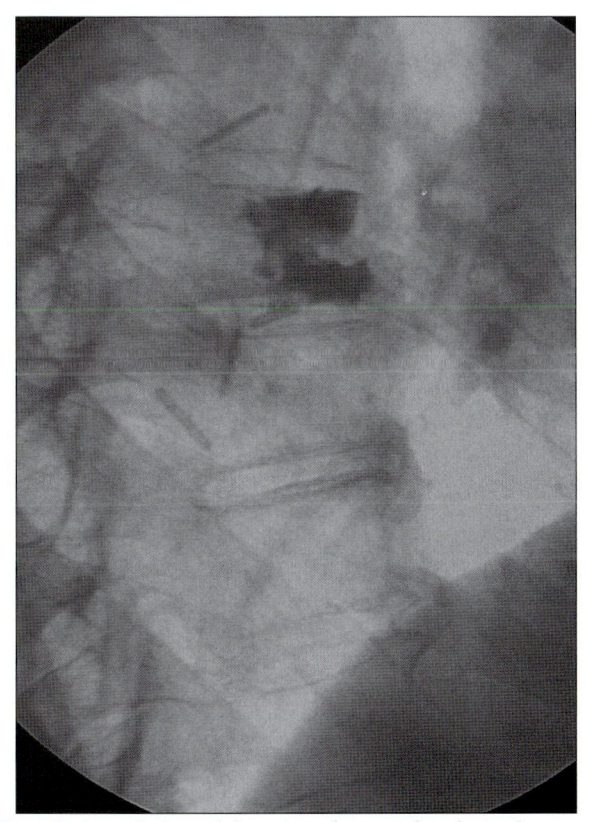

Figure 3. Lateral view of the spine after vertebroplasty shows cement within the anterior half of the T7 vertebral body.

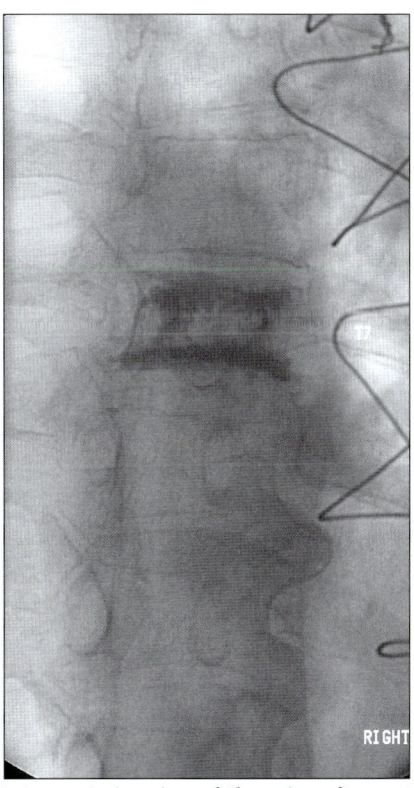

Figure 4. Anteroposterior view of the spine after vertebroplasty shows cement along the superior and inferior body end plates.

Case 259

DEMOGRAPHICS/CLINICAL HISTORY

A 62-year-old man with a history of non–small cell lung carcinoma and back pain, undergoing magnetic resonance imaging (MRI).

DISCUSSION

History/Indications for Procedure

A 62-year-old man has a history of non–small cell lung carcinoma and new-onset back pain. The pain is worse with movement and is not associated with radicular symptoms.

Procedure

Kyphoplasty

Pre-procedure Imaging

Contrast-enhanced MRI of the thoracic spine shows a compression fracture of the T5 vertebral body, with 40% loss of vertebral body height. There is increased T2-weighted MRI signal (Fig. 1) and enhancement after contrast administration.

Intraprocedural Findings

Bilateral, transpedicular accesses were obtained, and a vertebral biopsy was performed. The kyphoplasty balloon was inflated (Figs. 2 and 3), and polymethylmethacrylate was placed under fluoroscopy (Fig. 4).

Follow-up and Complications

The biopsy revealed no malignant cells. The patient's back pain significantly improved, and he was able to discontinue the use of oral analgesics.

Suggested Readings

Coumans JV, Reinhardt MK, Lieberman IH, et al: Kyphoplasty for vertebral compression fractures: 1-year clinical outcomes from a prospective study. J Neurosurg 99(Suppl):44-50, 2003.

Evans AJ, Jensen ME, Kip KE, et al: Vertebral compression fractures: Pain reduction and improvement in functional mobility after percutaneous polymethylmethacrylate vertebroplasty—retrospective report of 245 cases. Radiology 226:366-372, 2003.

Ledlie JT, Renfro M: Balloon kyphoplasty: One-year outcomes in vertebral body height restoration, chronic pain, and activity levels. J Neurosurg 98:36-42, 2003.

Mathis JM, Ortiz AO, Zoarski GH: Vertebroplasty versus kyphoplasty: A comparison and contrast. AJNR Am J Neuroradiol 25:840-845, 2004.

Ortiz AO, Zoarski GH, Beckerman M: Kyphoplasty. Tech Vasc Intervent Radiol 5:239-249, 2002.

Case 259   519

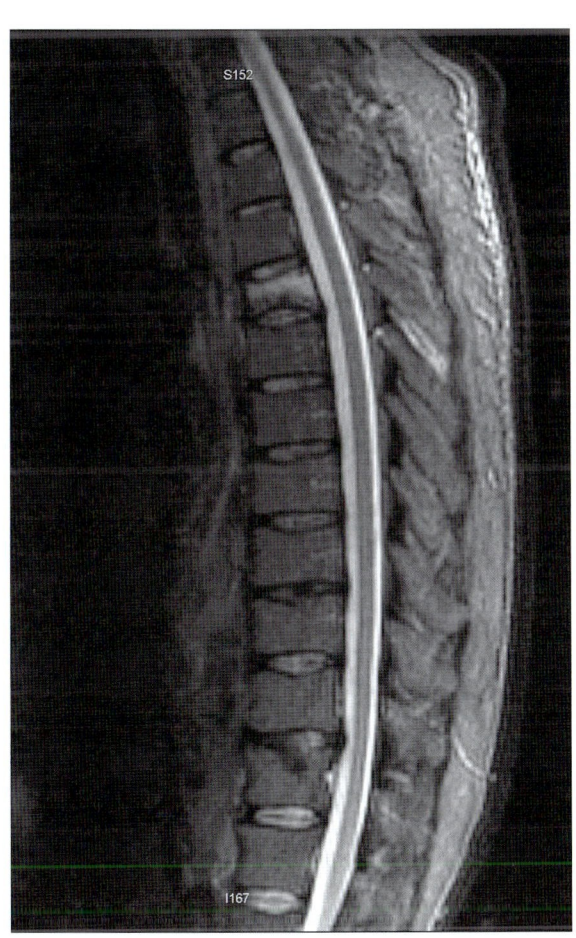

Figure 1. Sagittal, T2-weighted MRI through the thoracic spine shows a compression fracture of the T5 vertebral body. The vertebral body has increased T2-weighted signal intensity, indicating vertebral body edema.

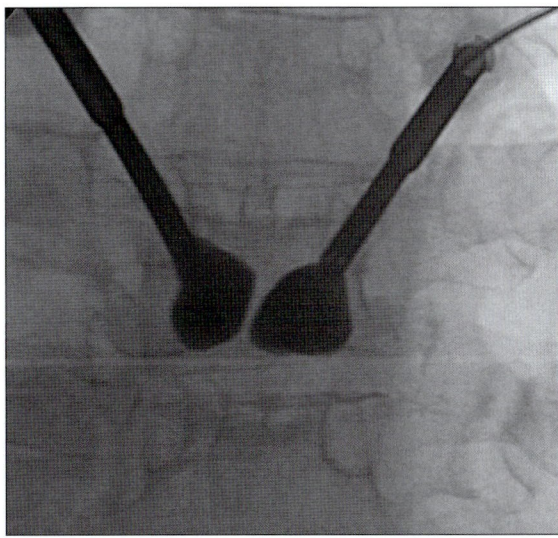

Figure 2. Anteroposterior radiograph obtained during the kyphoplasty procedure shows the presence of bilateral, 12-gauge cannulas. The kyphoplasty balloons have been inflated.

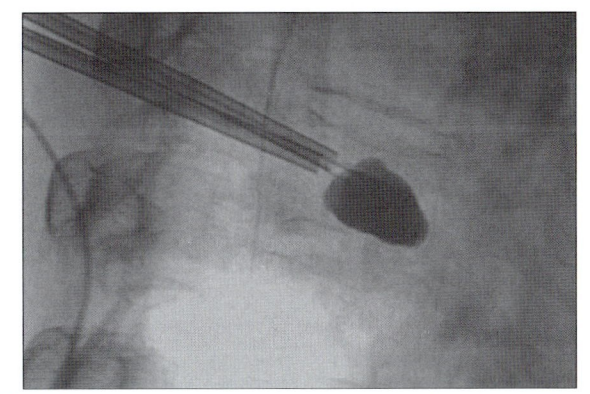

Figure 3. Lateral radiograph shows the inflated kyphoplasty balloons in the anterior one half of the vertebral body.

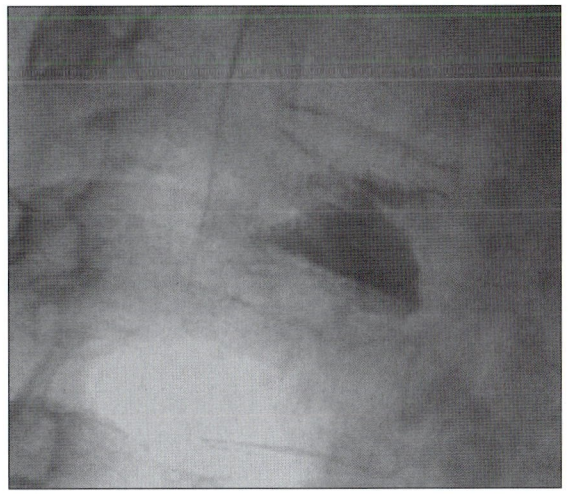

Figure 4. Lateral radiograph shows polymethylmethacrylate filling the cavity created by the kyphoplasty balloons.

Case 260

Charles Burke, MD, and Robert G. Dixon, MD

DEMOGRAPHICS/CLINICAL HISTORY

A 67-year-old woman with esophageal cancer after transhiatal esophagectomy, undergoing radiography and thoracic duct embolization.

DISCUSSION

History/Indications for Procedure
A 67-year-old woman with a persistent left chylothorax had more than 2000 mL/day of output from the chest tube. The high output persisted despite conservative measures.

Procedure
Percutaneous embolization of the thoracic duct

Pre-procedure Imaging
A chest radiograph showed expected postoperative changes after esophagectomy with gastric pull-through and with bilateral chest tubes in place.

Intraprocedural Findings
A lymphatic vessel was cannulated in the dorsum of the right foot with a 27-gauge needle and pedal lymphangiography opacifying the cisterna chyli, providing a target for percutaneous access (Figs. 1 and 2). The thoracic duct was catheterized and embolized with coils (Figs. 2 to 4).

Follow-up and Complications
The high-output chylothorax diminished rapidly over the next 2 days. The chest tubes were removed, and the patient was discharged to her home with no recurrent chylothorax on follow-up chest radiographs.

Suggested Readings
Cerfolio RJ, Allen MS, Deschamps C, et al: Postoperative chylothorax. J Thorac Cardiovasc Surg 112:1361-1366, 1996.

Cope C, Kaiser LR: Management of unremitting chylothorax by percutaneous embolization and blockage of retroperitoneal lymphatic vessels in 42 patients. J Vasc Intervent Radiol 13:1139-1148, 2002.

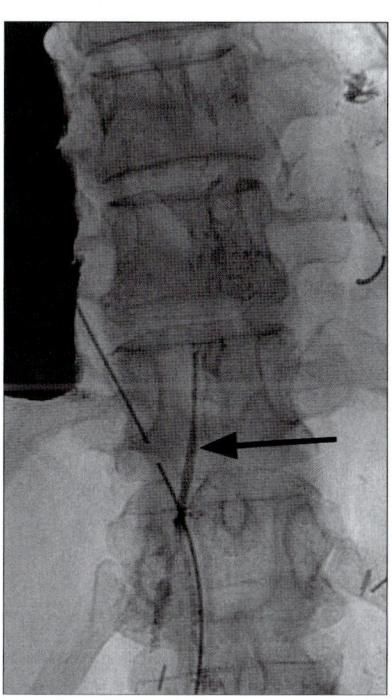

Figure 1. The cisterna chyli *(arrow)* is identified after right pedal lymphangiography. The nasogastric tube can be seen, as well as residual contrast in the stomach from a prior study.

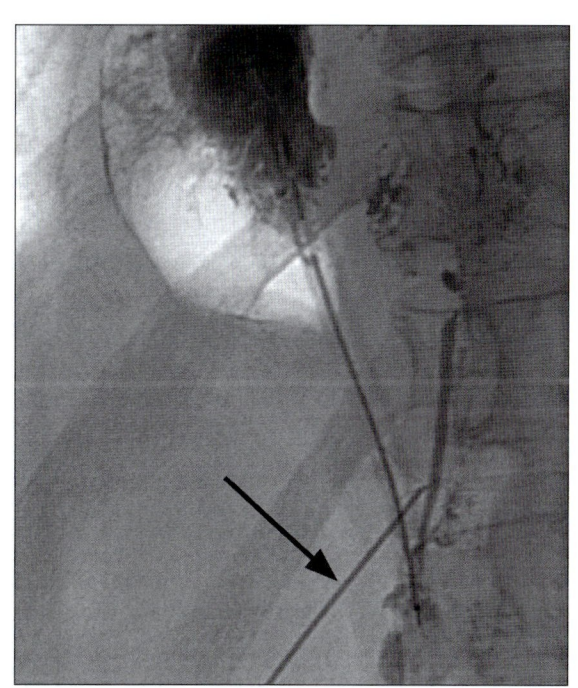

Figure 2. A 21-gauge needle *(arrow)* has been successfully advanced to the cisterna chyli from a slightly right anterior oblique approach under fluoroscopic guidance. After accessing the cisterna chyli, an 0.018-inch nitinol guidewire was used to exchange the needle for a 4-French catheter.

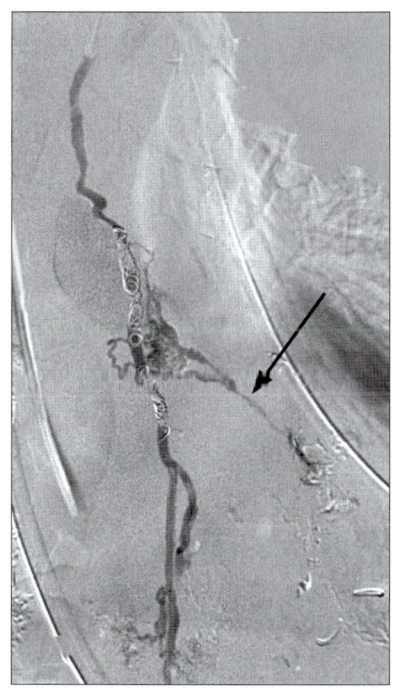

Figure 3. Subtracted thoracic duct injection identifies the leak *(arrow)* extending into the left hemithorax.

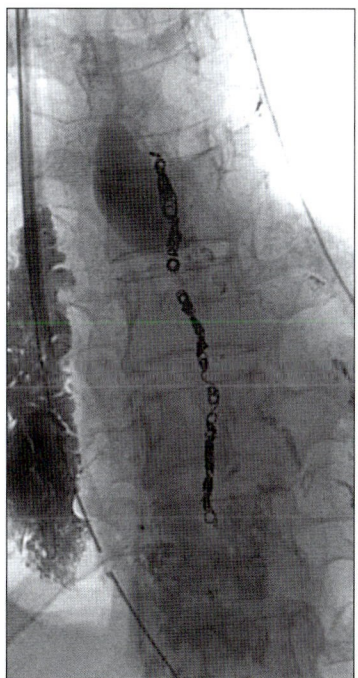

Figure 4. After coil embolization of the thoracic duct, residual contrast is seen adjacent to the coiled thoracic duct. No leak was identified on follow-up thoracic duct injection.

olysis bullosa and
chronic pelvic pain caused by indwelling suprapubic
catheter.

DISCUSSION

History/Indications for Procedure
A 24-year-old man with epidermolysis bullosa and chronic pelvic pain caused by indwelling suprapubic catheter.

Procedure
CT-guided sacral nerve block

Intraprocedural Findings
Using CT guidance, a 22-gauge Chiba needle was advanced into the dorsal S3-4 neural foramen (Fig. 1). Contrast was injected, opacifying the S3 nerve root; anesthetic and steroid were then injected (Figs. 2 and 3).

Follow-up and Complications
The patient's pain lessened after the procedure and remained under control for the next 10 weeks.

Suggested Readings
Gangi A, Dietemann JL, Mortazavi R, et al: CT-guided interventional procedures for pain management in the lumbosacral spine. Radiographics 18:621-633, 1998.
Wagner AL, Murtagh FR: Selective nerve root blocks. Tech Vasc Intervent Radiol 5:194-200, 2002.

Case 261   523

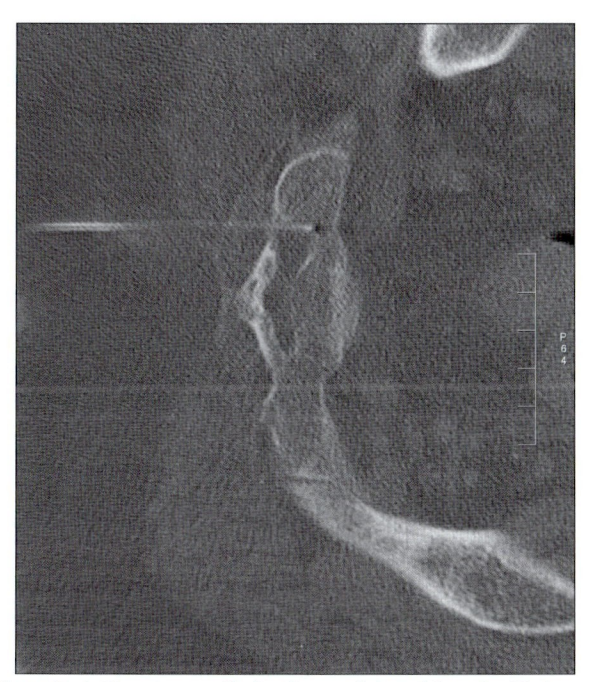

Figure 1. A 22-gauge needle has been advanced into the S3-4 neural foramen.

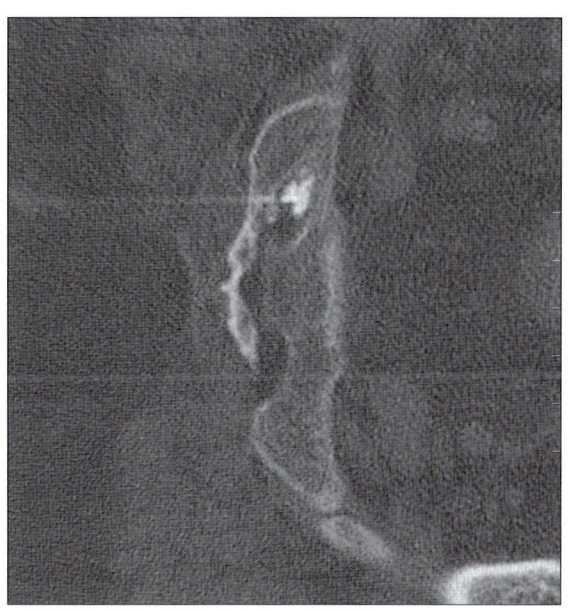

Figure 2. Contrast, 0.75 mL, has been injected and fills the neural foramen.

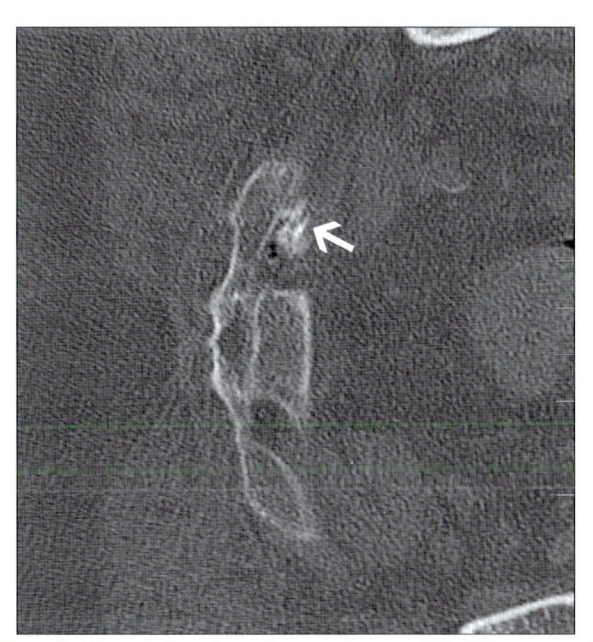

Figure 3. There is free flow of contrast around the S3 nerve root (arrow).

Case 262

DEMOGRAPHICS/CLINICAL HISTORY

An 83-year-old man with obstructive jaundice.

DISCUSSION

History/Indications for Procedure
An 83-year-old man with prior hepaticojejunostomy for gallbladder carcinoma presents with obstructive jaundice.

Procedure
Percutaneous transhepatic cholangiogram

Pre-procedure Imaging
Contrast-enhanced CT (not shown) shows marked intrahepatic biliary ductal dilatation. No mass is identified.

Intraprocedural Findings
Percutaneous cholangiogram shows dilated intrahepatic bile ducts with obstruction at the biliary-enteric anastomosis (Fig. 1). Bile duct brushing was performed, revealing atypical ductal cells.

Follow-up and Complications
Using a more peripheral duct for access, an internal-external biliary drain was placed for biliary decompression (Figs. 2–4).

Suggested Readings
Burke DR, Lewis CA, Cardella JF, et al. for the Society of Interventional Radiology Standards of Practice Committee: Quality improvement guidelines for percutaneous transhepatic cholangiography and biliary drainage. J Vasc Intervent Radiol 14:S243-S246, 2003.

Covey AM, Brown DT: Palliative percutaneous drainage in malignant biliary obstruction. Part 1: Indications and preprocedure evaluation. J Support Oncol 4:269-273, 2006.

Ferrucci JT Jr., Mueller PR, Harbin WP: Percutaneous transhepatic biliary drainage: Technique, results, and applications. Radiology 135:1-13, 1980.

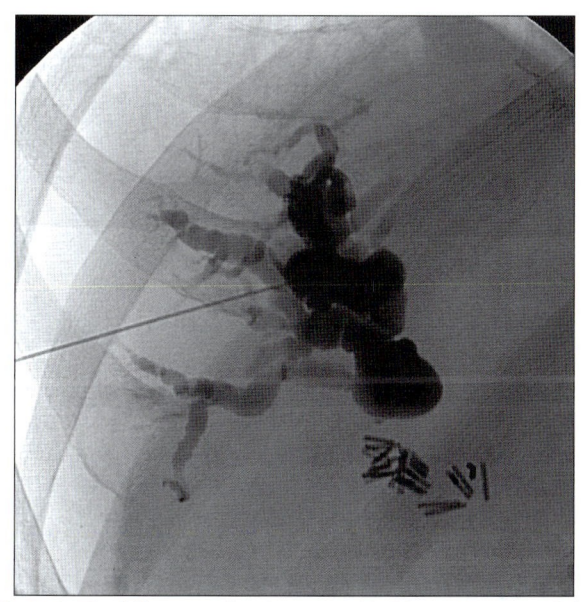

Figure 1. The biliary tree has been opacified by a 22-gauge Chiba needle. There is marked dilatation of the intrahepatic bile ducts. No contrast passes into the small bowel.

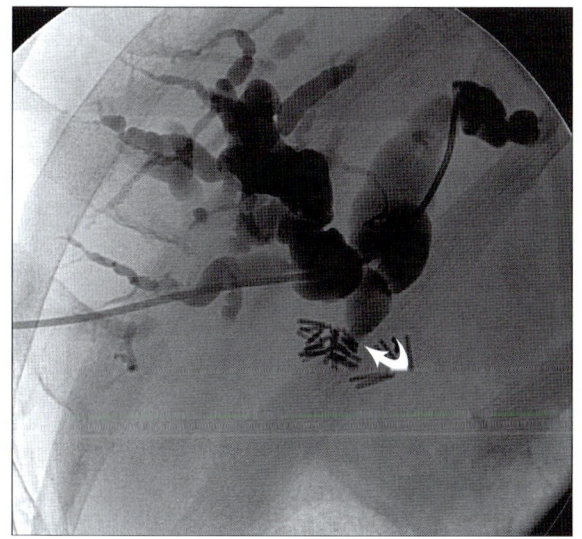

Figure 2. A more peripheral duct of the right lobe was accessed with a second needle. A 5-French catheter has been used to opacify the left-sided bile ducts. There is abrupt obstruction *(arrow)* at the confluence of the right and left hepatic ducts.

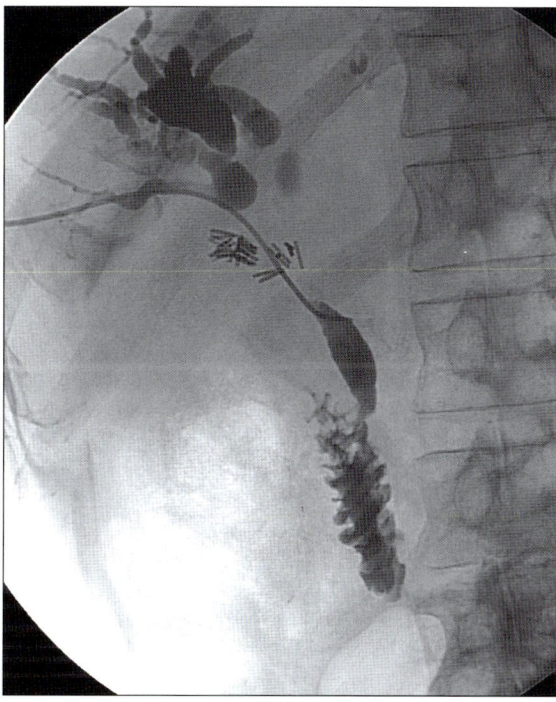

Figure 3. The 5-French catheter has been used to cross the point of obstruction. The distal common bile duct is patent.

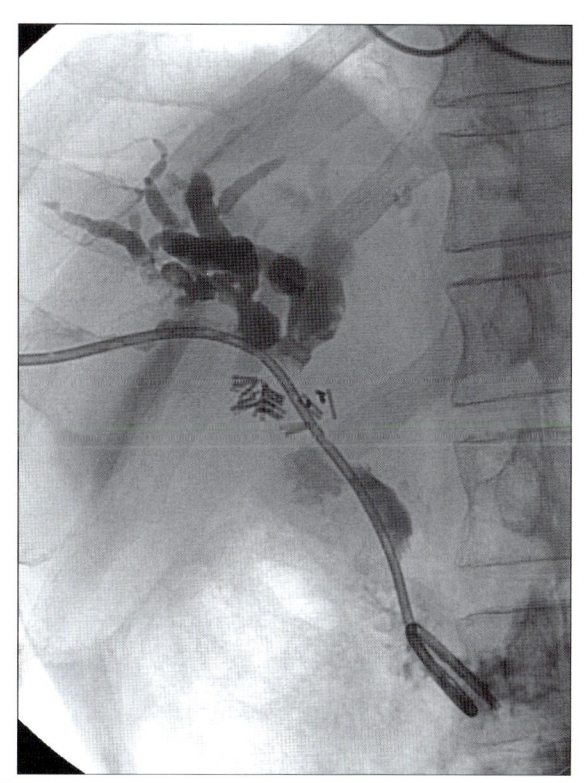

Figure 4. An 8-French internal-external drain was placed for biliary decompression.

Case 263

DEMOGRAPHICS/CLINICAL HISTORY

A 65-year-old man with a history of liver transplantation presenting with elevated bilirubin levels, undergoing percutaneous transhepatic cholangiography.

DISCUSSION

History/Indications for Procedure
A 65-year-old man underwent liver transplantation 11 years earlier for primary sclerosing cholangitis (PSC), and now presents with elevated bilirubin levels (8.8 mg/dL).

Procedure
Double needle technique, percutaneous transhepatic cholangiogram and biliary drain placement

Pre-procedure Imaging
MRI of the abdomen shows mild intrahepatic ductal dilation with ductal irregularity. The common bile duct is not dilated, but the wall is thickened and enhances after contrast administration.

Intraprocedural Findings
Percutaneous transhepatic cholangiography (PTC) shows opacification of mildly dilated and irregular intrahepatic bile ducts with filling of periductal lymphatics (Fig. 1). Using a double-needle technique (Fig. 2), a peripheral right-sided bile duct was accessed, and an 8-French internal-external biliary drain was placed (Figs. 3 and 4).

Follow-up and Complications
Based on the appearance of the biliary tree, recurrent PSC was suspected. The patient underwent percutaneous liver biopsy, which showed periportal fibrosis consistent with recurrent PSC.

Suggested Readings
Burke DR, Lewis CA, Cardella JF, et al; for the Society of Interventional Radiology Standards of Practice Committee: Quality improvement guidelines for percutaneous transhepatic cholangiography and biliary drainage. J Vasc Intervent Radiol 14:S243, 2003.

Ferrucci JT Jr, Mueller PR, Harbin WP: Percutaneous transhepatic biliary drainage: Technique, results, and applications. Radiology 135:1, 1980.

Graziadei IW: Recurrence of primary sclerosing cholangitis after liver transplantation. Liver Transpl 8:575, 2002.

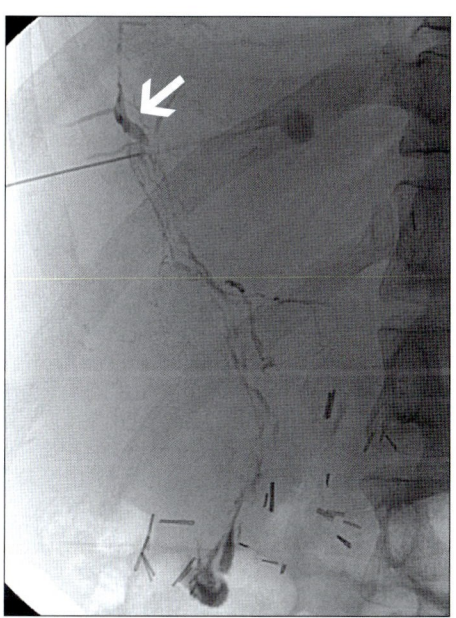

Figure 1. PTC shows 22-gauge Chiba needle has been used to opacify right-sided bile duct (*arrow*). There is also opacification of periductal lymphatics. On this image, it is unclear which duct is the common hepatic duct despite opacification of Roux-en-Y jejunal loop.

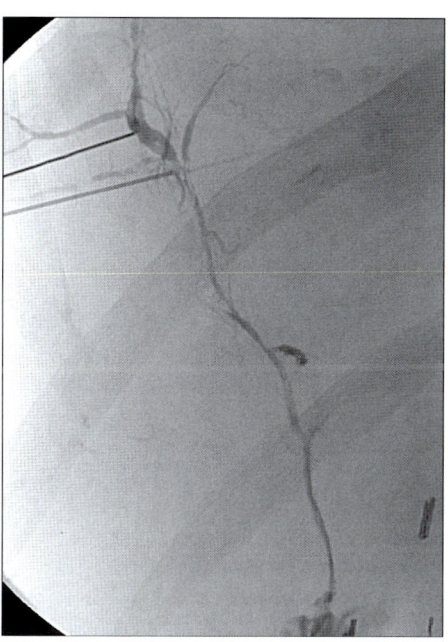

Figure 2. PTC shows second needle has been used to access opacified segment of right-sided bile duct.

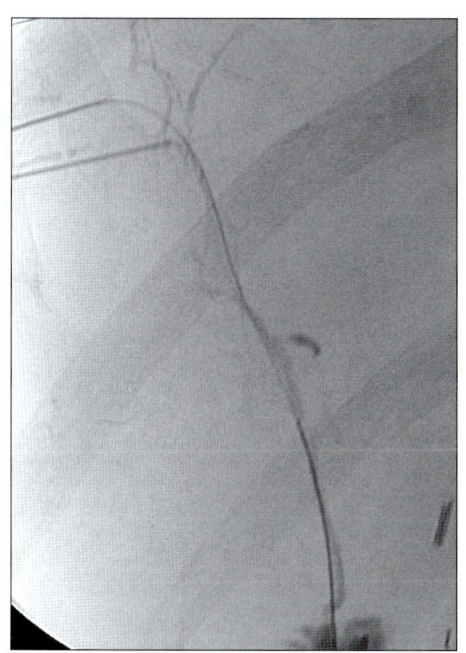

Figure 3. PTC shows guidewire has been inserted and has been passed down common hepatic duct.

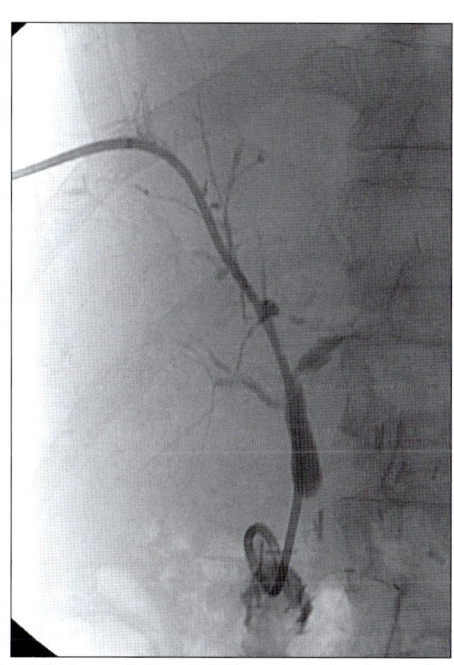

Figure 4. PTC shows 8-French biliary drain has been placed. Contrast injection shows diffuse irregularity of bile ducts, consistent with recurrent PSC.

Case 264

DEMOGRAPHICS/CLINICAL HISTORY

A 40-year-old woman with inadvertent right hepatic bile duct ligation during laparoscopic cholecystectomy.

DISCUSSION

History/Indications for Procedure
A 40-year-old woman with inadvertent ligation of the right hepatic bile duct during laparoscopic cholecystectomy.

Procedure
Percutaneous management of biliary obstruction secondary to clipped bile duct

Pre-procedure Imaging
MR cholangiopancreatography shows mild dilatation of the left and right intrahepatic bile ducts with abrupt obstruction at the level of the common hepatic duct. Percutaneous cholangiogram shows a surgical clip across the anterior right hepatic duct (Fig. 1).

Intraprocedural Findings
The common hepatic duct was opacified through a nasobiliary catheter (Fig. 2). Sharp recanalization was performed from the anterior right hepatic duct into the right hepatic duct using a 22-gauge Chiba needle. A guidewire was inserted into the common bile duct, and an 8-French internal-external biliary drain was placed (Fig. 3).

Follow-up and Complications
The patient underwent progressive balloon dilatation at the site of recanalization, and the biliary drain was progressively upsized to 12-French. Follow-up cholangiogram shows brisk drainage through the site of recanalization (Fig. 4); the percutaneous catheter was exchanged for an endoscopic stent 3 months after the recanalization for patient comfort.

Suggested Readings
Kocher M, Cerna M, Havlik R, et al: Percutaneous treatment of benign bile duct strictures. Eur J Radiol 62:170-174, 2007.
Trambert JJ, Bron KM, Zajko AB, et al: Percutaneous transhepatic balloon dilatation of benign biliary strictures. AJR Am J Roentgenol 149:945-948, 1987.

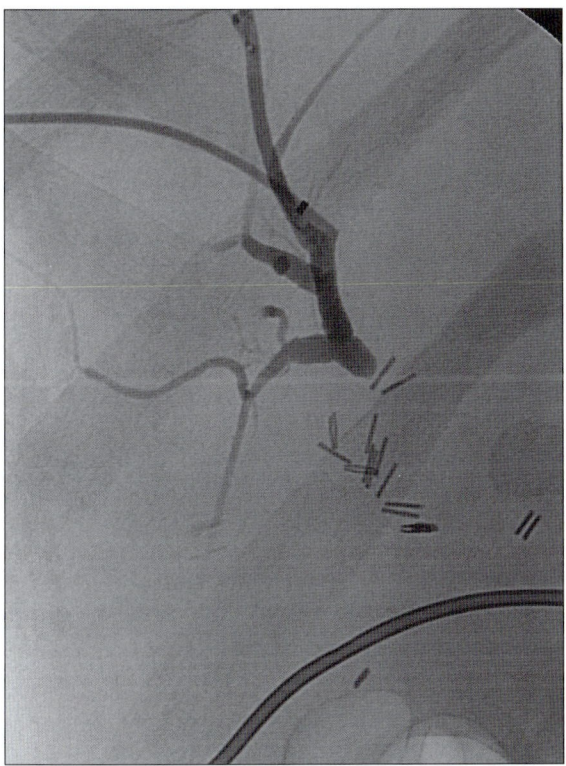

Figure 1. Single image from percutaneous cholangiogram shows opacification of the isolated bile duct as the result of surgical ligation.

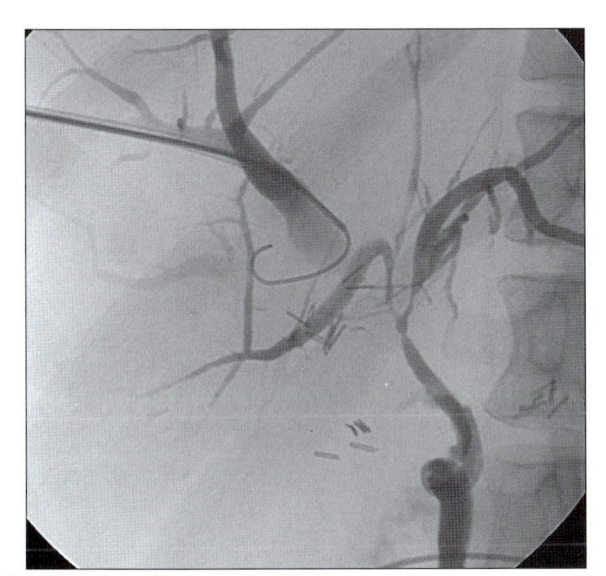

Figure 2. The common and right hepatic ducts were opacified by a nasobiliary catheter. Through a 6-French sheath, an 18-gauge needle has been inserted to the level of the surgical clip. Through this needle, a Chiba needle was used to perform a sharp recanalization of the obstructed bile duct.

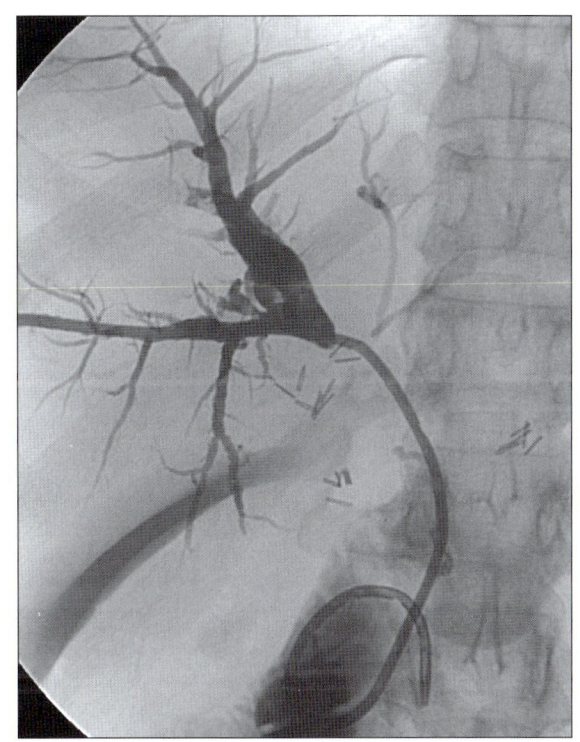

Figure 3. After successful recanalization, an 8-French internal-external biliary drain has been placed.

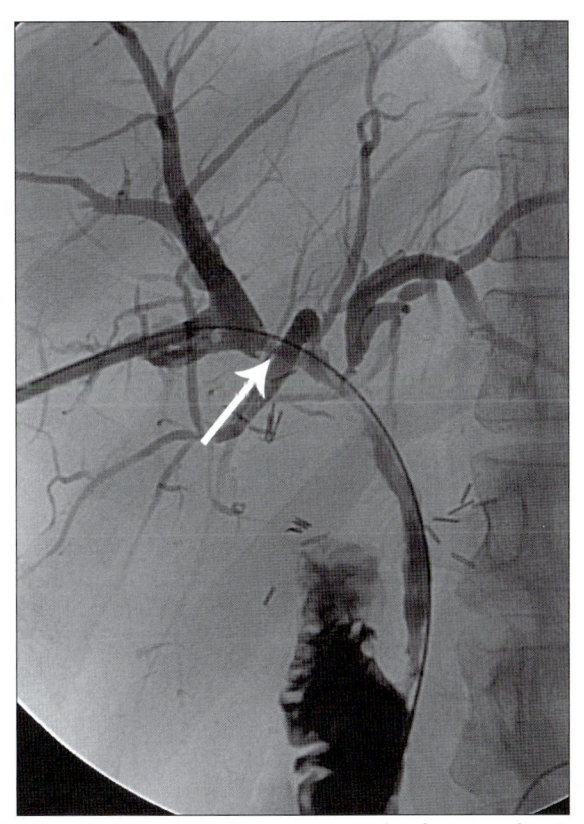

Figure 4. Follow-up cholangiogram 3 months after recanalization. A sheath cholangiogram shows good flow through the site of recanalization *(arrow)*.

Case 265

DEMOGRAPHICS/CLINICAL HISTORY

An 85-year-old woman with cholangititis and obstructing biliary stone.

DISCUSSION

History/Indications for Procedure
An 85-year-old woman with a 1-week history of nausea, vomiting, and severe abdominal pain. Blood cultures are positive for gram-negative bacteremia.

Procedure
Common bile duct stone removal

Pre-procedure Imaging
MRCP from the outside hospital shows a dilated biliary tree and a stone impacted in the common bile duct.

Intraprocedural Findings
Percutaneous cholangiogram confirmed the presence of a stone impacted in the distal common bile duct (Fig. 1). A percutaneous sphincteroplasty was performed with a 10-mm angioplasty balloon; the stone was then pushed into the duodenum with an 8-mm balloon (Fig. 2).

Follow-up and Complications
After stone removal, a 10-French internal-external biliary drain was placed (Fig. 3). Follow-up cholangiogram performed 1 week later showed decompression of the biliary tree and no further indication of biliary obstruction.

Suggested Readings
Garcia-Garcia L, Lanciego C: Percutaneous treatment of biliary stones: Spincteroplasty and occlusion balloon for the clearance of bile duct calculi. AJR Am J Roentgenol 182:663-670, 2004.

Garcia-Vila JH, Redondo-Ibanez M, Diaz-Ramon C: Balloon sphincteroplasty and transpapillary elimination of bile duct stones: 10 years' experience. AJR Am J Roentgenol 182:1451-1458, 2004.

Gil S, de la Iglesia P, Verdu JF, et al: Effectiveness and safety of balloon dilation of the papilla and the use of an occlusion balloon for clearance of bile duct calculi. AJR Am J Roentgenol 174:1455-1460, 2000.

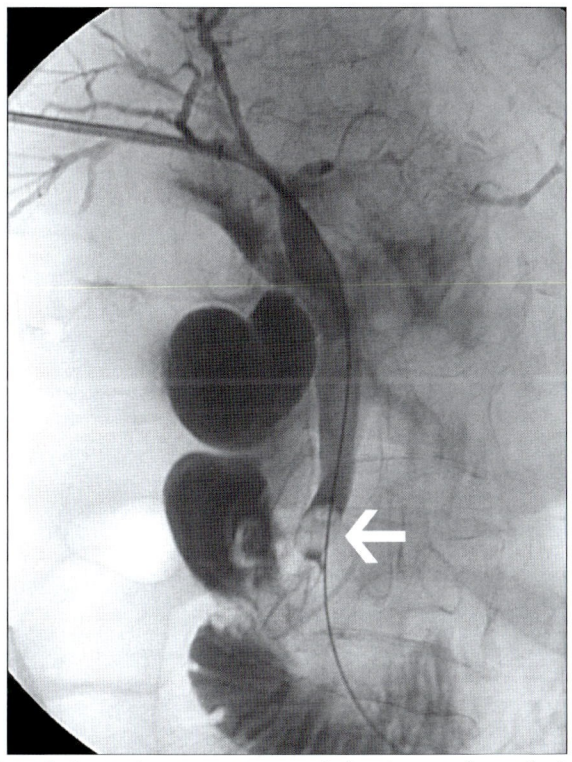

Figure 1. Image from percutaneous cholangiogram shows the impacted stone in the distal common bile duct *(arrow)*. Despite the impacted stone, a guidewire was successfully advanced into the duodenum.

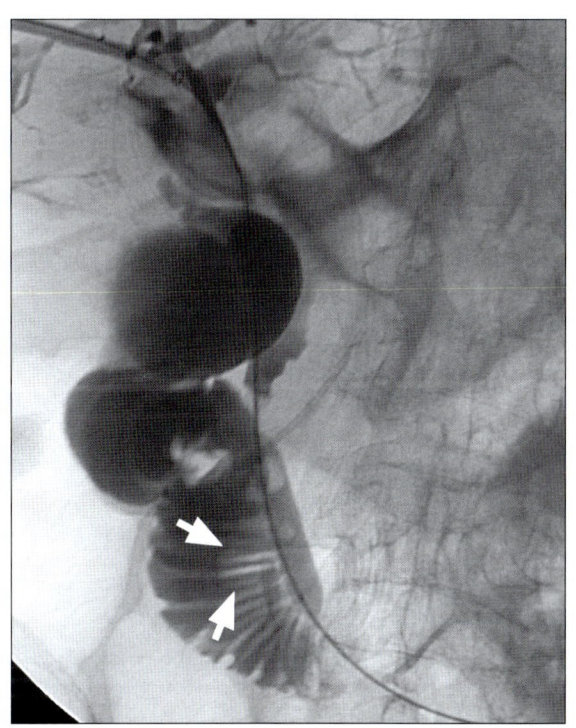

Figure 2. After balloon sphincterotomy, the stone was pushed into the duodenum *(arrows)* using an 8-mm balloon.

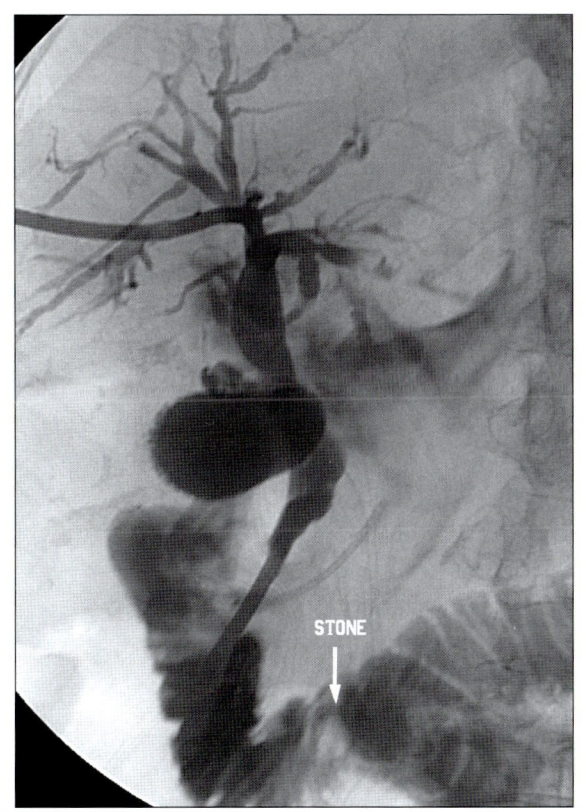

Figure 3. A 10-French internal-external biliary drain has been placed. The stone *(arrow)* has migrated to the third portion of the duodenum.

Case 266

DEMOGRAPHICS/CLINICAL HISTORY

A 56-year-old woman with cystic duct stump leak 1 week after laparoscopic cholecystectomy, undergoing nuclear medicine scanning, computed tomography (CT), and cholangiography.

DISCUSSION

History/Indications for Procedure

A 56-year-old woman had a persistent cystic duct leak 1 week after laparoscopic cholecystectomy. Attempts to cannulate the common bile duct at endoscopic retrograde choledochopancreatography (ERCP) were unsuccessful.

Procedure

Cystic duct stump leak

Pre-procedure Imaging

Nuclear medicine hepatobiliary scan shows radiotracer accumulation in the right lower quadrant and radiotracer accumulation in the right upper quadrant drainage catheter (Fig. 1). Contrast-enhanced CT showed a small fluid collection in the gallbladder fossa.

Intraprocedural Findings

Percutaneous cholangiogram shows extravasation of contrast from the cystic duct stump (Fig. 2). The cystic duct stump was embolized with coils (Fig. 3).

Follow-up and Complications

The biloma drainage output slowed after the biliary intervention. A follow-up cholangiogram performed 1 week after cystic duct embolization showed resolution of cystic duct leak with migration of one of the coils to the common bile duct; an internal-external biliary catheter was placed, and the coil was retrieved (Fig. 4).

Suggested Readings

Kaufman SL, Kadir S, Mitchell SE, et al: Percutaneous transhepatic biliary drainage for bile leaks and fistulas. AJR Am J Roentgenol 144:1055-1058, 1985.

Schelhammer F, Dahl SV, Heintges T, et al: A multimodal approach in coil embolization of a bile leak following cholecystectomy. Cardiovasc Intervent Radiol 30:529-530, 2007.

Society of Interventional Radiology Standards of Practice Committee: Quality guidelines for percutaneous transhepatic cholangiography and biliary drainage. J Vasc Intervent Radiol 14:S243-S246, 2003.

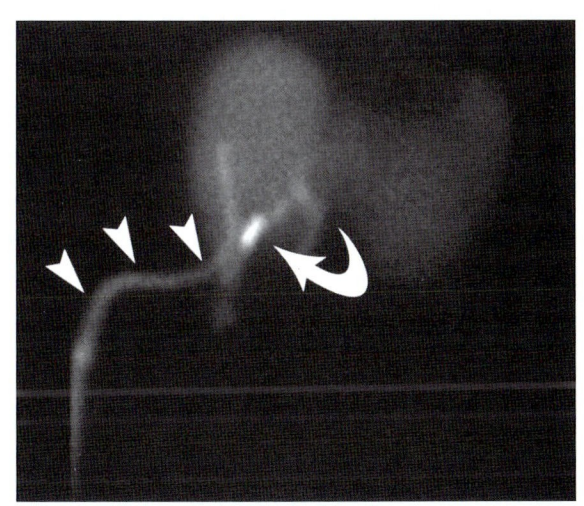

Figure 1. Nuclear medicine hepatobiliary scan with 5 mCi of technetium Tc-99m Choletec shows accumulation of radiotracer in the right upper quadrant *(curved arrow)* and in the drainage catheter *(arrowheads)*.

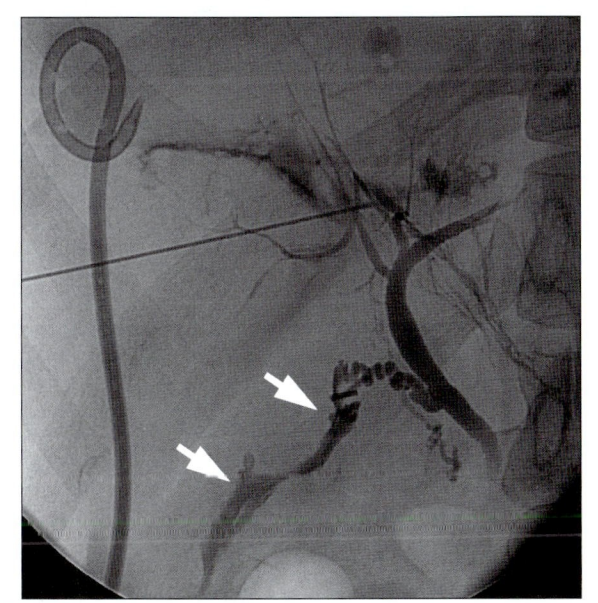

Figure 2. Percutaneous cholangiogram shows contrast extravasation from the cystic duct stump *(arrows)*.

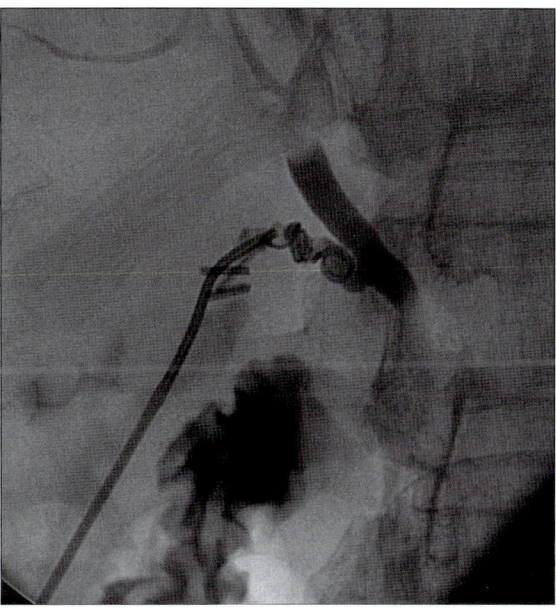

Figure 3. The cystic duct stump was cannulated from the gallbladder fossa and embolized with coils.

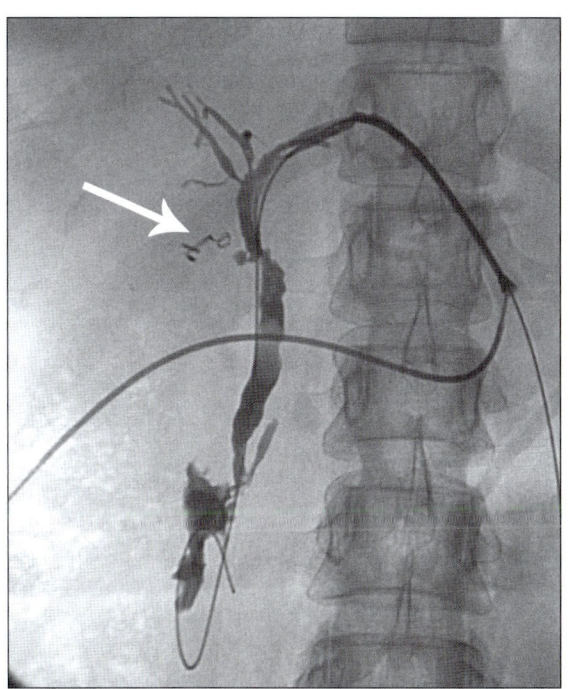

Figure 4. Follow-up cholangiogram 3 weeks after cystic duct embolization shows resolution of the cystic duct stump leak *(arrow)*. There is no ductal obstruction, and the biliary catheter was removed.

Case 267

DEMOGRAPHICS/CLINICAL HISTORY

A 48-year-old man with a self-inflicted gunshot wound to the abdomen, undergoing cholangiography.

DISCUSSION

History/Indications for Procedure
A 48-year-old man has a self-inflicted gunshot wound to the abdomen from a large-caliber handgun. The patient has severe pancreatic, duodenal, and renal injuries.

Procedure
Common bile duct injury

Intraprocedural Findings
The patient had an exploratory laparotomy with surgical repair of multiple abdominal injuries. The percutaneous transhepatic cholangiogram revealed laceration of the common bile duct, with leaking into the peritoneal cavity (Figs. 1 and 2). An internal-external biliary drain was placed (Fig. 3).

Follow-up and Complications
Two weeks after the initial cholangiogram, a biliary-arterial fistula was identified and embolized with coils. The patient had a biliary drain in place for a total of 3 months, after which the injury was healed, and the catheter was removed (Fig. 4).

Suggested Readings
Kaufman SL, Kadir S, Mitchell SE, et al: Percutaneous transhepatic biliary drainage for bile leaks and fistulas. AJR Am J Roentgenol 144:1055-1058, 1985.

Burke DR, Lewis CA, Cardella JF, et al, for the Society of Interventional Radiology Standards of Practice Committee: Quality guidelines for percutaneous transhepatic cholangiography and biliary drainage. J Vasc Intervent Radiol 14:S243-S246, 2003.

Vaccaro JP, Dorfman GS, Lambiase RE: Treatment of biliary leaks and fistulae by simultaneous percutaneous drainage and diversion. Cardiovasc Intervent Radiol 14:109-112, 1991.

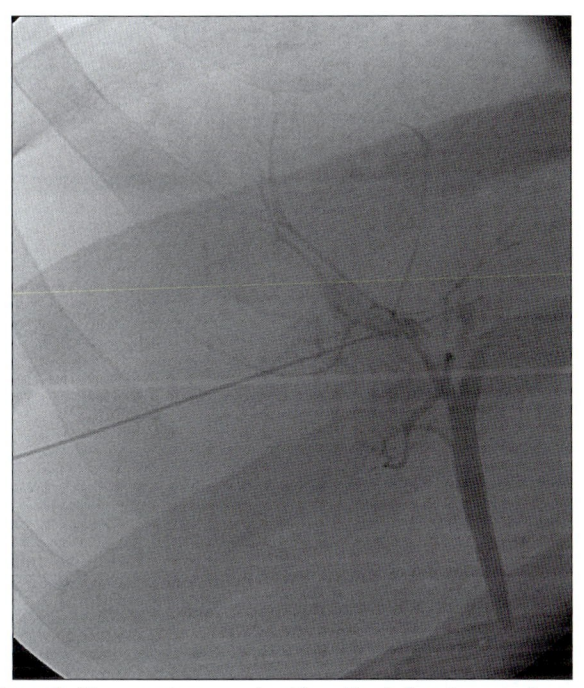

Figure 1. The percutaneous, transhepatic cholangiogram shows a nondilated biliary tree.

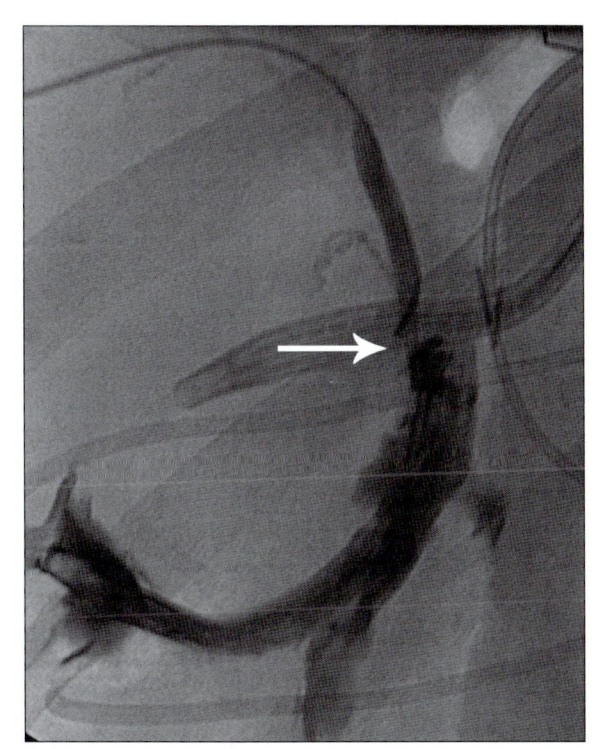

Figure 2. There is a laceration of the common bile duct *(arrow)*, with extravasation of contrast around the surgical drain.

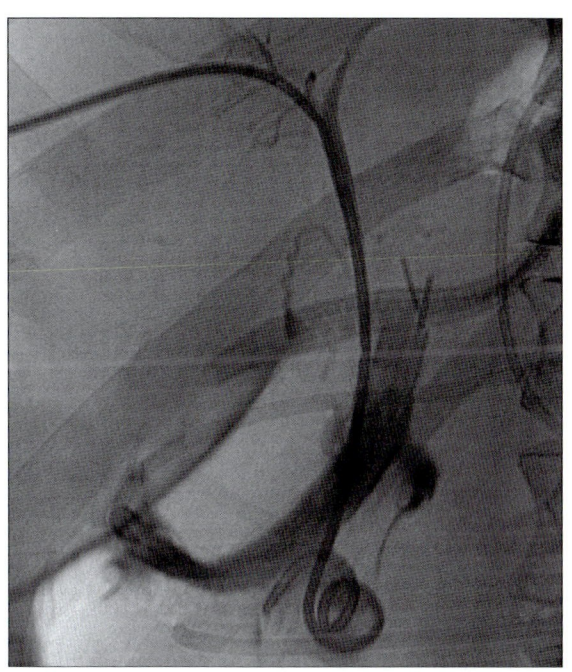

Figure 3. An 8-French internal-external biliary drain was placed.

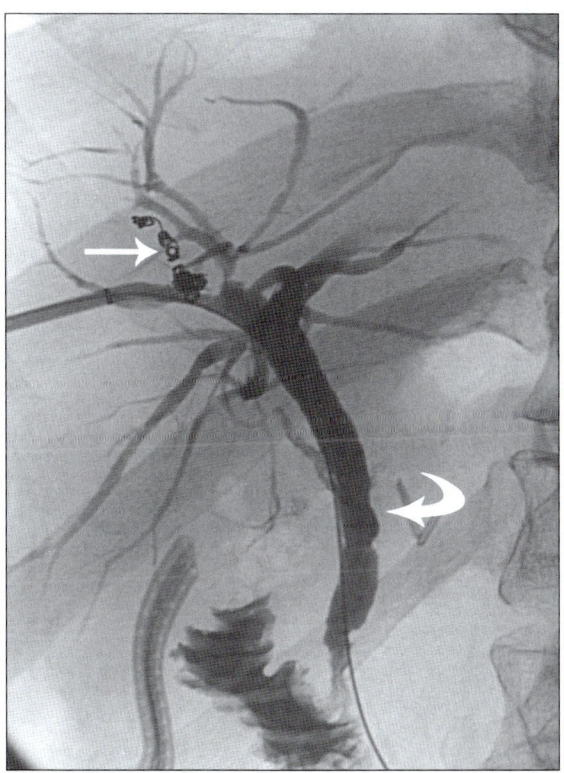

Figure 4. Sheath cholangiogram performed 3 months after the initial drain placement shows healing of the common bile duct injury. There is some irregularity of the duct at the site of injury *(curved arrow)*, but there is no obstruction. Coils from embolization of biliary-arterial fistula *(arrow)* can be seen.

Case 268

DEMOGRAPHICS/CLINICAL HISTORY

A 42-year-old man involved in a motor vehicle collision.

DISCUSSION

History/Indications for Procedure
A 42-year-old man who sustained a liver laceration in a motor vehicle collision. At laparotomy, a bile duct injury was identified.

Procedure
Management of traumatic bile duct laceration

Pre-procedure Imaging
CT scan of the abdomen shows a complex liver laceration involving the anterior right hepatic lobe and medial left hepatic lobe. A hepatobiliary scan shows diffuse abnormal radiotracer accumulation throughout the abdomen consistent with a biliary leak.

Intraprocedural Findings
The initial percutaneous cholangiogram shows a transected right bile duct (Fig. 1); the injured duct could not be crossed at this time and a left-sided biliary drain was placed (Fig. 2). At a later date, the biliary tree was opacified from the left-sided biliary drain, and an internal-external biliary drain was placed across the point of injury (Figs. 3,4).

Follow-up and Complications
The surgical drain output diminished after the biliary catheter was placed. The patient did experience hemobilia, most likely from a post-traumatic hepatic artery pseudoaneurysm; this was successfully embolized and the hemobilia resolved.

Suggested Readings

Bridges A, Wilcox CM, Varadarajulu S: Endoscopic management of traumatic bile leaks. Gastrointest Endosc 65:1081-1085, 2007.

Castagnetti M, Houben C, Patel S, et al: Minimally invasive management of bile leaks after blunt liver trauma in children. J Pediatr Surg 41:1539-1544, 2006.

Ernst O, Sergent G, Mizrahi D, et al: Biliary leaks: Treatment by means of percutaneous transhepatic biliary drainage. Radiology 211:345-348, 1999.

Kaufman SL, Dadir S, Mitchell SE, et al: Percutaneous transhepatic biliary drainage for bile leaks and fistulas. AJR Am J Roentgenol 144:1055-1058, 1985.

Case 268   537

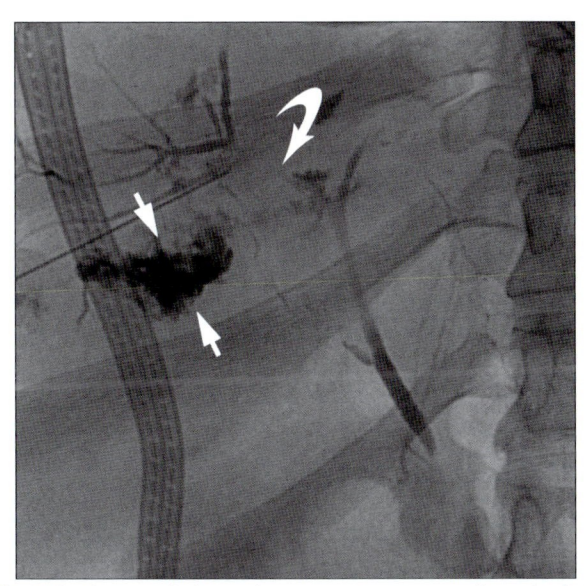

Figure 1. Fluroscopic image from percutaneous transhepatic cholangiogram shows disruption of the right hepatic duct *(curved arrow)*. Contrast is seen extravasating adjacent to the surgical drain *(arrows)*.

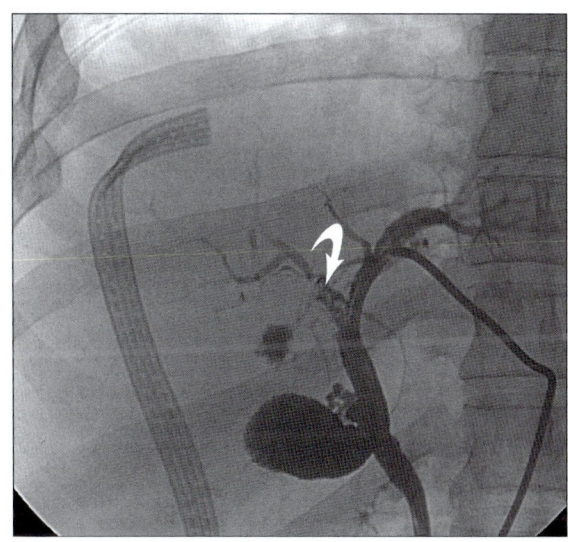

Figure 3. Follow-up cholangiogram. There continued to be high output from the surgical drain. Injection of the left-sided biliary catheter opacifies the injured right bile duct *(curved arrow)*.

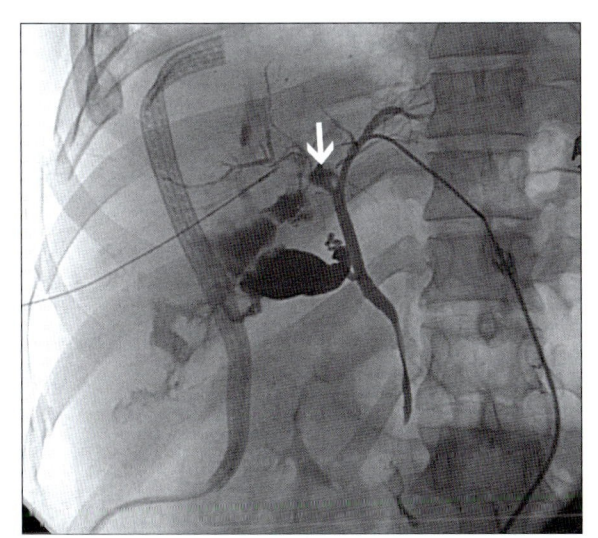

Figure 2. Attempts to cross the injured duct were not successful, so a left-sided drain was placed. (*arrow*—site of bile duct injury).

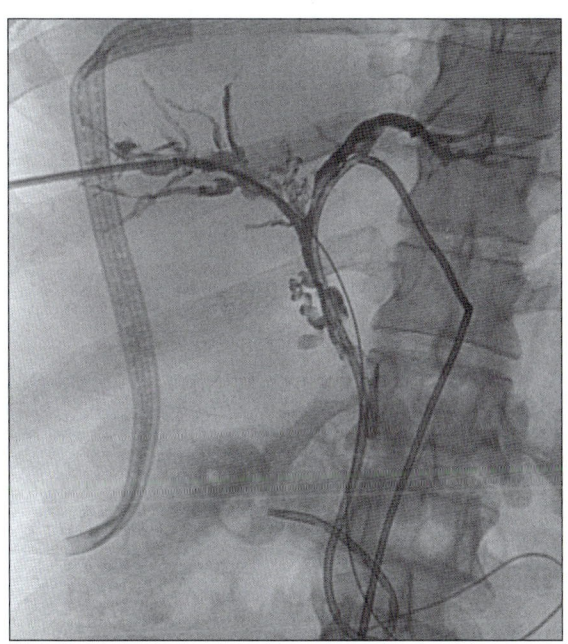

Figure 4. A peripheral branch of the right bile duct was accessed with fluoroscopy. The site of injury was successfully crossed, and an internal-external biliary drain was placed.

Case 269

DEMOGRAPHICS/CLINICAL HISTORY

A 45-year-old woman who underwent laparoscopic cholecystectomy 2 weeks earlier presents with abdominal pain and elevated liver enzyme levels, undergoing endoscopic retrograde pancreatoduodenography (ERCP) and fluoroscopy.

DISCUSSION

History/Indications for Procedure

A 45-year-old woman, who underwent an uncomplicated laparoscopic cholecystectomy 2 weeks prior, presented with abdominal pain. Ultrasound showed a perihepatic fluid collection, and a biloma was drained percutaneously.

Procedure

Management of bile leak

Pre-procedure Imaging

ERCP showed dilatation of the bile ducts, but no leak was seen. Contrast injection through the biloma catheter opacified an accessory bile duct (i.e., duct of Luschka) within the right hepatic lobe (Fig. 1).

Intraprocedural Findings

After opacifying the duct of Luschka by injecting the biloma catheter, the duct was accessed, and a 5-French sheath was placed (Fig. 2). The duct was sclerosed with 2 mL of ethanol and embolized with coils (Fig. 3).

Follow-up and Complications

Follow-up injection of the biloma drain showed complete occlusion of the accessory bile duct and continued leak into the cystic duct remnant (Fig. 4). The patient underwent endoscopic bile duct stent placement, and 4 months after the cholecystectomy, the cystic duct leak had healed, and the biloma drain was removed.

Suggested Readings

Kaufman SL, Kadir S, Mitchell SE, et al: Percutaneous transhepatic biliary drainage for bile leaks and fistulas. AJR Am J Roentgenol 144:1055-1058, 1985.

Sharif K, de Ville de Goyet J: Bile duct of Luschka leading to bile leak after cholecystectomy—revisiting the biliary anatomy. J Pediatr Surg 38:E21-E23, 2003.

Vaccaro JP, Dorfman GS, Lambiase RE: Treatment of biliary leaks and fistulae by simultaneous percutaneous drainage and diversion. Cardiovasc Intervent Radiol 14:109-112, 1991.

VanSonnenberg E, Ferrucci JT Jr, Mueller PR, et al: Percutaneous drainage of abscesses and fluid collections: Techniques, results, and applications. Radiology 142:1-10, 1982.

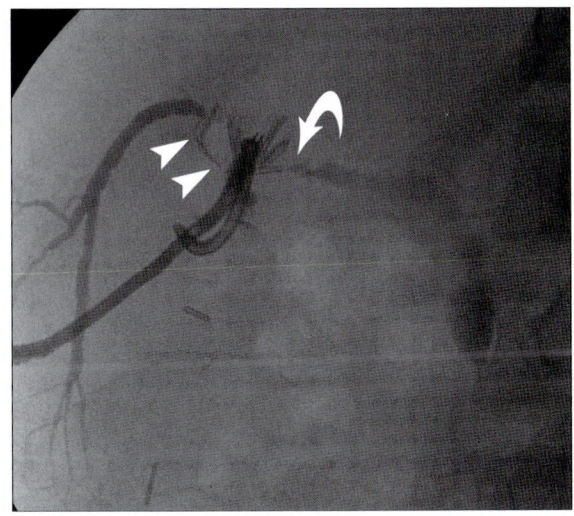

Figure 1. Biloma drain injection shows communication with a duct of Luschka *(arrowheads)*, and there is communication with the cystic duct remnant *(curved arrow)*.

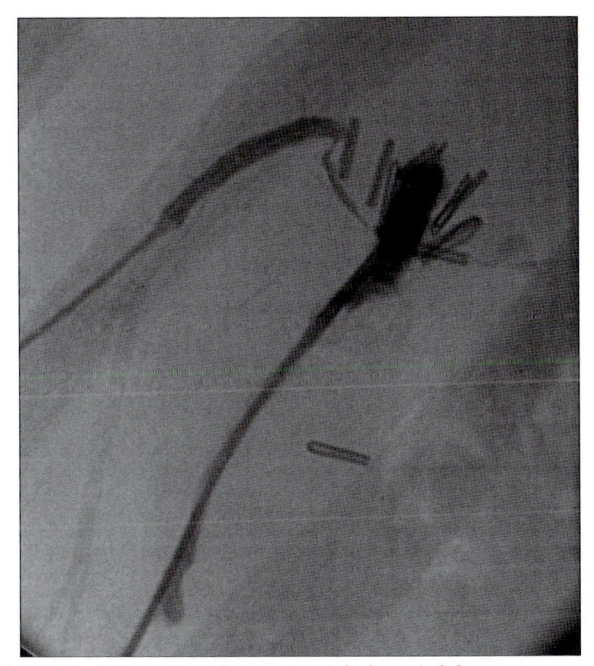

Figure 2. The accessory duct in the right hepatic lobe was accessed with a 5-French catheter. The duct of Luschka was sclerosed with alcohol.

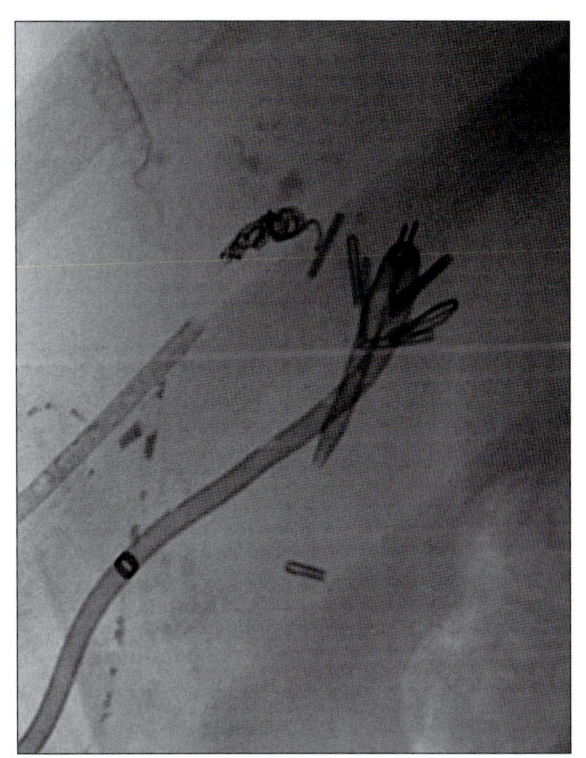

Figure 3. Spot fluoroscopic image after embolization shows that coils have been placed, occluding the accessory bile duct.

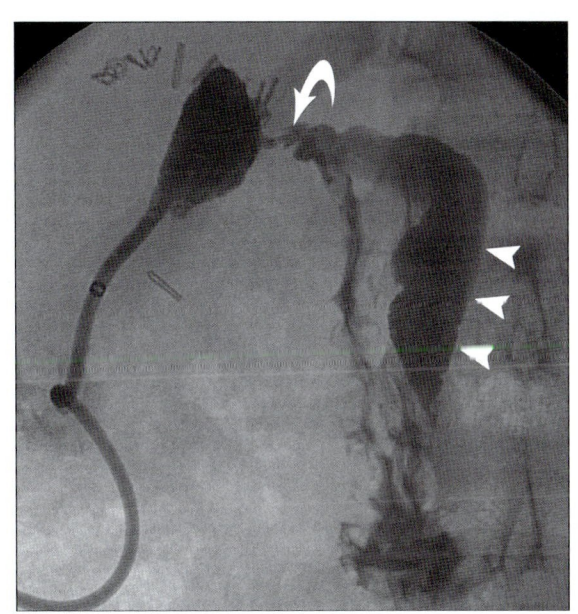

Figure 4. Follow-up biloma catheter injection occurred 1 week after intervention. The duct of Luschka no longer is seen. There is continued communication through the cystic duct stump *(curved arrow)* and dilatation of the common bile duct *(arrowheads)*. This was successfully managed with endoscopic stent placement.

Case 270

DEMOGRAPHICS/CLINICAL HISTORY

A 55-year-old man with bile leak after orthotopic liver transplant.

DISCUSSION

History/Indications for Procedure
A 55-year-old man with end-stage liver disease secondary to hepatitis C underwent orthotopic liver transplantation. Postoperatively, he developed abdominal pain and sepsis.

Procedure
Management of biliary leak after liver transplantation

Pre-procedure Imaging
Nuclear medicine hepatobiliary scan shows radiopharmaceutical activity tracking along the right abdomen, consistent with a biliary leak (Fig. 1). Ultrasound of the abdomen shows a large perihepatic fluid collection with internal septations; the collection was percutaneously drained, and bile was aspirated.

Intraprocedural Findings
A percutaneous transhepatic cholangiogram (PTC) was performed and shows decompression of the intrahepatic bile ducts and a large leak from the biliary anastomosis (Fig. 2). The leak was crossed with a guidewire, and an 8-French internal-external biliary drain was placed (Fig. 3).

Follow-up and Complications
The biliary drain was left in place for 6 weeks. At this time, follow-up cholangiogram showed no further leak from the biliary anastomosis, and the drainage catheter was removed (Fig. 4).

Suggested Readings
Kaufman SL, Kadir S, Mitchell SE, et al: Percutaneous transhepatic biliary drainage for bile leaks and fistulas. AJR Am J Roentgenol 144:1055-1058, 1985.
Letourneau JG, Castaneda-Zuniga WR: The role of radiology in the diagnosis and treatment of biliary complications after liver transplantation. Cardiovasc Intervent Radiol 13:278-282, 1990.
Sheng R, Sammon JK, Zajko AB, et al: Bile leak after hepatic transplantation: Cholangiographic features, prevalence, and clinical outcome. Radiology 192:413-416, 1994.
Society of Interventional Radiology Standards of Practice Committee: Quality guidelines for percutaneous transhepatic cholangiography and biliary drainage. J Vasc Intervent Radiol 14:S243-S246, 2003.

Case 270   541

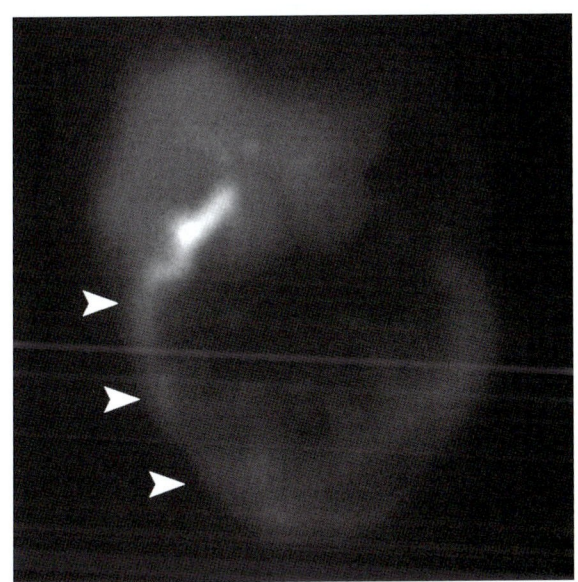

Figure 1. Nuclear medicine hepatobiliary scan shows radiotracer accumulation in the porta hepatis and tracking along the right abdomen *(arrowheads)*, consistent with a bile leak.

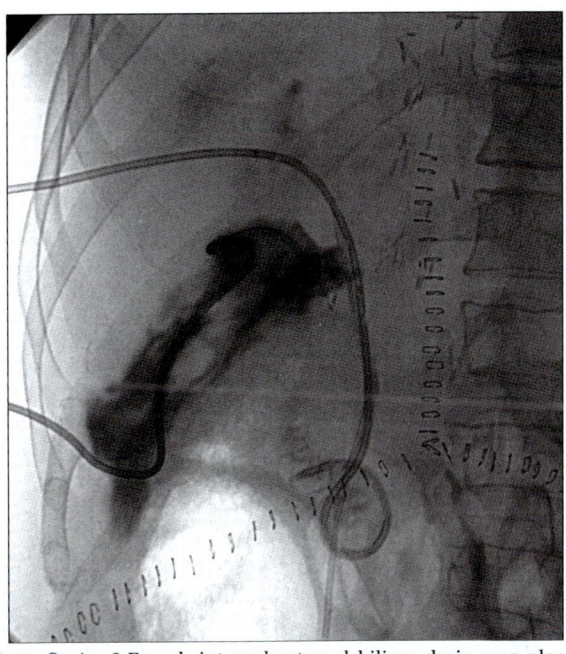

Figure 3. An 8-French internal-external biliary drain was placed across the leak.

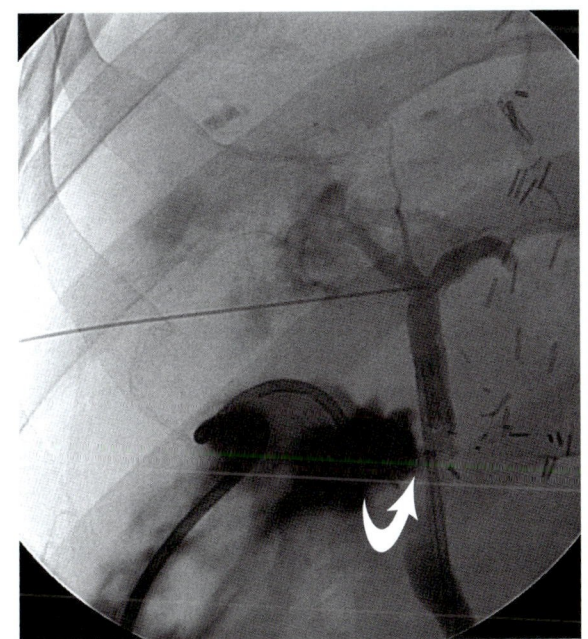

Figure 2. Percutaneous cholangiogram shows decompression of the intrahepatic biliary tree. There is irregularity at the biliary anastomosis with a large leak identified *(curved arrow)*. A catheter has previously been placed in perihepatic biloma.

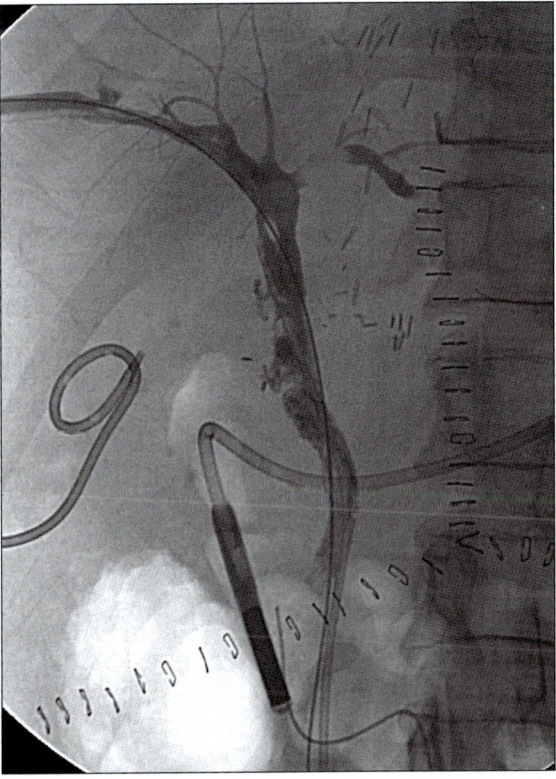

Figure 4. Follow-up sheath cholangiogram 6 weeks after biliary catheter placement shows irregularity at the biliary anastomosis. The leak is no longer present.

Case 271

DEMOGRAPHICS/CLINICAL HISTORY

A 60-year-old man with a postoperative biliary leak after liver transplantation, undergoing radiographic imaging.

DISCUSSION

History/Indications for Procedure

A 60-year-old man underwent liver transplantation because of liver disease attributed to nonalcoholic steatohepatitis (NASH). The patient had a persistent biliary leak postoperatively.

Procedure

Biliary leak after liver transplantation

Pre-procedure Imaging

The hepatobiliary scan demonstrates an accumulation of radiotracer in the porta hepatis that is consistent with a bile leak (Fig. 1). Endoscopic retrograde choledochopancreatography (ERCP) confirmed the presence of the leak from the cystic duct stump.

Intraprocedural Findings

The percutaneous transhepatic cholangiogram (PTC) demonstrates the extravasation of contrast from the cystic duct stump (Fig. 2). An 8-French internal-external biliary drain was placed.

Follow-up and Complications

A sheath cholangiogram performed 6 weeks after the original drain placement showed the leak had closed (Fig. 3). The drain was removed, and the patient required no further biliary interventions.

Suggested Readings

Letourneau JG, Castaneda-Zuniga WR: The role of radiology in the diagnosis and treatment of biliary complications after liver transplantation. Cardiovasc Intervent Radiol 13:278-282, 1990.

O'Connor TP, Lewis WD, Jenkins RL: Biliary tract complications after liver transplantation. Arch Surg 130:312-317, 1995.

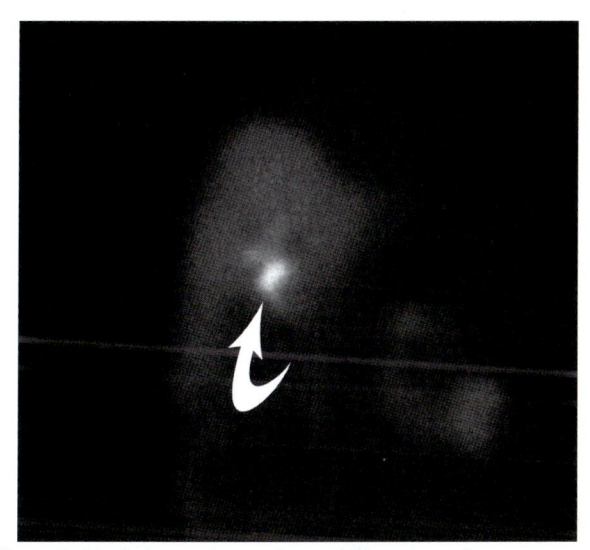

Figure 1. Single image from a hepatobiliary scan shows an accumulation of radiotracer in the porta hepatis *(curved arrow)* that is consistent with the presence of a bile leak.

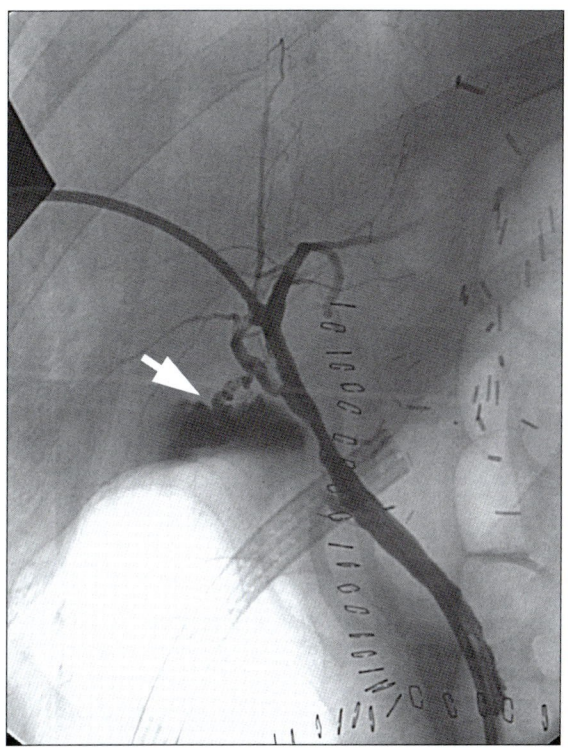

Figure 2. Image from the initial cholangiogram shows the leak arising from a cystic duct stump *(arrow)*.

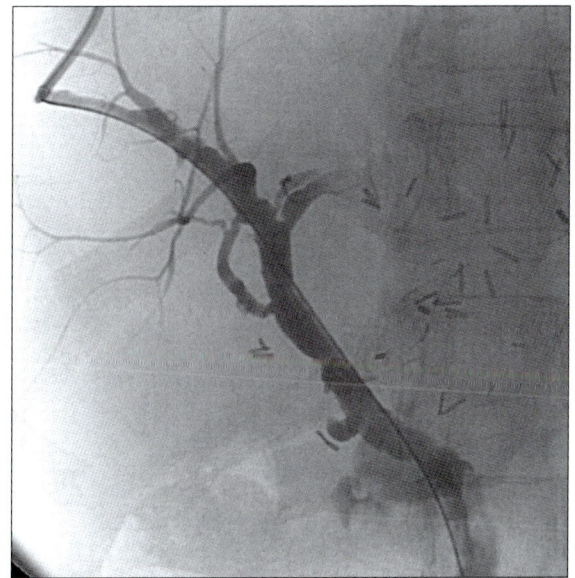

Figure 3. Image from the sheath cholangiogram performed 6 weeks after the initial drain placement demonstrates that the leak is no longer present.

Case 272

DEMOGRAPHICS/CLINICAL HISTORY

A 23-year-old woman after liver transplantation with hepatic artery thrombosis and biloma formation, undergoing arteriography and cholangiography.

DISCUSSION

History/Indications for Procedure
Three years after liver transplantation, a 23-year-old woman presented with elevated liver enzyme levels and right upper quadrant pain. An 8-French drain was placed into an intrahepatic fluid collection, and bilious fluid was aspirated.

Procedure
Biliary ischemia after liver transplantation

Pre-procedure Imaging
Doppler ultrasound of the liver was unable to identify blood flow within the common hepatic artery. Hepatic arteriogram confirmed occlusion of the common hepatic artery (Fig. 1).

Intraprocedural Findings
Percutaneous transhepatic cholangiogram shows the left biliary tree is diffusely irregular and contains a large amount of debris (Fig. 2). The common hepatic duct is diffusely narrowed.

Follow-up and Complications
An 8-French internal-external biliary drain was placed (Fig. 3); however, the left biliary system did not respond to conservative management, and the patient ultimately underwent resection of the left hepatic lobe with hepaticojejunostomy (Fig. 4). The patient has had no further biliary complications in the 4 years since the resection.

Suggested Readings
Cameron AM, Busuttil RW: Ischemic cholangiopathy after liver transplantation. Hepatobiliary Dis Int 4:495-501, 2005.

Kaplan SB, Zajko AB, Koneru B: Hepatic bilomas due to hepatic artery thrombosis in liver transplant recipients: Percutaneous drainage and clinical outcome. Radiology 174:1031-1035, 1990.

Karani JB, Yu DF, Kane PA: Interventional radiology in liver transplantation. Cardiovasc Intervent Radiol 28:271-283, 2005.

Orons PD, Sheng R, Zajko AB: Hepatic artery stenosis in liver transplant recipients: Prevalence and cholangiographic appearance of associated biliary complications. AJR Am J Roentgenol 165:1145-1149, 1995.

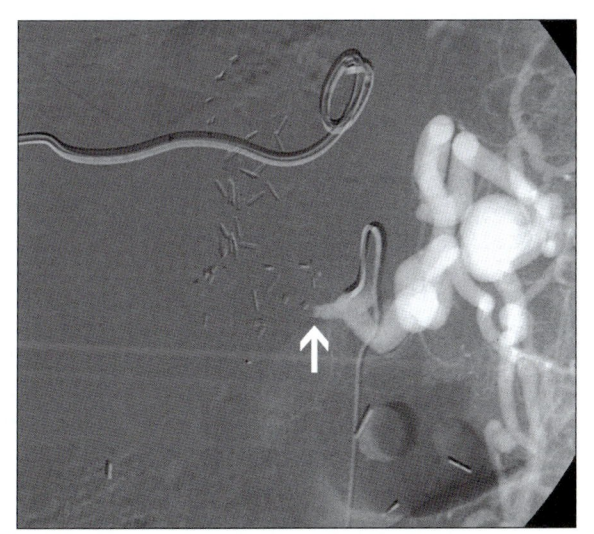

Figure 1. Celiac arteriogram shows abrupt occlusion of the proximal hepatic artery (arrow). No distal perfusion was seen.

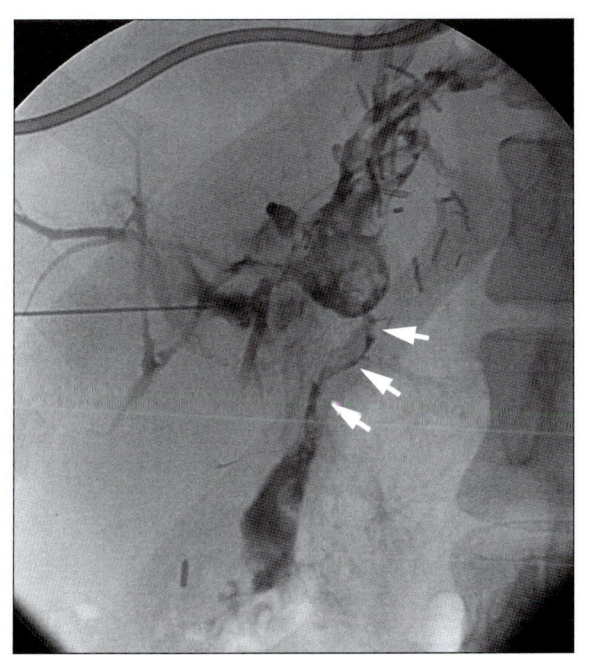

Figure 2. Percutaneous cholangiogram shows dilatation and irregularity of the left hepatic ducts. There is a large amount of intraductal debris. The common hepatic duct is diffusely narrowed (arrows).

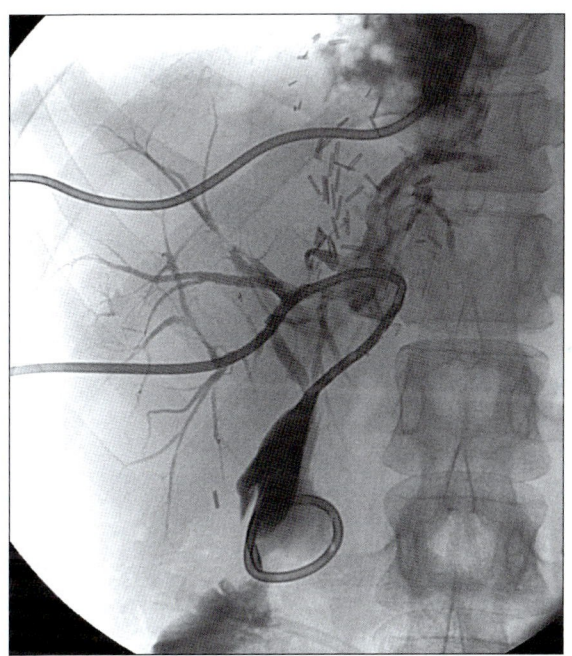

Figure 3. In a single image from the percutaneous cholangiographic study, retained contrast is present in the biliary system and around the biloma catheter. An internal-external biliary drain has been placed.

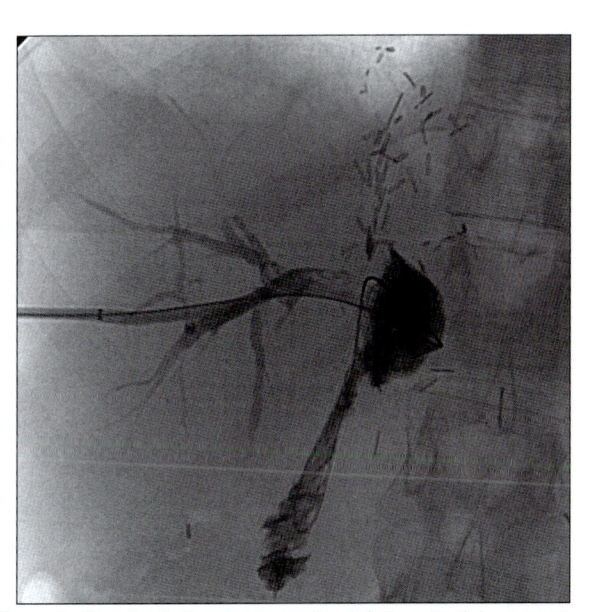

Figure 4. Sheath cholangiogram after left hepatic lobe resection shows that the hepaticojejunostomy anastomosis has healed. There is no leak into the resection bed, and the drain was removed at this time.

Case 273

DEMOGRAPHICS/CLINICAL HISTORY

A 67-year-old man with a pancreatic mass, undergoing computed tomography (CT), cholangiography, and stent placement.

DISCUSSION

History/Indications for Procedure
A 67-year-old man has a pancreatic mass causing biliary and gastric outlet obstruction.

Procedure
Endobiliary stent placement

Pre-procedure Imaging
Contrast-enhanced CT demonstrates a soft-tissue mass in the head of the pancreas (Fig. 1). There is marked distention of the stomach and duodenum.

Intraprocedural Findings
Percutaneous transhepatic cholangiogram demonstrates complete obstruction of the common bile duct with dilatation of the common hepatic duct (Fig. 2). The lesion was crossed and stented with a 10-mm × 10-cm Viabil stent-graft (Figs. 3 and 4).

Follow-up and Complications
After stent placement, the patient was discharged to a skilled nursing facility for palliative care.

Suggested Readings
Covey AM, Brown KT: Palliative percutaneous drainage in malignant biliary obstruction. Part 1. Indications and preprocedure evaluation. J Support Oncol 4:269-273, 2006.

Morgan RA, Adam AN: Malignant biliary disease: Percutaneous interventions. Tech Vasc Intervent Radiol 4:147-152, 2001.

Shoder M, Rossi P, Uflacker R, et al: Malignant biliary obstruction: Treatment with ePTFE-FEP-covered endoprostheses—initial technical and clinical experiences in a multicenter trial. Radiology 225:35-42, 2002.

Case 273   547

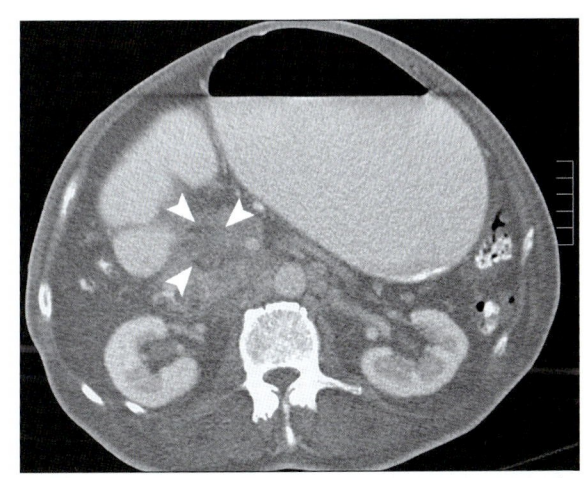

Figure 1. Contrast-enhanced, axial CT image demonstrates a large hypodense mass in the head of the pancreas (*arrowheads*)

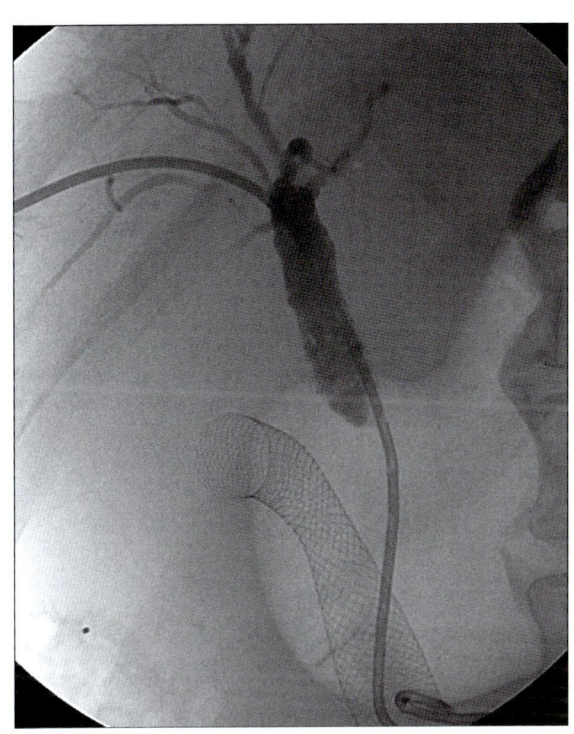

Figure 2. Percutaneous cholangiogram after internal and external drain placement demonstrates complete occlusion of the common bile duct. A duodenal stent has been placed endoscopically.

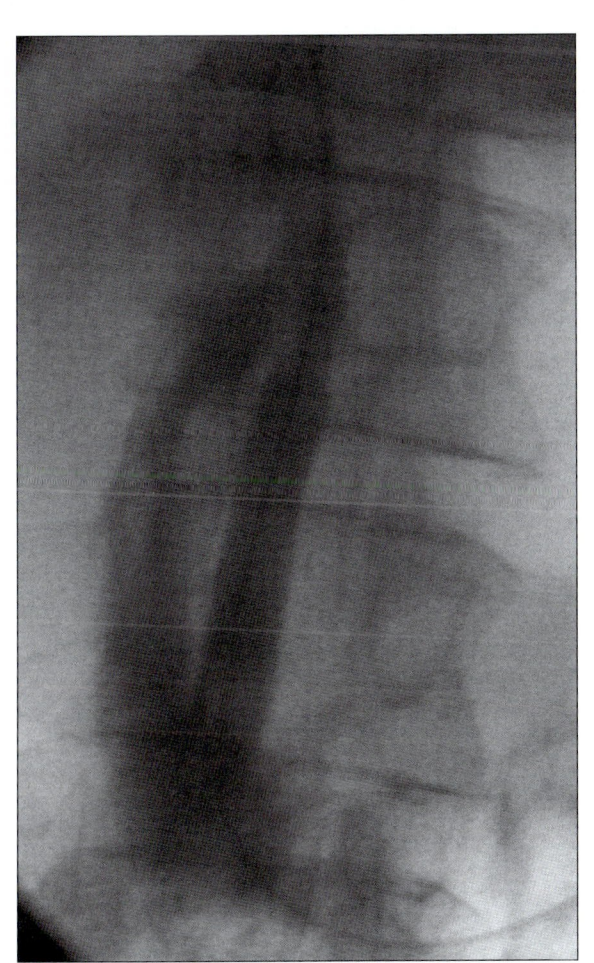

Figure 3. The duodenum was catheterized alongside the duodenal stent, and the stricture was predilated.

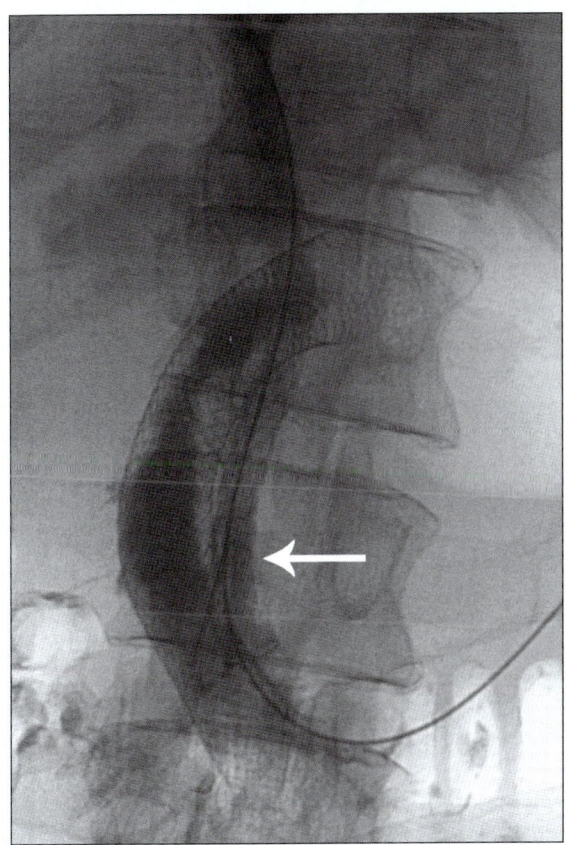

Figure 4. An expanded polytetrafluoroethylene-fluorinated ethylene propylene (ePTFE-FEP)–covered stent (Viabil, Gore & Associates, Flagstaff, AZ) has been placed (*arrow*). Markers indicate the proximal and distal ends of the fabric, and contrast injection shows good flow into the bowel.

Case 274

DEMOGRAPHICS/CLINICAL HISTORY

A 60-year-old man with abdominal pain and weight loss.

DISCUSSION

History/Indications for Procedure
A 60-year-old man with abdominal pain and weight loss. Abdominal CT and laparoscopy confirm metastatic pancreatic carcinoma.

Procedure
Biliary stent placement for malignant biliary obstruction

Pre-procedure Imaging
Contrast-enhanced CT of the abdomen shows a 6.3-cm mass in the head of the pancreas with intra- and extrahepatic biliary dilatation (Fig. 1). Diagnostic laparoscopy shows numerous small metastases in the right and left hepatic lobes.

Intraprocedural Findings
Percutaneous cholangiogram performed from a right intercostal approach shows marked dilation of the intrahepatic bile ducts with obstruction of the common bile duct (Figure 2). The point of obstruction was crossed, and an 860 Wallstent was placed across the area of obstruction (Figs. 3 and 4).

Follow-up and Complications
The biliary dilation had resolved on follow-up imaging. The patient required no further intervention until his demise from complications associated with the malignancy.

Suggested Readings
Lee BH, Choe DH, Lee JH, et al: Metallic stents in malignant biliary obstruction: Prospective long-term clinical results. AJR Am J Roentgenol 168:741-745, 1997.

Lee MJ, Dawson SL, Mueller PR, et al: Palliation of malignant bile duct obstruction with metallic biliary endoprostheses: Technique, results, and complications. J Vasc Intervent Radiol 3:665-671, 1992.

van Delden OM, Lameris JS: Percutaneous drainage and stenting for palliation of malignant bile duct obstruction. Eur Radiol 18:448-456, 2008.

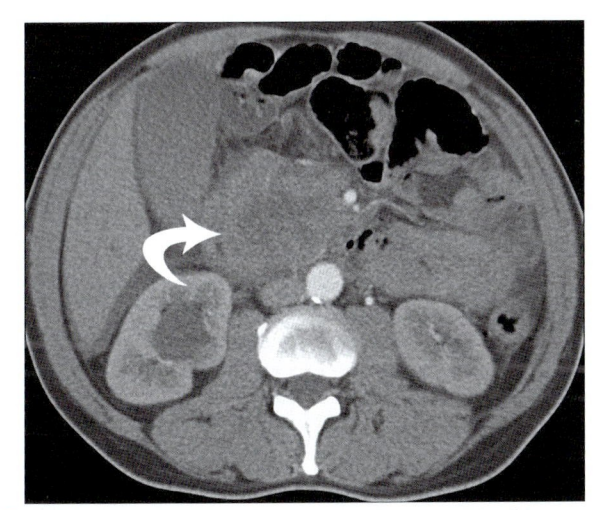

Figure 1. Contrast-enhanced CT shows a large mass in the pancreatic head *(curved arrow)*.

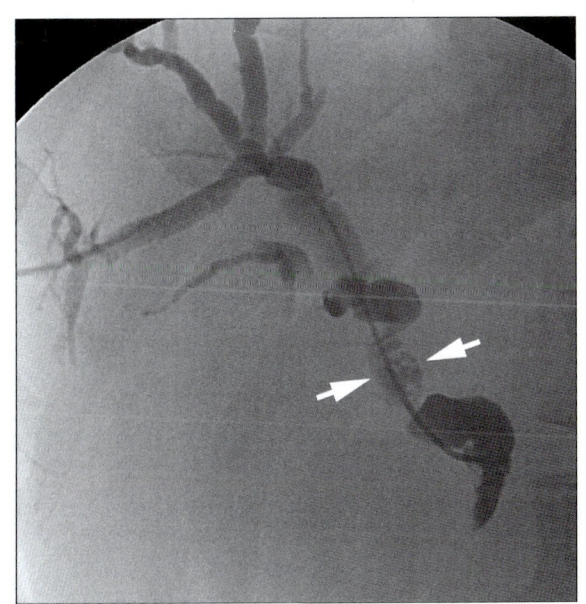

Figure 2. Single image from percutaneous cholangiogram. A catheter has been advanced into the distal common bile duct. There is narrowing and irregularity of the common bile duct at the level of the pancreatic head mass *(arrows)*. The intrahepatic bile ducts are dilated.

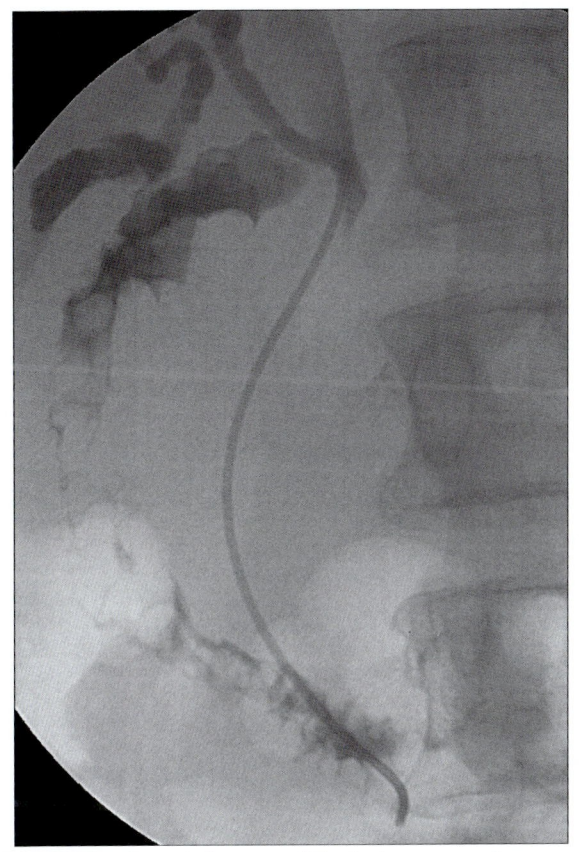

Figure 3. The obstructed common bile duct was crossed.

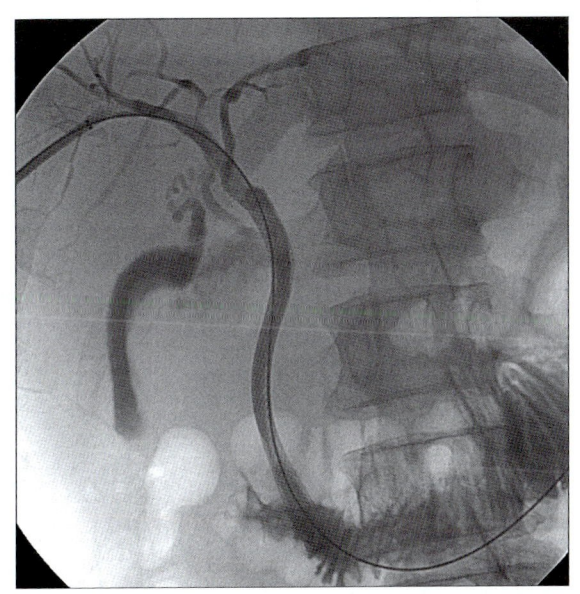

Figure 4. An 860 Wallstent was placed across the obstructed portion of the common bile duct into the duodenum. Sheath cholangiogram following stent placement shows good biliary drainage through the stent.

Case 275

DEMOGRAPHICS/CLINICAL HISTORY

A 57-year-old woman with biliary obstruction from metastatic colon carcinoma, undergoing cholangiography.

DISCUSSION

History/Indications for Procedure
A 57-year-old woman with metastatic colon carcinoma presents with new-onset jaundice and fatigue.

Procedure
Endobiliary stenting

Pre-procedure Imaging
Abdominal ultrasound shows dilation of the intrahepatic and extrahepatic bile ducts. A percutaneous cholangiogram shows biliary ductal dilation with obstruction at the level of the confluence of the right and left hepatic ducts (Fig. 1); an internal-external biliary drain was placed (Fig. 2).

Intraprocedural Findings
The left-sided bile ducts were opacified through the existing biliary drain, and a left-sided access was obtained. A Gore Viabil-covered stent (W.L. Gore & Associates, Flagstaff, AZ) was placed in the common bile duct (Fig. 3), and uncovered self-expanding nitinol stents (SMART, Cordis, Miami Lakes, FL) were deployed simultaneously across the obstruction at the confluence of the right and left hepatic ducts (Fig. 4).

Follow-up and Complications
The patient's bilirubin levels decreased from 7.1 mg/dL to 1.1 mg/dL after biliary drainage and stenting. She returned 4 months later with fever and elevated bilirubin levels. A percutaneous cholangiogram showed occlusion of the biliary stents, and bilateral biliary drains were placed.

Suggested Readings
Fanelli F, Orgera G, Bezzi M, et al: Management of malignant biliary obstruction: Technical and clinical results using an expanded polytetrafluoroethylene fluorinated ethylene propylene (ePTFE/PET)-covered metallic stent after 6-year experience. Eur Radiol 18:911, 2008.

Hatzidakis A, Krokidis M, Kalbakis K, et al: ePTFE/FEP-covered metallic stents for palliation of malignant biliary disease: Can tumor ingrowth be prevented? Cardiovasc Intervent Radiol 30:950, 2007.

Schoder M, Rossi P, Uflacker R, et al: Malignant biliary obstruction: Treatment with ePTFE-PET-covered endoprostheses initial technical and clinical experiences in a multicenter trial. Radiology 225:35-42, 2002.

Case 275   551

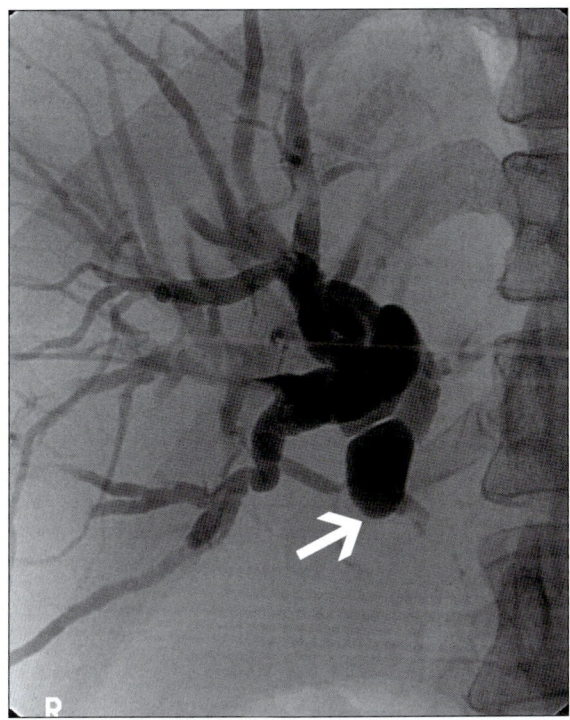

Figure 1. Percutaneous transhepatic cholangiogram from right-sided approach shows marked dilation of right-sided bile ducts. There is complete obstruction of right hepatic duct (*arrow*).

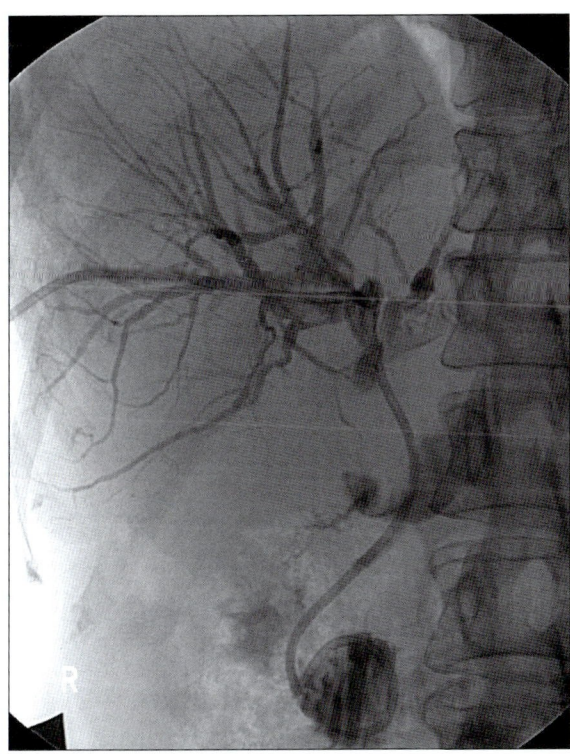

Figure 2. Cholangiogram shows 8-French internal-external biliary drain has been placed.

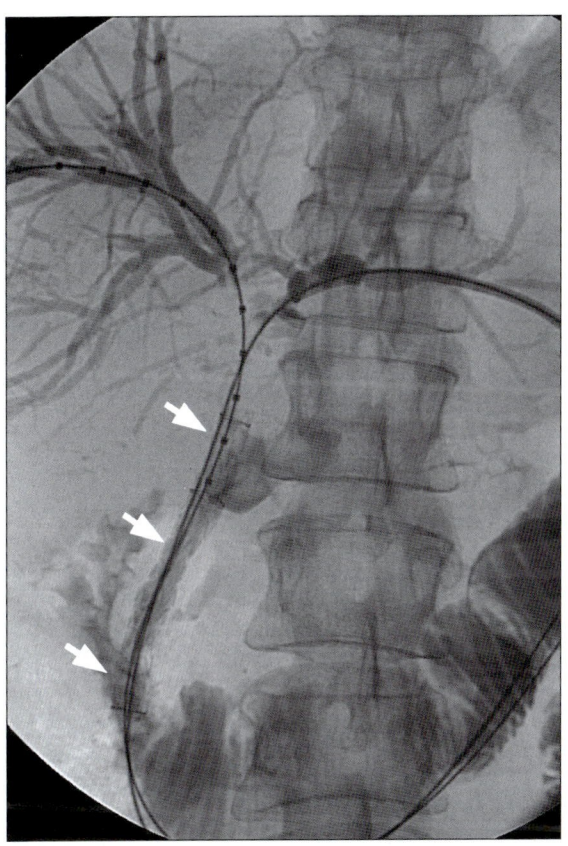

Figure 3. Left-sided access has been obtained. Viabil-covered stent has been placed in common bile duct (*arrows*).

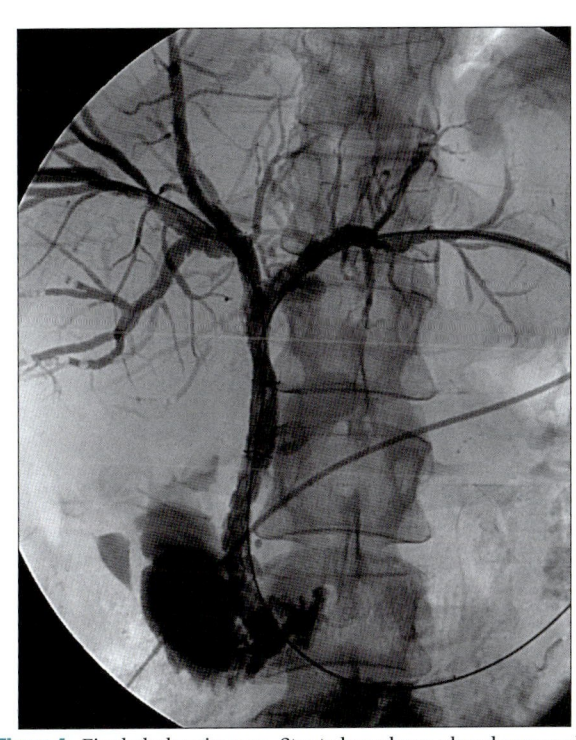

Figure 4. Final cholangiogram. Stents have been placed across obstruction at confluence of right and left hepatic ducts. Contrast material passes freely into small bowel, and intrahepatic bile ducts are decompressed.

Case 276

DEMOGRAPHICS/CLINICAL HISTORY

An 86-year-old man with recurrent gastric cancer and jaundice.

DISCUSSION

History/Indications for Procedure
An 86-year-old man with recurrent gastric cancer and jaundice. The patient reports a 4- to 5-day history of weakness and lethargy.

Procedure
Bilateral biliary stent placement

Pre-procedure Imaging
MRI of the abdomen shows a 6.6-cm × 3.3-cm mass in the porta hepatis. The mass is compressing the biliary system with resultant biliary dilation.

Intraprocedural Findings
The intrahepatic bile ducts are markedly dilated, with biliary obstruction at the confluence of the right and left bile ducts (Figs. 1 and 2). The occluded segment was crossed, and kissing biliary stents were placed (Figs. 3 and 4).

Follow-up and Complications
Follow-up cholangiogram 2 days after biliary stent placement shows decompression of the biliary tree; the biliary drains were removed.

Suggested Readings
Ferrucci JT Jr, Mueller PR, Harbin WP: Percutaneous transhepatic biliary drainage: Technique, results, and applications. Radiology 135:1-13, 1980.

Lee BH, Choe DH, Lee JH, et al: Metallic stents in malignant biliary obstruction: Prospective long-term clinical results. AJR Am J Roentgenol 168:741-745, 1997.

Lee MJ, Dawson SL, Mueller PR, et al: Palliation of malignant bile duct obstruction with metallic biliary endoprostheses: Technique, results, and complications. J Vasc Intervent Radiol 3:665-671, 1992.

Case 276   553

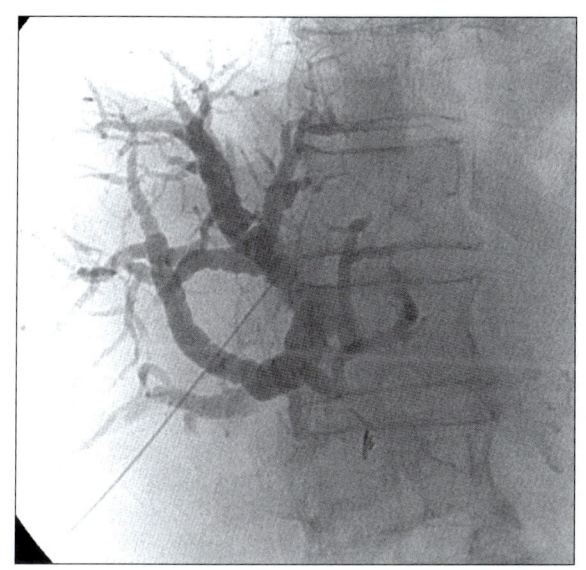

Figure 1. Single image from percutaneous transhepatic cholangiogram shows marked dilation of the right biliary tree. The right hepatic duct and common hepatic duct are not visualized.

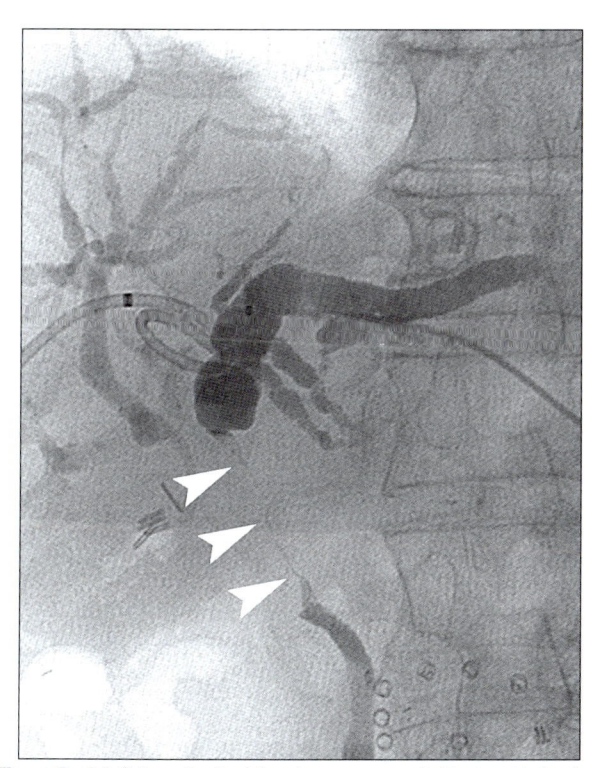

Figure 2. A left hepatic duct has been accessed. Contrast injection shows the level of obstruction just above the confluence of the right and left hepatic ducts. The common hepatic duct is extremely narrowed *(arrowheads)*.

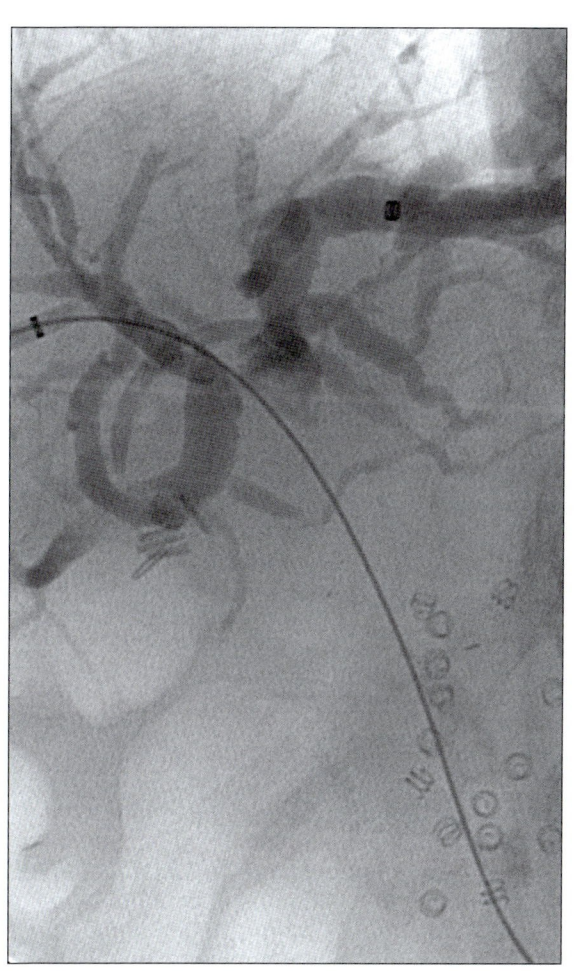

Figure 3. A guidewire has been placed across the level of obstruction.

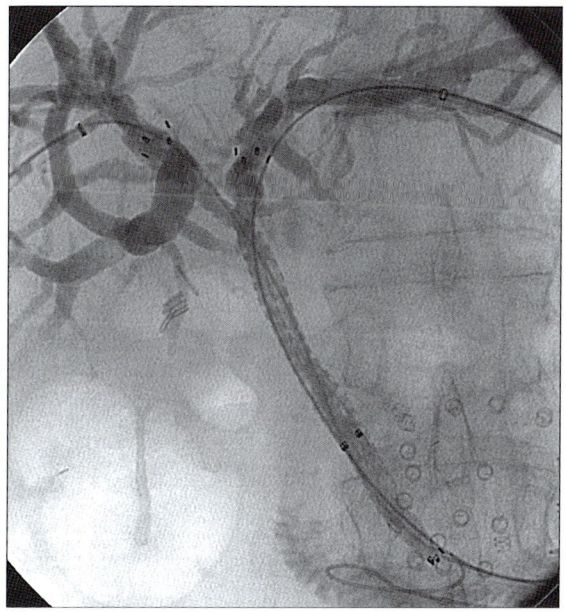

Figure 4. Bilateral self-expanding stents have been placed across the level of obstruction. The stents extend into the right and left hepatic ducts.

Case 277

DEMOGRAPHICS/CLINICAL HISTORY

A 36-year-old woman with right flank pain and intermittent fever, undergoing computed tomography (CT), ultrasonography, and fluoroscopy.

DISCUSSION

History/Indications for Procedure
A 36-year-old woman with a known right renal calculus presented with right flank pain and intermittent fever.

Procedure
Nephrostomy for xanthogranulomatous pyelonephritis

Pre-procedure Imaging
Contrast-enhanced CT of the abdomen shows an enlarged right kidney with a staghorn calculus (Fig. 1). There is marked hydronephrosis, poor enhancement, and perinephric inflammatory stranding of the right kidney.

Intraprocedural Findings
Intraprocedural ultrasound confirms severe hydronephrosis with a central obstructing calculus (Fig. 2). Two 8-French nephrostomy catheters were placed using ultrasound guidance (Fig, 3), and a total of 100 mL of pus was aspirated from the right kidney.

Follow-up and Complications
The patient was observed overnight and discharged to her home the next day. Six weeks later, she underwent open nephrectomy, and pathologic analysis confirmed the diagnosis of severe, chronic granulomatous pyelonephritis.

Suggested Readings
Bingol-Kologlu M, Ciftci AO, Senocak ME, et al: Xanthogranulomatous pyelonephritis in children: Diagnostic and therapeutic aspects. Eur J Pediatr 12:42-48, 2002.

Millward SF: Percutaneous nephrostomy: A practical approach. J Vasc Interv Radiol 11:955-964, 2000.

Parvati R, Cardella JF, Grassi CJ, et al: Quality improvement guidelines for percutaneous nephrostomy. J Vasc Intervent Radiol 14:S277-S281, 2003.

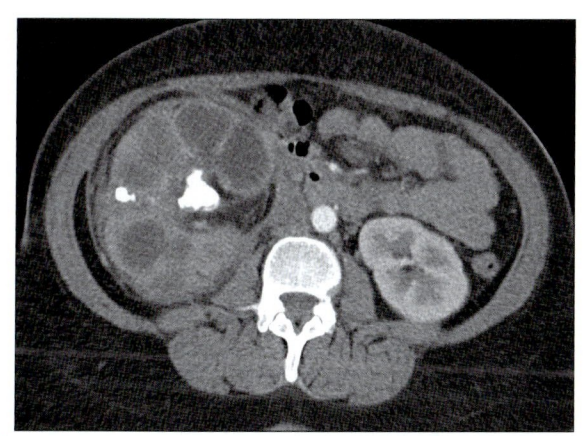

Figure 1. Contrast-enhanced CT of the abdomen shows a massively enlarged right kidney with a staghorn calculus in the renal pelvis. The kidney is poorly enhancing, and there is severe hydronephrosis.

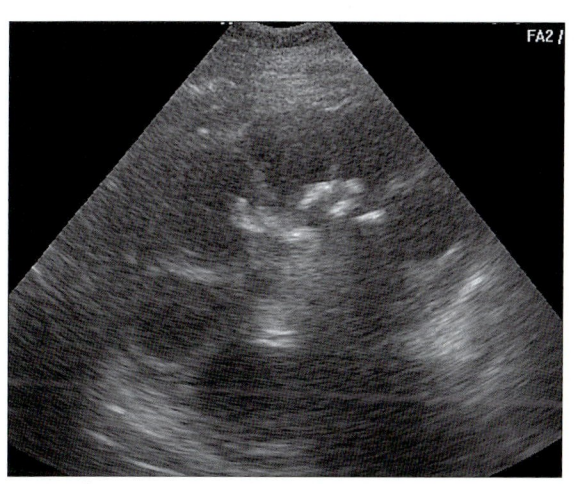

Figure 2. Ultrasound image of the right kidney at the time of nephrostomy placement shows massively dilated renal calyces. There is a central obstructing calculus.

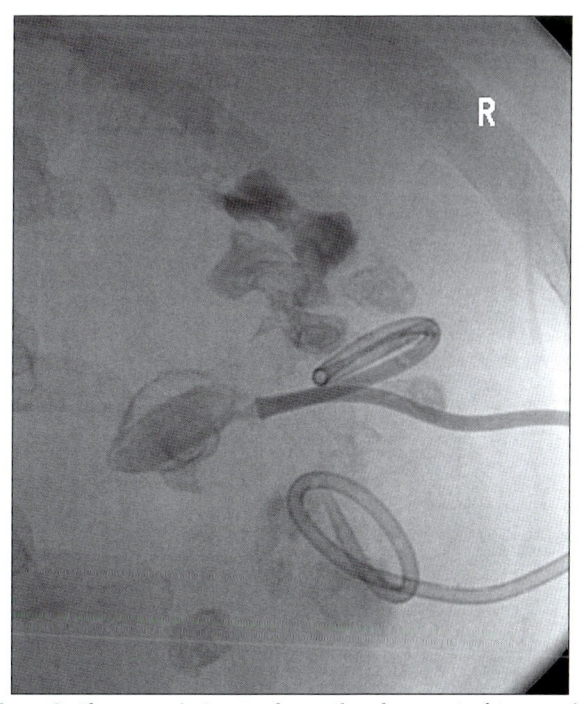

Figure 3. Fluoroscopic image shows the placement of two nephrostomy catheters, which were required because of the lack of communication between the upper and lower pole calyces. A total of 100 mL of pus was aspirated from the renal collecting system.

Case 278

DEMOGRAPHICS/CLINICAL HISTORY

A 55-year-old man with hydronephrosis who received a living, related renal transplant for end-stage renal disease, undergoing ultrasound and nephrostomy catheter placement.

DISCUSSION

History/Indications for Procedure
A 55-year-old man has a history of renal transplantation for end-stage renal disease resulting from polycystic kidney disease. He has elevated serum creatinine levels and hydronephrosis.

Procedure
Percutaneous nephrostomy placement

Pre-procedure Imaging
Ultrasound of the transplanted kidney demonstrated moderate to severe hydronephrosis with slight elevation of resistive indices.

Intraprocedural Findings
A mid-pole calyx was targeted with ultrasound (Fig. 1). With the return of clear urine, a wire was placed (Fig. 2), the tract was dilated, and an 8-French nephrostomy catheter was placed (Fig. 3).

Follow-up and Complications
Two days after nephrostomy placement, the patient returned for a nephrostogram. It revealed a focal stricture in the distal ureter (Fig. 4).

Suggested Readings
American College of Radiology (ACR): Practice guideline for the performance of percutaneous nephrostomy. ACR practice guideline, amended 2004 (res. 25). xxxx xx:463–471, 2004.

Farrell TA, Hicks ME: A review of radiologically guided percutaneous nephrostomies in 303 patients. J Vasc Intervent Radiol 8:769-774, 1997.

Millward SF: Percutaneous nephrostomy: A practical approach. J Vasc Intervent Radiol 11:955-964, 2000.

Ramchandani P, Cardella JF, Grassi CJ, et al: Quality improvement guidelines for percutaneous nephrostomy. J Vasc Intervent Radiol 14:S277-S281, 2003.

Case 278   557

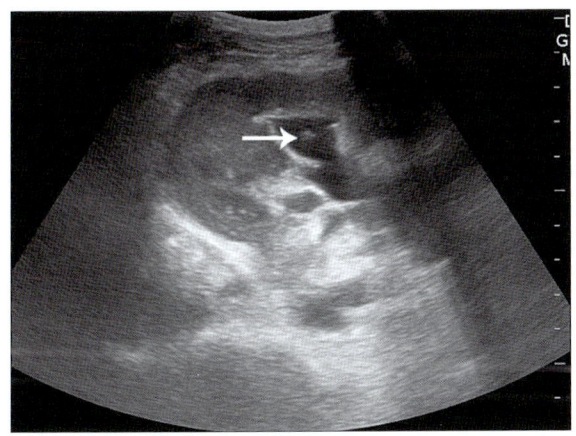

Figure 1. Ultrasound image during nephrostomy placement demonstrates moderate hydronephrosis of the transplanted kidney. A needle can be seen in a mid-pole calyx *(arrow)*.

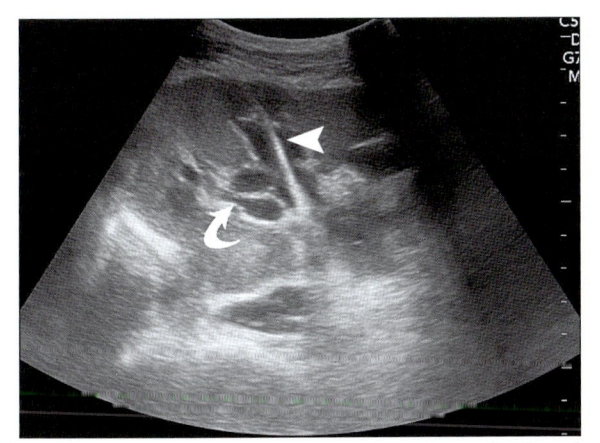

Figure 2. The guidewire is seen entering the mid-pole calyx *(arrowhead)* and looping into a lower pole calyx *(arrow)*.

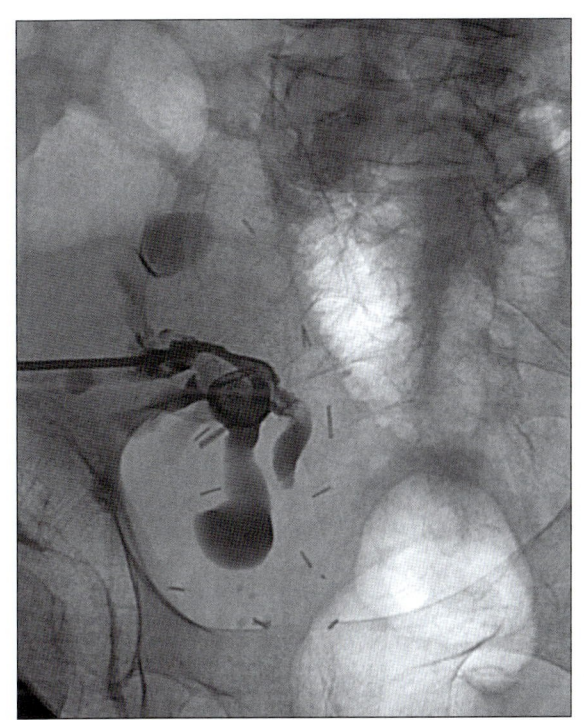

Figure 3. Contrast injected after nephrostomy placement confirms appropriate position.

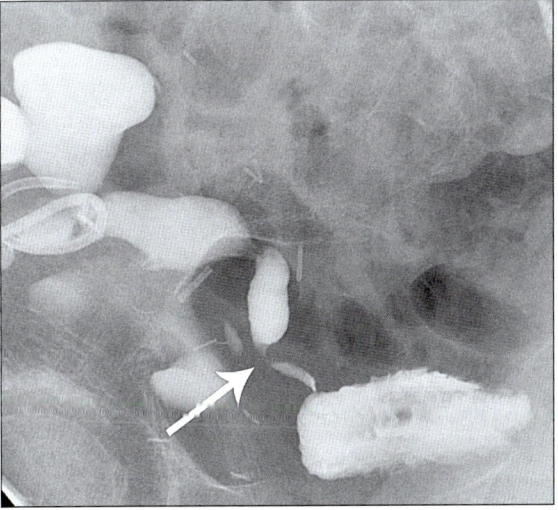

Figure 4. Follow-up nephrostogram demonstrates a focal stricture in the distal ureter *(arrow)*.

Case 279

DEMOGRAPHICS/CLINICAL HISTORY

A 58-year-old woman with fever and obstructing ureteral calculus, undergoing CT.

DISCUSSION

History/Indications for Procedure
This patient presented with fever and obstructing calculus at the right ureterovesical junction.

Procedure
CT-guided nephrostomy placement

Pre-procedure Imaging
Unenhanced CT of the abdomen and pelvis shows right hydronephrosis and perinephric stranding (Fig. 1). A 6-mm calculus is present at the right ureterovesical junction.

Intraprocedural Findings
The right renal collecting system could not be identified easily with ultrasound because of the patient's body habitus. CT was used to gain access and place a nephrostomy catheter (Figs. 2 to 4). Purulent urine was aspirated from the collecting system.

Follow-up and Complications
The obstructing calculus spontaneously passed, and the nephrostomy catheter was removed approximately 2 weeks after insertion. The patient was given a course of antibiotics for the infection.

Suggested Readings
American College of Radiology (ACR): Practice guideline for the performance of percutaneous nephrostomy. ACR Practice Guideline; Amended 2004 (Res.25), pp 463-471.
Matlaga BR, et al: Computerized tomography guided access for percutaneous nephrostolithotomy. J Urol 170:45-47, 2003.
Millward SF: Percutaneous nephrostomy: A practical approach. J Vasc Intervent Radiol 11:955-964, 2000.

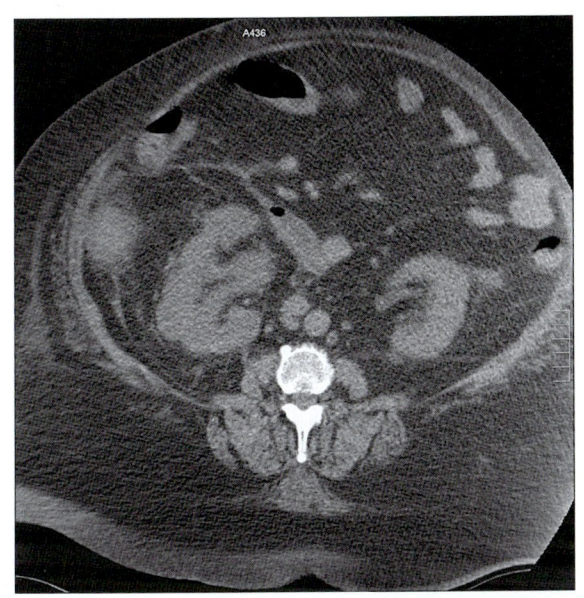

Figure 1. Unenhanced CT scan shows enlargement of the right kidney with perinephric stranding and hydronephrosis.

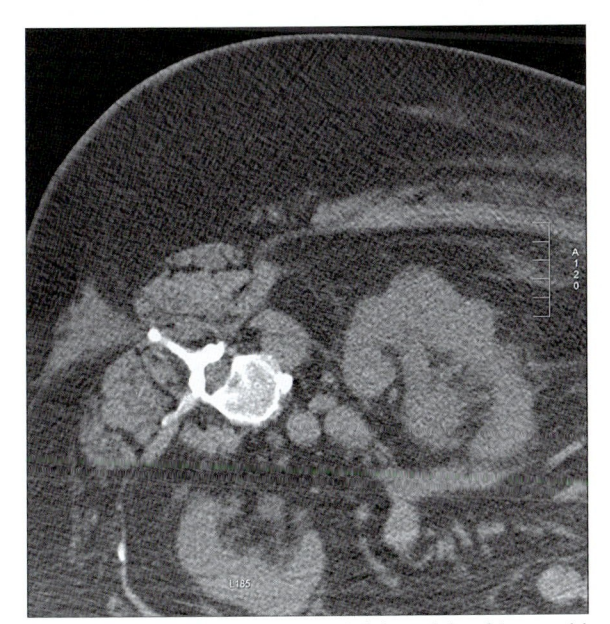

Figure 2. The patient was placed in a left lateral decubitus position for planning nephrostomy placement.

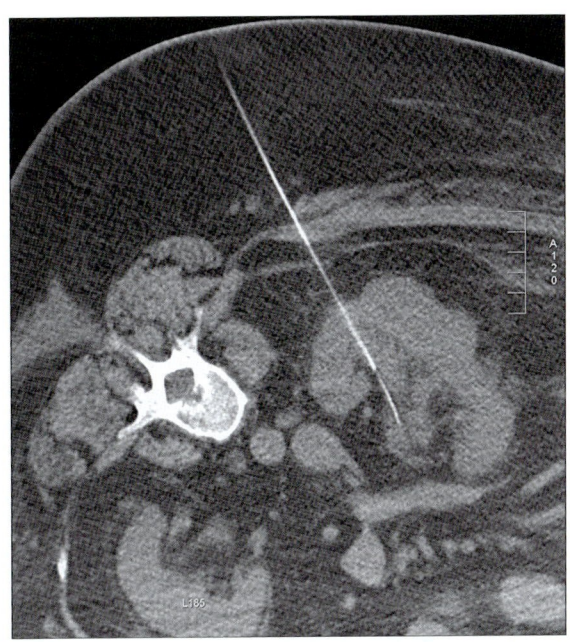

Figure 3. A horizontally oriented calyx was accessed, and a 0.018 inch guidewire was placed centrally.

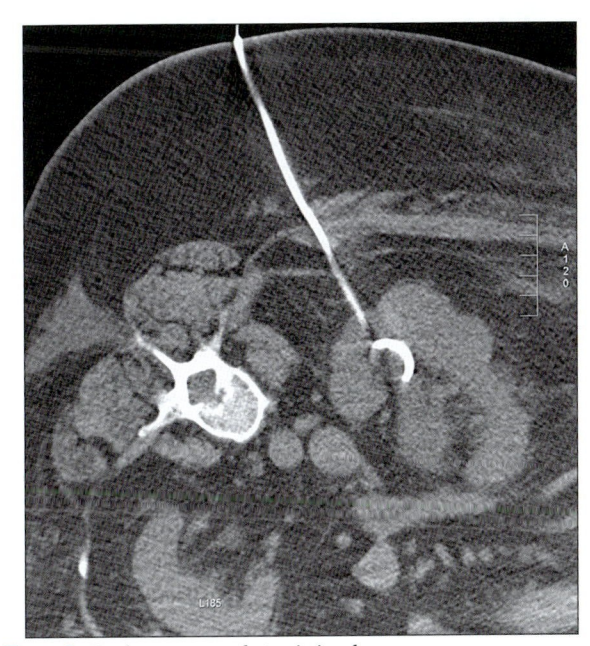

Figure 4. Nephrostomy catheter is in place.

Case 280

DEMOGRAPHICS/CLINICAL HISTORY

A 55-year-old man who underwent renal transplant and ureteroneocystoplasty presents with increasing creatinine and hydronephrosis.

DISCUSSION

History/Indications for Procedure
A 55-year-old man who underwent renal transplant for renal failure secondary to polycystic kidney disease and ureteroneocystoplasty for ureteral obstruction presents with increasing creatinine and hydronephrosis.

Procedure
Nephrostomy management in a renal transplant patient

Pre-procedure Imaging
Ultrasound of the transplanted kidney shows severe hydronephrosis (Fig. 1).

Intraprocedural Findings
An 8-French nephrostomy was placed under ultrasound guidance (Fig. 2); follow-up nephrostogram shows persistent hydronephrosis with diffuse narrowing of the ureter (Fig. 3). A Whitaker test was performed; the kidney-bladder gradient remained normal during the infusion.

Follow-up and Complications
Based on the findings of the Whitaker test, the nephrostomy catheter was removed. Since that time, the creatinine level and urine output have remained stable.

Suggested Readings
Jaffe RB, Middleton AW Jr: Whitaker test: Differentiation of obstructive from nonobstructive uropathy. AJR Am J Roentgenol 134:9-15, 1980.

Kashi SH, Irving HC, Sadek SA: Does the Whitaker test add to antegrade pyelography in the investigation of collecting system dilatation in renal allografts?. Br J Radiol 66:877-881, 1993.

Zollikofer CL, Bruhlmann WF, Baumgartner D, et al: Antegrade pyelography, percutaneous nephrostomy and ureteral perfusion (Whitaker test) for the renal transplant recipient. Rofo 142:193-200, 1985.

Case 280   561

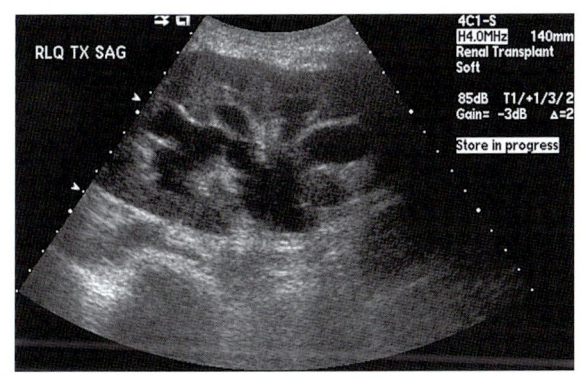

Figure 1. Ultrasound shows severe hydronephrosis of the transplanted kidney.

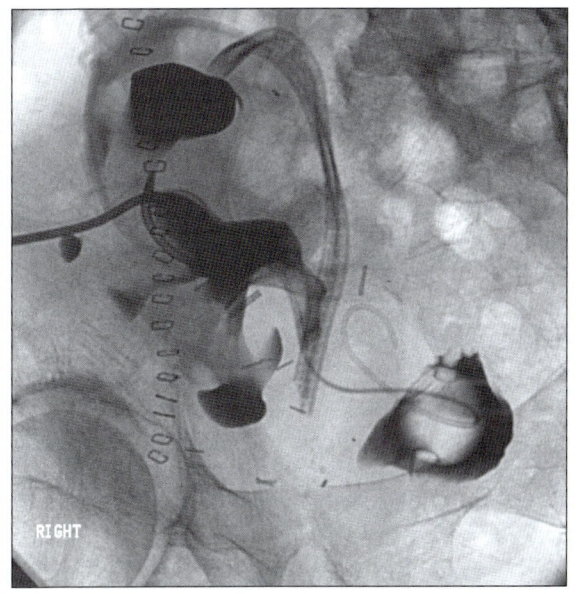

Figure 2. An 8-French nephrostomy has been placed via an upper pole calyx. There is moderate hydronephrosis on nephrostogram.

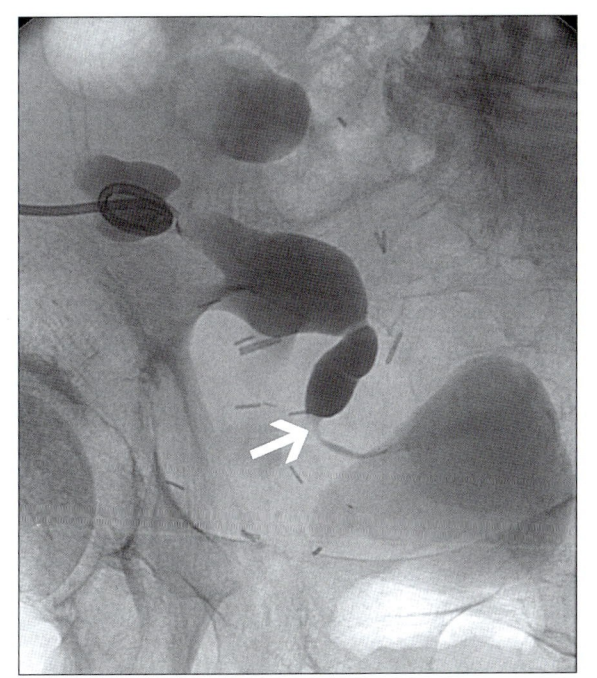

Figure 3. Follow-up nephrostogram shows persistent hydronephrosis. There is abrupt caliber change of the proximal ureter (*arrow*) with diffuse narrowing of the distal ureter.

Case 281

DEMOGRAPHICS/CLINICAL HISTORY

A 62-year-old man with a history of cystoprostatectomy for bladder carcinoma with new, right-sided hydronephrosis, undergoing magnetic resonance imaging (MRI) and ultrasonography.

DISCUSSION

History/Indications for Procedure
A 62-year-old man with a history of cystoprostatectomy and ileal conduit presented with new hydronephrosis of the right kidney.

Procedure
Ureteroileal anastomotic stricture

Pre-procedure Imaging
MRI of the abdomen and pelvis shows moderate hydronephrosis of the right kidney with layering debris in the right renal pelvis (Fig. 1). There is a focal stricture of the distal right ureter just before the site of insertion into the ileal conduit (Fig. 2).

Intraprocedural Findings
The right renal collecting system was accessed using ultrasound guidance, and an antegrade nephrostogram confirms moderate hydronephrosis with an obstructing stricture of the distal right ureter (Fig. 3). The point of obstruction was crossed, and an 8-French, 22-cm nephroureteral catheter was placed (Fig. 4).

Follow-up and Complications
The patient developed rigors after the procedure, for which he was treated with additional antibiotics and supportive management. The distal ureteral stricture did not respond to balloon dilation, and eventually, the patient underwent surgical reimplantation of the distal ureter.

Suggested Readings
Alago W Jr, Sofocleous CT, Covey AM, et al: Placement of transileal conduit retrograde nephroureteral stents in patients with ureteral obstruction after cystectomy: Technique and outcome. AJR Am J Roentgenol 19:1536-1539, 2008.

Hausegger KA: Percutaneous nephrostomy and antegrade ureteral stenting: Technique-indications-complications. Eur Radiol 16:2016-2030, 2006.

Richter F, Irwin RD, Watson RA, Lang EK: Endourologic management of benign ureteral strictures with and without compromised vascular supply. Urology 55:652-657, 2000.

Case 281   563

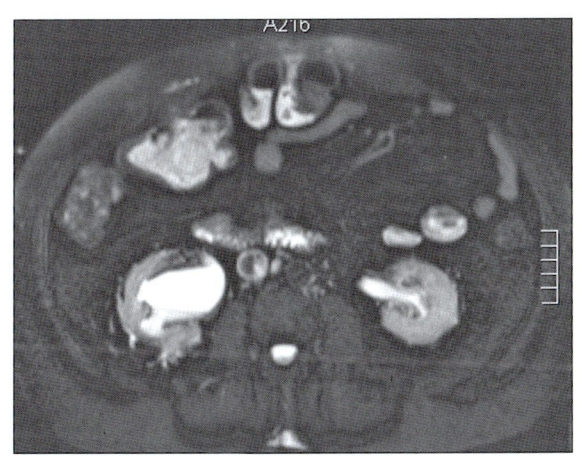

Figure 1. Axial, T2-weighted MRI through the kidneys shows moderate hydronephrosis of the right kidney. A small amount of layering debris is seen within the renal pelvis.

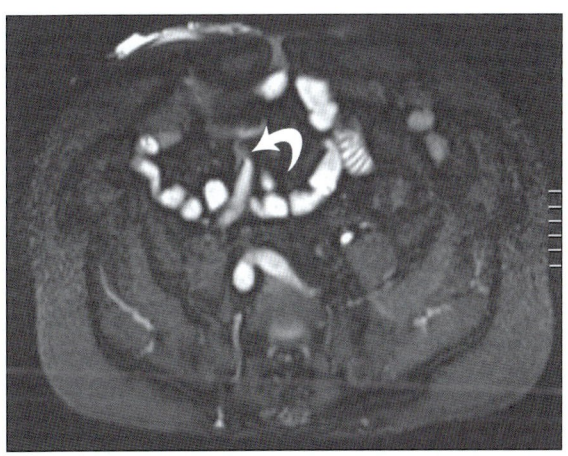

Figure 2. Axial, T2-weighted MRI through the lower abdomen shows a dilated distal right ureter with a focal stricture *(curved arrow)* just before the ureter enters the ileal conduit.

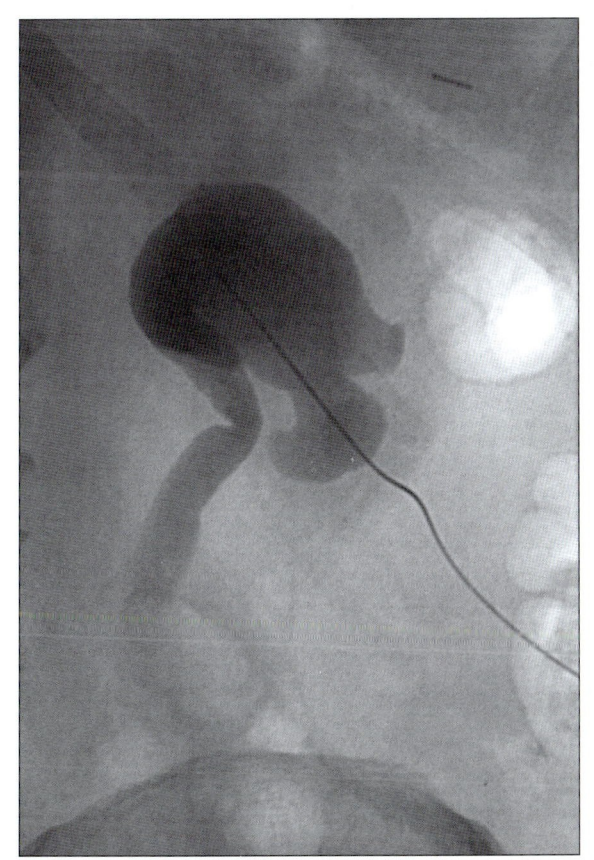

Figure 3. A lower pole calyx was accessed with ultrasound guidance. Contrast injection into the right kidney shows moderate hydronephrosis and hydroureter.

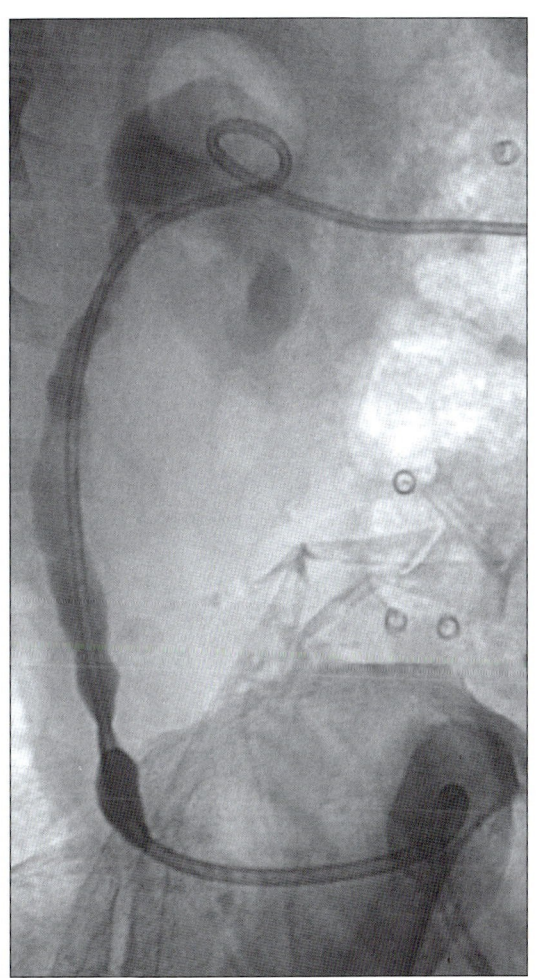

Figure 4. An 8-French, 22-cm nephroureteral catheter was placed, decompressing the renal collecting system. The distal loop is coiled in the ileal conduit.

Case 282

DEMOGRAPHICS/CLINICAL HISTORY

A 45-year-old man with a left-sided staghorn calculus, undergoing computed tomography (CT), fluoroscopy, and stent placement.

DISCUSSION

History/Indications for Procedure
A 45-year-old man has a left-sided staghorn calculus, for which a nephroureteral catheter is placed for percutaneous ultrasonic lithotripsy (PUL) access.

Procedure
Nephroureteral stent placement

Pre-procedure Imaging
Unenhanced axial CT of the abdomen demonstrates a staghorn calculus in the left renal pelvis that extends into the lower pole collecting system (Fig. 1).

Intraprocedural Findings
Under fluoroscopy, the stone-containing lower pole calyx was accessed (Fig. 2), and a 5-French pigtail nephroureteral catheter was placed. To provide additional mechanical advantage during PUL, a second nephroureteral catheter was placed in a mid-pole calyx (Fig. 3).

Follow-up and Complications
PUL was performed without complication. The follow-up CT scan performed 2 days after the procedure demonstrates several small residual calculi remaining in the renal collecting system (Fig. 4).

Suggested Readings
Hausegger KA, Portugaller HR: Percutaneous nephrostomy and antegrade ureteral stenting: Technique—indications—complications. Eur Radiol 16:2016-2030, 2005.
Sandhu C, Ansom KM, Patel U: Urinary tract stones. Part II, Current status of treatment. Clin Radiol 58:422-433, 2003.

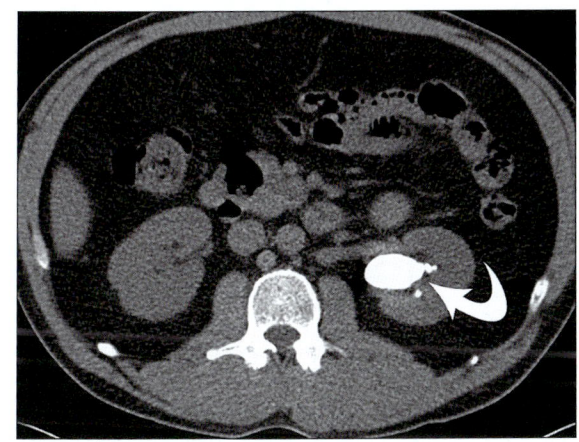

Figure 1. Unenhanced CT image demonstrates a large staghorn calculus in the left renal pelvis *(arrow)*.

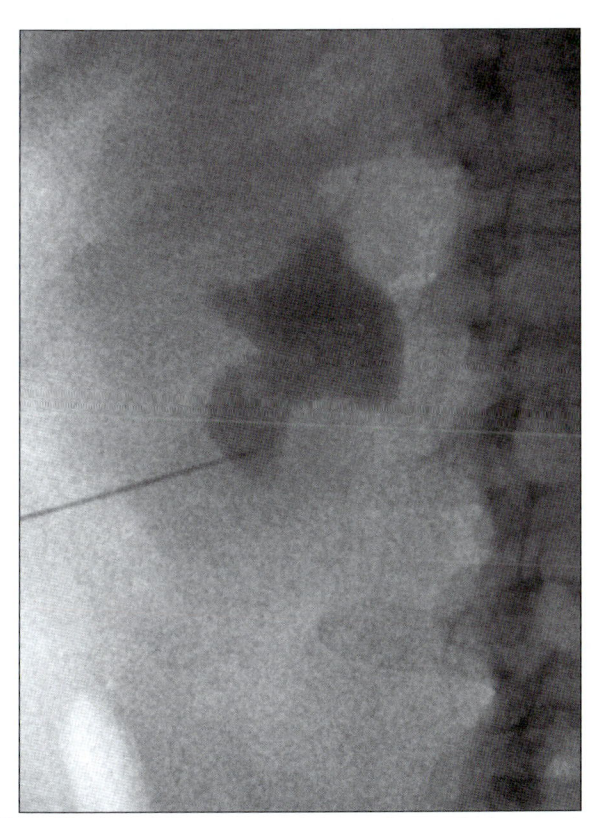

Figure 2. The inferior margin of the staghorn calculus was targeted with the use of fluoroscopy.

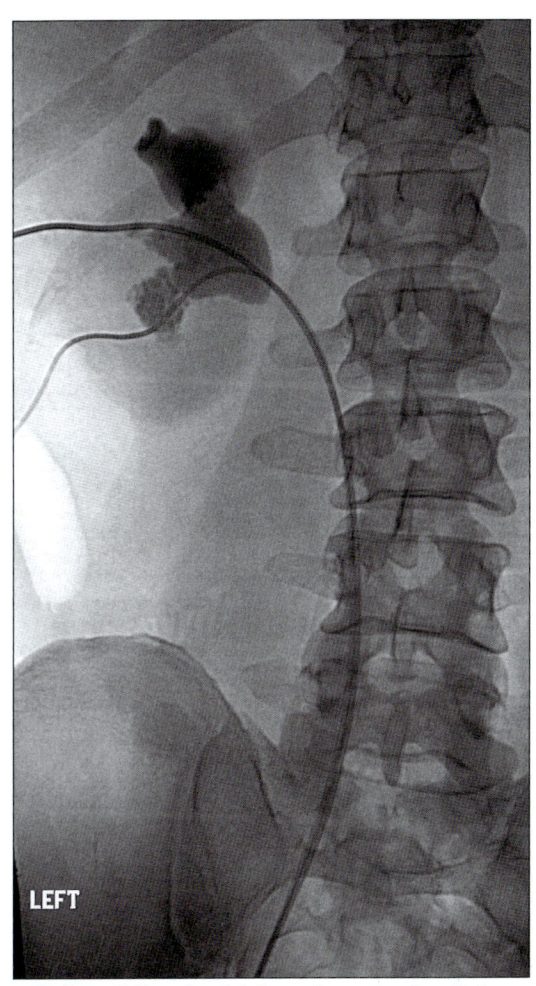

Figure 3. Two 5-French pigtail nephroureteral catheters were placed for PUL access.

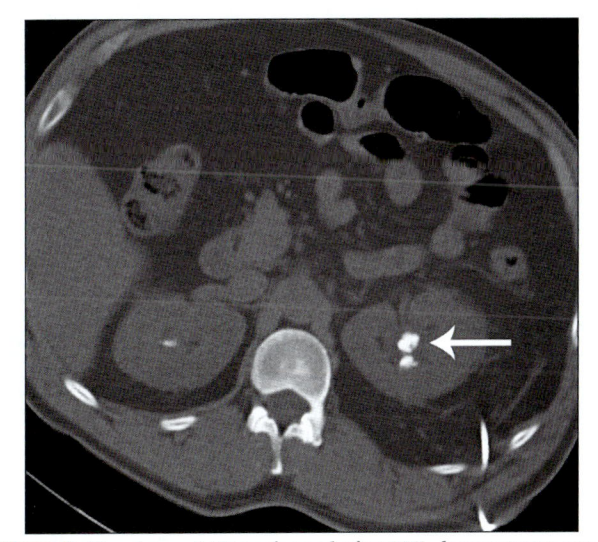

Figure 4. Unenhanced CT performed after PUL demonstrates several small residual calculi *(arrow)*.

Case 283

DEMOGRAPHICS/CLINICAL HISTORY

A 60-year-old woman with an obstructing bladder mass.

DISCUSSION

History/Indications for Procedure
A 60-year-old woman with squamous cell carcinoma of the bladder, locally invasive to the bladder base, causing left renal obstruction.

Procedure
Nephroureteral stent placement

Pre-procedure Imaging
Contrast-enhanced CT of the pelvis shows an enhancing mass along the posterior base of the bladder (Fig. 1).

Intraprocedural Findings
A lower-pole calyx was accessed with ultrasound, and the left ureter was catheterized (Fig. 2). The distal left ureter was dilated with a 5-mm angioplasty balloon, and an 8-French, 22-cm nephroureteral catheter was placed (Figs. 3 and 4).

Follow-up and Complications
The patient was observed overnight and was discharged home the following day. She was scheduled to return for routine catheter exchange 3 months after the catheter placement.

Suggested Readings
Hausegger KA: Percutaneous nephrostomy and antegrade ureteral stenting: Technique-indications-complications. Eur Radiol 16: 2016-2030, 2006.

Millward SF: Percutaneous nephrostomy: A practical approach. J Vasc Intervent Radiol 11:955-964, 2000.

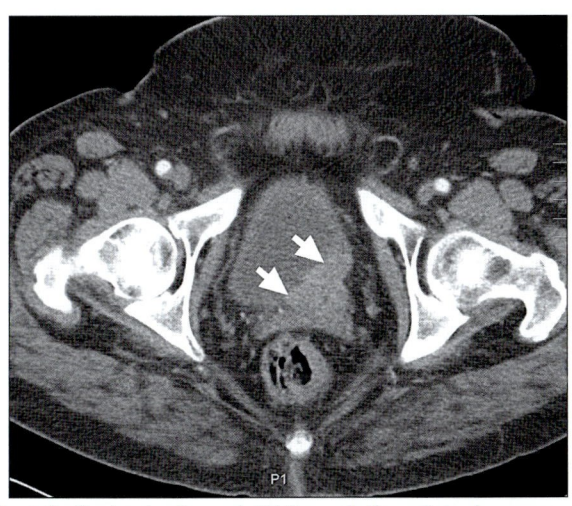

Figure 1. Contrast-enhanced CT through the pelvis shows an enhancing mass *(arrows)* of the bladder wall at the level of the left ureteral orifice.

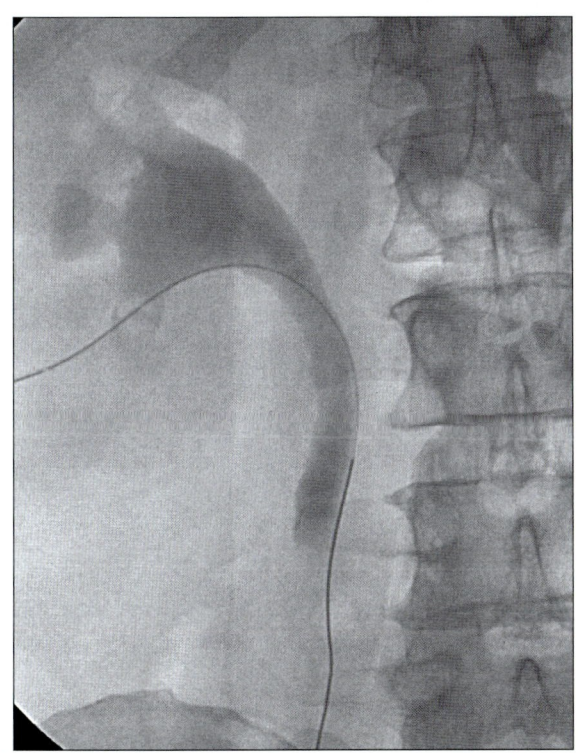

Figure 2. A lower-pole calyx was accessed with ultrasound, and the guidewire has been advanced in the left ureter.

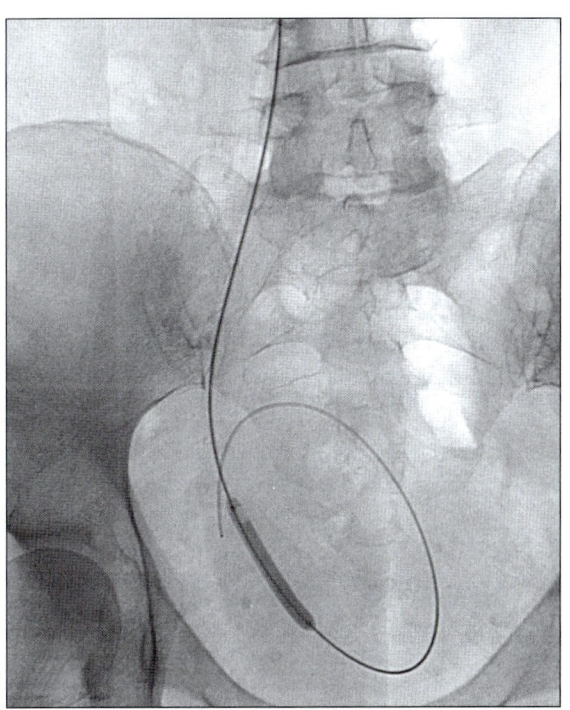

Figure 3. The distal left ureter was dilated with a 5-mm balloon in order to advance the nephroureteral catheter through the obstructing mass.

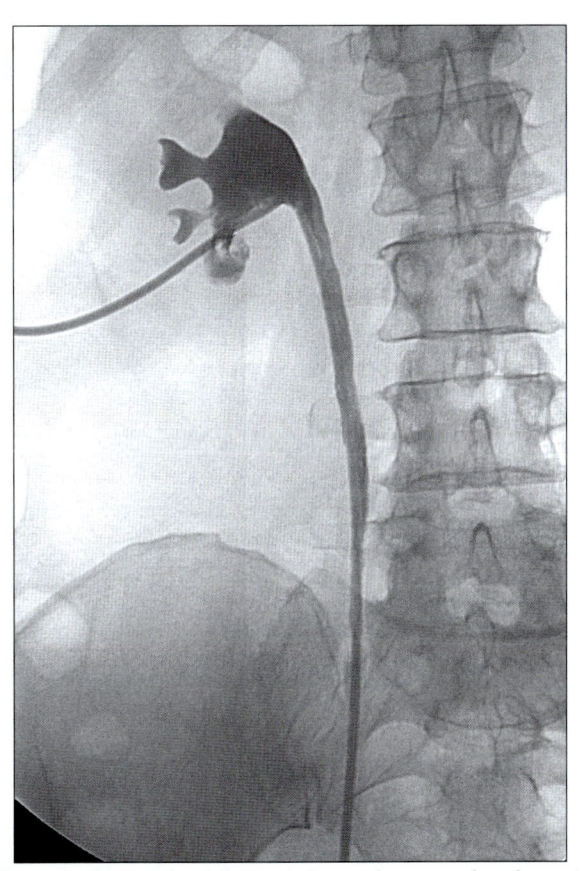

Figure 4. The proximal loop of the nephroureteral catheter is coiled in the renal pelvis. There is decompression of the renal collecting system.

Case 284

DEMOGRAPHICS/CLINICAL HISTORY

A 33-year-old man with horseshoe kidney and left renal calculus, undergoing ultrasound, computed tomography (CT), fluoroscopy, catheterization, and lithotripsy.

DISCUSSION

History/Indications for Procedure

A 33-year-old man has a horseshoe kidney and left renal calculus. The patient has occasional flank pain, and access is needed for percutaneous ultrasonic lithotripsy.

Procedure

Nephroureteral catheter in a horseshoe kidney

Pre-procedure Imaging

Unenhanced CT of the abdomen demonstrates a 1.4-cm stone at the left ureteropelvic junction of the horseshoe kidney (Fig. 1).

Intraprocedural Findings

The left ureteropelvic junction stone is visible fluoroscopically (Fig. 2). Using intravenous contrast to opacify the collecting system, a mid-pole calyx was accessed (Fig. 3), and a 5-French nephroureteral catheter was placed (Fig. 4).

Follow-up and Complications

The patient underwent percutaneous ultrasonic lithotripsy the next day, and the stone was completely removed.

Suggested Readings

Darabi Mahboub MR, Zolfaghari M: Ahanian A: Percutaneous nephrolithotomy of kidney calculi in horseshoe kidney. Urol J 4:147-150, 2007.

Hausegger KA: Percutaneous nephrostomy and antegrade ureteral stenting: Technique—indications—complications. Eur Radiol 16:2016-2030, 2005.

Sandhu C, Ansom KM, Patel U: Urinary tract stones. Part II. Current status of treatment. Clin Radiol 58:422-433, 2003.

Case 284   569

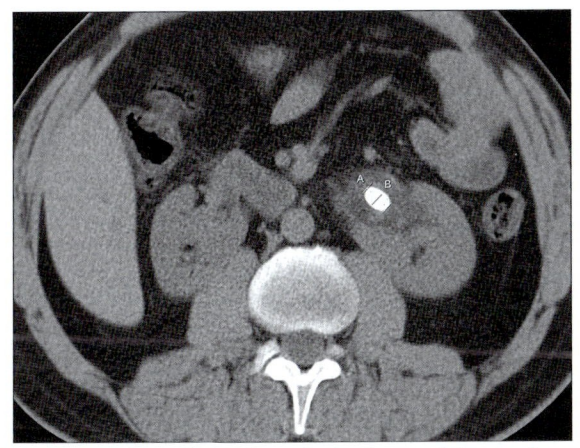

Figure 1. Unenhanced CT through the lower abdomen demonstrates a 1.4-cm stone in the region of the left ureteropelvic junction of the horseshoe kidney.

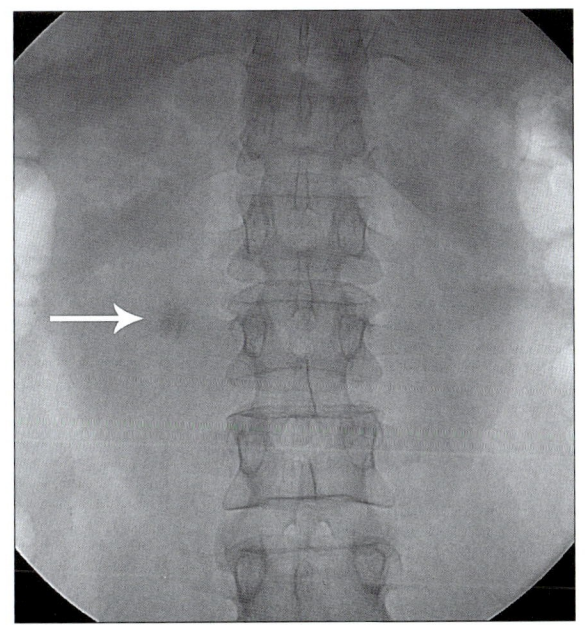

Figure 2. The calculus is visible fluoroscopically overlying the region of the left ureteropelvic junction *(arrow)*.

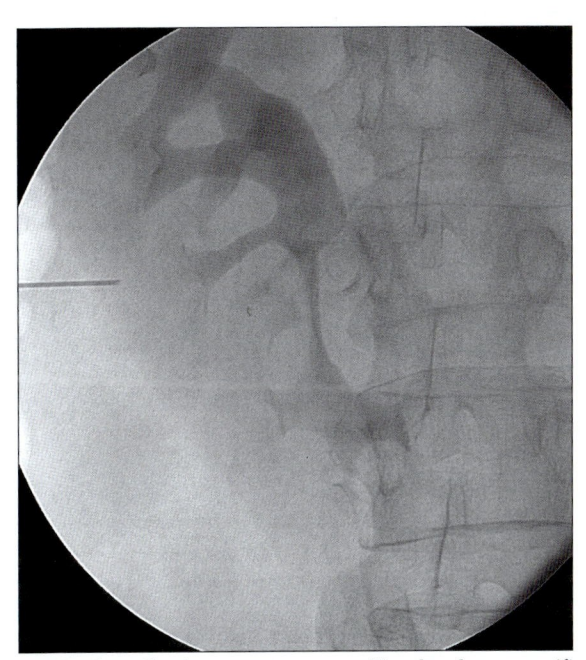

Figure 3. The collecting system was not dilated and was opacified by intravenous administration of contrast. A mid-pole calyx was then targeted.

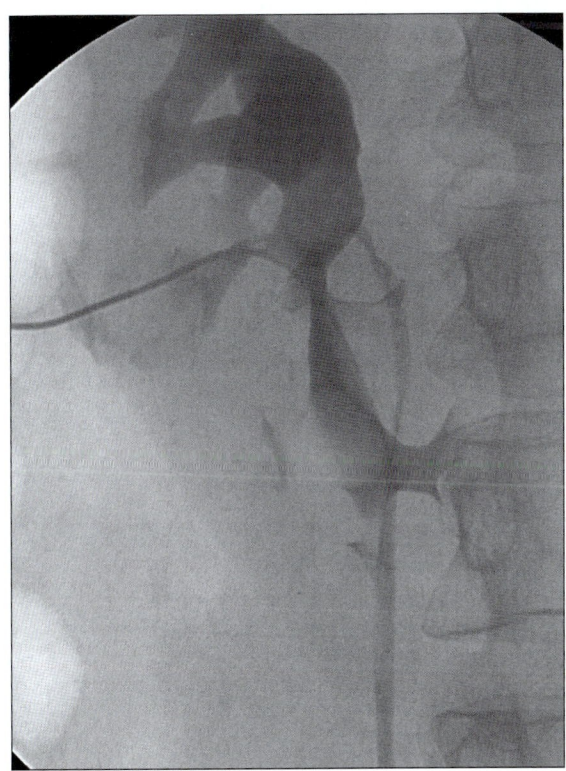

Figure 4. After the collection system was accessed, a 5-French nephroureteral catheter was placed.

Case 285

DEMOGRAPHICS/CLINICAL HISTORY

A 19-year-old woman with a large, left renal cyst, undergoing computed tomography (CT), ultrasonography, and alcohol sclerosis.

DISCUSSION

History/Indications for Procedure
A 19-year-old woman had a large renal cyst that recurred despite surgical deroofing.

Procedure
Renal cyst drainage and sclerosing

Pre-procedure Imaging
CT of the abdomen shows a 14.5-cm × 11.6-cm cystic mass arising from the lower pole of the left kidney (Fig. 1). The mass contains a single visible septation.

Intraprocedural Findings
Preliminary ultrasound showed a large cyst with a loculated component. Two drains were placed for complete cyst drainage (Fig. 2).

Follow-up and Complications
The patient returned intermittently over the next 2 months for follow-up drain studies and alcohol sclerosis of the cavity (Figs. 3 and 4). The drain was removed, and the patient did not return for recurrent symptoms over the next 5 years.

Suggested Readings
Chung BH, Kim JH, Hong CH, et al: Comparison of single and multiple sessions of percutaneous sclerotherapy for simple renal cyst. BJU Int 85:626-627, 2000.

Okeke AA, Mitchelmore AE, Keeley FX, Timoney AG: A comparison of aspiration and sclerotherapy with laparoscopic de-roofing in the management of symptomatic simple renal cysts. BJU Int 92: 610-613, 2003.

Zerem E, Imamovic G, Omerovic S: Symptomatic simple renal cyst: Comparison of continuous negative-pressure catheter drainage and single-session alcohol sclerotherapy. AJR Am J Roentgenol 190:1193-1197, 2008.

Case 285   571

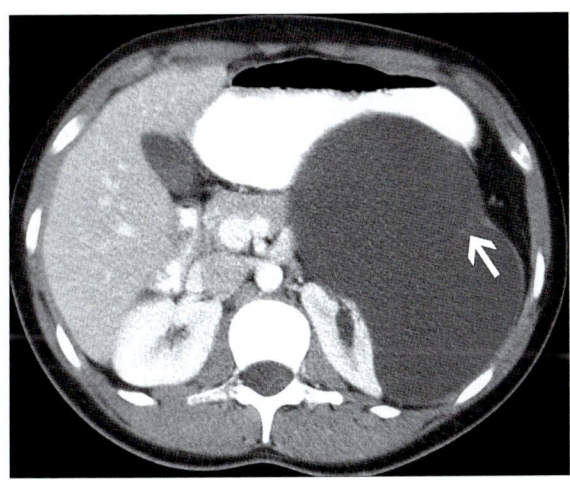

Figure 1. Contrast-enhanced CT shows a large hypodense cystic mass compressing the left kidney. The mass has a single septation *(arrow)*.

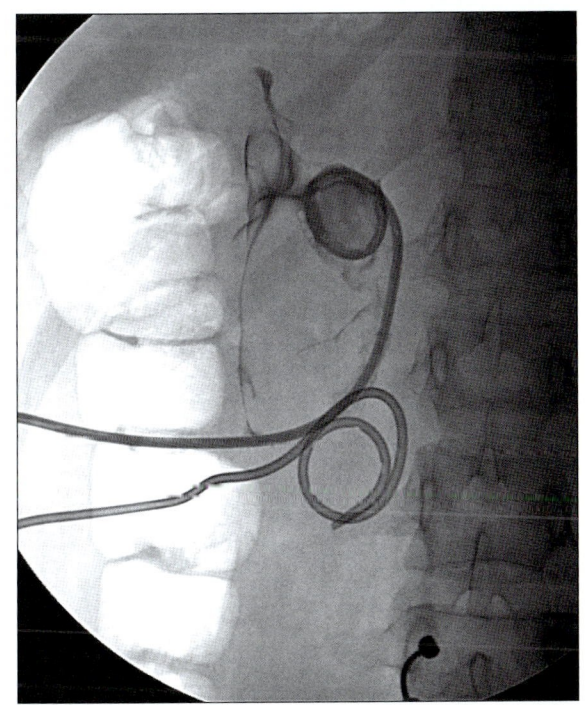

Figure 2. Two pigtail drainage catheters were placed in the two cyst compartments with ultrasound guidance.

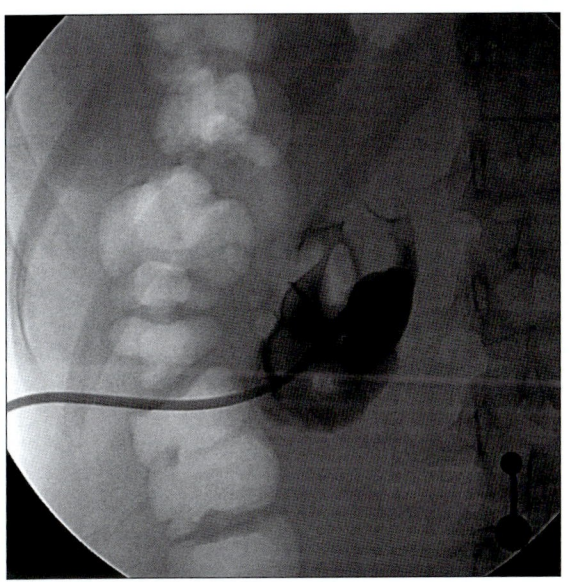

Figure 3. The upper catheter has been removed. Follow-up injection of the lower catheter shows a residual cavity. The patient returned for several attempts at alcohol cyst sclerosis.

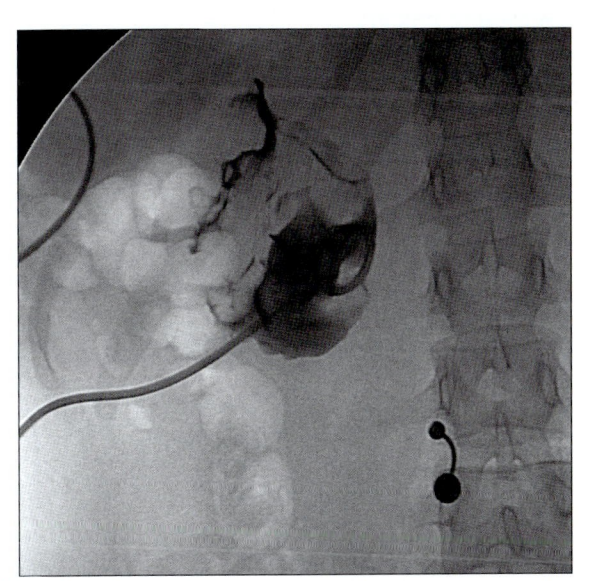

Figure 4. Follow-up drain study 2 months after placement shows very little change in the size of the cyst cavity. There had been minimal output from the catheter, and the drain was removed.

Case 286

DEMOGRAPHICS/CLINICAL HISTORY

A 54-year-old woman with a perinephric abscess, undergoing computed tomography (CT).

DISCUSSION

History/Indications for Procedure
A 54-year-old woman has flank pain and fever.

Procedure
Percutaneous drainage of perirenal abscess

Pre-procedure Imaging
Contrast-enhanced CT of the abdomen shows a 13-cm × 11-cm, heterogeneous fluid collection adjacent to the right kidney (Fig. 1).

Intraprocedural Findings
An 18-gauge needle was placed into the collection with ultrasound guidance, and pus was aspirated. A 10-French pigtail drainage catheter was placed (Fig. 2), and 100 mL of pus was aspirated.

Follow-up and Complications
The catheter continued to drain purulent material over the next 4 weeks. After the drainage ceased and the catheter was removed, repeat CT showed near-complete drainage of the collection (Fig. 3).

Suggested Readings
Lang EK: Renal, perirenal, and pararenal abscesses: Percutaneous drainage. Radiology 174:109-113, 1990.

Sacks D, Banner MP, Meranze SG, et al: Renal and related retroperitoneal abscesses: Percutaneous drainage. Radiology 167:447-451, 1988.

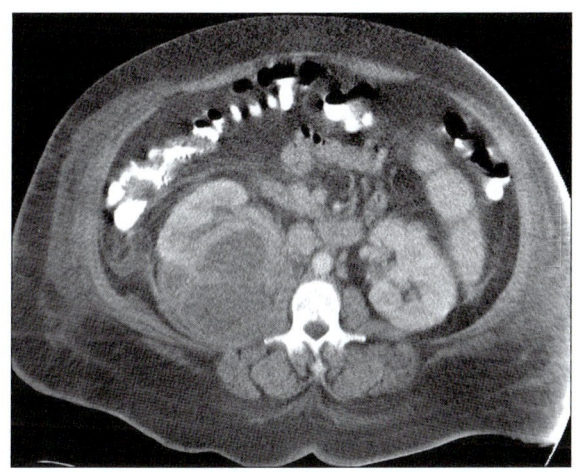

Figure 1. Contrast-enhanced CT shows a large heterogeneous fluid collection posterior to the right kidney. The collection displaces the right kidney anteriorly and involves the right psoas muscle.

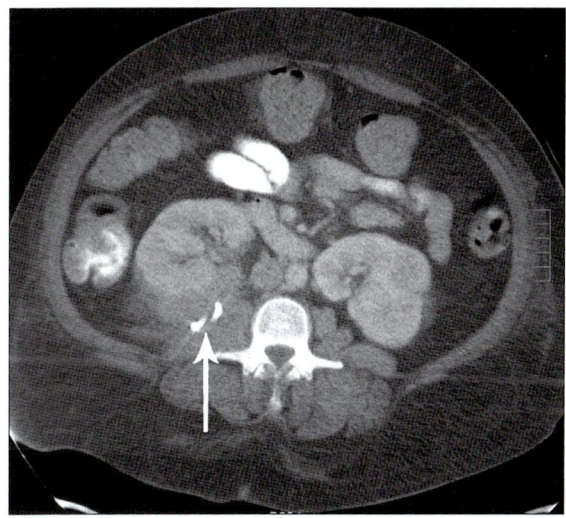

Figure 2. Follow-up CT shows a drainage catheter within the collection *(arrow)*, which has significantly decreased in size.

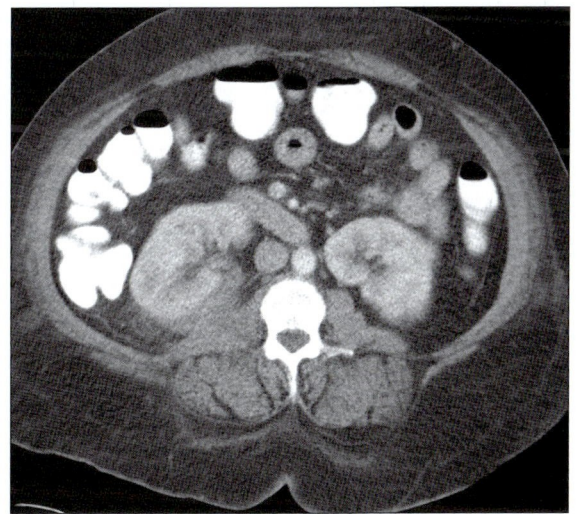

Figure 3. Follow-up CT after the drainage catheter was removed shows residual inflammatory changes posterior to the right kidney. Minimal fluid remains.

Case 287

DEMOGRAPHICS/CLINICAL HISTORY

A 70-year-old woman with an air-fluid collection within the kidney following embolization of a large angiomyolipoma.

DISCUSSION

History/Indications for Procedure
A 70-year-old woman who underwent embolization of an 8.5-cm angiomyolipoma 4 weeks earlier. She has had increasing left flank pain and fevers.

Procedure
Percutaneous drainage of renal abscess

Pre-procedure Imaging
Contrast-enhanced CT of the abdomen shows an air-fluid level within the angiomyolipoma consistent with abscess formation.

Intraprocedural Findings
An 18-gauge needle was placed into the collection with CT guidance and 100 ml of pus was aspirated (Fig. 3). An 8-French pigtail drainage catheter was placed (Fig. 4).

Follow-up and Complications
The drain remained in place for 7 weeks. At this point, there was no residual fluid on CT and minimal residual cavity on drain injection; thus, the drain was removed.

Suggested Readings
Bernardino ME, Baumgartner BR: Abscess drainage in the genitourinary tract. Radiol Clin North Am 24:539-549, 1986.
Lang EK: Renal, perirenal, and pararenal abscesses: Percutaneous drainage. Radiology 174:109-113, 1990.
Ozkara H, Ozkan B, Solok V: Management of renal abscess formation after embolization due to renal angiomyolipomas in two cases. Int Urol Nephrol 38:427-429, 2006.

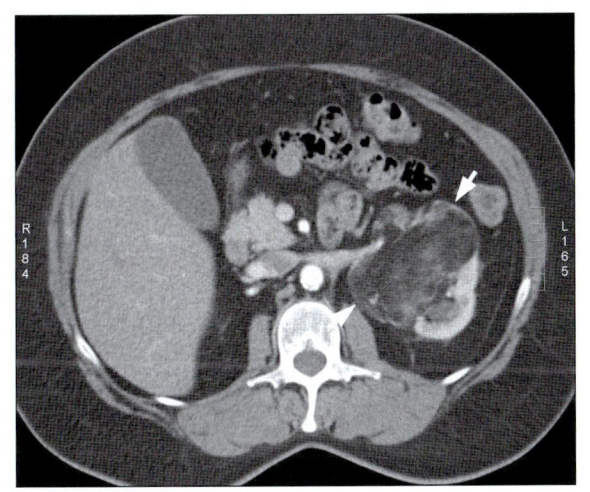

Figure 1. Contrast-enhanced CT shows an 8.5-cm × 8-cm mass arising from the left kidney *(arrows)*. The mass is predominantly fat attenuation, consistent with an angiomyolipoma.

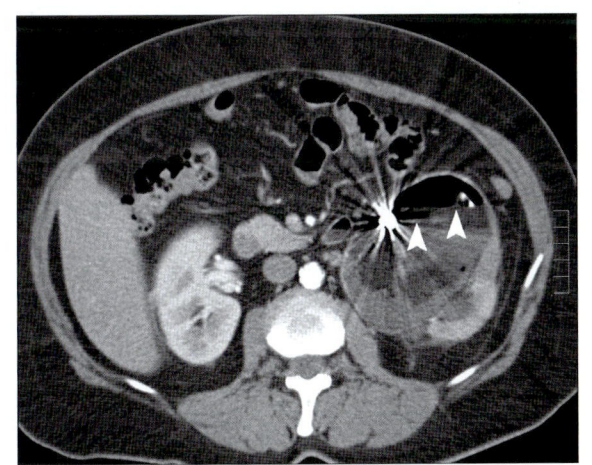

Figure 2. Follow-up CT 4 weeks after embolization shows enlargement of the mass and the presence of an air-fluid level *(arrowheads)*.

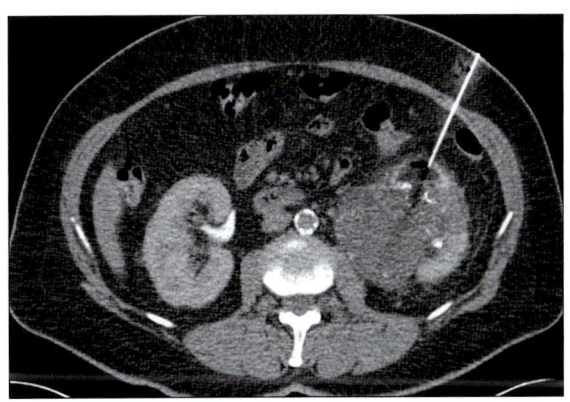

Figure 3. An 18-gauge needle has been placed into the abscess using CT guidance.

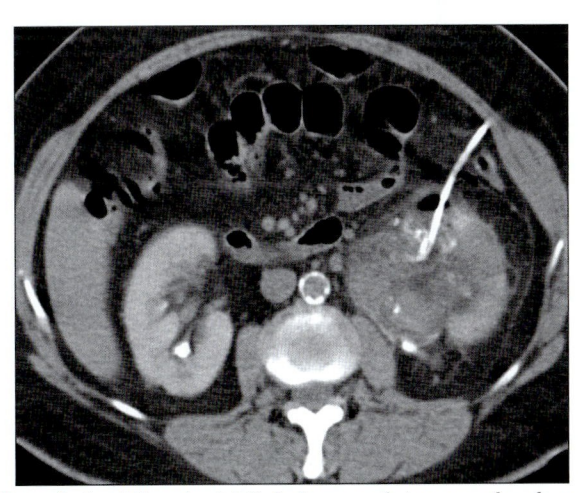

Figure 4. An 8-French pigtail drainage catheter was placed, and 100 ml of pus was aspirated from the lesion.

Case 288

DEMOGRAPHICS/CLINICAL HISTORY

A 73-year-old man with metastatic prostate carcinoma, undergoing computed tomography (CT), urography, and ultrasonography.

DISCUSSION

History/Indications for Procedure
A 73-year-old man had metastatic prostate cancer. The patient developed recurrence in the prostate bed 14 years after radical prostatectomy and required long-term catheterization to treat chronic hematuria and obstructin.

Procedure
Suprapubic cystostomy catheter placement

Pre-procedure Imaging
CT urography performed 8 months before the procedure shows increased soft tissue at the bladder base, which is consistent with recurrent tumor (Fig. 1).

Intraprocedural Findings
The bladder was distended with sterile water injected into the indwelling Foley catheter (Fig. 2). The bladder was accessed with ultrasound guidance, and an 8-French pigtail catheter was placed (Figs. 3 and 4).

Follow-up and Complications
The suprapubic catheter was placed for drainage. The hematuria resolved in the days after catheter placement, and the Foley catheter was removed shortly afterward.

Suggested Readings
Lee MJ, Papanicolaou N, Nocks BN, et al: Fluoroscopically guided percutaneous suprapubic cystostomy for long-term bladder drainage: An alternative to surgical cystostomy. Radiology 188:787-789, 1993.

Papanicolaou N, Pfister RC, Nocks B: Percutaneous large-bore suprapubic cystostomy: Technique and results. AJR Am J Roentgenol 152:303-306, 1989.

Case 288   577

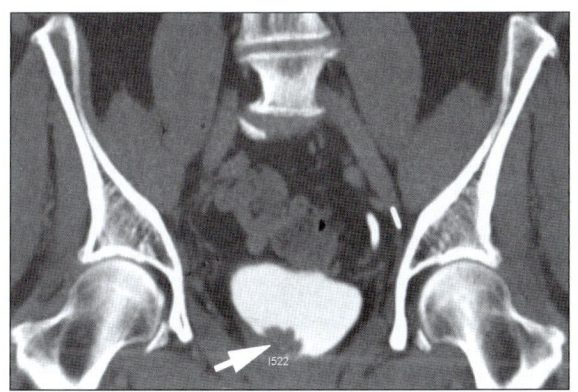

Figure 1. CT urography performed 8 months before the procedure shows a mass at the base of the bladder *(arrow)* that is consistent with prostate cancer recurrence.

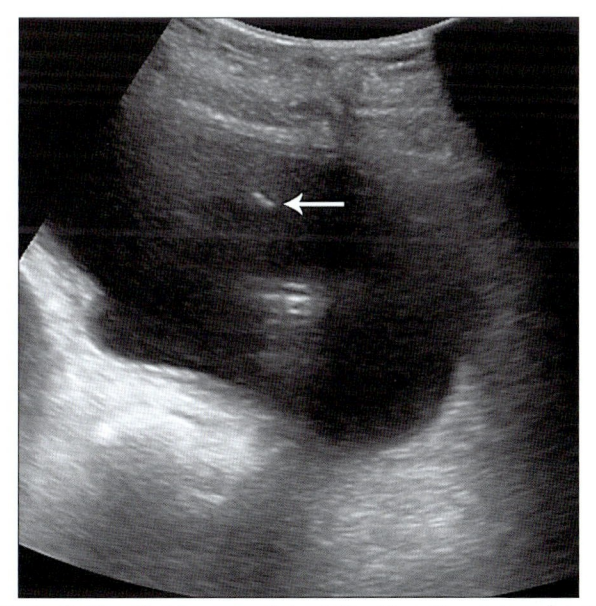

Figure 2. The bladder was distended with saline injected into the indwelling Foley catheter. Under ultrasound guidance, an 18-gauge needle was advanced into the bladder. The needle tip is visible with ultrasound *(arrow)*.

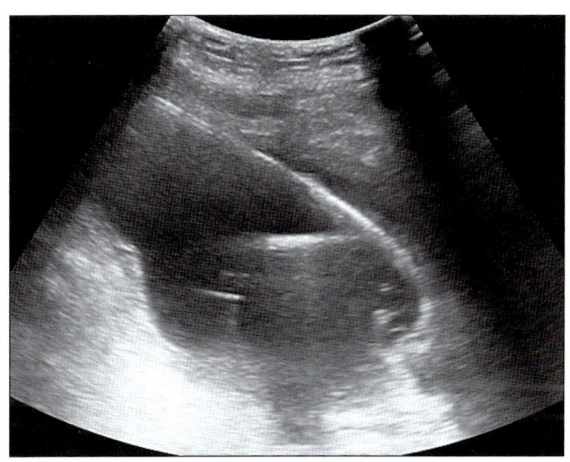

Figure 3. A 0.038-inch guidewire is coiled in the bladder.

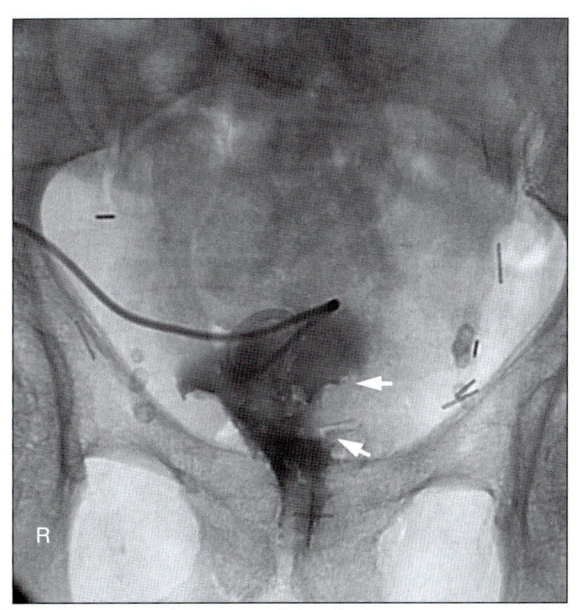

Figure 4. Cystography was performed after cystostomy catheter placement. The large mass along the left lateral wall of the bladder *(arrows)* is consistent with progression of the patient's prostate cancer.

Case 289

DEMOGRAPHICS/CLINICAL HISTORY

A 1-year-old boy with a history of esophageal atresia, undergoing balloon dilatation with fluoroscopic guidance.

DISCUSSION

History/Indications for Procedure
A 1-year-old boy has a history of esophageal atresia and has undergone a primary elongation procedure with a direct end-to-end anastomosis.

Procedure
Balloon dilatation of benign esophageal stricture

Intraprocedural Findings
A focal esophageal stricture in the region of the anastomosis (Fig. 1) was dilated with 18- and 20-mm balloons (Figs. 2 to 4).

Follow-up and Complications
The patient has returned for many additional esophageal dilatation procedures over the next 5 months. He has not returned for further intervention during the past 6 years.

Suggested Readings
Ferguson DD: Evaluation and management of benign esophageal strictures. Dis Esophagus 18:359-364, 2005.

Ko HK, Shin JH, Song HY, et al: Balloon dilatation of anastomotic strictures secondary to surgical repair of esophageal atresia in a pediatric population: Long-term results. J Vasc Intervent Radiol 17:1327-1333, 2006.

Lisý J, Hetková M, Snajdauf J, et al: Long-term outcomes of balloon dilatation of esophageal strictures in children. Acad Radiol 5:832-835, 1998.

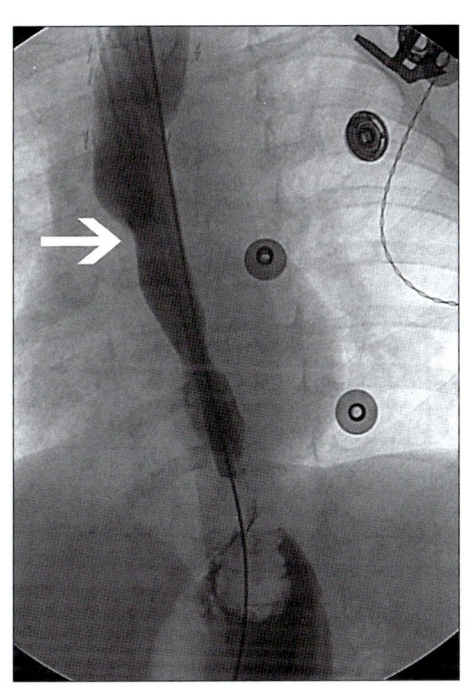

Figure 1. On the esophagram performed immediately before esophageal dilatation, there is narrowing of the middle esophagus in the region of the anastomosis *(arrow)*. Nissen fundoplication changes are evident in the gastric cardia.

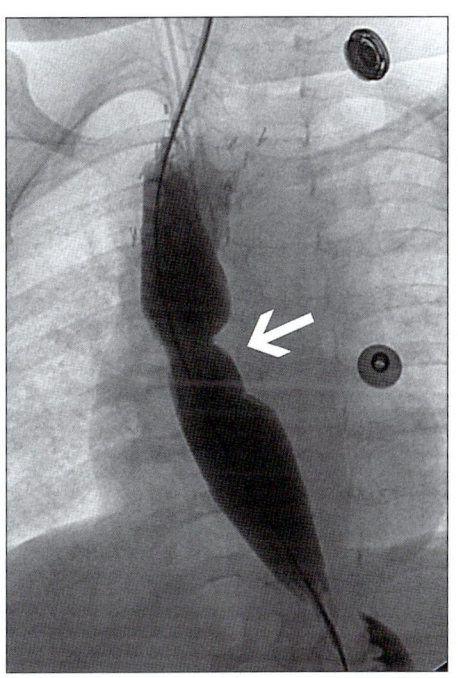

Figure 2. The mid-esophageal stricture was initially dilated with an 18-mm balloon. There is a focal waist in the balloon at the level of the stricture *(arrow)*.

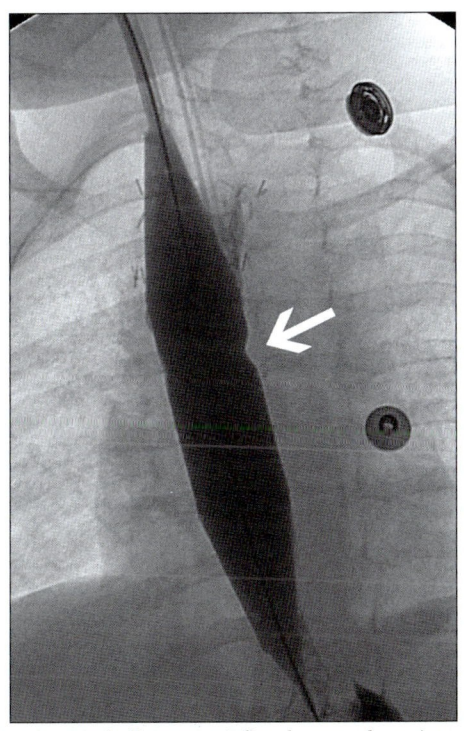

Figure 3. A 20-mm balloon was inflated across the stricture. There is a slight indentation in the balloon at the level of the stricture *(arrow)*.

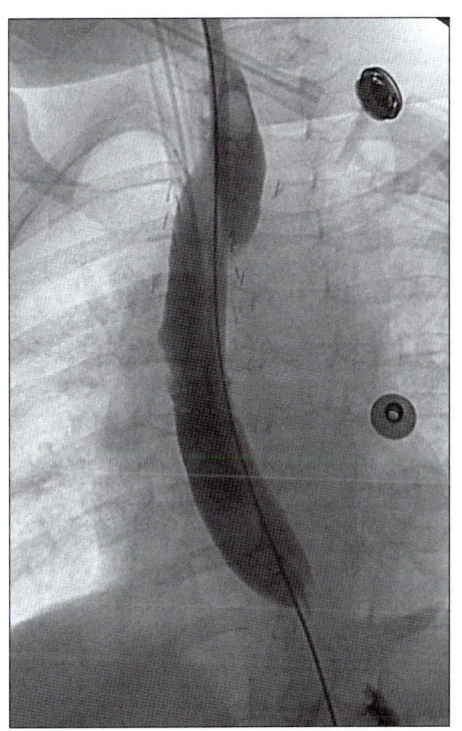

Figure 4. Follow-up esophagram after balloon dilatation shows significant improvement in the caliber of the esophagus at the level of the anastomosis.

Case 290

DEMOGRAPHICS/CLINICAL HISTORY
A 2-year-old boy with esophageal food foreign body.

DISCUSSION

History/Indications for Procedure
A 2-year-old boy with a history of surgical repair for esophageal atresia. The patient presents with an esophageal stricture and a piece of food stuck in the proximal esophagus.

Procedure
Esophageal foreign body retrieval

Pre-procedure Imaging
Barium esophagram shows dilation of the proximal esophagus and mild narrowing at the level of the surgical anastomosis. A piece of food is lodged in the esophagus just above the surgical anastomosis (Fig. 1).

Intraprocedural Findings
Under general anesthesia, a basket was advanced transorally into the proximal esophagus and used to remove the foreign body (Fig. 2); a small piece of food was retrieved. The esophageal anastomosis was dilated to 10 mm (Fig. 3).

Follow-up and Complications
Follow-up esophagram shows improved caliber of the esophagus at the surgical anastomosis (Fig. 4). Patient was able to eat without difficulty later the same day and has since returned for multiple repeat balloon dilatations.

Suggested Readings
Ko HK, Shin JH, Song HY, et al: Balloon dilation of anastomotic strictures secondary to surgical repair of esophageal atresia in a pediatric population: Long-term results. J Vasc Intervent Radiol 17:1327-1333, 2006.

Macpherson RI, Hill JG, Othersen HB, et al: Esophageal foreign bodies in children: Diagnosis, treatment, and complications. AJR Am J Roentgenol 166:919-924, 1996.

Weintraub JL, Eubig J: Balloon catheter dilatation of benign esophageal strictures in children. J Vasc Intervent Radiol 17:831-835, 2006.

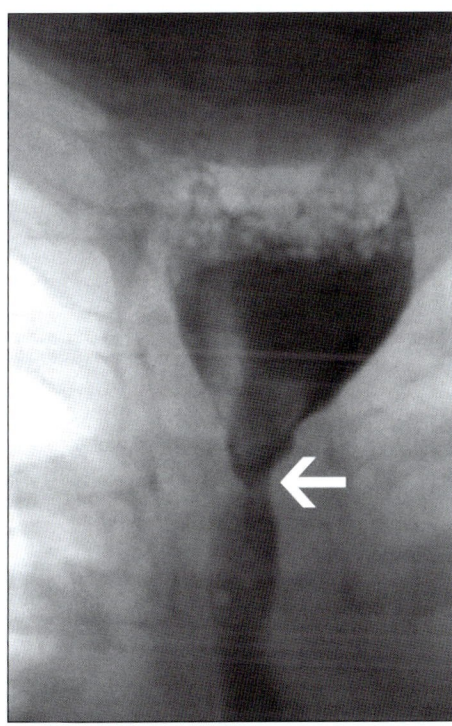

Figure 1. Barium esophagram shows a focal stricture in the proximal esophagus (arrow). There is a piece of food lodged in the esophagus at the level of the stricture.

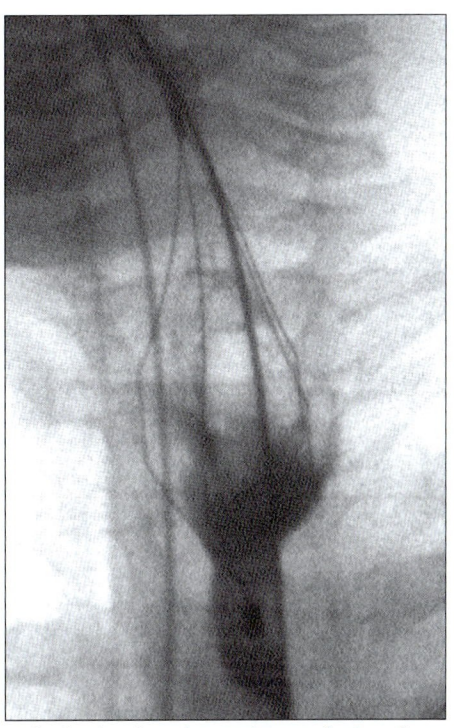

Figure 2. A basket has been inserted perorally into the esophagus and has been used to retrieve the piece of food.

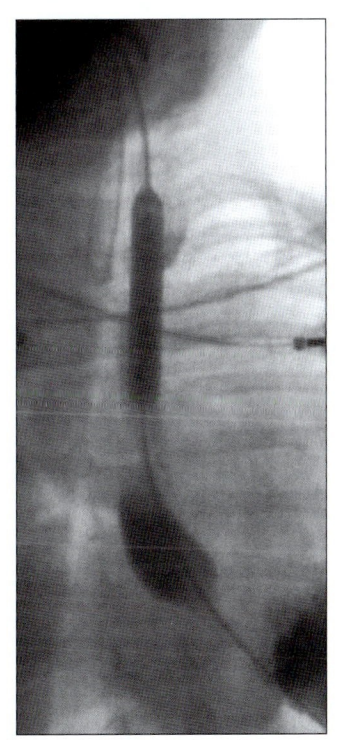

Figure 3. After foreign body extraction, the esophageal stricture is dilated using a 10-mm balloon.

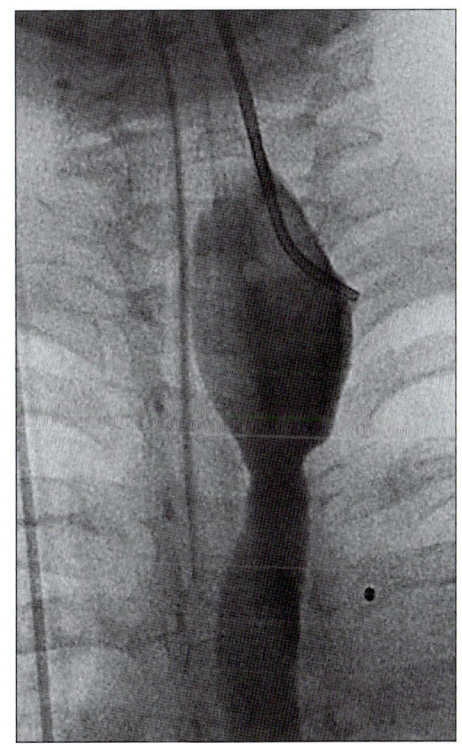

Figure 4. Final esophagram after esophageal dilatation. The piece of food has been removed, and there is only mild esophageal narrowing at the anastomosis.

Case 291

DEMOGRAPHICS/CLINICAL HISTORY

A 72-year-old man with quadriplegia from a spinal cord injury suffered after a fall.

DISCUSSION

History/Indications for Procedure

A 72-year-old man with quadriplegia from a spinal cord injury after a fall, needing a gastrostomy tube for enteral feeding.

Procedure

Percutaneous gastrostomy tube placement

Pre-procedure Imaging

Kidney-ureter-bladder (KUB) film obtained prior to gastrostomy tube placement shows the splenic flexure of the colon in the left upper quadrant, overlying the stomach (Fig. 1).

Intraprocedural Findings

The stomach was inflated with air, pushing the colon out of the way (Fig. 2). Two percutaneous t-fasteners were deployed for gastropexy (Fig. 3), and a 16-French MIC gastrostomy tube was placed through a peel-away sheath (Fig. 4).

Follow-up and Complications

The gastrostomy tube was placed to gravity drainage overnight, and the patient was able to begin tube feeds the next day without complication.

Suggested Readings

Funaki B, Peirce R. Lorenz J, et al.: Comparison of balloon- and mushroom-retained large-bore gastrostomy catheters. AJR Am J Roentgenol 177:359-362, 2001.

Kuo YC, Shlansky-Goldberg RD, Mondschein JI, et al.: Large or small bore, push or pull: A comparison of three classes of percutaneous fluoroscopic gastrostomy catheters. J Vasc Intervent Radiol 19:557-563, 2008.

Lyon SM, Pascoe DM: Percutaneous gastrostomy and gastrojejunostomy. Semin Intervent Radiol 21:181-189, 2004.

Case 291   583

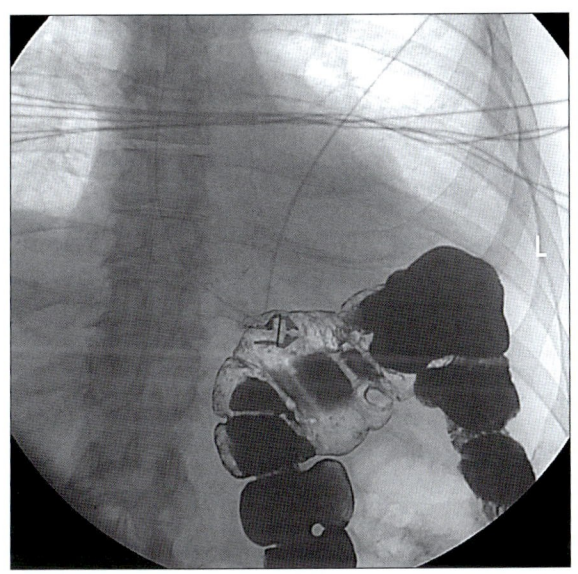

Figure 1. Fluoroscopic image obtained just prior to gastrostomy tube placement. The splenic flexure of the colon is outlined by barium administered the previous evening. The colon overlies the left upper quadrant and obscures the tip of the nasogastric tube that resides in the stomach.

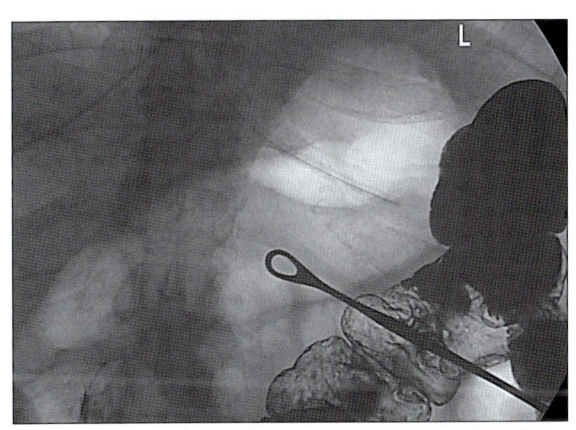

Figure 2. The stomach is inflated with air, pushing the colon out of the way.

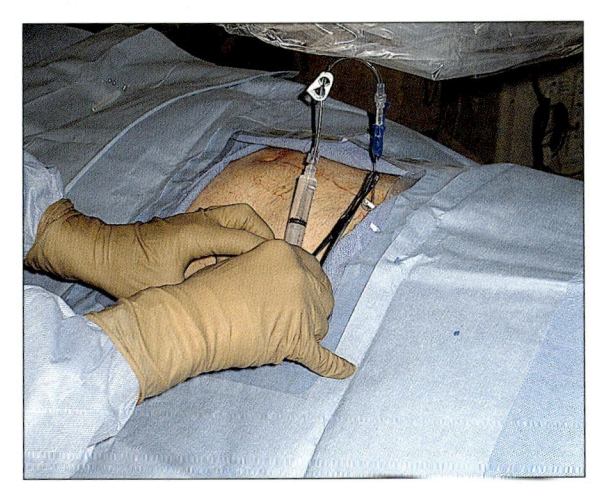

Figure 3. The t-fastener introducer needle is advanced into the stomach under fluoroscopy. Sponge forceps are used in order to avoid unnecessary radiation to the operator's hands.

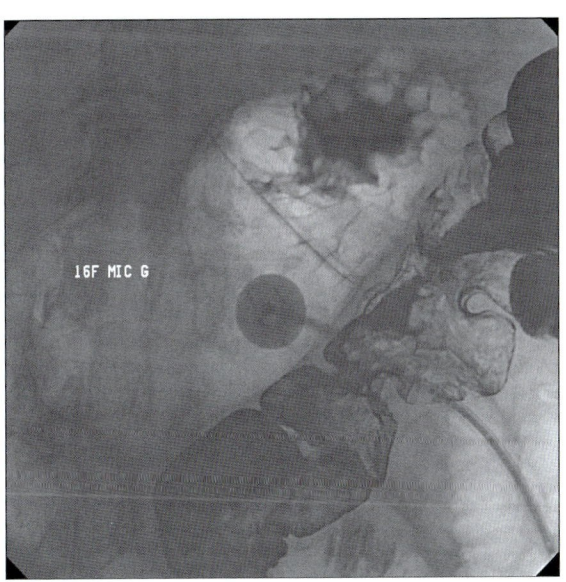

Figure 4. Final image. A 16-French MIC gastrostomy tube has been placed. Contrast injected to confirm intragastric location is pooling in the gastric fundus.

Case 292

DEMOGRAPHICS/CLINICAL HISTORY

A 61-year-old man with T3,N1,M0 squamous cell carcinoma of the supraglottis.

DISCUSSION

History/Indications for Procedure
A 61-year-old man with T3,N1,M0 squamous cell carcinoma of the supraglottis.

Procedure
Percutaneous gastrostomy tube placement

Pre-procedure Imaging
None

Intraprocedural Findings
The colon is opacified with barium given the previous evening and the stomach is insufflated with air through the nasogastric tube (Fig. 1). Two metal t-fasteners are deployed for gastropexy (Fig. 2), and a 12-French gastrostomy tube (Cook Inc, Bloomington, IN) is placed between the t-fasteners (Figs. 3,4).

Follow-up and Complications
The gastrostomy tube was placed to straight drainage for 24 hours, after which time the patient tolerated a test bolus feed and was able to begin routine use for feeding.

Suggested Readings
Kuo YC, Shlansky-Goldberg RD, Mondschein JI, et al: Large or small bore, push or pull: A comparison of three classes of percutaneous fluoroscopic gastrostomy catheters. J Vasc Intervent Radiol 19:557-563, 2008.

Lyon SM, Pascoe DM: Percutaneous gastrostomy and gastrojejunostomy. Semin Intervent Radiol 21:181-189, 2004.

O'Dowd M, Given MF, Lee MJ: New approaches to percutaneous gastrostomy. Semin Intervent Radiol 21:191-197, 2004.

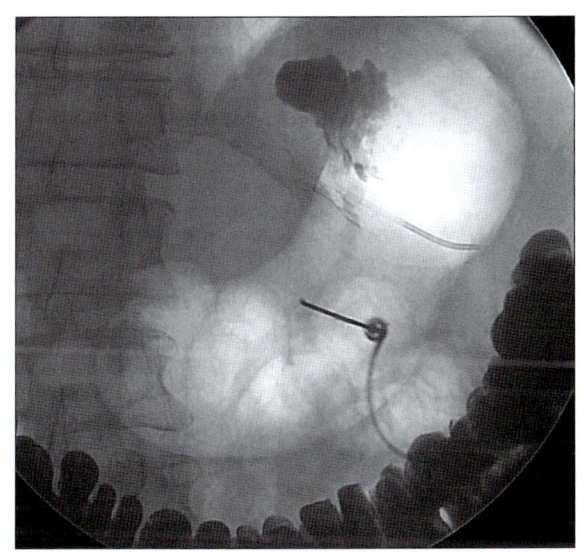

Figure 1. Fluoroscopic image during placement of the first t-fastener. The colon is well opacified with barium and out of the way. The stomach has been distended with air injected through a nasogastric tube. A small amount of contrast is seen pooling in the dependent portion of the gastric fundus, injected to confirm successful intragastric needle location prior to gastropexy.

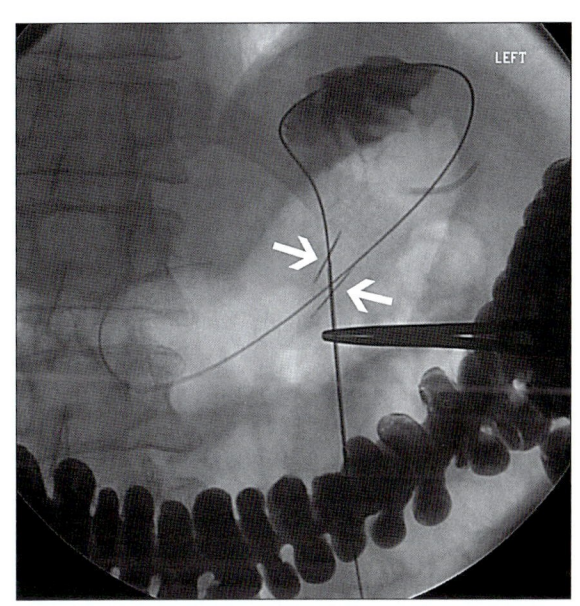

Figure 2. Two t-fasteners have been deployed, tacking the anterior wall of the stomach to the abdominal wall *(arrows)*. The gastric wall has been punctured between the t-fasteners and a wire is looped in the fundus.

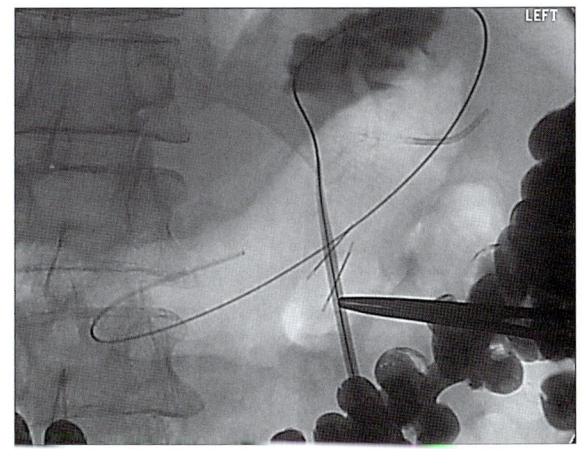

Figure 3. The tract is dilated with a 12-French dilator.

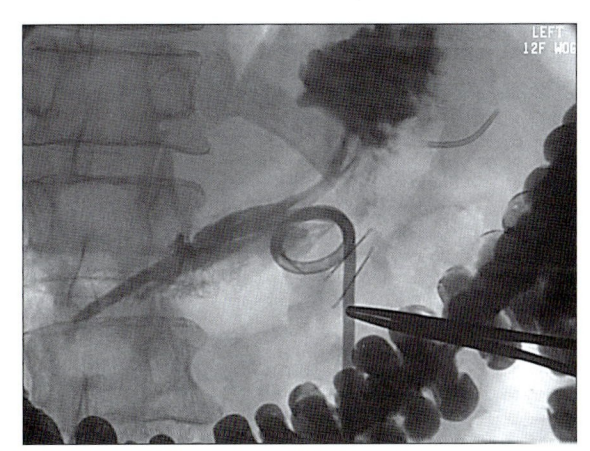

Figure 4. A 12-French Wills-Oglesby gastrostomy catheter has been placed. Additional contrast has been injected, confirming satisfactory placement.

Case 293

DEMOGRAPHICS/CLINICAL HISTORY

A 47-year-old woman with malnutrition after Roux-en-Y gastric bypass, undergoing computed tomography (CT).

DISCUSSION

History/Indications for Procedure
A 47-year-old woman had debilitating diarrhea after eating. She underwent Roux-en-Y gastric bypass at another hospital for obesity 1 year before presentation.

Procedure
CT-guided gastrostomy tube placement

Pre-procedure Imaging
A single-contrast upper gastrointestinal study showed a small gastric pouch and rapid passage through the gastrojejunal anastomosis (Fig. 1).

Intraprocedural Findings
Because of the complex anatomy, the procedure was performed with CT guidance. A 22-gauge needle was used to insufflate the gastric antrum (Fig. 2), and after tacking the stomach to the anterior abdominal wall with a percutaneous t-fastener (Fig. 3), a 12-French G-tube was placed (Fig. 4).

Follow-up and Complications
The patient was admitted to the hospital after the procedure for observation and to begin tube feedings. Tube feedings were initially started at 20 mL/hr and slowly advanced over the next 48 hours.

Suggested Readings
Lyon SM, Pascoe DM: Percutaneous gastrostomy and gastrojejunostomy. Semin Intervent Radiol 21:181-184, 2004.

O'Dowd M, Given MR, Lee MJ: New approaches to percutaneous gastrostomy. Semin Intervent Radiol 21:191-197, 2004.

Sanchez RB, vonSonnenberg E, D'Agnostino HB, et al: CT guidance for percutaneous gastrostomy and gastroenterostomy. Radiology 184:201-205, 1992.

Case 293   587

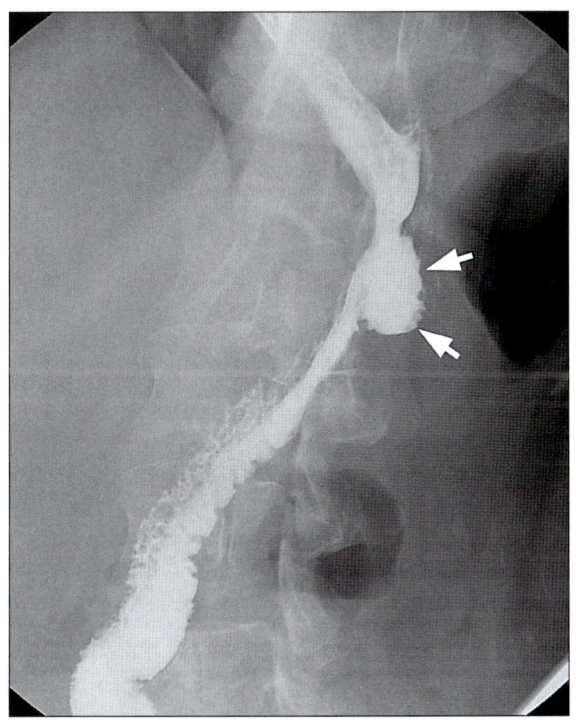

Figure 1. Single image from an upper gastrointestinal examination shows filling of the small gastric remnant (arrows). Contrast passed quickly across the gastrojejunal anastomosis into the small bowel.

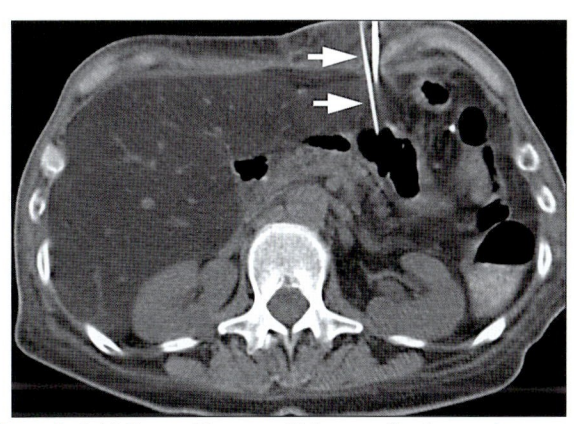

Figure 2. Initially, a 22-gauge Chiba needle (arrows) was advanced into the gastric antrum and used to insufflate the stomach with air.

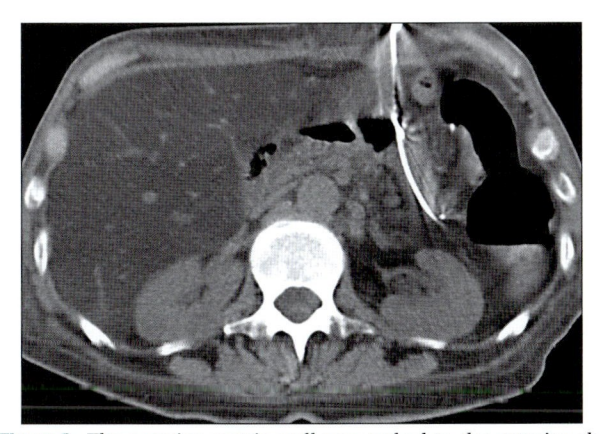

Figure 3. The anterior gastric wall was tacked to the anterior abdominal wall with a percutaneous t-fastener. The fastener was deployed by passing a guidewire through the delivery needle.

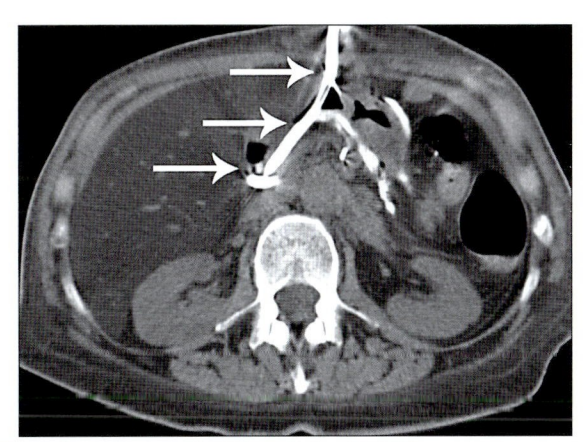

Figure 4. A 12-French Wills-Oglesby (WOGS) gastrostomy tube has been placed (arrows).

Case 294

DEMOGRAPHICS/CLINICAL HISTORY

A 68-year-old woman with necrotizing pancreatitis.

DISCUSSION

History/Indications for Procedure
A 68-year-old woman with necrotizing pancreatitis. A gastrostomy tube placed at an outside hospital appears to be extraluminal.

Procedure
Gastrojejunostomy tube placement

Pre-procedure Imaging
Contrast-enhanced CT of the abdomen shows a percutaneous gastrostomy tube positioned against the anterior gastric wall (Fig. 1).

Intraprocedural Findings
The existing gastrostomy tube was removed, and the proximal jejunum was catheterized using a 5-French angle-tipped catheter and guidewire (Fig. 2). A 22-French peel-away sheath was placed, through which an 18-French MIC gastrojejunostomy tube was advanced (Fig. 3).

Follow-up and Complications
Once the gastrojejunostomy tube was placed, tube feedings commenced without complication. CT scan obtained following tube placement to evaluate the pancreatic disease shows the gastrojejunostomy tube in appropriate position (Fig. 4).

Suggested Readings
Kerns SR. Coversion of gastrostomy tube to gastrojejunostomy tube by using a peel-away sheath. AJR Am J Roentgenol 160:206-207, 1993.

Lyon SM, Pascoe DM: Percutaneous gastrostomy and gastrojejunostmy. Semin Intervent Radiol 21:181-189, 2004.

Shin KH, Shin JH, Song HY, et al: Primary and conversion percutaneous gastrojejunostomy under fluoroscopic guidance: 10 years of experience. Clin Imaging 32:274-279, 2008.

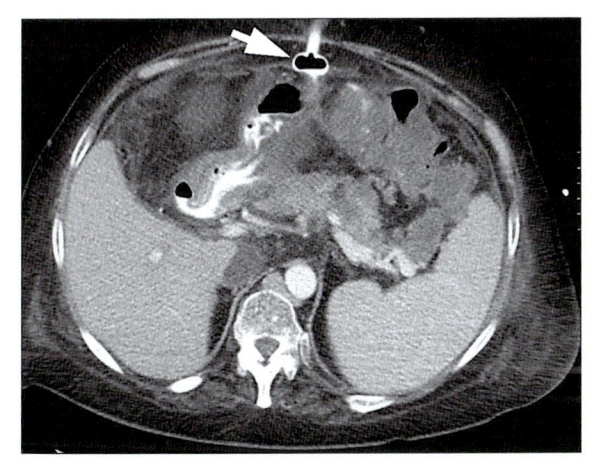

Figure 1. Contrast-enhanced CT shows the gastrostomy tube to reside outside the lumen of the stomach (*arrow*).

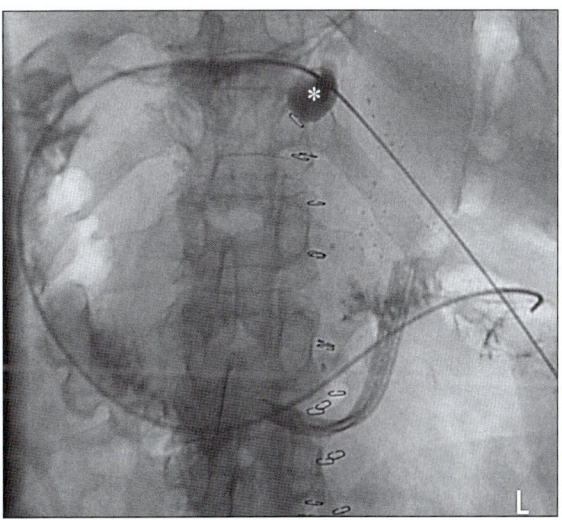

Figure 2. The gastrostomy tube was removed and the proximal jejunum was selectively catheterized (*asterisk* indicates contrast pooling in space previously occupied by the gastrostomy tube).

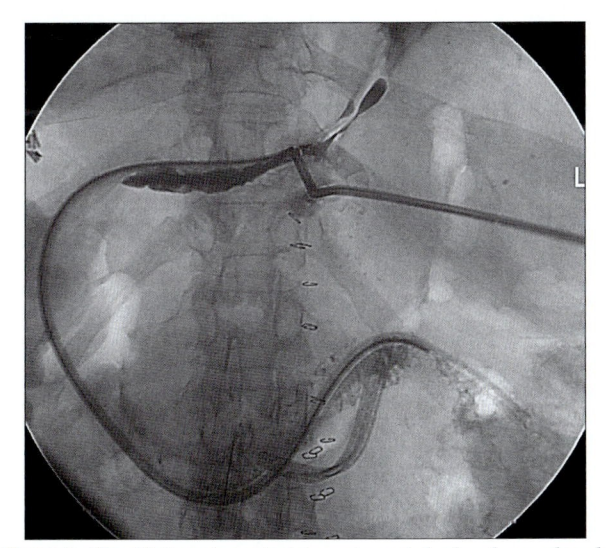

Figure 3. The 10-French gastrojejunostomy tube has been placed, and contrast injected through each lumen, confirming proper tube position.

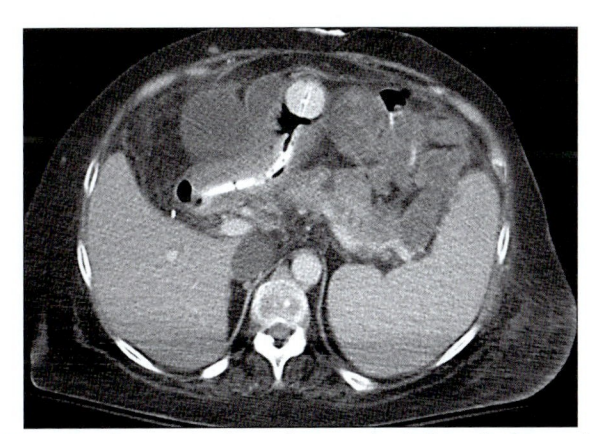

Figure 4. Follow-up CT shows the retention balloon in the gastric lumen, opposed to the anterior gastric wall. In this image, the tube is seen coursing into the duodenum.

Case 295

DEMOGRAPHICS/CLINICAL HISTORY

A 67-year-old man with pancreatic carcinoma obstructing the duodenum, undergoing computed tomography (CT) and stent placement.

DISCUSSION

History/Indications for Procedure
A 67-year-old man has a mass in the pancreatic head that is compressing the second portion of the duodenum, resulting in gastroduodenal outlet obstruction.

Procedure
Gastroduodenal outlet obstruction

Pre-procedure Imaging
Contrast-enhanced CT demonstrates a 5-cm × 6-cm mass in the pancreatic head that is compressing the second portion of the duodenum. There is marked distention of the stomach and proximal duodenum (Fig. 1).

Intraprocedural Findings
A 3- to 4-cm stricture was identified in the second portion of the duodenum that was thought to represent local invasion of the pancreatic mass. The stricture was stented with a 22-mm × 90-mm Wallstent (Fig. 2).

Follow-up and Complications
Unenhanced CT scan performed the day after the duodenal stent was placed shows decompression of the stomach, and a small amount of free air is visible adjacent to the stent (Fig. 3), suggesting a small perforation. No further intervention was required, and the patient was discharged to a skilled nursing facility for palliative care.

Suggested Readings
Dormann A, Meisner S, Verin N, et al: Self-expanding metal stents for gastroduodenal malignancies: Systematic review of their clinical effectiveness. Endoscopy 36:543-550, 2004.

Lopera JE, Brazzini A, Gonzales A, et al: Gastroduodenal stent placement: Current status. Radiographics 24:1561-1573, 2004.

Mauro MA, Koehler RE, Baron TH: Advances in gastrointestinal interventions: The treatment of gastroduodenal and colorectal obstructions with metallic stent. Radiology 215:659-669, 2000.

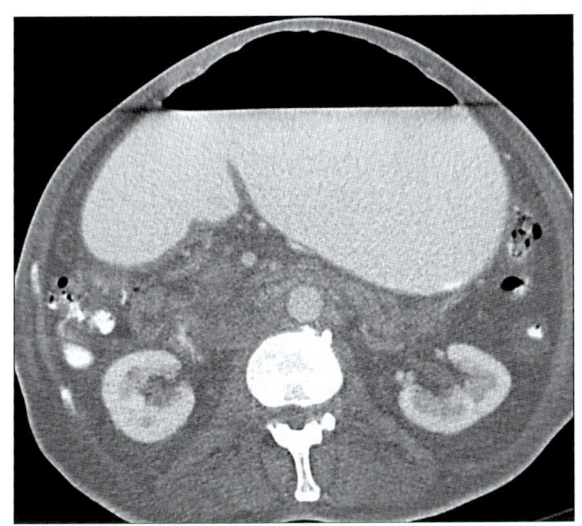

Figure 1. Contrast-enhanced CT through the upper abdomen demonstrates marked gastric distention.

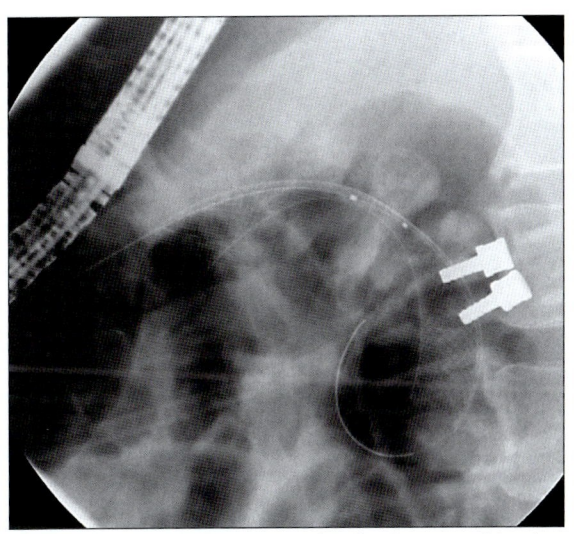

Figure 2. A 22-mm Wallstent was placed using a combination of endoscopic and fluoroscopic guidance.

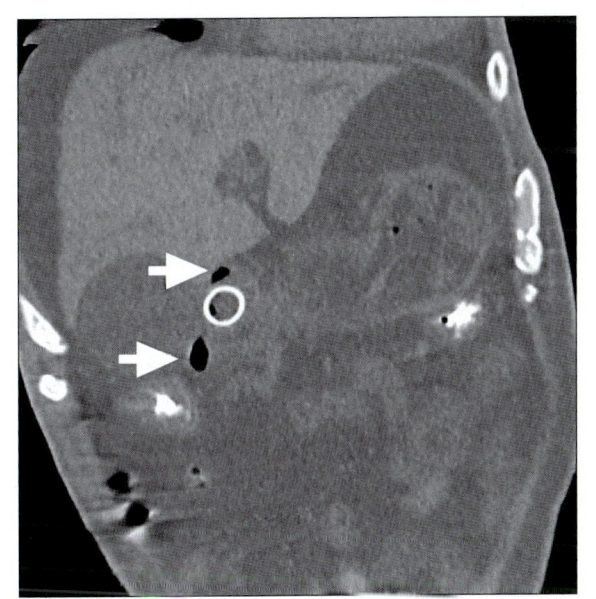

Figure 3. Coronal reconstruction from unenhanced CT performed the day after duodenal stent placement shows that there has been interval decompression of the stomach. Two small air lucencies are seen adjacent to the stent *(arrows)*, suggesting a small perforation.

Case 296

DEMOGRAPHICS/CLINICAL HISTORY

A 67-year-old man with necrotizing pancreatitis.

DISCUSSION

History/Indications for Procedure
A 67-year-old man with necrotizing pancreatitis.

Procedure
Percutaneous management of pancreatic pseudocyst

Pre-procedure Imaging
Endoscopic retrograde cholangiopancreatography (ERCP) shows multiple areas of disruption of the pancreatic duct (not shown). CT of the abdomen shows an 8-cm x 18-cm collection anterior to the body of the pancreas (Fig. 1).

Intraprocedural Findings
Using CT-guidance, an 18-gauge needle was placed into the collection from an anterior approach. A 10-French drain was placed (Fig. 2).

Follow-up and Complications
The patient returned for a follow-up drain study 2 weeks later, at which time no fistula to the pancreatic duct was identified (Fig. 3). The drain remained in place for several months, with eventual resolution of the fluid collection, but there was persistent high drain output because of fistulous connection with the pancreatic duct (Fig. 4).

Suggested Readings
Freeny PC, Hauptmann E, Althaus SJ, et al.: Percutaneous CT-guided drainage of infected acute necrotizing pancreatitis: Techniques and results. AJR Am J Roentgenol 170:969-975, 1998.

Segal D, Mortele KJ, Banks PA, Silverman SG: Acute necrotizing pancreatitis: Role of CT-guided percutaneous catheter drainage. Abdom Imaging 32:351-361, 2007.

Shankar S, vanSonnenberg E, Silverman SG, et al.: Imaging and percutaneous management of acute complicated pancreatitis. Cardiovasc Intervent Radiol 27:567-580, 2004.

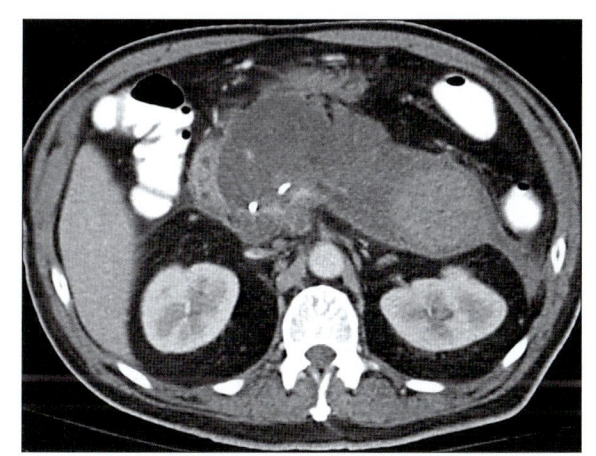

Figure 1. CT of the abdomen shows a large heterogeneous fluid collection anterior to the pancreas.

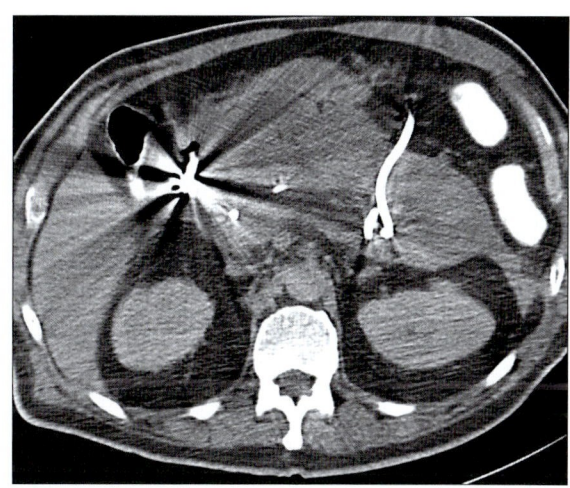

Figure 2. A 10-French drain was placed into the collection with CT guidance.

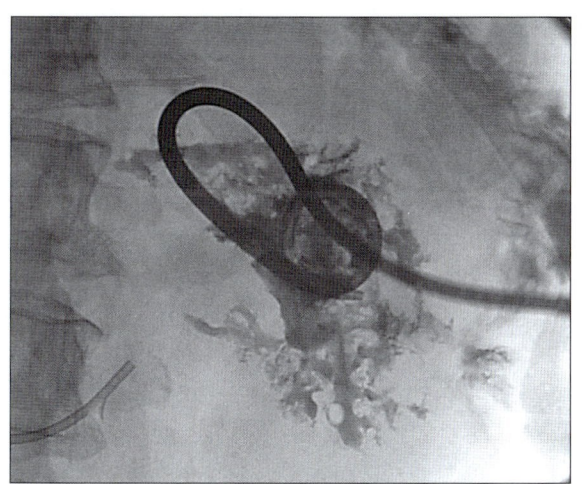

Figure 3. Follow-up drain study 2 weeks after placement. There is a large cavity with debris. The drain was upsized to 14 French. No fistula to the pancreatic duct was seen.

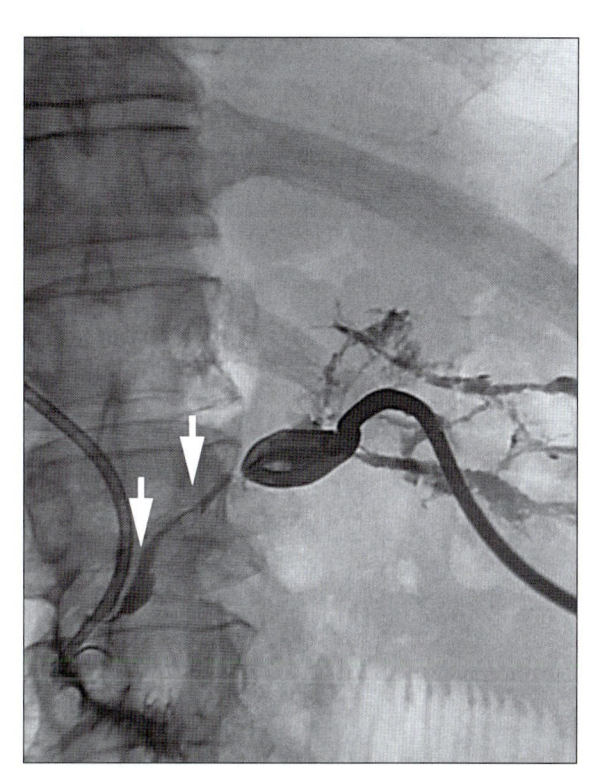

Figure 4. Follow-up drain study. The cavity has nearly completely resolved, but the patient continued to have large output from the drain. There is a fistula to the pancreatic duct *(arrows)* visualized.

Case 297

DEMOGRAPHICS/CLINICAL HISTORY

A 33-year-old woman with a history of pancreatitis during a hospitalization after a complicated post–cesarean section course, undergoing computed tomography (CT), endoscopic retrograde choledochopancreatography (ERCP), and stent placement.

DISCUSSION

History/Indications for Procedure
A 33-year-old woman developed pancreatitis while recovering in the hospital from a complicated post–cesarean section course.

Procedure
Pancreatic pseudocyst management

Pre-procedure Imaging
Contrast-enhanced CT scan demonstrates a large, rim-enhancing fluid collection in the left retroperitoneum (Fig. 1). The collection is adjacent to the tail of the pancreas, and the pancreatic duct is mildly dilated.

Intraprocedural Findings
The collection was percutaneously drained, and the drain was progressively upsized to a 20-French drain because of intracavitary debris clogging the catheter. ERCP demonstrated extravasation of contrast from the distal pancreatic duct (Fig. 2), and a pancreatic duct stent was placed (Fig. 3).

Follow-up and Complications
After placement of the pancreatic duct stent, the output from the drainage catheter became minimal, and the drain was removed (Fig. 4). Follow-up ERCP demonstrated that the pancreatic duct leak has healed, allowing removal of the pancreatic duct stent.

Suggested Readings
Balthazar EJ, Freeny PC, vanSonnenberg E: Imaging and intervention in acute pancreatitis. Radiology 193:297-306, 1994.

Freeny PC, Lewis GP, Traverso LW, Ryan JA: Infected pancreatic fluid collections: Percutaneous catheter drainage. Radiology 167:435-441, 1988.

Karlson B, Martin EC, Fankuchen EI, et al: Percutaneous drainage of pancreatic pseudocysts and abscesses. Radiology 142:619-624, 1984.

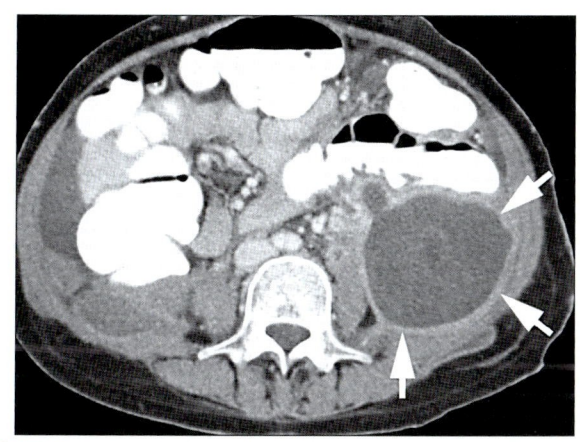

Figure 1. Contrast-enhanced CT demonstrates a hypodense fluid collection in the left lower quadrant *(arrows)* adjacent to the pancreatic tail.

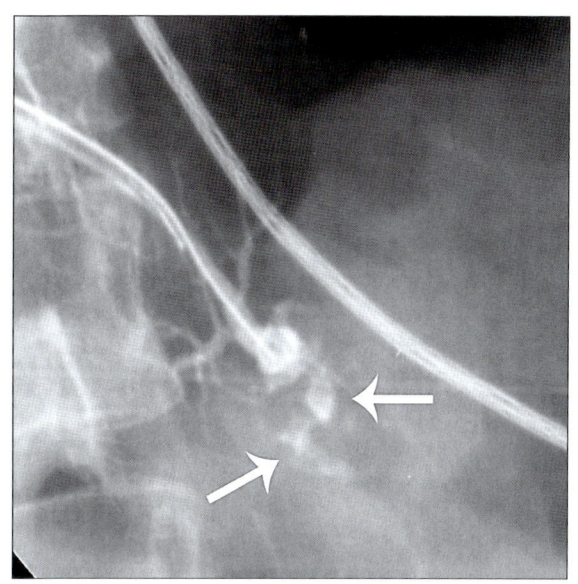

Figure 2. Selected image from ERCP demonstrates extravasation of contrast *(arrows)* from the distal pancreatic duct.

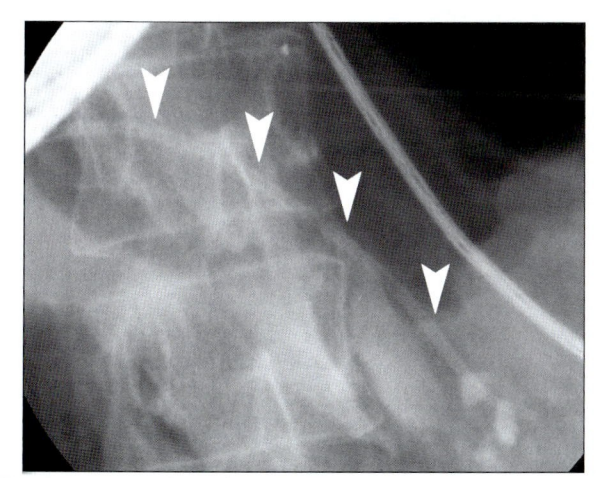

Figure 3. A stent *(arrowheads)* was placed in the pancreatic duct endoscopically.

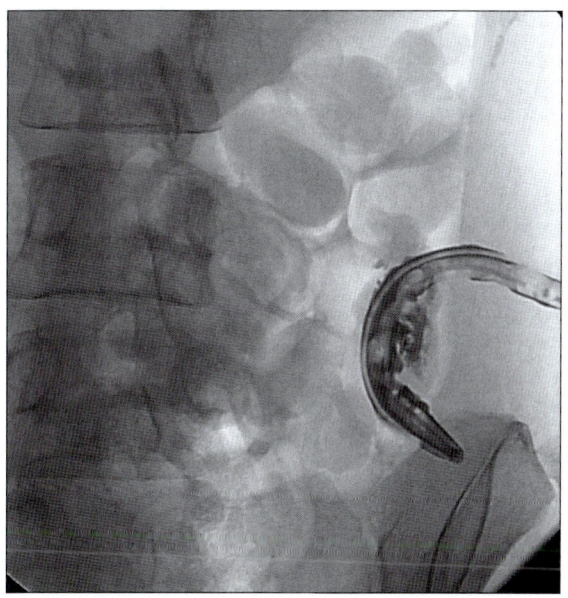

Figure 4. Follow-up catheter injection after pancreatic duct stent placement demonstrates no residual cavity or communication with the pancreatic duct. The drainage catheter was removed.

Case 298

DEMOGRAPHICS/CLINICAL HISTORY

A 49-year-old man with a history of pneumonia and loculated pleural fluid collection, undergoing computed tomography (CT).

DISCUSSION

History/Indications for Procedure
A 49-year-old man has a history of pneumonia and a loculated pleural fluid collection. The patient has had persistent cough and fevers despite antibiotic therapy.

Procedure
Empyema drainage

Pre-procedure Imaging
CT of the chest shows a loculated pleural fluid collection in the anterior left hemithorax that is 7.5 cm × 4.2 cm (Fig. 1). This collection does have associated thick pleural enhancement and contains small foci of air, findings suggesting empyema.

Intraprocedural Findings
Using CT guidance, an 8-French pigtail chest tube was placed into the empyema (Figs. 2 and 3), allowing aspiration of 20 mL of purulent fluid.

Follow-up and Complications
The patient was continued on antibiotics, and follow-up chest CT performed 4 days later showed complete drainage of the empyema (Fig. 4). The chest tube was removed, and the patient was discharged from the hospital to complete a 4-week course of antibiotics at home.

Suggested Readings
Moulton JS, Benkert RE, Weisiger KH, Chambers JA: Treatment of complicated pleural fluid collections with image-guided drainage and intracavitary urokinase. Chest 108:1252-1259, 1995.

vanSonnenberg E, Ferrucci JT Jr, Mueller PR, et al: Percutaneous drainage of abscesses and fluid collections: Technique, results, and applications. Radiology 142:1-10, 1982.

Wells RG, Havens PL: Intrapleural fibrinolysis for parapneumonic effusion and empyema in children. Radiology 228:370-378, 2003.

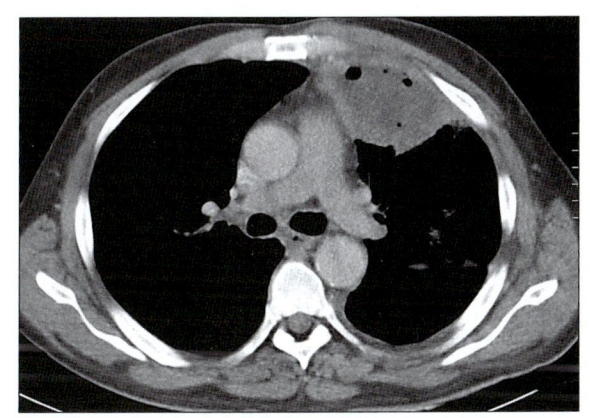

Figure 1. Single image from a contrast-enhanced CT study of the chest shows an enhancing, loculated pleural fluid collection in the anterior left hemithorax. The collection contains small locules of air, suggesting underlying infection.

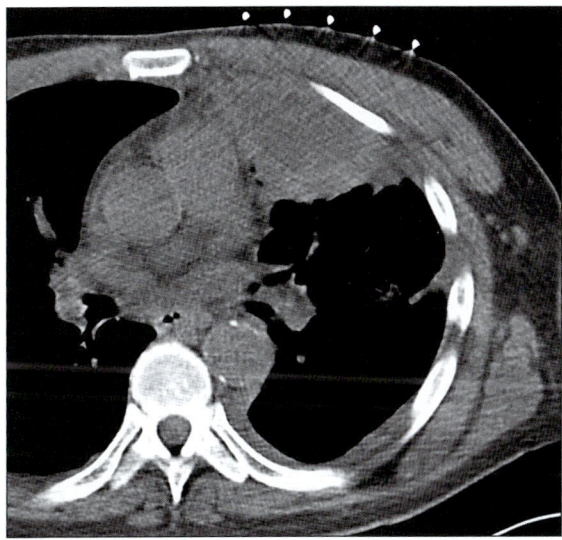

Figure 2. Image obtained during CT-guided chest tube placement shows localizing markers that were placed over the collection.

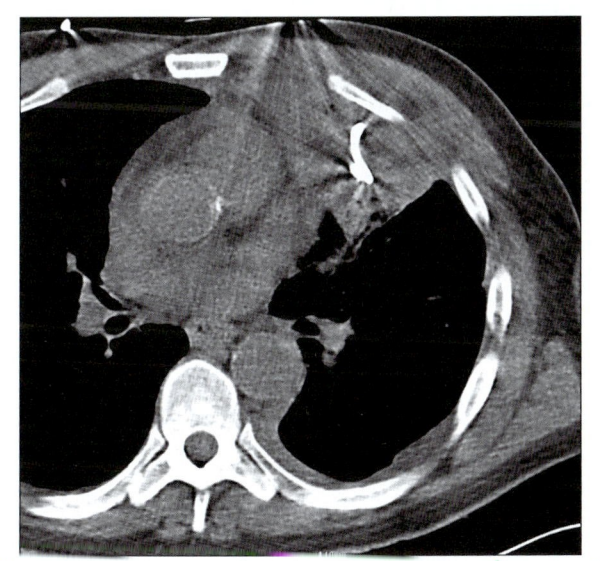

Figure 3. A pigtail chest tube has been placed within the center of the collection.

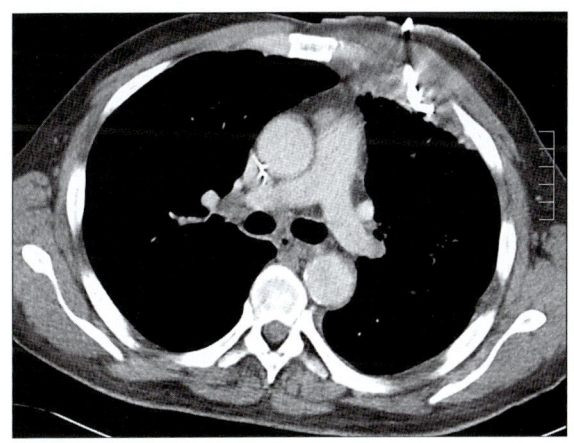

Figure 4. Chest CT scan performed 4 days after chest tube placement shows complete drainage of the empyema.

Case 299

DEMOGRAPHICS/CLINICAL HISTORY

A 57-year-old woman with a 5-day history of cough and fever.

DISCUSSION

History/Indications for Procedure
A 57-year-old woman with a 5-day history of cough and fever. Laboratory analysis shows leukocytosis.

Procedure
CT-guided empyema drainage

Pre-procedure Imaging
Chest radiograph shows right lower lobe consolidation with adjacent pleural fluid (Fig. 1). Chest CT shows dense consolidation in the right lower lobe with an adjacent loculated pleural fluid collection that has an enhancing wall (Fig. 2).

Intraprocedural Findings
The patient was placed prone on the CT table, a skin site was localized, and an 18-gauge needle was advanced into the empyema using intermittent CT guidance. After a sample of pus was aspirated, an 8-French pigtail chest tube was placed (Fig. 3).

Follow-up and Complications
The chest tube drained a total of 930 mL of fluid over the ensuing 5 days. Follow-up chest CT shows resolution of the empyema (Fig. 4). The chest tube was removed.

Suggested Readings
Akhan O, Ozkan O, Akinci D, et al: Image-guided catheter drainage of infected pleural effusions. Diagn Intervent Radiol 13:204-209, 2007.

Keeling AN, Leong S, Logan PM, et al: Empyema and effusion: Outcome of image-guided small-bore catheter drainage. Cardiovasc Intervent Radiol 31:135-141, 2008.

Moulton JS: Image-guided management of complicated pleural fluid collections. Radiol Clin North Am 38:345-374, 2000.

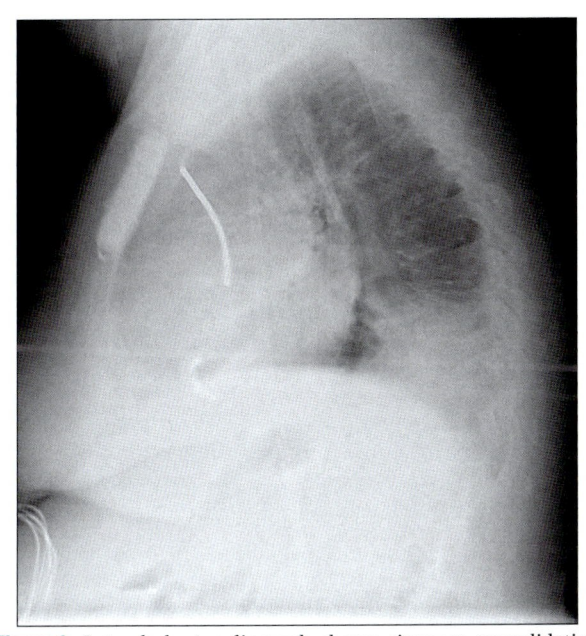

Figure 1. Lateral chest radiograph shows air-space consolidation in the right lower lobe.

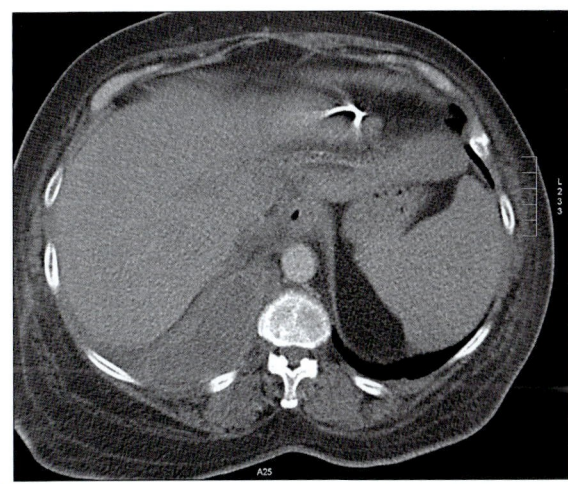

Figure 2. Contrast-enhanced CT shows a loculated right pleural fluid collection with an enhancing wall. The findings are consistent with an empyema.

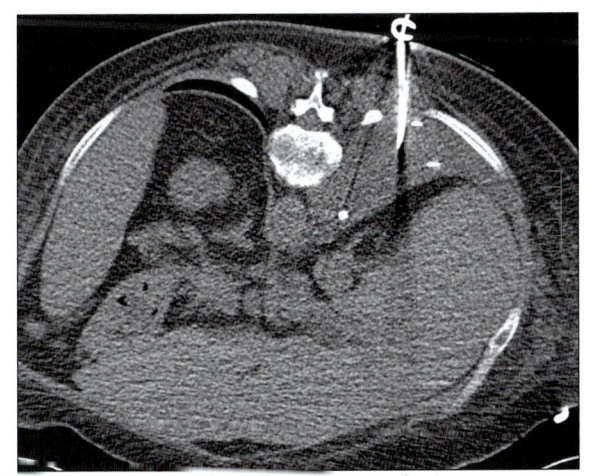

Figure 3. With the patient prone, an 8-French pigtail chest tube is placed using CT guidance.

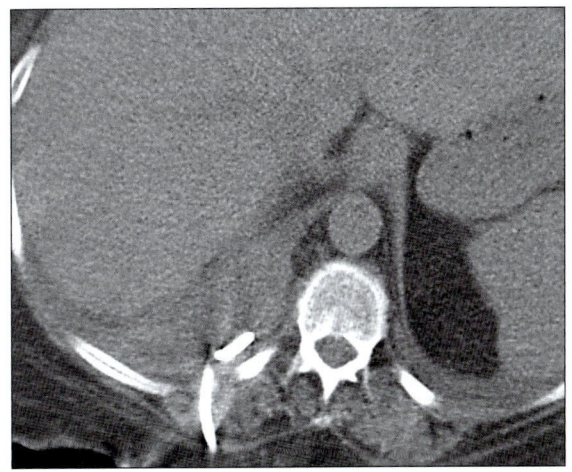

Figure 4. Follow-up unenhanced chest CT shows resolution of the empyema. There is persistent dense consolidation of the right lower lobe.

Case 300

DEMOGRAPHICS/CLINICAL HISTORY

A 38-year-old man with right upper quadrant abdominal pain and fever.

DISCUSSION

History/Indications for Procedure
A 38-year-old man with an 8-day history of right upper quadrant abdominal pain and fever. He reports a loss of appetite and 15-lb weight loss over this time period.

Procedure
Ultrasound-guided drainage of hepatic abscess

Pre-procedure Imaging
Contrast-enhanced MRI shows a 10- × 9- × 10-cm complex fluid collection in the posterior right hepatic lobe (Fig. 1). The collection has decreased T1 signal, heterogeneous T2 signal, and peripheral rim enhancement.

Intraprocedural Findings
There is a heterogeneous mass in the posterior right hepatic lobe on ultrasound (Fig. 2). Using ultrasound guidance, an 18-gauge needle was advanced into the abscess and pus was aspirated; a 10-French drain was placed (Figs. 3 and 4).

Follow-up and Complications
The drainage catheter remained in place for 4 weeks. At that time, the abscess cavity was resolved and there was minimal drainage from the catheter; the catheter was removed.

Suggested Readings
Ferraioli G, Garlaschelli A, Zanaboni D, et al: Percutaneous and surgical treatment of pyogenic liver abscesses: Observation over a 21-year period in 148 patients. Dig Liver Dis 40:690-696, 2008.

Rajak CL, Gupta S, Jain S, et al: Percutaneous treatment of liver abscesses: Needle aspiration versus catheter drainage. AJR Am J Roentgenol 170:1035-1039, 1998.

Zerem E, Hadzic A: Sonographically guided percutaneous catheter drainage versus needle aspiration in the management of pyogenic liver abscess. AJR Am J Roentgenol 189:W138-W142, 2007.

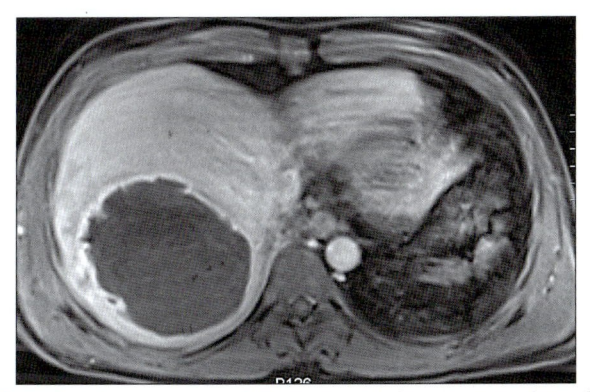

Figure 1. T1, post-contrast MR image with fat saturation through the liver shows a large low-signal mass with peripheral rim enhancement.

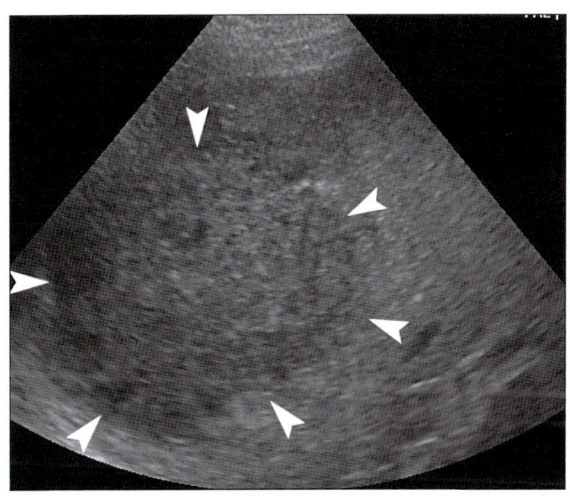

Figure 2. Ultrasound image obtained at the time of drainage shows a heterogeneous, slightly hyperechoic mass in the posterior right hepatic lobe (arrowheads).

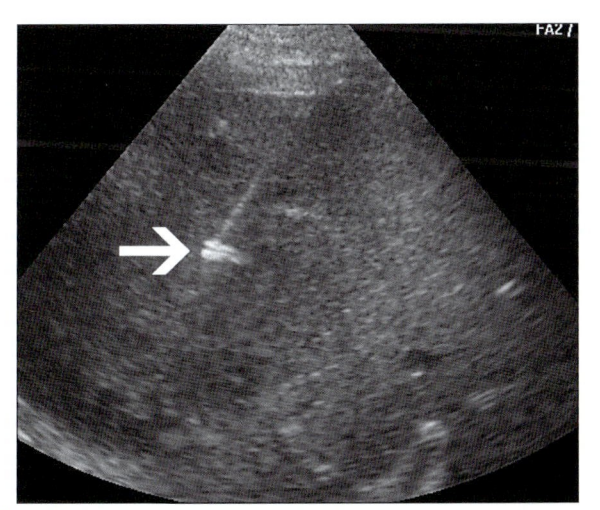

Figure 3. Ultrasound image showing the placement of an 18-gauge needle (arrow) into the collection.

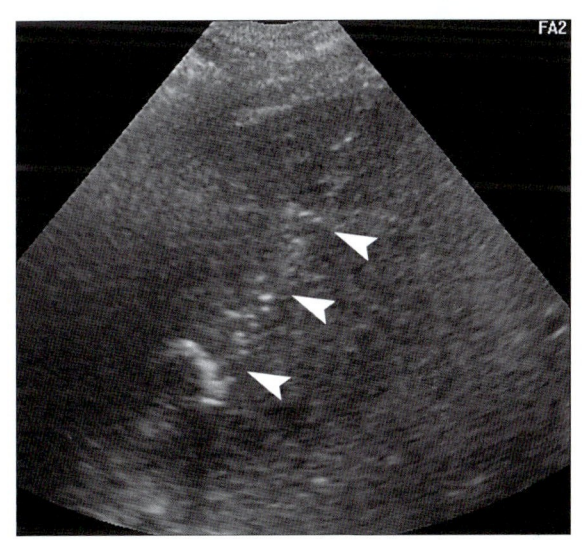

Figure 4. A 10-French pigtail drainage catheter (arrowheads) has been placed into the abscess.

Case 301

DEMOGRAPHICS/CLINICAL HISTORY

A 30-year-old woman status post-hysterectomy for endometriosis, undergoing CT and fluoroscopy.

DISCUSSION

History/Indications for Procedure
At the same time this patient underwent the hysterectomy, an endometrial implant was resected from the anterior rectal wall. On postoperative day 3, the patient developed a fever and elevated white blood cell count.

Procedure
Transvaginal abscess drain

Pre-procedure Imaging
Contrast-enhanced CT scan shows an extraluminal collection of gas and fluid just anterior to the rectum and superior to the vaginal cuff (Fig. 1).

Intraprocedural Findings
The fluid collection was identified using a transvaginal ultrasound probe (Fig. 2). The collection was accessed using an 18-gauge needle via a transvaginal approach; an 8-French drainage catheter was placed under fluoroscopy (Fig. 3).

Follow-up and Complications
The patient returned for follow-up drain study 3 days after the drain was placed (Fig. 4). A fistula to the anterior rectal wall was identified; the drain was left in place until the fistula closed.

Suggested Readings
American College of Radiology (ACR): Percutaneous catheter drainage of infected intra-abdominal fluid collections. ACR Appropriateness Criteria. Radiology 215:(Suppl), 2000.

VanDerKolk HL: Small, deep pelvic abscesses: Definition and drainage guided with an endovaginal probe. Radiology 181:283-284, 1991.

vanSonnenberg E, Mueller PR, Ferrucci JT Jr: Percutaneous drainage of 250 abdominal abscesses and fluid collections, part I: Results, failures, and complications. Radiology 151:337-341, 1984.

Case 301   603

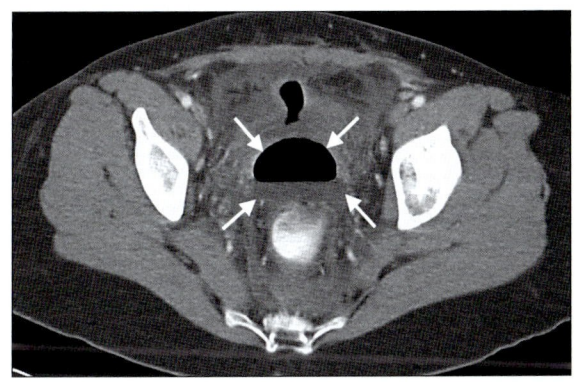

Figure 1. Image from pelvic CT scan shows an extraluminal collection of gas and fluid (arrows) anterior to the rectum.

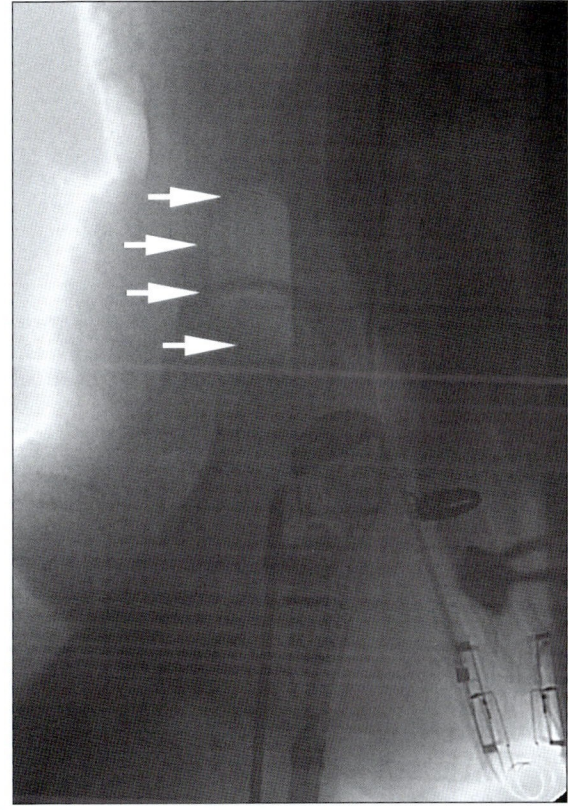

Figure 2. Spot fluoroscopic image shows the endovaginal probe with needle guide in place. The gas within the collection is visible fluoroscopically (arrows).

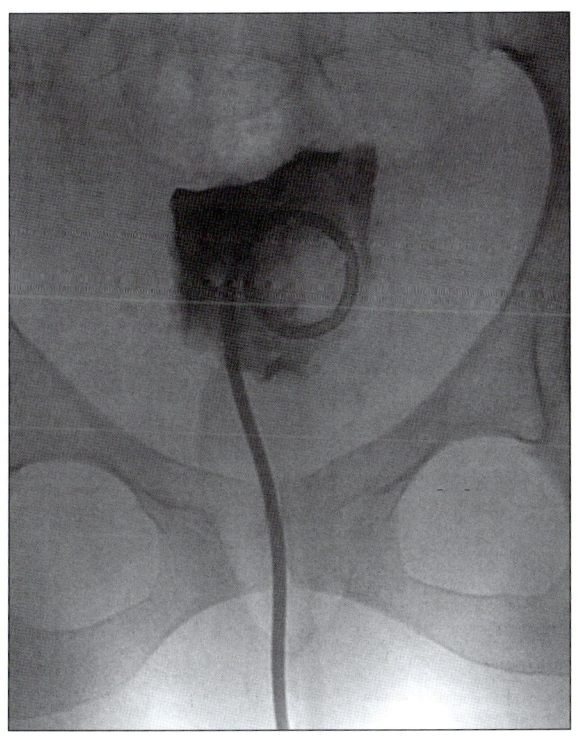

Figure 3. Spot fluoroscopic image after drain has been placed. A small amount of contrast agent has been injected into the cavity.

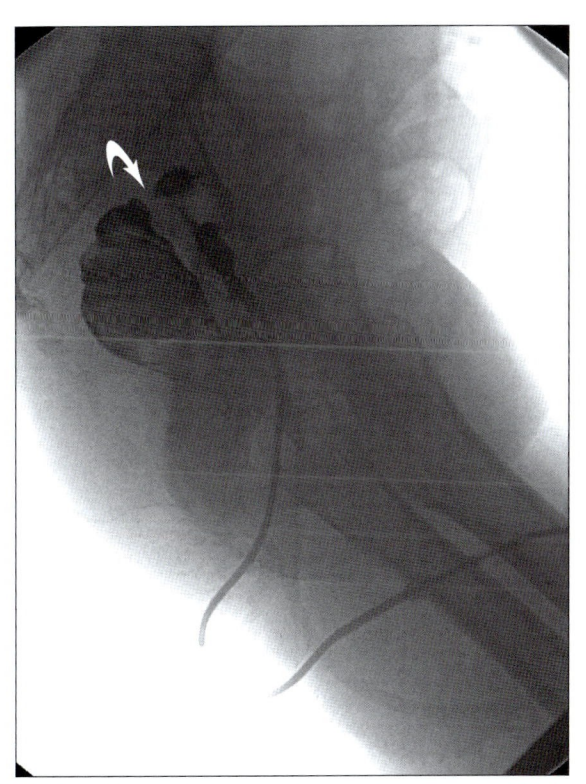

Figure 4. Follow-up drain study 3 days after placement shows a fistula to the rectum (arrow).

Case 302

DEMOGRAPHICS/CLINICAL HISTORY

A 74-year-old man with ulcerative colitis and pelvic fluid collection following proctocolectomy.

DISCUSSION

A 74-year-old man who underwent proctocolectomy with J-pouch anal anastomosis for dysplasia secondary to long-standing ulcerative colitis. On postoperative day 7, the patient developed an elevated white blood cell count.

Procedure
CT-guided abscess drainage

Pre-procedure Imaging
Contrast-enhanced CT of the pelvis shows a small, perianastomotic abscess (Fig. 1). The abscess contains some bowel contrast, suggesting an anastomotic leak.

Intraprocedural Findings
The patient was placed in a left-lateral decubitus position, and the leak was identified through the administration of rectal contrast. An 18-gauge needle was used to access the fluid collection from a right transgluteal approach (Fig. 2), and an 8-French pigtail drain was placed (Fig. 3).

Follow-up and Complications
The drainage catheter was left in place for 2 weeks. Follow-up drain study shows resolution of the abscess cavity and closure of the anastomotic leak (Fig. 4); the drain was removed.

Suggested Readings
Harisinghani MG, Gervais DA, Hahn PF, et al: CT-guided transgluteal drainage of deep pelvic abscesses: Indications, technique, procedure-related complications, and clinical outcomes. Radiographics 22:1353-1367, 2002.

Maher MM, Gervais DA, Kalra MK, et al: The inaccessible or undrainable abscess: How to drain it. Radiographics 24:717-735, 2004.

vanSonnenberg E, Ferrucci JT Jr, Mueller PR, et al: Percutaneous drainage of abscesses and fluid collections: Technique, results, and applications. Radiology 142:1-10, 1982.

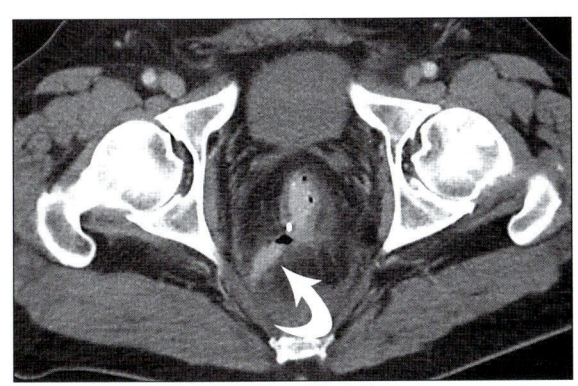

Figure 1. Contrast-enhanced CT of the pelvis shows a small collection of contrast posterolateral to the J-pouch anastomosis *(arrow)*. The collection contains bowel contrast, suggesting an anastomotic leak.

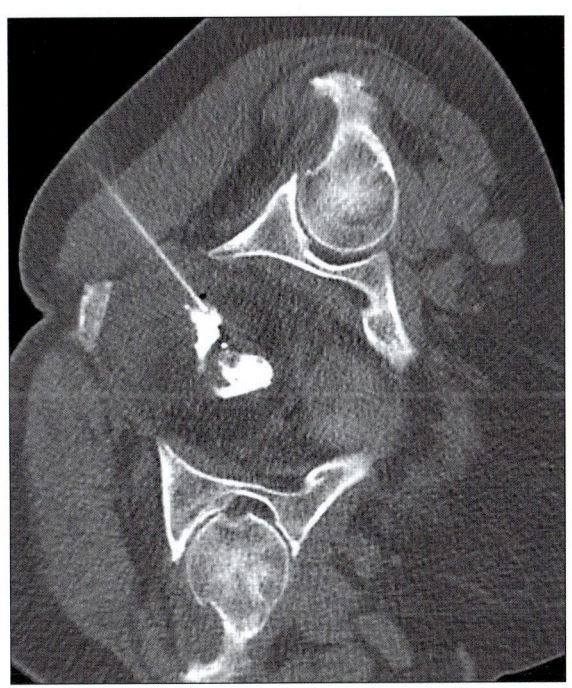

Figure 2. The collection was opacified by the administration of rectal contrast. An 18-gauge needle has been used to access the leak from a right transgluteal approach.

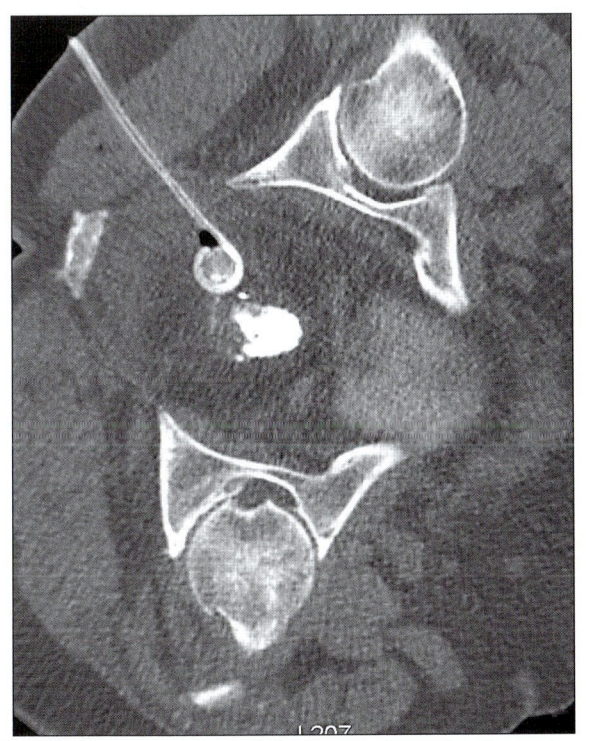

Figure 3. An 8-French pigtail drainage catheter has been placed into the collection.

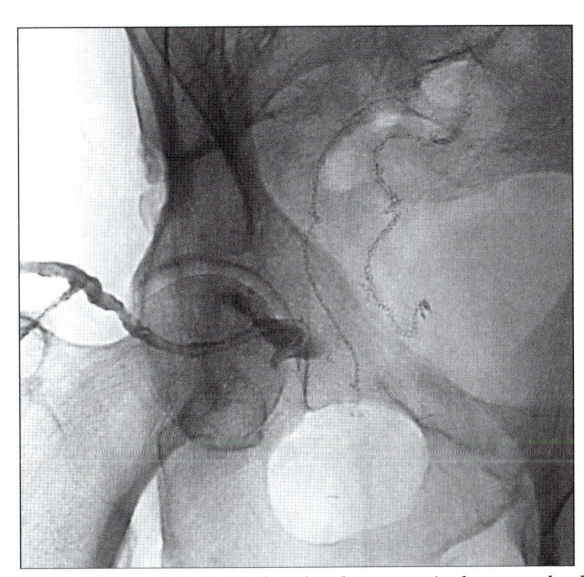

Figure 4. Follow-up drain study. The abscess cavity has completely resolved, and the anastomotic leak has healed.

Case 303

DEMOGRAPHICS/CLINICAL HISTORY

A 34-year-old man with ulcerative colitis, undergoing computed tomography (CT) and abscess drainage.

DISCUSSION

History/Indications for Procedure
A 34-year-old man with ulcerative colitis underwent total colectomy 10 years before presenting with increasing bowel movements.

Procedure
Presacral mucocele drainage

Pre-procedure Imaging
Contrast-enhanced CT through the pelvis demonstrates a 7-cm × 5-cm presacral fluid collection (Fig. 1). The collection has a thick, enhancing rim.

Intraprocedural Findings
CT-guided drainage was performed from a left transgluteal approach (Figs. 2 and 3), and 45 mL of thick, gelatinous fluid was aspirated.

Follow-up and Complications
The drain remained in place for a total of 2 weeks. The drain study at that time showed no residual cavity and no fistula to the pouch (Fig. 4).

Suggested Readings
Harisinghani MG, Gervais DA, Hahn PF, et al: CT-guided transgluteal drainage of deep pelvic abscesses: Indications, technique, procedure-related complications, and clinical outcome. Radiographics 22:1353-1367, 2002.

Mueller PR, vanSonnenberg E, Ferrucci JT Jr: Percutaneous drainage of 250 abdominal abscesses and fluid collections. Part II. Current procedural concepts. Radiology 151:343-347, 1984.

vanSonnenberg E, Mueller PR, Ferrucci JT Jr: Percutaneous drainage of 250 abdominal abscesses and fluid collections. Part I. Results, failures, and complications. Radiology 151:337-341, 1984.

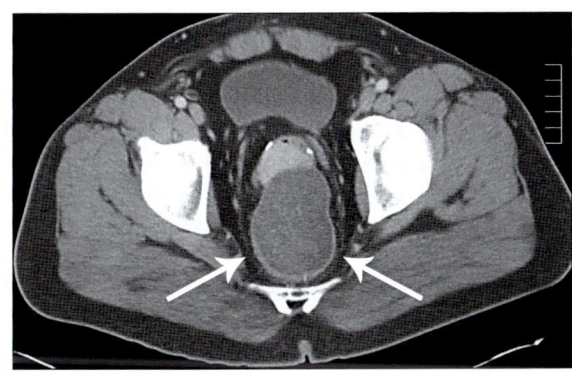

Figure 1. Single image from a contrast-enhanced pelvic CT scan demonstrates a heterogeneous fluid collection in the presacral space *(arrows)*. The collection has a thick, enhancing rim.

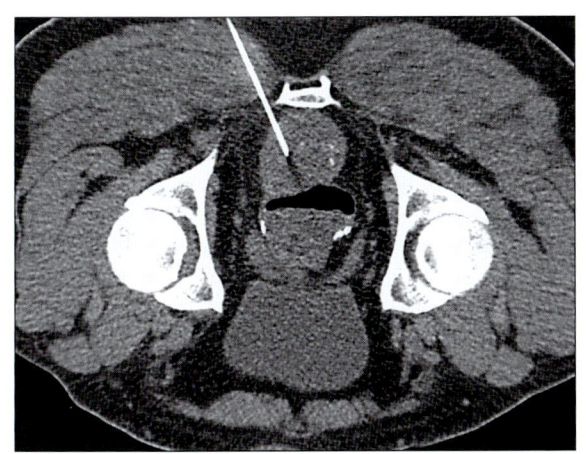

Figure 2. Using a left transgluteal approach, an 18-gauge needle was advanced into the collection under CT guidance.

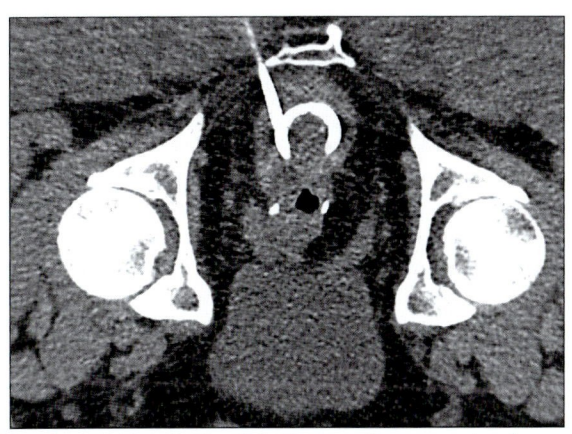

Figure 3. A 10-French pigtail drainage catheter was placed.

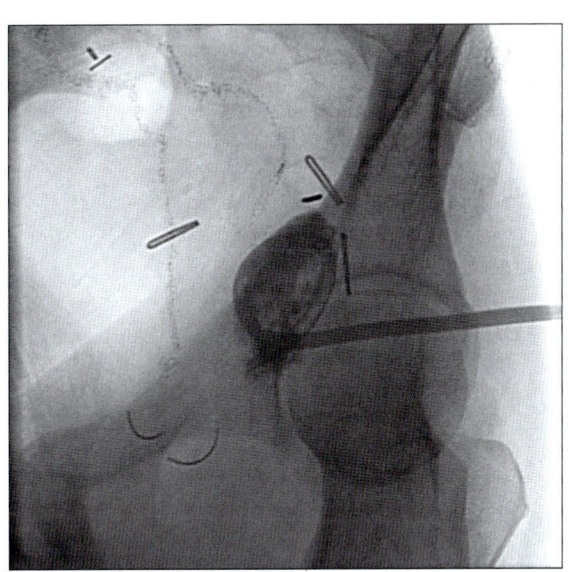

Figure 4. The follow-up drain study 2 weeks after the initial drain placement shows only a very small residual cavity remains. There is no fistulous communication with the adjacent rectal pouch.

Case 304

DEMOGRAPHICS/CLINICAL HISTORY

A 61-year-old man who underwent percutaneous abscess drainage following left hemicolectomy.

DISCUSSION

History/Indications for Procedure

A 61-year-old man who underwent left hemicolectomy for colon cancer. Percutaneous drainage of postoperative abscess was performed at an outside hospital.

Procedure

Percutaneous closure of anastomotic fistula following hemicolectomy

Pre-procedure Imaging

Contrast-enhanced CT shows the drainage catheter to reside in a collection of fluid and gas within the anterior lower abdomen (Fig. 1). Gas is seen tracking to the left, just anterior to the large bowel anastomosis.

Intraprocedural Findings

Abscess catheter injection shows contrast passing freely into the sigmoid colon, indicating an anastomotic leak (Fig. 2). The fistulous connection to the large bowel was closed with two collagen matrix plugs (Surgisis, Cook, Bloomington, IN), extending from the bowel wall to the skin (Figs. 3,4).

Follow-up and Complications

At 6-week follow-up, the site of the enterocutaneous fistula has completely healed; the patient reports no further drainage.

Suggested Readings

Cristoforidis D, Etzioni DA, Goldberg SM, et al.: Treatment of complex anal fistulas with the collagen fistula plug. Dis Colon Rectum 2008 [Epub ahead of print].

Ky AJ, Sylla P, Steinhagen R, et al: Collagen fistula plug for the treatment of anal fistulas. Dis Colon Rectum 51:838-843, 2008.

The Surgisis AFP anal fistula plug Report of a consensus conference. Colorectal Dis 10:17-20, 2008.

Case 304   609

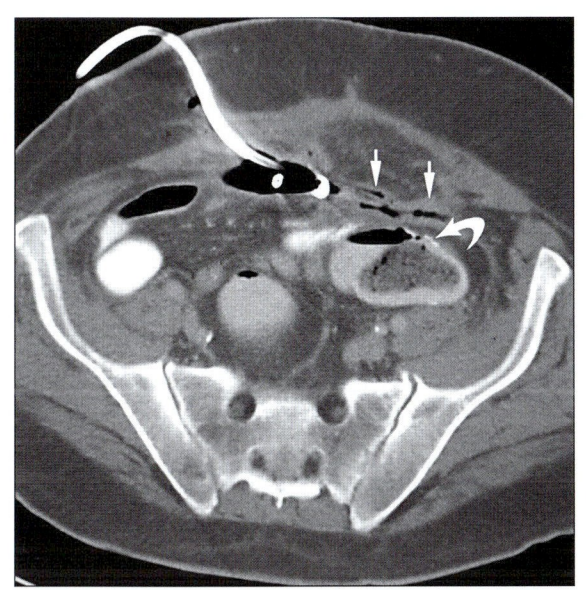

Figure 1. Contrast-enhanced CT of the pelvis shows the percutaneous drainage catheter in a collection of fluid and gas. Small gas lucencies extend from this collection just anterior to the sigmoid colon *(arrows)*. Radioopaque suture material is seen in the bowel wall at the anastomosis *(curved arrow)*.

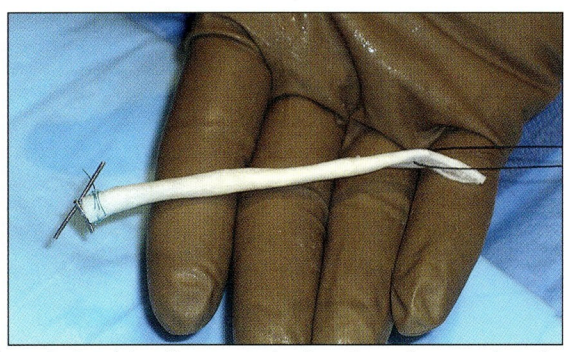

Figure 3. Surgisis collagen matrix plug. Two t-fasteners have been sutured on one end for securing the plug to the bowel wall. The other end of the plug is sutured to the skin.

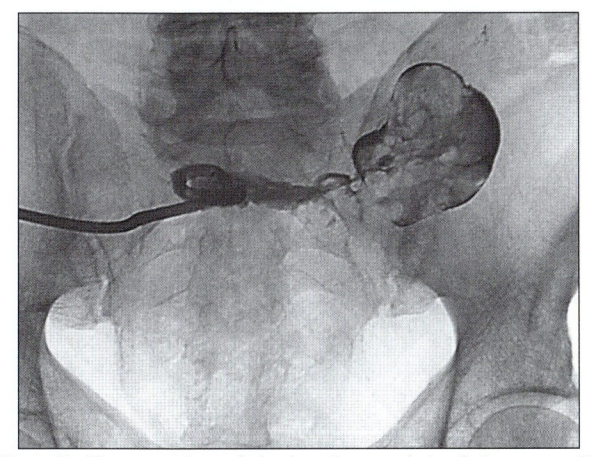

Figure 2. Abscess catheter injection shows minimal abscess cavity with direct communication to the large bowel.

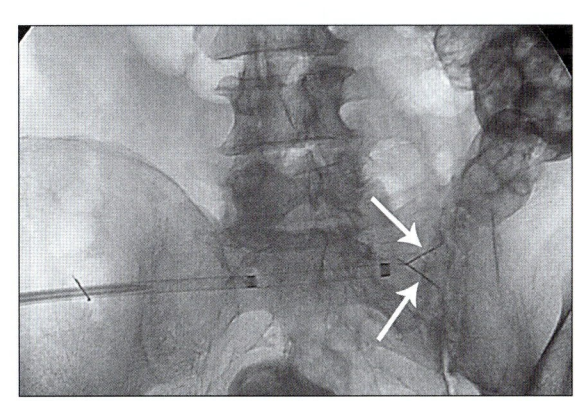

Figure 4. The large bowel fistula was closed with the placement of two collagen plugs. T-fasteners are used to secure the plug to the bowel *(arrows)*.

Index of Cases

1. Bilateral Common Iliac Artery Stenoses
2. Aortic revascularization
3. Endovascular Treatment of Aortic Stenosis
4. Endovascular Treatment of Subclavian Artery Stenosis
5. Right Subclavian Artery Occlusion
6. Percutaneous Treatment of Right Brachiocephalic Artery Stenosis
7. Left Subclavian Artery Stenting
8. Endovascular Management of Subclavian Steal
9. Brachial Artery Angioplasty
10. Brachial Artery Angioplasty
11. Thrombolysis for Hypothenar Hammer Syndrome
12. Acute Superficial Femoral Artery Thrombosis
13. Laser Atherectomy of Chronically Occluded Superficial Femoral Artery
14. Left Lower Extremity Arterial Recanalization
15. Atherosclerotic Disease of the Superficial Femoral Artery
16. Subintimal Recanalization of Lower Extremity
17. Recanalization of Chronic Superficial Femoral and Popliteal Artery Occlusion
18. Cryoplasty of Superficial Femoral Artery Stenosis
19. Subintimal Recanalization of the Posterior Tibial Artery
20. Tibioperoneal Stenosis Angioplasty
21. Anterior Tibial Artery Recanalization
22. Recanalization of Occluded Posterior Tibial Artery
23. Percutaneous Atherectomy for Anterior Tibial Artery Stenosis
24. Complication with Arterial Closure Device
25. Complication with Arterial Closure Device
26. Renal Artery Thrombosis
27. Management of Acute Post-traumatic Renal Ischemia
28. Renal Artery Stenting
29. Renal Artery Stenting in the Presence of Aortic Dissection
30. Renal Artery Angioplasty
31. Angioplasty for Renal Artery Stenosis
32. Renal Angioplasty in a Pediatric Patient with Hypertension
33. Management of Renovascular Hypertension in a Patient with Williams Syndrome
34. Percutaneous Thrombectomy or Thrombolysis of Superior Mesenteric Artery Embolus
35. Management of Acute Superior Mesenteric Artery Embolus
36. Chronic Mesenteric Ischemia
37. Superior Mesenteric Artery Stent Placement
38. Left subclavian Artery Stenosis Secondary to Takayasu's Arteritis
39. Chronic Mesenteric Ischemia
40. Management of Post-traumatic Popliteal Arterial Injury
41. Endovascular Management of Arteriovenous Fistula
42. Coil Embolization for Traumatic Lower Extremity Arteriovenous Fistula
43. Endovascular Repair of Traumatic Upper Extremity Arterial Injury
44. Embolization of Post-traumatic Anterior Tibial Artery Pseudoaneurysm
45. Embolization of Post-traumatic Dorsalis Pedis Artery Pseudoaneurysm
46. Percutaneous Stent Placement in the Setting of Lower Extremity Traumatic Dissection
47. Pelvic Hemorrhage Caused by Trauma
48. Endovascular Management of Thyrocervical Aneurysm
49. Endovascular Repair of Subclavian Artery Aneurysm
50. Stent-Graft Placement for Arterial Pseudoaneurysm Secondary to Pelvic Radiation
51. Endovascular Management of Celiac Trunk Pseudoaneurysm
52. Splenic Artery Aneurysm
53. Percutaneous Thrombin Injection of Hepatic Artery Pseudoaneurysm
    By Robert G. Dixon, MD
54. Endovascular Repair of Abdominal Aortic Aneurysm
55. Endovascular Repair of Ruptured Abdominal Aortic Aneurysm
56. Endograft Placement, Aortoenteric Fistula Repair
57. Endovascular Repair of Juxtarenal Aortic Aneurysm
58. Endovascular Repair of Juxtarenal Abdominal Aortic Aneurysm

Index of Cases

59 Management of abdominal Endoleak after Endovascular Abdominal Aortic Aneurysm Repair
60 Type II Endoleak Repair
61 Translumbar Embolization of Type II Endoleak
62 Transarterial Embolization of Type II Endoleak
63 Diagnosis and Management of Type Ib Endoleak
64 Late Endovascular Management of Endograft Failure
65 Endovascular Repair for Diverticulum of Kommerell Aneurysm
66 Endovascular Management of Acute Traumatic Aortic Injury
67 Thoracic Endograft for Acute Traumatic Aortic Injury
68 Endovascular Repair of Acute Traumatic Aortic Injury
69 Stent-Graft Placement for Lower Extremity Ischemia Secondary to Dissection
70 Endograft for Type B Aortic Dissection
71 Endovascular Stent Graft Placement for Type B Aortic Dissection
72 Endovascular Repair of Chronic Thoracic Aortic Pseudoaneurysm
73 Carotid Artery Stenting
74 Placement of Carotid Stent
75 Carotid Artery Stenting for Recurrent Stenosis after Endarterectomy
76 Carotid Dissection
77 Endovascular Management of Internal Carotid Artery Dissecting Aneurysm
78 Internal Carotid Artery Embolization
79 Endovascular Management of Carotid Blowout
80 Embolization of Juvenile Nasal Angiofibroma
81 Embolization of Mandibular Mass
82 Vertebral Artery Stenting
83 Intracranial Stent Placement
84 Intracranial Angioplasty
85 Middle Cerebral Artery Angioplasty
86 Percutaneous Angioplasty for Middle Cerebral Artery Stenosis
87 Endovascular Stroke Management
88 Endovascular Management of Basilar Artery Thrombosis
89 Diagnosis and Management of Subarachnoid Hemorrhage
90 Endovascular Treatment of Intracranial Aneurysm
91 Embolization for Epistaxis Secondary to HHT
92 Endovascular Management of Epistaxis
93 External Carotid Artery Embolization in Trauma
94 External Carotid Artery Embolization in the Trauma Setting
95 Stent Placement for External Carotid Pseudoaneurysm
96 Bronchial Artery Embolization
97 Bronchial Artery Embolization
98 Bronchial Artery Embolization for Invasive Pulmonary Aspergillosis
99 Bronchial Artery Embolization
100 Bronchial Artery Embolization
101 Bronchial Artery Embolization
102 Embolization of Renal Angiomyolipoma
103 Embolotherapy for Iatrogenic Renal Arteriovenous Fistula
104 Renal Artery Embolization in Trauma
105 Selective Embolization for Hemorrhagic Cyst in a Patient with Polycystic Kidney Disease
106 Transarterial Ablation of the Kidney
107 Acute Upper Gastrointestinal Hemorrhage
108 Acute Upper Gastrointestinal Hemorrhage
109 Management of Gastrointestinal Hemorrhage
110 Endovascular Management for Massive Hemobilia Secondary to Hepatic Artery Pseudoaneurysm
111 Lower Gastrointestinal Bleeding
112 Superselective Embolization for Acute Lower Gastrointestinal Hemorrhage
113 Endovascular Management of Lower Gastrointestinal Hemorrhage
114 Management of Acute Lower Gastrointestinal Hemorrhage
115 Superselective Embolization for Lower Gastrointestinal Hemorrhage
116 Embolization of Forearm Arteriovenous Malformation
117 Management of Large, High-Flow Shoulder Arteriovenous Malformation (AVM)
118 Embolization of Large Pelvic Arteriovenous Malformation
119 Arteriovenous Malformation in the Hand
120 Direct Puncture Embolization of Arteriovenous Malformation of the Foot
121 Endovascular Management of Renal Arteriovenous Fistula
122 Endovascular Management of Iatrogenic Injury to LIMA Graft
123 Endovascular Management of Thoracic Arteriovenous Fistula
124 Endovascular Treatment of Pelvic Arteriovenous Fistula
125 Endovascular Treatment of Venous Malformation
126 Percutaneous Sclerotherapy for Lower-Extremity Venous Malformation
127 Management of Cervical Lymphangioma

Index of Cases

128 Percutaneous Management of Soft-Tissue Hemangioma
129 Percutaneous Sclerotherapy for Kaposiform Hemangioendothelioma of the Extremity
130 Chemoembolization for Hepatocellular Carcinoma
131 Transarterial Chemoembolization (TACE) for Hepatocellular Carcinoma
132 Transarterial Chemoembolization of Hepatocellular Carcinoma
133 Chemoembolization for Hepatocellular Carcinoma
134 Transarterial Chemoembolization for Hepatocellular Carcinoma
135 Hepatic Chemoembolization for Metastatic Melanoma
136 Bland Embolization for Metastatic Carcinoid Tumor
137 Bland Embolization of Hepatocellular Carcinoma
138 Hepatic Adenoma Embolization
139 Embolization of Hepatic Hemangioendothelioma
140 Bland Embolization for Hepatic Malignancies
141 Radioembolization for Hepatocellular Carcinoma
142 Intra-arterial Radioembolization for Hepatocellular Carcinoma
143 Radioembolization for Metastatic Liver Gastrinoma
144 Radioembolization for Metastatic Carcinoid
145 Portal Vein Embolization
146 Hemorrhage after Cholecystostomy Catheter Placement
147 Endovascular Management for Traumatic Liver Laceration
148 Hepatic Artery Embolization for Traumatic Liver Laceration
149 Embolization for Hepatic Artery Trauma
150 Liver Trauma
151 Management of Post-traumatic Splenic Pseudoaneurysm and Arteriovenous Fistula
152 Endovascular Management of Splenic Trauma
153 Splenic Artery Embolization
154 Embolization, Splenic, for Thrombocytopenia
155 Splenic Artery Embolization for Management of Gastric Varices
156 Uterine Fibroid Embolization
157 Uterine Fibroid Embolization
158 Uterine Artery Embolization for Cervical Leiomyomas
159 Pelvic Embolization for Postpartum Hemorrhage
160 Uterine Artery Embolization for Management of Placenta Percreta
161 Percutaneous Angioplasty for Hepatic Artery Stenosis
162 Hepatic Artery Stenosis Management in the Liver Transplant Patient
163 Hepatic Artery Stenosis after Liver Transplantation
164 Percutaneous Angioplasty for Hepatic Artery Stenosis in a Liver Transplant Patient
165 Celiac Artery Stent Placement for Arterial Steal Syndrome in a Liver Transplant Patient
166 Portal Vein Stenosis after Liver Transplantation
167 Management of Portal Vein Stenosis in a Liver Transplant Patient
168 Portal Vein Thrombosis in a Liver Transplant Recipient
169 Inferior Vena Cava (IVC) Stenting in a Liver Transplant Patient
170 Inferior Vena Cava Stenosis in a Liver Transplant Patient
171 Inferior Vena Cava Stent Placement in a Liver Transplant Patient
172 Hepatic Vein Stenting Following Liver Transplantation
173 Embolization of Pulmonary Arteriovenous Malformation (AVM)
174 Endovascular Management of Large Pulmonary Arteriovenous Malformation (AVM)
175 Embolization of Pulmonary Arteriovenous Malformation
176 Pulmonary Artery Thrombolysis
177 Superior Vena Cava Filter Placement
178 Management of Inferior Vena Cava Filter Migration
179 Removal of Chronically Embedded Inferior Vena Cava Filter
180 Management of Acute Lower Extremity Deep Venous Thrombosis
181 Management of Acute Lower Extremity Deep Venous Thrombosis
182 Thrombolysis for Acute Lower Extremity Deep Venous Thrombosis
183 Management of Chronic Iliac Vein and IVC Thrombosis
184 Endovascular Treatment for Chronic Lower Extremity Deep Venous Thrombosis
185 Management of Chronic Inferior Vena Cava Occlusion
186 Chronic Lower Extremity Deep Venous Thrombosis
187 Recanalization of Chronically Occluded Venous Stent
188 Management for Acute Upper Extremity Deep Venous Thrombosis
189 Endovascular Management of Catheter-Related Superior Vena Cava Stenosis
190 Percutaneous Stent for Superior Vena Cava Stenosis,
191 Upper Extremity Deep Venous Thrombosis

Index of Cases

192 Chronic Right Upper Extremity Venous Occlusion Management
193 Endovascular Management of Chronic Upper Extremity Deep Venous Thrombosis
194 Portal-Mesenteric Venous Thrombosis
195 Percutaneous Management for Portal Vein Thrombosis after Hepatectomy
196 Transjugular Intrahepatic Portosystemic Shunt (TIPSS) Placement
197 Transjugular Intrahepatic Portosystemic Shunt (TIPSS) Reduction
198 Embolization of Hepatic Artery as a Complication of Transjugular Intrahepatic Portosystemic Stent Shunt (TIPSS) Placement
199 Retrograde Balloon Occlusion Variceal Ablation
200 Balloon-Occluded Retrograde Transvenous Obliteration of Gastric Varices
201 Retrograde Occlusion of Stomal Varices
202 Renal Vein Sampling
203 Adrenal Vein Sampling
204 Adrenal Venous Sampling
205 Parathyroid Venous Sampling
206 Parathyroid Venous Sampling
207 Hemodialysis Graft Management
208 Management of Recurrent Dialysis Graft Stenosis
209 Dialysis Graft Maintenance
210 Nonmaturing Fistula
211 Cephalic Vein Stent Placement for Hemodialysis Fistula Maintenance
212 Clotted Hemodialysis Fistula
213 Dialysis Fistula Declot
214 Management of Dialysis Graft Pseudoaneurysms
215 Shunt Declot
216 Management of Thrombosed Femoral Dialysis Graft
217 Clotted Necklace Hemodialysis Graft
218 Placement of Transhepatic Dialysis Catheter
219 Placement of Transhepatic Dialysis Catheter
220 Translumbar Dialysis Catheter Placement
221 Peripherally Inserted Central Catheter (PICC) Placement with Left-Sided Superior Vena Cava (SVC)
222 Intra-arterial Central Venous Catheter Removal
223 Management of Inadvertent Placement of Central Venous Catheter in the Vertebral Artery
224 Subclavian Vein Port Insertion
225 "Pinch-Off Syndrome"—Foreign Body Retrieval
   By Robert G. Dixon, MD
226 Retrieval of Lost Guidewire
227 Management of Malpositioned Intravascular Stent
228 Retrieval of Lost Embolization Coil
229 Varicocele Embolization
230 Varicocele Embolization
231 Gonadal Vein Embolization for the Treatment of a Left-Sided Varicocele
232 Gonadal Vein Embolization, Pelvic Varicosities
233 Bilateral Ovarian Vein Embolization for Pelvic Congestion Syndrome
234 Endovenous Laser Ablation of the Great Saphenous Vein
   By Susan Weeks, MD
235 Transjugular Liver Biopsy
236 Transvenous Biopsy of Inferior Vena Cava Mass
237 Ultrasound-Guided Liver Biopsy
238 CT-Guided Pelvic Mass Biopsy
239 Stereotactic Breast Biopsy
240 Stereotactic Breast Biopsy
241 Breast Biopsy, MRI Guidance
242 Percutaneous Biopsy of the Lung
243 Percutaneous Biopsy of the Lung
244 Radiofrequency Ablation of Hepatocellular Carcinoma
245 Ultrasound and CT-Guided Microwave Ablation of Hepatocellular Carcinoma
246 Ultrasound-Guided Microwave Ablation of Hepatocellular Carcinoma
247 Cryoablation of Hepatocellular Carcinoma
248 Radiofrequency Ablation of Colorectal Liver Metastasis
249 Radiofrequency Ablation of Metastatic Sarcoma to Liver
250 Radiofrequency Ablation of Recurrent Adrenal Corticocarcinoma
251 Radiofrequency Ablation of Renal Cell Carcinoma
252 Radiofrequency Ablation of Renal Tumors
   By Charles Burke, MD, and Robert G. Dixon, MD
253 Cryoablation for Renal Cell Carcinoma
254 Cryoablation of Renal Cell Carcinoma
255 Radiofrequency Ablation for Osteoid Osteoma
256 Radiofrequency Ablation of Osteoid Osteoma
257 Radiofrequency Ablation for Painful Acetabular Metastasis
258 Thoracic Vertebroplasty
259 Kyphoplasty
260 Percutaneous Embolization of the Thoracic Duct
   By Charles Burke, MD, and Robert G. Dixon, MD
261 CT-Guided Sacral Nerve Block
262 Percutaneous Transhepatic Cholangiogram
263 Double Needle Technique, Percutaneous Transhepatic Cholangiogram and Biliary Drain Placement
264 Percutaneous Management of Biliary Obstruction Secondary to Clipped Bile Duct
265 Common Bile Duct Stone Removal
266 Cystic Duct Stump Leak

267	Common Bile Duct Injury	286	Percutaneous Drainage of Perirenal Abscess
268	Management of Traumatic Bile Duct Laceration	287	Percutaneous Drainage of Renal Abscess
269	Management of Bile Leak	288	Suprapubic Cystostomy Catheter Placement
270	Management of Biliary Leak after Liver Transplantation	289	Balloon Dilatation of Benign Esophageal Stricture
271	Biliary Leak after Liver Transplantation	290	Esophageal Foreign Body Retrieval
272	Biliary Ischemia after Liver Transplantation	291	Percutaneous Gastrostomy Tube Placement
273	Endobiliary Stent Placement	292	Percutaneous Gastrostomy Tube Placement
274	Biliary Stent Placement for Malignant Biliary Obstruction	293	CT-Guided Gastrostomy Tube Placement
275	Endobiliary Stenting	294	Gastrojejunostomy Tube Placement
276	Bilateral Biliary Stent Placement	295	Gastroduodenal Outlet Obstruction
277	Nephrostomy for Xanthogranulomatous Pyelonephritis	296	Percutaneous Management of Pancreatic Pseudocyst
278	Percutaneous Nephrostomy Placement	297	Pancreatic Pseudocyst Management
279	CT-Guided Nephrostomy Placement	298	Empyema Drainage
280	Nephrostomy Management in a Renal Transplant Patient	299	CT-Guided Empyema Drainage
		300	Ultrasound-Guided Drainage of Hepatic Abscess
281	Ureteroileal Anastomotic Stricture	301	Transvaginal Abscess Drain
282	Nephroureteral Stent Placement	302	CT-Guided Abscess Drainage
283	Nephroureteral Stent Placement	303	Presacral Mucocele Drainage
284	Nephroureteral Catheter in a Horseshoe Kidney	304	Percutaneous Closure of Anastamotic Fistula Following Hemicolectomy
285	Renal Cyst Drainage and Sclerosing		

Index

A

Abdominal aortic aneurysm
　assessment of, 108
　endograft in, 108, 109f
　endoleak management in, 118, 119f
　　access to, 118, 119f
　　catheterization in, 120
　　classification of, 118
　　embolization of, 118, 120, 121f, 122, 123f
　　obliteration of, 118, 119f
　　occlusion of, 120, 121f
　　streak artifact in, 122, 123f
　　translumbar access to, 122, 123f
　　type II, 121f, 122, 123f
　intervention indication, 108, 109f
　post-procedure assessment of, 108, 109f
　ruptured
　　hematoma in, 110, 111f
　　resolution of, 111f
　　stent graft in, 110, 111f
　　symptoms, 110
Abscess drainage, 604, 605f
　hepatic, 600, 601f
　perirenal, 572, 573f
　presacral mucocele, 606, 607f
　renal, 574, 575f
　transvaginal, 602, 603f
Acalculous cholecystitis, 292
Accessory bile duct leak, 538, 539f
Acculink stent, in internal carotid artery stenosis, 146, 147f, 148, 149f, 150, 151f
Acetabular metastasis, radiofrequency ablation of, 514, 515f
Adenoma, hepatic
　embolization of, 276, 277f
　hypervascularity in, 276, 277f
　masses in, 276, 277f
Adrenal corticocarcinoma, radiofrequency ablation of, 500, 501f
Adrenal vein sampling, 407f
　aldosterone levels in, 406, 407f, 408
　catheterization in, 408, 409f
　indications, 406, 408
Anastomotic fistula closure, 608, 609f
Angiofibroma, nasal
　arterial supply to, 160, 161f
　embolization of, 160, 161f
　mass in, 160, 161f
　symptoms, 160
Angiomyolipoma, renal
　embolization of, 204, 205f
　hypervascularity in, 204, 205f
　mass in, 204, 205f
Angio-Seal closure device
　filling-defect after use of, 48, 49f
　stenosis after use of, 48, 49f
Ankle/brachial index
　in aortic stenosis, 4, 6
　in atherosclerotic disease of superficial femoral artery, 30
　in chronic superficial femoral artery occlusion, 26
　in posterior tibial artery obstruction, 38
　in posterior tibial artery obstruction follow-up, 38, 39f, 44

Ankle/brachial index (Continued)
　in superficial femoral artery stenosis, 36
　in tibial artery with nonpulsatile flow, 28
Anterior tibial artery
　aberrant origin of, 47f
　percutaneous atherectomy for stenosis of
　　ankle/brachial index before, 46
　　catheter in, 46
　　indications, 46
　　stenosis in, 46, 47f
　post-traumatic pseudoaneurysm in, 89f
　　occlusion of, 88, 89f
　　symptoms, 88
　recanalization
　　angioplasty in, 42, 43f
　　indications, 42
　　runoff disease in, 42, 43f
Antiphospholipid antibody syndrome, 384, 392
Aortic aneurysm
　abdominal
　　assessment of, 108
　　endograft in, 108, 109f
　　endoleak management in, 118, 119f
　　intervention indication, 108, 109f
　endoleak management in
　　access to, 118, 119f
　　catheterization in, 120
　　classification of, 118
　　embolization of, 118, 120, 121f, 122, 123f
　　obliteration of, 118, 119f
　　occlusion of, 120, 121f
　　streak artifact in, 122, 123f
　　translumbar access to, 122, 123f
　　type II, 121f, 122, 123f
　juxtarenal, 114, 115f
　　endograft in, 114, 115f
　　endovascular repair of
　　　exclusion in, 116, 117f
　　　stent graft in, 116, 117f
　　　stenting in, 116, 117f
　　exclusion of, 114, 115f
　　iliac artery in, 114
Aortic arch aneurysm, in diverticulum of Kommerell
　bypass prior to, 130
　dilation in, 130, 131f
　embolization in, 130
　occlusion of, 130, 131f
Aortic dissection
　from aortic arch to left common iliac artery, 139f
　flap extension into renal artery, 58, 59f
　lower extremity ischemia secondary to
　　stenting in, 138, 139f
　　symptoms, 138
　renal artery narrowing from, 58, 59f
　renal artery stenting in, 58, 59f
　type B, 141f, 142, 143f
　　aneurysm in, 140, 141f
　　bypass in, 142
　　debranching in, 140, 141f
　　endograft in, 140, 141f
　　false lumen in, 142, 143f
　　resolution of, 143f
　　stenting in, 142

Aortic injury
　hematoma resolution in, 132, 133f
　intimal hyperplasia from, 136, 137f
　leak from, 134, 135f
　pseudoaneurysm in, 132, 133f
　stent grafting in, 132, 133f, 134, 135f, 136, 137f
Aortic pseudoaneurysm, chronic, 144, 145f
　resolution of, 144, 145f
　stenting in, 144, 145f
Aortic revascularization, 5f
　ankle/brachial index in, 4
　indications, 4
　stent placement in, 5f
Aortic stenosis
　aortic revascularization for, 5f
　ankle/brachial index in, 4
　indications, 4
　stent placement in, 5f
　endovascular treatment of
　　ankle/brachial index in, 6
　　balloon expandable stent in, 6, 7f
Aortic stent graft, in aortoenteric fistula repair, 112, 113f
Aortoenteric fistula
　gas in endograft for, 112, 113f
　pseudoaneurysm in, 112, 113f
　stent graft in, 112, 113f
　symptoms, 112
Arc of Riolen, in superior mesenteric artery stenosis, 74, 75f
Arterial closure device
　dissection after use of, 50, 51f
　filling defect after use of, 48, 49f, 50, 51f
　stenosis after use of, 48, 49f
Arterial recanalization, left lower extremity
　indications, 28
　through superior femoral artery, 29f
Arterial steal syndrome, in transplant patient, 330, 331f
Arteriovenous fistula
　coil embolization for
　　indications, 84
　　pseudoaneurysm in, 84, 85f
　　of sural artery, 83f
　endovascular treatment of
　　pseudoaneurysm in, 82, 83f
　　stenting in, 82, 83f
　of internal jugular vein, 86
　pelvic
　　iliac veins in, 248, 249f
　　situation of, 248, 249f
　　stenting in, 248, 249f
　　symptoms, 248
　renal
　　embolization of, 242, 243f
　　in left kidney hilum, 242, 243f
　renal iatrogenic
　　embolization of, 206, 207f
　　symptoms, 206, 207f
　splenic
　　embolization of, 302, 303f
　　laceration in, 302, 303f
　　symptoms, 302
Arteriovenous malformation
　in foot
　　embolization of, 240, 241f

Note: Page numbers followed by f indicate figures.

617

Arteriovenous malformation *(Continued)*
  puncturing of, 238, 239f
  supply of, 240, 241f
 in forearm
  embolization of, 232, 233f
  supply of, 232, 233f
 in hand
  arterial steal in, 238, 239f
  embolization of, 238, 239f
  internal flow voids in, 238, 239f
  supply of, 238, 239f
  symptoms, 238
 pelvic
  continued flow in, 236, 237f
  selective embolization of, 236, 237f
  supply of, 236, 237f
 pulmonary, 346, 347f, 350, 351f
  aneurysm in, 348, 349f
  embolization of, 348, 349f, 350, 351f
 in shoulder
  arteriovenous shunting in, 234, 235f
  embolization of, 234, 235f
  enlargement of, 234, 235f
  subclavian vein in, 234
Ascending cervical artery, embolization of, for subclavian artery aneurysm, 98, 99f
Aspergillosis, 196, 197f
Atherectomy
 for anterior tibial artery stenosis
  ankle/brachial index before, 46
  catheter in, 46
  indications, 46
  stenosis in, 46, 47f
 for chronic superficial femoral artery occlusion, 26, 27f
Atherosclerotic disease, of superficial femoral artery
  ankle/brachial index in, 30
  intrastent stenosis in, 30, 31f
  stenosis in, 30, 31f
  Viabahn stent in, 30, 31f
Autosomal dominant polycystic kidney disease
  cysts in, 210, 211f
  embolization in, 210, 211f
  hemorrhages in, 210, 211f
Axillary vein stenosis, 434, 435f

B
Balloon angioplasty
 for brachial artery stenosis, 18, 19f, 20, 21f
 for brachial vein stenosis, 414, 415f
 for cephalic vein stenosis, 420, 421f, 422, 423f, 426, 427f
 for deep vein thrombosis, 372, 373f, 383f
 for dialysis graft stenosis, 416, 417f
 of dorsalis pedis artery, 42, 43f
 for fibromuscular dysplasia of renal artery, 61f
 for hepatic artery stenosis, 322, 323f, 324, 325f, 328, 329f
 for hepatic vein stenosis, 438, 439f
 for internal carotid artery occlusion, 168, 169f
 for middle cerebral artery occlusion, 170, 171f
 for middle cerebral artery stenosis, 172, 173f
 for portal vein stenosis, 332, 333f, 334
 for posterior tibial artery occlusion, 44
 for renal artery stenosis in pediatric patient, 64, 65f
 for renal artery stenosis in transplant patient, 62, 63f
 for restenosis, 12, 13f
 for subclavian artery stenosis secondary to Takayasu's arteritis, 76, 77f
 for superficial femoral artery occlusion, 32, 33f
 of tibioperoneal stenosis, 40, 41f
Balloon dilatation, of esophageal stricture, 578, 579f
Balloon expandable stent
 in aortic stenosis, 6, 7f
 in basilar artery thrombosis, 176
 in carotid artery stenosis, 166, 167f
 in celiac artery stenosis, 72, 73f, 330, 331f
 in celiac trunk pseudoaneurysm, 102, 103f
 in hepatic artery stenosis, 326, 327f
 in juxtarenal aortic aneurysm, 116, 117f
 in mesenteric ischemia with Takayasu's vasculitis, 78, 79f

Balloon expandable stent *(Continued)*
 in post-traumatic renal ischemia, 54, 55f
 in renal artery stenosis, 56, 57f
  from aortic dissection, 58, 59f
 in subclavian artery aneurysm, 98, 99f
 in subclavian artery occlusion, 10, 11f
 in subclavian artery stenosis, 8, 9f
 in subclavian steal syndrome, 16, 17f
 in superficial femoral artery dissection, 92, 93f
 in superior mesenteric artery stenosis, 74, 75f
 in Williams syndrome management, 66, 67f
Basilar artery thrombosis
 flow absence in, 176, 177f
 occlusion in, 176, 177f
 stenosis in, 176, 177f
 stenting in, 176
 symptoms, 176
 tPA for, 176, 177f
Basilic vein thrombosis, 424, 425f
Bilateral common iliac artery stenoses
 ankle/brachial index in, 2
 kissing stents in, 2, 3f
 narrowing in, 2, 3f
 self-expanding stent in, 2, 3f
Bile duct laceration, 534, 535f, 536, 537f
Bile duct leak, 538, 539f, 540, 541f, 542, 543f
Bile duct stone, 530, 531f
Biliary-arterial fistula, 534, 535f
Biliary drain placement, 524, 525f, 526, 527f, 528, 529f
Biliary ischemia, after liver transplant, 544, 545f
Biliary stent placement, bilateral, 552, 553f
Biopsy
 breast
  MRI-guided, 482, 483f
  stereotactic, 478, 479f, 480, 481f
 inferior vena cava, 472, 473f
 liver
  transjugular, 470, 471f
  ultrasound-guided, 474, 475f
 lung, 484, 485f, 486
 pelvic, 476, 477f
Bland embolization
 for hepatocellular carcinoma, 274, 275f
 for metastatic carcinoid tumor, 272, 273f
Blue toe syndrome, 5f
 ankle/brachial index in, 4
 stent placement in, 5f
 symptoms in, 4
Brachial artery angioplasty
 balloon in, 18, 19f, 20, 21f
 Doppler ultrasound in, 20
 fistula anastomosis in, 20, 21f
 indications in, 18, 20
 residual stenosis in, 20, 21f
 stenosis in, 18, 19f
Brachial vein stenosis, 414, 415f
Brachiocephalic artery stenosis, percutaneous treatment of
 balloon angioplasty for restenosis in, 12, 13f
 indications, 12
 intrastent stenosis in, 12
 pressure gradient in, 12
 stenting in, 12, 13f
Brachiocephalic vein occlusion, 384, 385f
Breast biopsy
 MRI-guided, 482, 483f
 stereotactic, 478, 479f, 480, 481f
Bronchial artery
 embolization, 192, 193f, 194, 195f, 196, 197f, 198, 200, 201f, 202, 203f
 in hyperemia, 200, 201f
 hypertrophy of, 192, 193f
 in hypervascularity, 198, 199f
 in invasive pulmonary aspergillosis, 196, 197f
 in *Mycobacterium* complex disease, 194, 195f
Budd-Chiari syndrome, 392

C
Carcinoid tumor, metastatic to liver
 embolization of, 272, 273f
 lesions in, 272, 273f

Carcinoma
 hepatocellular
  bland embolization of, 274, 275f
  catheterization in, 264, 265f
  chemoembolization of, 260, 261f, 262, 263f, 264, 265f, 266, 267f
  cryoablation of, 494, 495f
  hypervascularity in, 262, 263f, 274, 275f, 282, 283f
  intra-arterial radioembolization of, 284, 285f
  lesions in, 262, 263f
  lung shunt in, 282
  mass in, 260, 261f, 264, 265f, 266, 267f, 274, 275f
  microwave ablation of, 490, 491f, 492, 493f
  radioembolization of, 282, 283f
  radiofrequency ablation of, 268, 269f, 488, 489f
  supply of, 260, 261f
  symptoms, 266
 renal cell
  cryoablation of, 506, 507f, 508, 509f
  radiofrequency ablation of, 502, 503f, 504, 505f
Carotid artery, internal, pseudoaneurysm after endarterectomy, 156, 157f
 embolization in, 156, 157f
 occlusion balloon test of, 156, 157f
Carotid artery dissection, internal
 in aneurysm
  on brain MRI, 154
  fibromuscular dysplasia in, 154, 155f
  stenting in, 154, 155f
  symptoms, 154
 stenosis in, 152, 153f
 stenting in, 152, 153f
 symptoms, 152
Carotid artery occlusion, internal
 balloon angioplasty of, 168, 169f
 dilation of, 168
 symptoms, 168
Carotid artery pseudoaneurysm, external, 186, 187f, 190, 191f
 exclusion of, 190, 191f
 stenting of, 190, 191f
 symptoms, 190
Carotid artery stenosis, internal, 146, 147f, 148, 149f
 angioplasty of, 166, 167f
 distal projection device in, 146, 147f
 recurrent, after endarterectomy, 150, 151f
  distal projection device in, 150, 151f
  stenting in, 150, 151f
  vasospasm in, 150, 151f
 stenting in, 146, 147f, 148, 149f, 166, 167f
Carotid blowout
 embolization of, 158, 159f
 lingual artery in, 158, 159f
 in oropharyngeal cancer, 158
Catheter-related superior vena cava stenosis, 378, 379f
Celiac artery stenosis
 in liver transplant patient, 331f
  stenting in, 330, 331f
 in mesenteric ischemia, 71f, 72
 in Takayasu's vasculitis, 78, 79f
Celiac trunk pseudoaneurysm, 102, 103f
 embolization of, 102, 103f
 at splenic artery, 102, 103f
 stenting of, 102, 103f
Central catheter
 in left-sided superior vena cava, 442, 443f
 removal of aberrant, 444, 445f
 in vertebral artery, 446, 447f
Cephalic vein stenosis, 420, 421f, 422, 423f, 426, 427f
Cerebral salt wasting syndrome, 178
Cervical artery, embolization of, for subclavian artery aneurysm, 98, 99f
Cervical fibroids, 317f
 embolization of, 316
 supply of, 316, 317f
Cervical lymphangioma, 254, 255f
 cystic, 254, 255f
 sclerosing of, 254, 255f

Index

Cesarean section, 320, 321f
Chemoembolization
  of hepatocellular carcinoma, 260, 261f, 262, 263f, 264, 265f, 266, 267f, 268, 269f
  of hepatocellular metastatic melanoma, 270, 271f
Cholangiogram, percutaneous transhepatic, 524, 525f, 526, 527f
Cholecystectomy catheter, hemorrhage from, 292, 293f
Chronic aortic pseudoaneurysm, 144, 145f
  resolution of, 144, 145f
  stenting in, 144, 145f
Chronic mesenteric ischemia
  stenosis in, 71f, 72
  stenting in, 72, 73f
  symptoms, 72
Chronic occlusion of superficial femoral artery
  ankle/brachial index in, 26
  arteriogram of, 26, 27f
  atherectomy for, 26, 27f
  popliteal artery in, 27f
Chylothorax, 520
Closure device
  dissection from, 50, 51f
  filling defect after use of, 48, 49f, 50, 51f
  stenosis after use of, 48, 49f
Colorectal liver metastasis, radiofrequency ablation of, 496, 497f
Common bile duct stone, 530, 531f
Common femoral artery, distal right
  dissection from closure device in, 50, 51f
  filling defect after arteriotomy closure in, 48, 49f, 50, 51f
  stenosis after arteriotomy closure in, 48, 49f
Common iliac artery stenoses, bilateral
  ankle/brachial index in, 2
  kissing stents in, 2, 3f
  narrowing in, 2, 3f
  self-expanding stent in, 2, 3f
Covered stent
  for aortic dissection, 138, 139f
  for biliary obstruction, 550, 551f
  for external carotid pseudoaneurysm, 188, 189f
  for iliac artery pseudoaneurysm, 100, 101f
  for left internal mammary artery injury, 244, 245f
Cryoablation
  of hepatocellular carcinoma, 494, 495f
  of renal cell carcinoma, 506, 507f, 508, 509f
Cryoplasty, of superficial femoral artery stenosis
  ankle/brachial index before, 36
  balloon in, 36, 37f
  dissection after, 36, 37f
  indications, 36
  stenosis in, 36, 37f
CT-guided empyema drainage, 597f, 598
CT-guided gastrostomy placement, 586, 587f
CT-guided nephrostomy placement, 558, 559f
CT-guided pelvic biopsy, 476, 477f
CT-guided sacral nerve block, 522, 523f
Cystic duct stump embolization, 532, 533f
Cystic fibrosis, 442

D

Deep venous thrombosis
  lower extremity
    Angiojet catheter for, 364
    balloon angioplasty of, 372, 373f
    8-French Trellis device for, 360
    femoral vein in, 368, 369f
    iliac veins in, 363f, 368, 369f
    May-Thurner lesion in, 372, 373f
    stenting in, 363f
    symptoms, 360
    thrombolysis for, 364, 365f
    thrombus in, 361f, 363f, 365f
    venous expansion in, 365f
  upper extremity
    balloon angioplasty for, 383f
    brachiocephalic vein in, 386, 387f
    occlusion in, 383f
    stenting in, 386, 387f

Deep venous thrombosis (Continued)
  subclavian and axillary veins in, 376, 377f
  symptoms, 376, 382, 386
  thrombolysis of, 376, 377f
Dialysis catheter
  transhepatic
    balloon angioplasty in, 438, 439f
    brachiocephalic vein occlusion in, 436, 437f
    hepatic vein stenosis in, 438, 439f
    placement of, 436, 437f
    superior vena cava occlusion in, 438
    vena cava occlusion in, 436, 437f
  translumbar
    IVC access in, 440, 441f
    placement of, 440, 441f
Dialysis graft. See also Dialysis catheter
  axillary vein stenosis in, 434, 435f
  balloon angioplasty in, 414, 415f, 416, 417f, 418, 419f, 420, 421f, 422, 423f, 426, 427f
  basilic vein thrombosis in, 424, 425f
  brachial vein stenosis in, 414, 415f
  cephalic vein stenosis in, 420, 422, 423f, 426, 427f
  embolization in, 420, 421f
  nonmaturing fistula in, 420
  outflow vein stenosis in, 418
  pseudoaneurysms in, 418, 428, 429f
    enlargement of, 428, 429f
    stenting of, 428, 429f
  stenting of, 416, 417f, 422, 423f, 424, 425f, 434, 435f
  thrombectomy in, 426, 427f
  thrombolysis in, 430, 431f, 432, 433f, 434, 435f
  venous anastomosis stenosis in, 416, 417f
Diamondback atherectomy catheter, 46
Digital artery occlusion, in hypothenar hammer syndrome, 22, 23f
Dissection
  aortic
    from aortic arch to left common iliac artery, 139f
    flap extension into renal artery, 58, 59f
    lower extremity ischemia secondary to
      stenting in, 138, 139f
      symptoms, 138
    renal artery narrowing from, 58, 59f
    renal artery stenting in, 58, 59f
    type B, 141f, 142, 143f
      aneurysm in, 140, 141f
      bypass in, 142
      debranching in, 140, 141f
      endograft in, 140, 141f
      false lumen in, 142, 143f
      resolution of, 143f
      stenting in, 142
  carotid
    in aneurysm
      on brain MRI, 154
      fibromuscular dysplasia in, 154, 155f
      stenting in, 154, 155f
      symptoms, 154
    stenosis in, 152, 153f
    stenting of, 152, 153f
    symptoms, 152
  of superficial femoral artery
    stenosis in, 92, 93f
    stenting in, 92, 93f
Distal projection device, in internal carotid artery stenosis, 146, 147f, 150, 151f
Distal right common femoral artery
  filling defect after arteriotomy closure in, 48, 49f
  stenosis after arteriotomy closure in, 48, 49f
Diverticulum of Kommerell aneurysm
  bypass prior to, 130
  dilation in, 130, 131f
  embolization in, 130
  occlusion of, 130, 131f
Dorsalis pedis artery
  balloon angioplasty of, 42, 43f
  post-traumatic pseudoaneurysm of, 90, 91f
  embolization of, 90, 91f
  occlusion in, 90, 91f
Duct of Luschka leap, 538, 539f

E

Embolization coil, lost, 456, 457f
Empyema drainage, 596, 597f, 598
Endarterectomy
  carotid artery pseudoaneurysm after, 156, 157f
    embolization in, 156, 157f
    occlusion balloon test of, 156, 157f
  recurrent internal carotid artery stenosis after, 150, 151f
    distal projection device in, 150, 151f
    stenting in, 150, 151f
    vasospasm in, 150, 151f
Endobiliary stenting, 550, 551f
Endobiliary stent placement, 546, 547f
Endograft
  in abdominal aortic aneurysm, 108, 109f
  in aortic dissection, 140, 141f
  in aortoenteric fistula repair, 112, 113f
  in biliary obstruction, 546, 547f, 548, 549f
  failure
    occlusion in, 128, 129f
    sac pressure in, 128, 129f
    thrombolysis in, 128
    Wallgraft for, 128, 129f
  gas in, 112, 113f
  in juxtarenal aortic aneurysm, 114, 115f, 116, 117f
Endoleak
  in abdominal aortic aneurysm repair, 118, 119f
  access to, 118, 119f
  classification of, 118
  embolization of, 118
  obliteration of, 118, 119f
  type II, 121f, 122, 123f
    catheterization in, 120
    embolization of, 120, 121f, 122, 123f
    occlusion of, 120, 121f
    streak artifact in, 122, 123f
    translumbar access to, 122, 123f
  type II, 124, 125f
    arc of Riolan in, 124, 125f
    catheterization in, 124, 125f
    embolization of, 124, 125f
    occlusion of, 124, 125f
    type Ib vs., 126, 127f
  type III, 128
Epistaxis
  catheterization in, 184
  maxillary artery embolization in, 184, 185f
  secondary to hemorrhagic hereditary telangiectasia
    arterial embolization for, 182
    hyperemia and, 182
    hypervascularity in, 183f
  traumatic, 188
Esophageal foreign body removal, 580, 581f
Esophageal stricture, dilatation of, 578, 579f
Excluder stent graft
  in aortic pseudoaneurysm, 144, 145f
  in ruptured aortic aneurysm, 110, 111f
External carotid artery pseudoaneurysm, 186, 187f, 190, 191f
  exclusion of, 190, 191f
  stenting of, 190, 191f
  symptoms, 190
External iliac artery, in renal transplant anastomosis, 62, 63f

F

Failure, of endograft
  occlusion in, 128, 129f
  sac pressure in, 128, 129f
  thrombolysis in, 128
  Wallgraft for, 128, 129f
Femoral artery
  distal right common
    filling defect after arteriotomy closure in, 48, 49f
    stenosis after arteriotomy closure in, 48, 49f
  left superior, occlusion of, 29f
  right common
    dissection with closure device in, 50, 51f
    filling defect with closure device in, 50, 51f

Femoral artery (Continued)
  superficial
    acute thrombosis of
      occlusion in, 24, 25f
      stenting in, 24, 25f
      symptoms in, 24
      thrombolysis for, 24
      ultrasound of, 24
    atherosclerotic disease of
      ankle/brachial index in, 30
      intrastent stenosis in, 30, 31f
      stenosis in, 30, 31f
      Viabahn stent in, 30, 31f
    chronic occlusion of
      ankle/brachial index in, 26
      arteriogram of, 26, 27f
      atherectomy for, 26, 27f
      popliteal artery in, 27f
    cryoplasty of stenosis in
      ankle/brachial index before, 36
      balloon in, 36, 37f
      dissection after, 36, 37f
      indications, 36
      stenosis in, 36, 37f
    dissection of
      stenosis in, 92, 93f
      stenting in, 92, 93f
    subintimal recanalization for chronic occlusion of
      arteriogram in, 34, 35f
      indications, 34
      ultrasound in, 34
  superior, recanalization through, 29f
Fibromuscular dysplasia
  in carotid artery dissecting aneurysm, 154, 155f
  in renal artery, 60, 61f
  pediatric patient, 64, 65f
Fluency covered stent, in arteriovenous fistula, 82, 83f
Foot, arteriovenous malformation in
  embolization of, 240, 241f
  puncturing of, 238, 239f
  supply of, 240, 241f
Forearm arteriovenous malformation
  embolization of, 232, 233f
  supply of, 232, 233f
Foreign body removal
  embolization coil, 456, 457f
  esophageal, 580, 581f
  of lost guidewire, 452, 453f
  in subclavian vein port, 450, 451f

G
Gallbladder hemorrhage, 292, 293f
  cholecystectomy catheter in, 292, 293f
Gastric artery embolization, 218, 219f
Gastric bypass surgery, 356
Gastric varices, 310, 398, 399f, 400, 401f
Gastrinoma, metastatic liver
  masses in, 286, 287f
  radioembolization of, 286, 287f
Gastroduodenal artery embolization, 216, 217f
Gastroduodenal outlet stenting, 590, 591f
Gastrohepatic varices, 310, 311f
Gastrointestinal hemorrhage
  acute lower
    in ascending colon, 228, 229f
    catheterization in, 228, 229f, 230, 231f
    in cecum, 230, 231f
    embolization of, 228, 229f
    selective embolization of, 224, 225f, 230, 231f
  acute upper
    bleeding ulcer in, 216, 217f
    embolization in, 215f, 216, 217f, 218, 219f
    gastric artery in, 218, 219f
    gastroduodenal artery in, 216, 217f
    splenic artery in, 214, 215f
    symptoms in, 214, 216
  lower
    embolization in, 226, 227f
    hepatic flexure in, 226, 227f
    transverse colon in, 226, 227f

Gastrointestinal hemorrhage (Continued)
  recurrent lower
    embolization in, 220, 221f
    tPA in, 220
Gastrojejunostomy tube placement, 588, 589f
Gastrostomy tube placement
  CT-guided, 586, 587f
  percutaneous, 582, 583f, 584, 585f
Giantcuro stent
  for hepatic vein stenosis, 344, 345f
  for inferior vena cava stenosis, 338, 339f
  for superior vena cava stenosis, 380, 381f
Gonadal vein
  in varicocele, 460, 461f, 462, 463f
  varicose, 464, 465f
Great saphenous vein
  laser ablation of, 468, 469f
  occlusion of, 468, 469f
  reflux in, 468, 469f
Guidewire, lost, 452, 453f

H
Hand, arteriovenous malformation in
  arterial steal in, 238, 239f
  embolization of, 238, 239f
  internal flow voids in, 238, 239f
  puncturing of, 240, 241f
  symptoms, 238
Hemangioendothelioma
  hepatic
    ascites in, 277f, 278
    embolization of, 278
    vascularity of, 277f, 278, 279f
  kaposiform, 258, 259f
    sclerosing of, 258, 259f
    sequelae, 258
Hemangioma, in shoulder
  catheterization of, 256, 257f
  mass in, 256, 257f
  sclerosing of, 256, 257f
Hemicolectomy, anastomotic fistula closure after, 608, 609f
Hemobilia, secondary to hepatic artery pseudoaneurysm, 220, 221f
  catheterization of, 220, 221f
  embolization of, 220, 221f
Hemodialysis graft. See also Dialysis catheter
  axillary vein stenosis in, 434, 435f
  balloon angioplasty in, 414, 415f, 416, 417f, 418, 419f, 420, 421f, 422, 423f, 426, 427f
  basilic vein thrombosis in, 424, 425f
  brachial vein stenosis in, 414, 415f
  cephalic vein stenosis in, 420, 422, 423f, 426, 427f
  embolization in, 420, 421f
  nonmaturing fistula in, 420
  outflow vein stenosis in, 418
  pseudoaneurysms in, 418, 428, 429f
    enlargement of, 428, 429f
    stenting of, 428, 429f
  stenting of, 416, 417f, 422, 423f, 424, 425f, 434, 435f
  thrombectomy in, 426, 427f
  thrombolysis in, 430, 431f, 432, 433f, 434, 435f
  venous anastomosis stenosis in, 416, 417f
Hemorrhagic hereditary telangiectasia, epistaxis in, 182
Hepatectomy, portal vein thrombosis after
  thrombectomy in, 390, 391f
  thrombolysis in, 391f
  thrombus in, 390, 391f
Hepatic abscess drainage, 600, 601f
Hepatic adenoma
  embolization of, 276, 277f
  hypervascularity in, 276, 277f
  masses in, 276, 277f
Hepatic artery
  embolization as complication of TIPSS, 396, 397f
  pseudoaneurysm, 107f, 220, 221f
    catheterization of, 220, 221f
    embolization of, 220, 221f
    hemoperitoneum in, 107f

Hepatic artery (Continued)
    thrombin injection for, 106, 107f
    thrombosis of, 106, 107f
  stenosis, 322, 323f, 325f, 327f, 329f
    balloon angioplasty in, 322, 323f, 324, 325f, 328, 329f
    resistive indices in, 322, 324, 326
    stenting in, 326, 327f
  trauma
    embolization in, 298, 299f, 300, 301f
    lacerations in, 298, 299f
Hepatic duct recanalization, 528, 529f
Hepatic hemangioendothelioma
  ascites in, 277f, 278
  embolization of, 278
  vascularity of, 277f, 278, 279f
Hepatic vein
  shunt placement in stented, 392, 393f
  stenosis, 344, 345f
  stenting of, 344, 345f
Hepatitis C-related cirrhosis, 264
Hepatocellular carcinoma
  bland embolization of, 274, 275f
  catheterization in, 264, 265f
  chemoembolization of, 260, 261f, 262, 263f, 264, 265f, 266, 267f, 268, 269f
  cryoablation of, 494, 495f
  hypervascularity in, 262, 263f, 274, 275f, 282, 283f
  intra-arterial radioembolization of, 284, 285f
  lesions in, 262, 263f
  lung shunt in, 282
  mass in, 260, 261f, 264, 265f, 266, 267f, 268, 269f, 274, 275f
  microwave ablation of, 490, 491f, 492, 493f
  radioembolization of, 282, 283f
  radiofrequency ablation of, 268, 269f, 488, 489f
  supply of, 260, 261f
  symptoms, 268
Horseshoe kidney, nephroureteral catheter in, 568, 569f
Hypertension
  malignant, renal artery stenosis in, 56, 57f
  in pediatric patient, from renal artery stenosis, 64, 65f
  renovascular, in Williams syndrome, 66, 67f
Hypervascularity
  in hepatocellular carcinoma, 262, 263f, 274, 275f
  mucosal, 183f
  pulmonary, 198, 199f
Hypothenar hammer syndrome
  occlusions in, 22, 23f
  palmar arch aneurysm in, 22, 23f
  symptoms in, 22
  tPA for, 22

I
Iatrogenic arteriovenous fistula, renal
  embolization of, 206, 207f
  symptoms, 206, 207f
Iatrogenic left internal mammary artery injury
  arteriovenous fistula in, 244, 245f
  in dobutamine stress test, 244
  pseudoaneurysm in, 244, 245f
  stenting in, 244, 245f
  symptoms, 244
Iliac artery
  in cesarean section, 320, 321f
  hypertrophy of, 202, 203f
  in juxtarenal aortic aneurysm, 114
  in pelvic fracture, 94, 95f
  pseudoaneurysm of, 100, 101f
  in renal transplant anastomosis, 62, 63f
Iliac artery stenoses, bilateral common
  ankle/brachial index in, 2
  kissing stents in, 2, 3f
  narrowing in, 2, 3f
  self-expanding stent in, 2, 3f
Iliac vein thrombosis, 366, 367f
Inferior vena cava
  biopsy, 472, 473f
  chronic occlusion of, 370, 371f

Index 621

Inferior vena cava *(Continued)*
  filter migration, 356, 357f
  filter removal, 358, 359f
  mass in, 472, 473f
  recannulation, 370, 371f
  recurrent stenosis, 342, 343f
  stenosis, 338, 339f, 340, 341f
  stenting, 338, 339f, 340, 370, 371f
Infraorbital artery embolization, 186, 187f
Internal carotid artery dissection
  in aneurysm
    on brain MRI, 154
    fibromuscular dysplasia in, 154, 155f
    stenting in, 154, 155f
    symptoms, 154
  stenosis in, 152, 153f
  stenting in, 152, 153f
  symptoms, 152
Internal carotid artery occlusion
  balloon angioplasty of, 168, 169f
  dilation of, 168
  symptoms, 168
Internal carotid artery pseudoaneurysm, 156, 157f
  embolization in, 156, 157f
  occlusion balloon test of, 156, 157f
Internal carotid artery stenosis, 146, 147f, 148, 149f
  angioplasty of, 166, 167f
  distal projection device in, 146, 147f
  recurrent, after endarterectomy, 150, 151f
    distal projection device in, 150, 151f
    stenting in, 150, 151f
    vasospasm in, 150, 151f
  stenting in, 146, 147f, 148, 149f, 166, 167f
Internal iliac artery
  hypertrophy of, 202, 203f
  in juxtarenal aortic aneurysm, 114
  in pelvic fracture, 94, 95f
Internal mammary artery, embolization of for subclavian artery aneurysm, 98, 99f
Intimal hyperplasia, from aortic trauma, 136, 137f
Intra-arterial radioembolization
  for hepatocellular carcinoma, 284, 285f
  for small bowel carcinoid metastatic to liver, 288, 289f
Intracranial aneurysm
  embolization of, 180, 181f
  subarachnoid hemorrhage in, 180, 181f
Intracranial angioplasty
  balloon in, 168, 169f
  guidewire in, 168, 169f
  indications, 168
Intracranial stenting, 166, 167f
Intrastent stenosis, in brachiocephalic artery stenosis, 12
Invasive pulmonary aspergillosis, 196, 197f
Ischemia
  chronic mesenteric
    stenosis in, 71f, 72
    stenting in, 72, 73f
    symptoms, 72
  lower extremity, secondary to aortic dissection
    stenting in, 138, 139f
    symptoms, 138
  renal, acute post-traumatic
    renal artery catheterization in, 54, 55f
    stenting in, 54, 55f
    thrombosis in, 54
    vascular pedicle injury in, 54, 55f

J

Jugular vein occlusion, 384, 385f
Juvenile nasal angiofibroma
  arterial supply to, 160, 161f
  embolization of, 160, 161f
  mass in, 160, 161f
  symptoms, 160
Juxtarenal aortic aneurysm, 114, 115f
  endograft in, 114, 115f
  endovascular repair of
    exclusion in, 116, 117f
    stent graft in, 116, 117f
    stenting in, 116, 117f

Juxtarenal aortic aneurysm *(Continued)*
  exclusion of, 114, 115f
  iliac artery in, 114

K

Kaposiform hemangioendothelioma, 258, 259f
  sclerosing of, 258, 259f
  sequelae, 258
Kasabach-Meritt syndrome, 256
Kidney ablation, transarterial
  embolization in, 212, 213f
  mass in, 212, 213f
Kissing stents
  in bilateral common iliac artery stenoses, 2, 3f
  in biliary dilation, 552, 553f
  in iliac vein occlusion, 366, 367f
Kyphoplasty, 518, 519f

L

Laser ablation, of great saphenous vein, 468, 469f
Left hepatic artery pseudoaneurysm, 107f
  hemoperitoneum in, 107f
  thrombin injection for, 106, 107f
  thrombosis of, 106, 107f
Left internal mammary artery injury, iatrogenic
  arteriovenous fistula in, 244, 245f
  in dobutamine stress test, 244
  pseudoaneurysm in, 244, 245f
  stenting in, 244, 245f
  symptoms, 244
Left lower extremity arterial recanalization
  indications, 28
  through superior femoral artery, 29f
Left-sided superior vena cava, 442, 443f
Left superior femoral artery, occlusion of, 29f
Leiomyoma, uterine, 312, 313f
Lingual artery, in carotid blowout, 158, 159f
Liver biopsy
  transjugular, 470, 471f
  ultrasound-guided, 474, 475f
Liver laceration, 294, 295f
  embolization in, 294, 295f, 296, 300, 301f
  grade V, 300, 301f
  with hemoperitoneum, 295f, 296
  hepatic artery in, 294, 295f, 296
Liver transplantation, 322
  arterial steal syndrome in, 330, 331f
  biliary ischemia after, 544, 545f
  biliary leak after, 540, 541f, 542, 543f
  hepatic artery stenosis after, 322, 323f, 325f, 327f, 329f
    balloon angioplasty in, 322, 323f, 324, 325f, 328, 329f
    resistive indices in, 322, 324, 326
    stenting in, 326, 327f
  hepatic vein stenosis after, 344, 345f
  inferior vena cava stenosis after, 338, 339f, 340, 341f, 342, 343f
  portal vein stenosis after, 332, 333f, 334
  portal vein thrombosis after, 336, 337f
Lost embolization coil, 456, 457f
Lost guidewire, 452, 453f
Lower extremity deep venous thrombosis
  Angiojet catheter for, 364
  chronic
    balloon angioplasty of, 372, 373f
    May-Thurner lesion in, 372, 373f
  8-French Trellis device for, 360
  femoral vein in, 368, 369f
  iliac veins in, 363f, 368, 369f
  stenting in, 363
  symptoms, 360
  thrombolysis for, 364, 365f
  thrombus in, 361f, 363f, 365f
  venous expansion in, 365f
Lower extremity ischemia, secondary to aortic dissection
  stenting in, 138, 139f
  symptoms, 138

Lower extremity venous malformation
  access to, 252, 253f
  phlebolith in, 252, 253f
  puncturing of, 250, 251f
  sclerosing of, 250, 251f, 252, 253f
  situation of, 250
  symptoms, 250, 252
Lung biopsy, 484, 485f, 486
Lymphangioma, cervical, 254, 255f
  as cystic, 254, 255f
  sclerosing of, 254, 255f

M

Magnetic resonance angiography (MRA), of subclavian artery stenosis, 9f
Magnetic resonance imaging (MRI)-guided breast biopsy, 482, 483f
Malignant biliary obstruction, 548, 549f
Malignant hypertension, renal artery stenosis in, 56, 57f
Malpositioned stent, 454, 455f
Mammary artery
  embolization of for subclavian artery aneurysm, 98, 99f
  iatrogenic injury of
    arteriovenous fistula in, 244, 245f
    in dobutamine stress test, 244
    pseudoaneurysm in, 244, 245f
    stenting in, 244, 245f
    symptoms, 244
Mandibular mass, embolization of, 162, 163f
Maxillary sinus hemorrhage, 188, 189f
May-Thurner lesion, 372, 373f
Melanoma, hepatic metastatic
  chemoembolization of, 270, 271f
  mass in, 270, 271f
Merci Retriever, middle cerebral artery thrombectomy with, 173f, 174, 175f
Mesenteric artery, superior
  stenosis of
    arc of Riolen in, 74, 75f
    in mesenteric ischemia, 71f, 72
      in Takayasu's vasculitis, 78, 79f
    stenting in, 72, 73f, 74, 75f
  thromboembolism in
    filling defect in, 70, 71f
    occlusion in, 68, 69f
    symptoms, 68, 70
    tPA for, 70
    treatment of, 68, 69f
Mesenteric ischemia, chronic
  stenosis in, 71f, 72
  stenting in, 72, 73f
  symptoms, 72
Metastatic liver gastrinoma
  masses in, 286, 287f
  radioembolization of, 286, 287f
Metastatic melanoma, hepatic
  chemoembolization of, 270, 271f
  mass in, 270, 271f
Microwave ablation, of hepatocellular carcinoma, 490, 491f, 492, 493f
Middle cerebral artery angioplasty
  balloon in, 170, 171f
  indications, 170
  stenosis in, 170, 171f
Middle cerebral artery occlusion, 173f, 174
Middle cerebral artery stenosis
  balloon angioplasty in, 172, 173f
  symptoms, 172
Middle cerebral artery thrombectomy, 173f, 174, 175f
Mucocele drainage, 606, 607f
Mucosal hypervascularity, 183f
Mycobacterium complex disease, 194, 195f

N

Nasal angiofibroma
  arterial supply to, 160, 161f
  embolization of, 160, 161f

Nasal angiofibroma *(Continued)*
    mass in, 160, 161f
    symptoms, 160
Nephrostomy
    CT-guided placement of, 558, 559f
    percutaneous placement of, 556, 557f
    in renal transplant patient, 560, 561f
    for xanthogranulomatous pyelonephritis, 554, 555f
Nephroureteral catheter, in horseshoe kidney, 568, 569f
Nephroureteral stent, 564, 565f, 566, 567f
Neuroform stent, in carotid artery dissecting aneurysm, 154, 155f
Non-alcoholic steatohepatitis, 268
Nonmaturing fistula, in hemodialysis grafting, 420

O

Osteoid osteoma, radiofrequency ablation of, 510, 511f, 512, 513f
Ovarian veins, in pelvic congestion syndrome, 466, 467f

P

Palmar arch aneurysm, in hypothenar hammer syndrome, 22, 23f
Palmar arch occlusion, in hypothenar hammer syndrome, 22, 23f
Palmaz balloon expandable stent, in aortic revascularization, 5f
Palmaz 204 stent, in brachiocephalic artery stenosis, 12, 13f
Pancreatic cancer, biliary obstruction in, 548, 549f
Pancreatic pseudocyst, 592, 593f, 594, 595f
Parasplenic varices, 310, 311f
Parathyroid venous sampling, 411f, 413f, 421f
    hormone levels in, 410, 412
    indications, 410, 412
Pediatric nasal angiofibroma
    arterial supply to, 160, 161f
    embolization of, 160, 161f
    mass in, 160, 161f
    symptoms, 160
Pelvic arteriovenous fistula
    iliac veins in, 248, 249f
    situation of, 248, 249f
    stenting in, 248, 249f
    symptoms, 248
Pelvic arteriovenous malformation
    continued flow in, 236, 237f
    selective embolization of, 236, 237f
    supply of, 236, 237f
Pelvic biopsy, 476, 477f
Pelvic congestion syndrome
    embolization in, 466, 467f
    ovarian veins in, 466, 467f
    symptoms, 466
Pelvic embolization, for postpartum hemorrhage, 318
Pelvic fracture, 94, 95f
    embolization in, 94, 95f
    hemorrhage in, 94, 95f
Pelvic varicosities
    gonadal veins in, 464, 465f
    in pelvic congestion syndrome, 466, 467f
    sclerosing of, 464, 465f
    symptoms, 464
Percutaneous atherectomy, for anterior tibial artery stenosis
    ankle/brachial index before, 46
    catheter in, 46
    indications, 46
    stenosis in, 46, 47f
Percutaneous lung biopsy, 484, 485f, 486
Percutaneous nephrostomy placement, 556, 557f
Percutaneous thoracic duct embolization, 520, 521f
Percutaneous transhepatic cholangiogram, 524, 525f, 526, 527f

Peripherally inserted central catheter, in left-sided superior vena cava, 442, 443f
Perirenal abscess, drainage of, 572, 573f
Peristomal varices, 402, 403f
Peroneal artery, as dominant run-off vessel, 40
"Pinch-off syndrome," 450, 451f
Placenta percreta, 320, 321f
Polyvinyl alcohol microspheres
    in bronchial artery embolization, 198, 200, 201f
    in carotid blowout embolization, 158, 159f
    in mandibular mass embolization, 162, 163f
Popliteal artery
    in chronic superficial femoral artery occlusion, 27f
    occlusion of, 29f
    post-traumatic injury to
        pseudoaneurysm in, 80, 81f
        stenting in, 80, 81f
        symptoms in, 80
    reconstitution of, 32, 33f
    subintimal recanalization for chronic occlusion of
        arteriogram in, 34, 35f
        indications, 34
        ultrasound in, 34
Portal-mesenteric venous thrombosis
    after hepatectomy
        thrombectomy in, 390, 391f
        thrombolysis in, 391f
        thrombus in, 390, 391f
    symptoms, 388
    thrombolysis in, 388, 389f
    thrombus in, 388, 389f
Portal vein embolization
    access for, 290, 291f
    coils in, 290, 291f
Portal vein stenosis, 332, 333f, 334
Portal vein thrombosis, 308, 336, 337f
Port insertion
    "pinch off syndrome" and, 450, 451f
    subclavian vein, 448, 449f
Posterior tibial artery, recanalization of
    ankle/brachial index after, 38, 39f, 44
    ankle/brachial index before, 38
    balloon angioplasty in, 44
    guidewire access in, 44
    indications, 38, 44
    reconstitution before, 38, 39f, 44, 45f
    restoration of flow in, 38, 39f, 44, 45f
Postpartum hemorrhage, 318
Post-traumatic dorsalis pedis artery
    pseudoaneurysm, 90, 91f
    embolization of, 90, 91f
    occlusion in, 90, 91f
Post-traumatic popliteal artery injury
    pseudoaneurysm in, 80, 81f
    stenting in, 80, 81f
    symptoms in, 80
Post-traumatic pseudoaneurysm, in anterior tibial artery, 89f
    occlusion of, 88, 89f
    symptoms, 88
Post-traumatic renal ischemia, acute
    renal artery catheterization in, 54, 55f
    stenting in, 54, 55f
    thrombosis in, 54
    vascular pedicle injury in, 54, 55f
Presacral mucocele drainage, 606, 607f
Pseudoaneurysm
    aortic chronic, 144, 145f
        resolution of, 144, 145f
        stenting in, 144, 145f
    in aortoenteric fistula, 112, 113f
    in arteriovenous fistula, 82, 83f, 84, 85f
    at celiac trunk, 102, 103f
        embolization of, 102, 103f
        at splenic artery, 102, 103f
        stenting of, 102, 103f
    in dialysis graft, 418
    external carotid artery, 186, 187f, 190, 191f
        exclusion of, 190, 191f
        stenting of, 190, 191f
        symptoms, 190
    in hemodialysis graft, 418, 428, 429f

Pseudoaneurysm *(Continued)*
    enlargement of, 428, 429f
    stenting of, 428, 429f
    hepatic artery, 220, 221f
        catheterization of, 220, 221f
        embolization of, 220, 221f
    in hepatic artery, 107f
        hemoperitoneum in, 107f
        thrombin injection for, 106, 107f
        thrombosis of, 106, 107f
    internal carotid artery, after endarterectomy, 156, 157f
        embolization in, 156, 157f
        occlusion balloon test of, 156, 157f
    in pelvic radiation therapy, 100, 101f
        in iliac artery, 100, 101f
        stenting of, 100, 101f
    in popliteal artery injury, 80, 81f
    post-traumatic, in anterior tibial artery, 89f
        occlusion of, 88, 89f
        symptoms, 88
    post-traumatic dorsalis pedis artery, 90, 91f
        embolization of, 90, 91f
        occlusion in, 90, 91f
    splenic, 306, 307f
        embolization of, 302, 303f, 306, 307f
        laceration in, 302, 303f
        symptoms, 302
        thrombosis of, 306, 307f
Pseudocyst, pancreatic, 592, 593f, 594, 595f
Pulmonary arteriovenous malformation, 346, 347f, 350, 351f
    aneurysm in, 348, 349f
    embolization of, 348, 349f, 350, 351f
Pulmonary artery
    embolus, 352, 353f
    thrombolysis, 352, 353f
Pyelonephritis, xanthogranulomatous, nephrostomy for, 554, 555f

R

Radiation therapy, pseudoaneurysm secondary to, 100, 101f
    in iliac artery, 100, 101f
    stenting of, 100, 101f
Radioembolization
    of hepatocellular carcinoma, 282, 283f
    intra-arterial, of hepatocellular carcinoma, 284, 285f
    of metastatic liver gastrinoma, 286, 287f
    of small bowel carcinoid metastatic to liver, 288, 289f
Radiofrequency ablation
    of acetabular metastasis, 514, 515f
    of colorectal liver metastasis, 496, 497f
    of hepatocellular carcinoma, 268, 269f, 488, 489f
    of metastatic sarcoma to liver, 498, 499f
    of osteoid osteoma, 510, 511f, 512, 513f
    of recurrent adrenal corticocarcinoma, 500, 501f
    of renal cell carcinoma, 502, 503f, 504, 505f
Recanalization
    of anterior tibial artery
        angioplasty in, 42, 43f
        indications, 42
        runoff disease in, 42, 43f
    of chronic occlusion in superficial femoral and popliteal arteries
        arteriogram in, 34, 35f
        indications, 34
        ultrasound in, 34
    left lower extremity arterial
        indications, 28
        through superior femoral artery, 29f
    of posterior tibial artery
        ankle/brachial index after, 38, 39f, 44
        ankle/brachial index before, 38
        balloon angioplasty in, 44
        guidewire access in, 44
        indications, 38, 44
        reconstitution before, 38, 39f, 44, 45f
        restoration of flow in, 38, 39f, 44, 45f

Index   623

Recanalization *(Continued)*
   right lower extremity
      balloon angioplasty in, 32, 33f
      indications, 32
      stent in, 32, 33f
Rectal adenocarcinoma, metastatic to liver,
   embolization of, 290, 291f
Recurrent internal carotid artery stenosis, after
   endarterectomy, 150, 151f
   distal projection device in, 150, 151f
   stenting in, 150, 151f
   vasospasm in, 150, 151f
Renal abscess, drainage of, 574, 575f
Renal angiomyolipoma
   embolization of, 204, 205f
   hypervascularity in, 204, 205f
   mass in, 204, 205f
Renal arteries
   embolization of, 208, 209f
   trauma to, 208, 209f
Renal arteriovenous fistula
   embolization of, 242, 243f
   iatrogenic
      embolization of, 206, 207f
      symptoms, 206, 207f
   in left kidney hilum, 242, 243f
Renal artery
   aortic dissection flap extension into, 58, 59f
   fibromuscular dysplasia in, 60, 61f
   in pediatric patient, 64, 65f
Renal artery angioplasty, indications, 60
Renal artery stenosis
   in aortic dissection, 58, 59f
   balloon-expandable stent in, 56, 57f
      from aortic dissection, 58, 59f
   in malignant hypertension, 56, 57f
   in pediatric patient, 64, 65f
      fibromuscular dysplasia in, 64, 65f
   in renal artery thrombosis, 52, 53f
   in transplant patient, 62, 63f
      balloon angioplasty for, 62, 63f
   vasospasm after stenting of, 66, 67f
   in Williams syndrome, 66, 67f
Renal artery thrombosis
   decreased kidney perfusion in, 52, 53f
   in post-traumatic renal ischemia, 54
   stenosis in, 52, 53f
Renal cell carcinoma
   cryoablation of, 506, 507f, 508, 509f
   metastatic to acetabulum, radiofrequency ablation
      of, 514, 515f
   radiofrequency ablation of, 502, 503f, 504, 505f
Renal cyst
   drainage of, 570, 571f
   sclerosing of, 570, 571f
Renal ischemia, acute post-traumatic
   renal artery catheterization in, 54, 55f
   stenting in, 54, 55f
   thrombosis in, 54
   vascular pedicle injury in, 54, 55f
Renal obstruction, stenting for, 566, 567f
Renal transplant
   nephrostomy management in, 560, 561f
   renal artery stenosis after, 62, 63f
Renal vein sampling, 405f
   indications, 404
   renin levels in, 404
Renovascular hypertension, in Williams syndrome,
   66, 67f
Restenosis, balloon angioplasty for, 12, 13f
Right brachiocephalic artery stenosis, percutaneous
   treatment of
   balloon angioplasty for restenosis in, 12, 13f
   indications, 12
   intrastent stenosis in, 12
   pressure gradient in, 12
   stenting in, 12, 13f
Right common femoral artery, distal
   dissection from closure device in, 50, 51f
   filling defect after arteriotomy closure in, 48, 49f,
      50, 51f
   stenosis after arteriotomy closure in, 48, 49f
Right infraorbital artery embolization, 186, 187f

Right internal iliac artery
   in juxtarenal aortic aneurysm, 114
   in pelvic fracture, 94, 95f
Right lower extremity subintimal recanalization
   balloon angioplasty in, 32, 33f
   indications, 32
   stent in, 32, 33f
Right subclavian artery occlusion
   angiogram of, 11f
   balloon expandable stent in, 10, 11f
   symptoms in, 10
Ruptured abdominal aortic aneurysm
   hematoma in, 110, 111f
   resolution of, 111f
   stent graft in, 110, 111f
   symptoms, 110

S

Sacral nerve block, CT-guided, 522, 523f
Sarcoma, metastatic liver, radiofrequency ablation
   of, 498, 499f
Sclerotherapy
   of cervical lymphangioma, 254, 255f
   of gastric varices, 398, 399f, 400, 401f
   of hemangioendothelioma, kaposiform, 258, 259f
   of lower extremity venous malformation, 250,
      251f, 252, 253f
   of pelvic varicosities, 464, 465f, 466, 467f
   of renal cyst, 570, 571f
   of stomal varices, 402, 403f
Segmental arteries
   embolization of, 208, 209f
   trauma to, 208, 209f
Self-expanding stent, 96
   in acute superficial femoral artery thrombosis,
      24, 25f
   in basilic vein stenosis, 424, 425f
   in bilateral common iliac artery stenoses, 2, 3f
   in carotid dissection, 152, 153f
   in deep venous thrombosis, 384, 385f, 386, 387f
   in dialysis graft stenosis, 416, 417f, 422, 423f,
      434, 435f
   in lower extremity subintimal recanalization, 32,
      33f
   in subclavian artery stenosis, 14, 15f
   in superior vena cava stenosis, 378, 379f
Shoulder arteriovenous malformation
   arteriovenous shunting in, 234, 235f
   embolization of, 234, 235f
   enlargement of, 234, 235f
   subclavian vein in, 234
Shoulder hemangioma
   catheterization of, 256, 257f
   mass in, 256, 257f
   sclerosing of, 256, 257f
Soft-tissue hemangioma, in shoulder
   catheterization of, 256, 257f
   mass in, 256, 257f
   sclerosing of, 256, 257f
Sphenopalatine artery occlusion, 188, 189f
Splenic artery
   aneurysm, 105f
      catheterization of, 104
      embolization of, 104, 105f
      splenic infarction in, 104
   celiac trunk pseudoaneurysm at, 102, 103f
   embolization, 215f, 304, 305f
   in gastrointestinal hemorrhage, 214, 215f
Splenic embolization, 308, 309f, 310, 311f
Splenic pseudoaneurysm, 306, 307f
   embolization of, 302, 303f, 306, 307f
   laceration in, 302, 303f
   symptoms, 302
   thrombosis of, 306, 307f
Splenic trauma
   hematoma in, 304, 305f
   parenchyma in, 304, 305f
   splenic artery embolization in, 304, 305f
Splenomegaly, 309f, 310, 311f
Staghorn calculus, 554, 555f, 564, 565f
Steatohepatitis, 268

Stent(s)
   Acculink, in internal carotid artery stenosis, 146,
      147f, 148, 149f
   balloon expandable
      in aortic revascularization, 5f
      in aortic stenosis, 6, 7f
      in basilar artery thrombosis, 176
      in carotid stenosis, 166, 167f
      in celiac artery stenosis, 72, 73f, 330, 331f
      in celiac trunk pseudoaneurysm, 102, 103f
      in hepatic artery stenosis, 326, 327f
      in juxtarenal aortic aneurysm, 116, 117f
      in mesenteric ischemia with Takayasu's
         vasculitis, 78, 79f
      in post-traumatic renal ischemia, 54, 55f
      in renal artery stenosis, 56, 57f
         from aortic dissection, 58, 59f
      in subclavian artery aneurysm, 98, 99f
      in subclavian artery occlusion, 10, 11f
      in subclavian artery stenosis, 8, 9f
      in subclavian steal syndrome, 16, 17f
      in superficial femoral artery dissection, 92, 93f
      in superior mesenteric artery stenosis, 74, 75f
      in Williams syndrome management, 66, 67f
   covered
      for aortic dissection, 138, 139f
      for biliary obstruction, 550, 551f
      for external carotid artery pseudoaneurysm,
         188, 189f
      for iliac artery pseudoaneurysm, 100, 101f
      for left internal mammary artery injury,
         iatrogenic, 244, 245f
   Fluency covered, in arteriovenous fistula, 82, 83f
   Giantcuro
      for hepatic vein stenosis, 344, 345f
      for inferior vena cava stenosis, 338, 339f
      for superior vena cava stenosis, 380, 381f
   graft
      in abdominal aortic aneurysm, 108, 109f
      in aortic dissection, 142
      in aortic injury, 134, 135f, 136, 137f
      in aortic pseudoaneurysm, 132, 133f, 144, 145f
      in aortoenteric fistula repair, 112, 113f
      in biliary obstruction, 546, 547f, 548, 549f
      in diverticulum of Kommerell aneurysm, 130, 131f
      failure of
         occlusion in, 128, 129f
         sac pressure in, 128, 129f
         thrombolysis in, 128
         Wallgraft for, 128, 129f
      in juxtarenal aortic aneurysm, 114, 115f
      in pelvic arteriovenous fistula, 248, 249f
      in ruptured abdominal aortic aneurysm, 110, 111f
   kissing
      in bilateral common iliac artery stenoses, 2, 3f
      in biliary dilation, 552, 553f
      in iliac vein stenosis, 366, 367f
   malpositioned, 454, 455f
   Neuroform, in carotid artery dissecting aneurysm,
      154, 155f
   Palmaz204, in brachiocephalic artery stenosis,
      12, 13f
   recanalization of, 374, 375f
   self-expanding
      in acute superficial femoral artery thrombosis,
         24, 25f
      in basilic vein stenosis, 424, 425f
      in bilateral common iliac artery stenoses, 2, 3f
      in carotid dissection, 152, 153f
      in chronic deep venous thrombosis, 386, 387f
      in chronic venous occlusion, 384, 385f
      in dialysis graft stenosis, 416, 417f, 422, 423f
      in lower extremity subintimal recanalization,
         32, 33f
      in subclavian artery stenosis, 14, 15f
      in superior vena cava stenosis, 378, 379f
   Viabahn covered
      in atherosclerosis of superficial femoral artery,
         30, 31f
      in post-traumatic popliteal pseudoaneurysm,
         80, 81f
   Wingspan, in vertebral artery stenosis, 164, 165f
Stereotactic breast biopsy, 478, 479f, 480, 481f

Stomal varices, 402, 403f
Streak artifact, in type II endoleak, 122, 123f
Subarachnoid hemorrhage, 178, 179f
　aneurysm in, 178, 179f
　embolization for, 178, 179f
　symptoms, 178
Subclavian artery aneurysm, 98, 99f
　embolization of arteries surrounding, 98, 99f
　stenting in, 98, 99f
Subclavian artery occlusion, right
　angiogram of, 11f
　balloon expandable stent in, 10, 11f
　symptoms in, 10
Subclavian artery stenosis
　after thoracic aorta stenting
　　improvement of, 15f
　　stenting in, 14, 15f
　angiogram of, 9f
　balloon expandable stent in, 8, 9f
　improvement after stenting for, 15f
　magnetic resonance angiography of, 9f
　in subclavian steal syndrome, 16, 17f
　in Takayasu's arteritis
　　balloon angioplasty in, 76, 77f
　　stenosis in, 76, 77f
　　symptoms, 76
Subclavian artery trauma, stenting of, 86, 87f
Subclavian steal syndrome. *See also* Subclavian artery stenosis
　endovascular management of
　　indications, 16
　　subclavian artery stenosis in, 16, 17f
　　vertebral artery in, 16, 17f
Subclavian vein port insertion, 448, 449f
Subintimal recanalization
　of anterior tibial artery
　　angioplasty in, 42, 43f
　　indications, 42
　　runoff disease in, 42, 43f
　of chronic occlusion in superficial femoral and popliteal arteries
　　arteriogram in, 34, 35f
　　indications, 34
　　ultrasound in, 34
　left lower extremity arterial
　　indications, 28
　　through superior femoral artery, 29f
　of posterior tibial artery
　　ankle/brachial index after, 38, 39f
　　ankle/brachial index before, 38
　　indications, 38
　　reconstitution before, 38, 39f
　　restoration of flow in, 38, 39f
　right lower extremity
　　balloon angioplasty in, 32, 33f
　　indications, 32
　　stent in, 32, 33f
Superficial femoral artery
　acute thrombosis of
　　occlusion in, 24, 25f
　　stenting in, 24, 25f
　　symptoms in, 24
　　thrombolysis for, 24
　　ultrasound of, 24
　atherosclerotic disease of
　　ankle/brachial index in, 30
　　intrastent stenosis in, 30, 31f
　　stenosis in, 30, 31f
　　Viabahn stent in, 30, 31f
　chronic occlusion of
　　ankle/brachial index in, 26
　　arteriogram of, 26, 27f
　　atherectomy for, 26, 27f
　　popliteal artery in, 27f
　cryoplasty of stenosis in
　　ankle/brachial index before, 36
　　balloon in, 36, 37f
　　dissection after, 36, 37f
　　indications, 36
　　stenosis in, 36, 37f
　dissection of
　　stenosis in, 92, 93f
　　stenting in, 92, 93f

Superficial femoral artery *(Continued)*
　occlusion of distal right, 32, 33f
　subintimal recanalization for chronic occlusion of
　　arteriogram in, 34, 35f
　　indications, 34
　　ultrasound in, 34
Superior femoral artery
　occlusion of left, 29f
　recanalization through, 29f
Superior mesenteric artery
　stenosis of
　　arc of Riolen in, 74, 75f
　　in mesenteric ischemia, 71f, 72
　　in Takayasu's vasculitis, 78, 79f
　　stenting in, 72, 73f, 74, 75f
　thromboembolism in
　　filling defect in, 70, 71f
　　occlusion in, 68, 69f
　　symptoms, 68, 70
　　tPA for, 70
　　treatment of, 68, 69f
Superior vena cava
　filter, 354, 355f
　left-sided, central catheter in, 442, 443f
Superior vena cava stenosis, catheter-related, 378, 379f, 380, 381f
Suprapubic cystostomy catheter, 576, 577f
Sural artery coil embolization, 83f
Syndrome of inappropriate antidiuretic hormone secretion, 198

T

TAG thoracic stent graft
　in aortic dissection, 142
　in aortic injury, 134, 135f
　in aortic pseudoaneurysm, 132, 133f
　in diverticulum of Kommerell aneurysm, 130, 131f
Takayasu's arteritis
　mesenteric ischemia in
　　stenosis in, 78, 79f
　　stenting in, 78, 79f
　　symptoms, 78
　subclavian artery stenosis in
　　balloon angioplasty in, 76, 77f
　　stenosis in, 76, 77f
　　symptoms, 76
Testicular vein, in varicocele, 458, 459f
Thoracic aortic pseudoaneurysm, chronic, 144, 145f
　resolution of, 144, 145f
　stenting in, 144, 145f
Thoracic arteriovenous fistula
　occlusion of, 246, 247f
　situation of, 246, 247f
　supply of, 246
　symptoms, 246
Thoracic duct embolization, 520, 521f
Thoracic vertebroplasty, 516, 517f
Thrombectomy, middle cerebral artery, 173f, 174, 175f
Thrombin injection, for hepatic artery pseudoaneurysm, 104, 107f
Thrombolysis
　for acute superficial femoral artery thrombosis, indications, 24
　for hemodialysis graft clotting, 430, 431f, 432, 433f, 434, 435f
　for hepatic artery pseudoaneurysm, 106, 107f
　for hypothenar hammer syndrome
　　indications for, 22
　　tPA in, 22
　for portal-mesenteric venous thrombosis, 388, 389f
　for portal vein thrombosis, 336, 337f
　for renal artery thrombosis, stenosis in, 52, 53f
　for superior mesenteric artery embolism, 70
　for upper extremity deep venous thrombosis, 376, 377f

Thrombosis
　acute superficial femoral artery
　　occlusion in, 24, 25f
　　stenting in, 24, 25f
　　symptoms in, 24
　　thrombolysis for, 24
　　ultrasound of, 24
　basilar artery
　　flow absence in, 176, 177f
　　occlusion in, 176, 177f
　　stenosis in, 176, 177f
　　stenting in, 176
　　symptoms, 176
　　tPA for, 176, 177f
　portal-mesenteric venous
　　symptoms, 388
　　thrombectomy in, 390, 391f
　　thrombolysis in, 388, 389f, 391f
　　thrombus in, 388, 389f, 390, 391f
　portal vein, 336, 337f
　renal artery
　　decreased kidney perfusion in, 52, 53f
　　in post-traumatic renal ischemia, 54
　　stenosis in, 52, 53f
　superior mesenteric artery
　　filling defect in, 70, 71f
　　occlusion in, 68, 69f
　　symptoms, 68, 70
　　tPA for, 70
　　treatment of, 68, 69f
Thyrocervical aneurysm, endovascular management of
　coil packing in, 96, 97f
　embolization in, 96, 97f
　extravasation in, 96, 97f
　indications, 96
Thyrocervical trunk, embolization of, for subclavian artery aneurysm, 98, 99f
Tibial artery
　anterior
　　aberrant origin of, 47f
　　percutaneous atherectomy for stenosis of
　　　ankle/brachial index before, 46
　　　catheter in, 46
　　　indications, 46
　　　stenosis in, 46, 47f
　　post-traumatic pseudoaneurysm in, 89f
　　　occlusion of, 88, 89f
　　　symptoms, 88
　　recanalization of
　　　angioplasty in, 42, 43f
　　　indications, 42
　　　runoff disease in, 42, 43f
　occlusion of anterior, 40, 41f
　posterior, recanalization of
　　ankle/brachial index after, 38, 39f, 44
　　ankle/brachial index before, 38
　　balloon angioplasty in, 44
　　guidewire access in, 44
　　indications, 38, 44
　　reconstitution before, 38, 39f, 44, 45f
　　restoration of flow in, 38, 39f, 44, 45f
Tibioperoneal stenosis angioplasty
　balloon in, 40, 41f
　indications, 40
　outcome in, 40, 41f
Tissue plasminogen activator (tPA). *See also* Thrombolysis
　in basilar artery thrombosis, 176, 177f
　in deep venous thrombosis, 360
　in hypothenar hammer syndrome, 22
　in pulmonary artery thrombosis, 352, 353f
　in renal artery thrombosis, 54
　in superior mesenteric artery embolus, 70
Transarterial chemoembolization, of hepatocellular carcinoma, 260, 261f, 262, 263f, 264, 265f, 266, 267f, 268, 269f
Transarterial kidney ablation
　embolization in, 212, 213f
　mass in, 212, 213f
Transhepatic cholangiogram, percutaneous, 524, 525f, 526, 527f

Index

Transhepatic dialysis catheter
  balloon angioplasty in, 438, 439f
  brachiocephalic vein occlusion in, 436, 437f
  hepatic vein stenosis in, 438, 439f
  placement of, 436, 437f
  superior vena cava occlusion in, 438
  vena cava occlusion in, 436, 437f
Transjugular intrahepatic portosystemic shunt
  hepatic artery embolization as complication of, 396, 397f
  reduction, 394, 395f
Transjugular intrahepatic portosystemic shunt reduction, 394, 395f
Transjugular liver biopsy, 470, 471f
Translumbar dialysis catheter
  IVC access in, 440, 441f
  placement of, 440, 441f
Translumbar embolization, of type II endoleak, 122, 123f
Transplant
  liver
    arterial steal syndrome in, 330, 331f
    biliary ischemia after, 544, 545f
    biliary leak after, 540, 541f, 542, 543f
    hepatic artery stenosis after, 322, 323f, 325f, 327f, 329f
      balloon angioplasty in, 322, 323f, 324, 325f, 328, 329f
      resistive indices in, 322, 324, 326
      stenting in, 326, 327f
    hepatic vein stenosis after, 344, 345f
    inferior vena cava stenosis after, 338, 339f, 340, 341f, 342, 343f
    portal vein stenosis after, 332, 333f, 334
    portal vein thrombosis after, 336, 337f
  renal
    nephrostomy placement in, 560, 561f
    renal artery stenosis after, 62, 63f
Transvaginal abscess drain, 602, 603f
Trauma
  acute renal ischemia from
    renal artery catheterization in, 54, 55f
    stenting in, 54, 55f
    thrombosis in, 54
    vascular pedicle injury in, 54, 55f
  aortic
    hematoma resolution in, 132, 133f
    intimal hyperplasia from, 136, 137f
    leak from, 134, 135f
    pseudoaneurysm in, 132, 133f
    stent grafting in, 132, 133f, 134, 135f, 136, 137f
  bile duct, 534, 535f, 536, 537f
  dissection of superficial femoral artery from
    stenosis in, 92, 93f
    stenting in, 92, 93f
  dorsalis pedis artery pseudoaneurysm of, 90, 91f
    embolization of, 90, 91f
    occlusion in, 90, 91f
  hepatic artery
    embolization in, 298, 299f
    lacerations in, 298, 299f
  liver laceration from, 294, 295f
    embolization in, 294, 295f, 296, 300, 301f
    grade V, 300, 301f
    with hemoperitoneum, 295f, 296
    hepatic artery in, 294, 295f, 296

Trauma (Continued)
  pelvic fracture from, 94, 95f
    embolization in, 94, 95f
    hemorrhage in, 94, 95f
  popliteal artery injury from
    pseudoaneurysm in, 80, 81f
    stenting in, 80, 81f
    symptoms in, 80
  splenic
    hematoma in, 304, 305f
    parenchyma in, 304, 305f
    splenic artery embolization in, 304, 305f
  splenic arteriovenous fistula from
    embolization of, 302, 303f
    laceration in, 302, 303f
    symptoms, 302
  splenic pseudoaneurysm from, 306, 307f
    embolization of, 306, 307f
    thrombosis of, 306, 307f
  to subclavian artery
    arteriovenous fistula in, 86
    stenting in, 86, 87f
Type B aortic dissection, 141f, 142, 143f
  aneurysm in, 140, 141f
  bypass in, 142
  debranching in, 140, 141f
  endograft in, 140, 141f
  false lumen in, 142, 143f
  resolution of, 143f
  stenting in, 142
Type Ib endoleak, type II vs., 126, 127f
Type II endoleak, 124, 125f
  in abdominal aortic aneurysm, 121f, 122, 123f
  catheterization in, 120
  embolization of, 120, 121f, 122, 123f
  occlusion of, 120, 121f
  streak artifact in, 122, 123f
  translumbar access to, 122, 123f
  arc of Riolan in, 124, 125f
  catheterization in, 124, 125f
  embolization of, 124, 125f
  occlusion of, 124, 125f
  type Ib vs., 126, 127f
Type III endoleak, 128

U

Ultrasound-guided hepatic abscess drainage, 600, 601f
Ultrasound-guided liver biopsy, 474, 475f
Ultrasound-guided microwave ablation, 492, 493f
Upper extremity deep venous thrombosis
  balloon angioplasty for, 383f
  chronic
    brachiocephalic vein in, 386, 387f
    stenting in, 386, 387f
    symptoms, 386
  occlusion in, 383f
  subclavian and axillary veins in, 376, 377f
  symptoms, 376, 382
  thrombolysis of, 376, 377f
Ureteral obstruction, stenting for, 566, 567f
Ureteroileal anastomotic stricture, 562, 563f
Uterine artery embolization, 312, 313f
  in placenta percreta, 320, 321f
Uterine fibroid embolization, 312, 313f, 314

V

Varicocele
  embolization of, 458, 459f, 460, 461f, 462, 463f
  gonadal vein in, 460, 461f, 462, 463f
  pampiniform plexus in, 460, 461f
  testicular vein in, 458, 459f
Varicosities, pelvic
  gonadal veins in, 464, 465f
  in pelvic congestion syndrome, 466, 467f
  sclerosing of, 464, 465f
  symptoms, 464
Venous malformation, in lower extremity
  access to, 252, 253f
  phlebolith in, 252, 253f
  puncturing of, 250, 251f
  sclerosing of, 250, 251f, 252, 253f
  situation of, 250
  symptoms, 250, 252
Venous sampling
  adrenal, 407f
    aldosterone levels in, 406, 407f, 408
    catheterization in, 408, 409f
    indications, 406, 408
  parathyroid, 411f, 413f
    hormone levels in, 410, 412
    indications, 410, 412
  renal, 405f
    indications, 404
    renin levels in, 404
Ventriculoperitoneal shunt, 448
Vertebral artery
  central venous catheter in, 446, 447f
  predilation of, 164, 165f
  stenosis, 164, 165f
  stenting, 164, 165f
  in subclavian steal syndrome, 16, 17f
Vertebral kyphoplasty, 518, 519f
Vertebroplasty, thoracic, 516, 517f
Viabahn covered stent
  in atherosclerosis of superficial femoral artery, 30, 31f
  in post-traumatic popliteal pseudoaneurysm, 80, 81f

W

Wallgraft, in endograft failure management, 128, 129f
Williams syndrome, renal stenosis in, 66, 67f
Wingspan stent, in vertebral artery stenosis, 164, 165f

X

Xanthogranulomatous pyelonephritis, nephrostomy for, 554, 555f

Z

Zenith stent graft
  in abdominal aortic aneurysm, 108, 109f
  in juxtarenal aortic aneurysm, 116, 117f
Zollinger-Ellison syndrome, 286

KEISER UNIVERSITY
2400 Interstate Drive
Lakeland, FL 33805